IMMUNOLOGY
Clinical Case Studies
and Disease Pathophysiology

IMMUNOLOGY
Clinical Case Studies
and Disease Pathophysiology

Warren Strober
Laboratory of Host Defenses
National Institute of Allergy and Infectious Diseases/NIH

Susan R.S. Gottesman
Department of Pathology
SUNY Downstate Medical Center

✸WILEY-BLACKWELL

A JOHN WILEY & SONS, INC., PUBLICATION

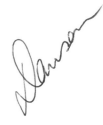

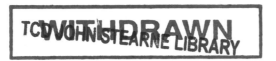

Published by John Wiley & Sons, Inc., Hoboken, New Jersey
Published simultaneously in Canada

For general information on our other products and services or for technical support, please contact our Customer Care Department within the United States at (800) 762-2974, outside the United States at (317) 572-3993 or fax (317) 572-4002.

Wiley also publishes its books in a variety of electronic formats. Some content that appears in print may not be available in electronic formats. For more information about Wiley products, visit our web site at www.wiley.com.

Library of Congress Cataloging-in-Publication Data:

Immunology : clinical case studies and disease pathophysiology / [edited by] Warren Strober, Susan Gottesman.
        p. ; cm.
    Companion to: Immunology / Richard Coico, Geoffrey Sunshine. 6th ed. c2008.
    Includes bibliographical references and index.
    ISBN 978-0-471-32659-5 (pbk.)
    1. Immunologic diseases. 2. Immunologic diseases–Case studies. 3. Clinical immunology. I. Strober, Warren. II. Gottesman, Susan.
      III. Coico, Richard. Immunology.
    [DNLM: 1. Immune System Diseases–diagnosis–Case Reports. 2. Immune System Diseases–physiopathology–Case Reports.
      3. Immune System Diseases–therapy–Case Reports. WD 300 I3315 2009]
    RC582.I473 2009
    616.97–dc22
                                                                                      2009000198

Printed in the United States of America

10 9 8 7 6 5 4 3 2 1

In memory of Hyam Gottesman.

Dedicated to our children, David, Lena, and Matthew.

With special thanks to Richard Coico and the hundreds of medical students, graduate students, and residents at SUNY Downstate Medical Center who have taught me how to teach.

Susan R. S. Gottesman

Dedicated to my wife, Heather Birnie.

Warren Strober

CONTENTS

Preface, ix

Contributors, xi

Index of Lessons in Normal Immunity, xiii

○ INTRODUCTION TO CASE STUDIES: A GUIDE TO USING THIS BOOK, 1

Unit I IMMUNODEFICIENCY DISEASES, 3

○ INTRODUCTION: ORGANIZATION OF THE IMMUNE SYSTEM AND EVALUATION OF THE IMMUNODEFICIENT PATIENT, 5

○ 1 X-LINKED AGAMMAGLOBULINEMIA (BRUTON'S AGAMMAGLOBULINEMIA), 15

○ 2 SEVERE COMBINED IMMUNODEFICIENCY DISEASE, 27

○ 3 DiGEORGE SYNDROME (CONGENITAL THYMIC APLASIA), 41

○ 4 HYPER-IgM SYNDROME, 53

○ 5 COMMON VARIABLE IMMUNODEFICIENCY DISEASE, 67

○ 6 AUTOIMMUNE LYMPHOPROLIFERATIVE SYNDROME (ALPS), 81

○ 7 X-LINKED LYMPHOPROLIFERATIVE SYNDROME, 91

○ 8 HEREDITARY ANGIOEDEMA, 101

○ 9 ACQUIRED IMMUNODEFICIENCY SYNDROME, 111

Unit II IMMEDIATE HYPERSENSITIVITY AND MAST CELL DISORDERS, 125

○ INTRODUCTION: WHEN ANTIGENS BECOME ALLERGENS, 127

○ 10 MASTOCYTOSIS, 129

○ 11 ANAPHYLAXIS, 137

○ 12 ASTHMA, 147

○ 13 THE VASCULITIDES, 161

Unit III AUTOIMMUNE DISORDERS, 173

○ INTRODUCTION: OVERVIEW OF AUTOIMMUNE DISORDERS AND MECHANISMS OF TOLERANCE, 175

○ 14 MYASTHENIA GRAVIS, 183

15 MULTIPLE SCLEROSIS, 195

16 DIABETES MELLITUS TYPE 1, 207

17 CELIAC DISEASE, 219

18 INFLAMMATORY BOWEL DISEASE, 231

19 PSORIASIS, 245

20 IgA NEPHROPATHY AND KIDNEY TRANSPLANTATION, 255

21 RHEUMATOID ARTHRITIS, 269

22 SYSTEMIC LUPUS ERYTHEMATOSUS, 283

23 SCLERODERMA, 299

Unit IV   MALIGNANCIES OF THE LYMPHOID SYSTEM, 309

INTRODUCTION: CLASSIFICATION OF LYMPHOID MALIGNANCIES, 311

24 CHRONIC LYMPHOCYTIC LEUKEMIA/SMALL LYMPHOCYTIC LYMPHOMA, 317

25 FOLLICULAR LYMPHOMA, 327

26 PLASMA CELL NEOPLASMS, 337

Unit V   349

LABORATORY TESTS USED IN THE WORKUP OF PATIENTS WITH IMMUNOLOGIC DISEASES, 351

Index, 369

PREFACE

This book consisting of clinical case studies of immunologically-related diseases is a companion volume to "Immunology, A Short Course" by Coico and Sunshine. The idea for the book grew out of our belief that the understanding of the complicated and sometimes confusing subject of immunology would be greatly facilitated by a study of the diseases of the immune system in which normal immune processes go awry. This view was strengthened by the complementary belief that the diseases of the immune system can be best understood through a firm grasp of normal immune mechanisms. The editors and authors have therefore created reality-based cases of typical patients with immunologic diseases and lead the reader through a detailed and logical clinical course based on both standard of care medical principles and a thorough knowledge of the underlying immunologic defect.

In addition, each case is accompanied by an in-depth discussion of the normal and pathological immunological processes related to the disease state being discussed. In effect, a careful reading of the cases as a whole provides the reader with an alternative course in immunology that amplifies and complements the various sections of the companion "Short Course." Overall, we hope this somewhat unique way of learning about immunology and its associated diseases will offer an effective path to the mastery of a difficult subject and, at the same time, deepen your knowledge of clinical medicine.

Susan R.S. Gottesman and Warren Strober
Authors/Editors

Richard Coico and Geoffrey Sunshine
Consulting Editors

CONTRIBUTORS

Cem Akin
Department of Internal Medicine
University of Michigan
Ann Arbor, MI

Smita Baid
Reproductive Endocrinology Section
National Institute of Child Health and Human Development
National Institutes of Health
Bethesda, MD

Milan Basta
National Institute of Neurological Disorders and Stroke
National Institutes of Health
Bethesda, MD

Camilla Buckley
Department of Clinical Neurology
Weatherall Institute of Molecular Medicine
Radcliffe Hospital
Oxford, United Kingdom

Fabio Candotti
Genetics and Molecular Biology Branch
National Human Genome Research Institute
National Institutes of Health
Bethesda, MD

Jeffrey I. Cohen
Medical Virology Section
National Institute of Allergy and Infectious Diseases
National Institutes of Health
Bethesda, MD

Thomas A. Fleisher
Department of Laboratory Medicine
Clinical Center
National Institutes of Health
Bethesda, MD

Susan R. S. Gottesman
Department of Pathology
SUNY Downstate Medical Center
Brooklyn, NY

Robert G. Hamilton
Division of Allergy and Clinical Immunology
Johns Hopkins University School of Medicine
Baltimore, MD

Keith Hull
Division of Therapeutic Biological Internal
    Medicine Products
U.S. Food and Drug Administration
Bethesda, MD

Gabor Illei
Sjögren's Syndrome Clinic
National Institute of Dental and Craniofacial Branch
National Institutes of Health
Bethesda, MD

Atsushi Kitani
Laboratory of Host Defenses
National Institute of Allergy and Infectious Diseases
National Institutes of Health
Bethesda, MD

Carol A. Langford
Center for Vasculitis Care and Research
Department of Rheumatic and Immunologic Diseases
Cleveland Clinic
Cleveland, OH

Frank Maldarelli
HIV Drug Resistance Program
National Cancer Institute
National Institutes of Health
Bethesda, MD

Peter Mannon
Division of Gastroenterology and Hepatology
University of Alabama at Birmingham
Birmingham, AL

Roslyn B. Mannon
Alabama Transplant Center
University of Alabama at Birmingham
Birmingham, AL

Roland Martin
Department of Neurology
University of Tübingen Medical School
Tübingen, Germany

Barbara Mittleman
National Institute of Arthritis and Musculoskeletal
    and Skin Disorders
National Institutes of Health
Bethesda, MD

Caryn G. Morse
Laboratory of Immunoregulation
National Institute of Allergy and Infectious Diseases
National Institutes of Health
Bethesda, MD

Kari C. Nadeau
Allergy and Immunology Clinic
Stanford University School of Medicine
Palo Alto, CA

Luigi D Notarangelo
Research and Molecular Diagnosis Program
    in Primary Immunodeficiencies
Children's Hospital of Boston
Boston, MA

Deric M. Park
Cellular Immunology Section
Neuroimmunology Branch
National Institute of Neurological Disorders and Stroke
National Institutes of Health
Bethesda, MD

Koneti Rao
Laboratory of Clinical Infectious Diseases
National Institute of Allergy and Infectious Diseases
National Institutes of Health
Bethesda, MD

Kristina I. Rother
Clinical Immunology Division
National Institute of Diabetes and Digestive
    and Kidney Diseases
National Institutes of Health
Bethesda, MD

Michael C. Sneller
Immunologic Diseases Section
Laboratory of Immunoregulation
National Institute of Allergy and Infectious Diseases
National Institutes of Health
Bethesda, MD

Bruce Strober
Department of Dermatology
New York University School of Medicine
New York, NY

Warren Strober
Laboratory of Host Defenses
Mucosal Immunity Section
National Institute of Allergy and Infectious Diseases
National Institutes of Health
Bethesda, MD

Dale T. Umetsu
Department of Pediatrics
Harvard University School of Medicine
Children's Hospital of Boston
Boston, MA

Angela Vincent
Department of Clinical Neurology
Weatherall Institute of Molecular Medicine
Radcliffe Hospital
Oxford, United Kingdom

INDEX OF LESSONS IN NORMAL IMMUNITY

Each of the case studies contains a discussion of one or more normal immunologic processes that is relevant to the disease under discussion. In this way the abnormalities of the immune response occurring in the individual diseases is contrasted with normal immunologic function. Below is a list of the normal immune functions discussed in the various case studies; these discussions can serve as a review of the principles of immunology.

Receptor Structure:

Antigen receptor gene rearrangement: Severe combined immunodeficiency disease

Cytokine receptor structure and signaling: Severe combined immunodeficiency disease

B Cells/Humoral Immunity

B-cell development in bone marrow: X-linked agamma-globulinemia

Isotype class switching: Hyper-IgM syndrome

Heavy-chain constant regions: Hyper-IgM syndrome

Memory B-cell formation: Common variable immunodeficiency disease

B-cell anergy during B-cell development: Systemic lupus erythematosus

B-cell subsets: Chronic lymphocytic leukemia

Oral tolerance and mucosal immunity: Celiac disease

Germinal center events: Follicular lymphoma

Plasma cell development: Plasma cell neoplasms

Plasma cell–stromal cell crosstalk: Plasma cell neoplasms

Immunoglobulin structure: Plasma cell neoplasms, Anaphylaxis

Monoclonal antibody production for therapy: Follicular lymphoma

IgE biology: Anaphylaxis

T Cells:

T-cell differentiation in the thymus summary: Severe combined immunodeficiency disease

T-cell differentiation in the thymus: DiGeorge syndrome

    Negative selection

    T-cell receptor gene rearrangement

    CD4/CD8 subset commitment

Central T-cell tolerance and AIRE: DiGeorge syndrome
Autoimmunity introduction, Diabetes mellitus

T_H2 response and T_H2 cytokines: Asthma

$CD4^+$ T-subset differentiation: Multiple Sclerosis

T_H1/T_H17 subsets: Multiple Sclerosis, Inflammatory bowel disease

Delayed-type hypersensitivity: Multiple Sclerosis

T-cell-mediated cytotoxicity: Diabetes mellitus

T_{reg} cells: Autoimmunity introduction, Celiac disease, Inflammatory bowel disease

Fas-FasL apoptotic pathway: Autoimmune lymphoproliferative syndrome

Superantigen: Vasculitides, Psoriasis

Innate Immunity:

Innate immunity: Inflammatory bowel disease

Fc receptors: Systemic lupus erythematosus

Mast cell biology: Mastocytosis

Complement pathway: Hereditary angioedema

Viruses:

EBV: X-linked lymphoproliferative syndrome

HIV life cycle: Acquired immunodeficiency syndrome

Miscellaneous:

Major histocompatibility complex: Diabetes mellitus

Epitopes and epitope spreading: Myasthenia gravis

Molecular mimicry: Multiple sclerosis

Allogeneic organ transplantation: IgA nephropathy

Immunosuppressive therapy: IgA nephropathy

Steroid effects: Myasthenia gravis

INTRODUCTION TO CASE STUDIES: A GUIDE TO USING THIS BOOK

This book is designed to pique your interest in and increase your understanding of the immune system in normal individuals by showing you what happens when it goes awry in disease states. This book contains a series of clinical vignettes. Each is based on one or more real patients suffering from one of the main types of immunologic disorders. You follow each patient through the initial workup and laboratory studies to observe how the diagnosis and treatment plan are developed. You then follow the patient's subsequent course to learn how the disease typically evolves and, at times, how it requires changes in therapy.

Each clinical story has been calibrated to illustrate the main features of the disease under study and to discuss the disorders of normal function that result in these features. However, the disease manifestations presenting in a single patient usually do not encompass all of the manifestations of a particular disease entity that can occur in a large number of patients. Thus, where appropriate, we have included a section describing the characteristics of the disease in the entire patient population. Finally, each vignette morphs into a discussion of the normal immune system and the defects that have led to disease, that is, the mechanism of the disease as we now understand it. This provides a platform for discussion of many of the major immunologic processes that collectively make up the immune system.

You will encounter several recurrent themes as you read the vignettes. One theme that will become apparent to you is that immunologic disease of almost any type has some genetic basis. This is quite obvious in the congenital immunodeficiency diseases that are most often due to a single gene mutation. This is also true of autoimmune disease and malignant disease; however, in these cases the diseases are multigenic. It is apparent that the genetic abnormalities associated with autoimmune diseases consist of gene polymorphisms that are also present in large numbers of normal individuals. In order to give rise to disease, these polymorphisms must be present with other, additional gene polymorphisms and the genetic abnormalities in autoimmunity actually consist of multiple polymorphisms acting in tandem. Thus, one of the key challenges of research into the cause of multigenic diseases is to understand how each of the component polymorphisms contributes to a pathologic change in immune function. In malignant transformations of cells of the immune system, the neoplasm is the result of mutations in one or more key genes, usually involved in cell cycle control and thus affecting cell proliferation. The effects of these mutations combine with the individual's inherent (genetic) ability to control that proliferation. In malignant disease, in contrast to the situation in immunodeficiency or autoimmunity, the mutation is a somatic mutation that occurs in a very limited number of

Immunology: Clinical Case Studies and Disease Pathophysiology, By Warren Strober and Susan R. S. Gottesman
Copyright © 2009 John Wiley & Sons, Inc.

at least partially differentiated cells in the body. In immunodeficiency or autoimmune diseases, the genetic mutation or genetic susceptibility polymorphism is inherited in the germline and is therefore present in all the body's cells.

A second theme emerges from the inherent complexity of the immune response. Since the immune system consists of an astonishing array of different cell types and subtypes, understanding immune processes often involves dissecting the functions of each of these cells as well as their complex interactions. In studying immunologic diseases, one finds again and again that the key to understanding the mechanisms of immunologic disorders is to identify the specific cell subtypes initiating disease and how each one functions in the normal immune response as well as in the disease state. A related theme is really a testament to the economy of cell biology in general in that cells of the immune system with different phenotypes and functions often use identical intracellular signaling pathways and transcription control mechanisms. Therefore, characterization of diseases that affect many different cell types frequently leads to the identification of abnormalities of intracellular molecular processes occurring in those cells.

Our third theme, and one that should give clinicians pause in their approach to treating patients, evolves from the realization that the immune system is finely tuned to act as a totality. Therefore, any breakdown or manipulation of one function of the immune system inevitably affects another immune function. A consequence of this is evidenced in the fact that a deficiency in one arm of the immune system may lead to dysregulation of another arm, resulting in an overexuberant response against self or autoimmune disorder or, alternatively, even allowing the proliferation of mutated cells (neoplasms). One should not be surprised therefore to learn that seemingly disparate disease manifestations—immunodeficiency, autoimmunity, and malignancy—not infrequently appear together in the same patient.

The first section of this book (Unit I) is devoted to immunodeficiency diseases. In most cases these are congenital immunodeficiency diseases. In that primary immunodeficiency diseases involve, for the most part, a defect in a discrete component of the immune system, they have provided immunologists with an unparalleled opportunity to study and understand the function of these discrete components in humans. These diseases, some uncommon and some rare, are true "experiments of nature," and by learning about them you will enhance your understanding of the normal development of the immune system. This section also con-

tains a chapter devoted to one of the most important secondary immunodeficiency disorders of our time, acquired immunodeficiency syndrome (AIDS). Analysis of AIDS, a disease in which the immune defect develops predominantly from the elimination of mature cells, has allowed immunologists to assess the immune system as a totality in which most of the immune system becomes dysfunctional. In this book we follow in the footsteps of these immunologists in that we use these various immunodeficiencies to teach about the specific as well as the general functions of the human immune system.

Units II (Immediate Hypersensitivity and Mast Cell Disorders) and III (Autoimmune Disorders) illustrate the consequences of dysregulation of the immune system whether due to responses to outside (exogenous) agents such as allergens or infectious organisms, to internal self-antigens as a result of the breakdown of tolerance, or to a combination of the two.

Lastly, Unit IV Malignancies of the Lymphoid System, demonstrates what happens when the internal cellular controls of lymphocytes fail to properly regulate their life cycle. Here again it becomes apparent that the inability of even a subset of lymphocytes to function normally (because of malignant transformation) leads to poor regulation of the remaining nonneoplastic cells, often resulting in the clinical sequelae of immunodeficiency (infection) and loss of tolerance (autoimmunity).

We envision this book to be used at a variety of levels based on the background and needs of the reader. The presentation in most chapters is based on two current methods of medical school teaching. One is block learning, in which all aspects of an organ system or disease are studied together: pathophysiology, epidemiology, biochemistry, and treatment or pharmacology. The second is the method of case-based learning, in which students take an active role in dissecting, learning, and teaching a case. In many ways this mimics real life, in which you analyze the problem in front of you, be it in diagnosing and treating a patient or in developing a research project to better understand a disease. By incorporating into each chapter up-to-date research and theories and freely admitting what is unknown, the reader can easily appreciate the uncharted intellectual territory ahead and the possibility of personally contributing to new knowledge through further research. We therefore hope that this book will motivate a new generation of scientists to study immunology through the lens of disease. Enjoy!

Susan R. S. Gottesman and Warren Strober

Unit I

IMMUNODEFICIENCY DISEASES

INTRODUCTION: ORGANIZATION OF THE IMMUNE SYSTEM AND EVALUATION OF THE IMMUNODEFICIENT PATIENT

SUSAN R. S. GOTTESMAN and WARREN STROBER

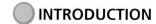 ## INTRODUCTION

This first unit examines several inherited immunodeficiency diseases as well as the acquired immunodeficiency syndrome (AIDS). As stated in the introduction, the study of congenital immunodeficiency diseases (and their animal models) has provided scientists with an unparalleled opportunity to define the function of the individual components of the immune system. Such an opportunity was in fact encountered by immunologists in the 1960s and 1970s who were conducting the initial series of investigations of patients with X-linked or Bruton's agammaglobulinemia (Case 1), severe combined immunodeficiency diseases (SCID; Case 2), and DiGeorge syndrome (Case 3). In analyzing children with these congenital immunodeficiency disorders and in the development of animal models with similar findings, it became apparent to immunologists that the adaptive immune system consists of two main compartments, one populated by T lymphocytes and the other by B lymphocytes. In this way, one of the main organizing principles of modern immunology became established. Students approaching the study of these rare diseases are encouraged to adopt the approach of the early investigators in realizing that a thorough understanding of these diseases will lead to an in-depth understanding of the immune system as a whole.

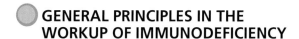 ## GENERAL PRINCIPLES IN THE WORKUP OF IMMUNODEFICIENCY

The following description of the differential diagnosis and workup of patients with possible immunodeficiency is based on broad principles concerning organization of the immune system as well as specific approaches to evaluation of immune function. Nevertheless, it is not designed to give you computer algorithms into which you can simply plug in data and arrive at a correct diagnosis. Much of what is known in medicine, and in immunology in particular, would never have been discovered if physicians had restricted themselves to prescribed algorithms. However, orderly thinking and a framework for problem solving are needed as an approach to understanding these patients, along with the realization that each patient is sufficiently unique that arrival at a diagnosis will usually require some creative thinking.

Primary and Secondary Immunodeficiency Diseases

Immunodeficiency diseases may be divided into two categories: primary and secondary. In *primary immunodeficiency diseases*, which are either inherited or acquired, the immunodeficiency is the underlying abnormality.

Secondary immunodeficiency disorders are those that arise from a nonimmunologic abnormality that has collateral effects on the immune system. This distinction thus separates inherited immunodeficiencies and their usual complication, recurrent infection, from the infectious disease caused by the human immunodeficiency virus (HIV), in which the infection itself is the cause of the immunodeficient state. It should be borne in mind that primary immunodeficiency diseases are infrequent (with one or two exceptions) and thus one must always search for a nonimmunologic cause of frequent infections; for example, one must rule out secondary immunodeficiency before an expensive and difficult immunologic workup is undertaken.

Whether primary or secondary, the immunodeficiency, almost by definition, will lead to impaired host defense and therefore increased susceptibility to infection. This leads to the axiom that an immunodeficiency disease should be suspected in any patient with recurrent infections who does not have predisposing factors and should particularly be suspected in a patient with unusual infections.

Two Systems

The first level of characterization of immunodeficiency disorders can be based on which of the two major branches of the immune system is defective: the innate immune system or the adaptive immune system. The approach to the evaluation of these systems may differ considerably.

Innate Immune System.   Our innate immune system starts with the physical or anatomic barriers that protect us from the outside world. These include our skin and epithelial barriers and protective secretory molecules such as mucus. We will not discuss these in this section but do touch upon them in the section on autoimmune diseases (see Unit III).

After breaching these physical barriers, the body stands ready to respond to insult with antigen-nonspecific cells and molecules that do not require prior sensitization or have memory. The former include granulocytes (predominantly neutrophils and eosinophils), macrophages, and natural killer (NK) cells whereas the latter include the complex of molecules comprising the complement system and secreted molecules such as lactoferrin and defensins. The cells of our innate immune system have evolved from similar cells found in lower organisms: phagocytes are present in species as primitive as sponges and sea anemones. However, in contrast to these organisms, our innate immune elements have a dual role. On one hand, they mount a defensive response by themselves while allowing the body the time to generate a specific adaptive immune response to the challenge; on the other hand, they interact with and facilitate the response of the adaptive immune system in both its afferent and efferent phases.

In recent years it has been discovered that the cells of the innate immune system have an elaborate system of receptors with which they recognize and respond to categories of molecules associated with potential pathogens. These molecules, called *pathogen-associated molecular patterns (PAMPs)*, are general molecular signatures of classes of organisms identifying the type of infectious agent (e.g., bacteria, parasite) invading the body. They are recognized by *pattern recognition molecules* which serve as receptors for the PAMPs. The most widely studied of this group of receptors are the *Toll-like receptors (TLRs)* of the innate immune system. These receptors recognize and mount responses to the prototypic molecules associated with both pathogens and commensal organisms. Signaling through these receptors initiates activation of intracellular signaling, stimulation of phagocytosis, secretion of small molecules (particularly cytokines of the interferon family), and other innate immune responses. These responses provide host defense on their own and communicate with the adaptive immune system.

Adaptive Immune System.   Our adaptive immune system is designed to respond to a specific challenge, usually that of a foreign organism. In addition, it has memory for that antigenic challenge, a property lacking in the innate immune system. Immune memory allows a more rapid and effective response on second encounter with the organism. The adaptive immune system may be subdivided into two arms, the humoral immune response and the cell-mediated immune response (see below).

Two Arms of Adaptive Immunity

The two arms constituting adaptive immunity are the *humoral* or *antibody immune response* and the *cell-mediated immune response*. The final effector cell of the humoral response is the B cell or its differentiated counterpart, the plasma cell, and the product of these cells is immunoglobulin or antibody. In contrast, the cell-mediated immune response is mediated in its final step by one of the many types of T cells. In actuality, interactions among different cell types are required for both responses, and these include cells of the innate immune system such as dendritic cells and macrophages, which serve as antigen-presenting cells. Of course, as we will see, the humoral immune response, a prototypic B-cell response, reaches full capability only with assistance (help) provided by T cells. In addition to direct cell–cell interaction, much of the communication among cells is achieved through the local release of small protein molecules, cytokines and chemokines, which are products of cells of both the innate and adaptive immune systems.

Immunodeficiency diseases (Table UI.1) can be categorized on the basis of the branch that is defective: the innate immune system or the adaptive immune system. For the innate immune system the possible defective components include (1) nonspecific effector cells, for example, phagocytic cells, including defects in their ability to migrate to sites of infection, the TLR signaling pathway, or their soluble products of defense and (2) complement components. For the adaptive immune system the defect may lie within the (3) T-cell or cell-mediated immune response, (4) B-cell or antibody-mediated immune response, or (5) both T and B cells or combined cell-mediated and humoral immunity. Mutations resulting in the defective functioning of cytokines and chemokines (the protein molecules by which the cells communicate) and/or their receptors may underlie some of these diseases and are therefore incorporated into the above listed categories based on which cell lineage is dependent on these molecules for cell differentiation and function.

The above categorization of immunodeficiency is simplistic since it does not fully incorporate the fundamental reality that the immune system has an elaborate network of intercommunication as well as some redundancy in the use of small molecules. For example, a "pure" T-cell defect may affect both the humoral and cell-mediated immune responses. Even both the innate and adaptive immune systems can be perturbed by a deficiency in a single molecule. This cross–talk and interdependence are part of what drives the need for an orderly approach to the analysis of the patient with possible immunodeficiency.

● PRACTICAL APPROACH TO THE WORKUP OF IMMUNODEFICIENCY PATIENTS

History and Physical Examination

When a patient presents with recurrent and/or unusual infections, the types of infections usually govern the approach to analysis. However, the details of the history and physical examination are of paramount importance in the investigation of possible immunodeficiency. The obvious first consideration is the *patient's age*. Many of the more severe immunodeficiency diseases are congenital (present at birth) and/or genetic (inherited), and patients present as infants or young children. Other primary immunodeficiencies are influenced by environmental factors and may thus become evident at a later age (teens or twenties) for unclear reasons. Of course, secondary immunodeficiencies are the consequence of non–immune system abnormalities and their age at presentation is dictated by the underlying disease.

Another age-related distinction arises from the fact that the infectious consequences of humoral immunodeficiencies do not become apparent until after six months of age when the maternal antibodies protecting the newborn disappear. On the other hand, cell-mediated immunodeficiencies will present at birth or very soon thereafter and may result in

failure to thrive. Finally, patients with defects in phagocytes or the complement system may present at any age.

Given the fact that most primary immunodeficiencies have a genetic component, a *family history* is another important element in the analysis of these diseases. A relevant family history may reinforce the perception that this child is having more than his or her share of the usual childhood infections and may also suggest a pattern of inheritance, either autosomal or X-linked. Questions about early deaths in an extended family, particularly those from repeated infections, need to be specifically asked since an inherited immunodeficiency disorder may have gone previously unrecognized.

An essential aspect of the patient's history is the *pattern* (location and type) *of infections* that the individual has experienced since this will help identify the particular arm of the immune system which would be required for host defense against that category of organism (Table UI.2). In particular, it is critical to know if the patient has been subject primarily to bacterial infections or to viral, protozoan, and fungal infections. Patients with recurrent infections caused by **pyogenic** (pus-forming) bacteria, usually targeting the respiratory or gastrointestinal tract, will most often be suffering from a B-cell or humoral immune abnormality, since the primary means of fighting extracellular bacterial organisms rests with the synthesis of specific antibodies to that organism. By contrast, patients with viral, protozoan, and fungal infections are more likely to have a T-cell-mediated immunodeficiency since T cells are the primary defenders against intracellular organisms and are also required for defense against large fungal organisms. These include **opportunistic infections**, the clinical consequences of organisms that do not cause disease in immunologically intact individuals. Finally, recurrent skin infections and impaired wound healing will be more suggestive of a phagocytic cell deficiency, whereas systemic infection with encapsulated organisms and autoimmunity in older individuals will prompt consideration of a complement deficiency (Table UI.2).

The physical examination of the patient will likely yield two pieces of information. First, it will direct your attention to the presence of a currently ongoing acute or chronic infection. In addition, examination may provide evidence of preceding infections, that is, their location, severity or frequency, and consequences, which the patient (or in the case of children, the patient's parents) may have forgotten to mention. For example, repeated severe ear infections (otitis media) can result in scarring of the tympanic membrane. Second, a complete physical examination will provide information on possible structural abnormalities and their underlying causes. The sizes of the **secondary lymphoid organs**—the lymph nodes, spleen, and tonsils—are of particular importance. A clinical "pearl" is the observation of underdeveloped tonsils in any patient inherently incapable of generating germinal

TABLE UI.1. Summary of Major Immunodeficiency Disorders

Adaptive Immune System
Severe combined immunodeficiency diseases
   Cytokine receptor γ-chain defect: X-linked SCID
   JAK3 deficiency
   Interleukin-7Rα chain defect
   Recombination activating gene defect
   Artemis deficiency
   Adenosine deaminase deficiency
   Purine nucleoside phosphorylase deficiency
   Wiskott–Aldrich syndrome
   Ataxia telangiectasia
   SLAM-Associated Protein (SAP) mutation (X-linked lymphoproliferative syndrome)
T-cell deficiencies
   DiGeorge syndrome
   Zap-70 deficiency (presents as SCID)
   CD3 chain defect
   Bare lymphocyte syndrome (on antigen-presenting cells; some may present as SCID)
      MHC[a] class 1 deficiency
      MHC class 2 deficiency
   Fas mutation (autoimmune lymphoproliferative syndrome)
B-cell deficiencies
   X-linked agammaglobulinemia: Bruton's agammaglobulinemia
   Hyper-IgM syndromes
      Type I: X–linked: CD40L defect
      Type II: activation-induced cytidine deaminase defect
      Type III: CD40 defect
      Type IV: NEMO defect
      Type V: Uracil–DNA glycosylase defect
   Common variable immunodeficiency disorder
   IgA deficiency
   IgG subclass deficiency
Innate Immune System
Neutrophil disorders
   Leukocyte adhesion deficiency
      Type 1: integrin β-chain defect
      Type 2: selectin ligand defect
      Type 3: integrin signaling defect
   Chronic granulomatous disease
   Hyper IgE syndrome
Complement deficiencies
   Early components:
      C1, C4, or C2 defect
      C3 deficiency
   Late components: C5–C9
   Glycosyl phosphatidyl inositol deficiency: leads to red blood cell lysis
   Hereditary angioedema: C1 esterase inhibitor deficiency; leads to uncontrolled complement activation

[a]MHC: major histocompatibility complex

TABLE UI.2. Major Clinical Manifestations of Immune Disorders

Deficiency	Associated Diseases
B-lymphocyte deficiency: deficiency in antibody-mediated immunity	Recurrent bacterial infections, e.g., otitis media, recurrent pneumonia
T-lymphocyte deficiency: deficiency in cell-mediated immunity	Increased susceptibility to viral, fungal, and protozoal infections
T- and B-lymphocyte deficiency: combined deficiency of antibody and cell-mediated immunity	Acute and chronic infections with viral, bacterial, fungal, and protozoal organisms
Phagocytic cell deficiency	Systemic infections with bacteria of usually low virulence; infections with pyogenic bacteria; impaired pus formation and wound healing
NK cell deficiency	Viral infections, associated with several T-cell disorders and X-linked lymphoproliferative syndromes
Complement component deficiency	Bacterial infections; autoimmunity

centers (the structure necessary for high-affinity antibody formation). The presence of other anomalies, such as craniofacial or cardiac malformations or abnormalities of pigmentation, will suggest certain associated immunodeficiency syndromes. Failure to thrive, a symptom particularly prominent in T-cell defects, can be determined simply from the infant's pattern of growth in height and weight.

While a thorough history and physical examination are critical in suggesting and guiding evaluation of an immunodeficiency syndrome, in the final analysis, with a suspicion of an immunodeficiency disorder based on recurrent and/or unusual infections, a laboratory workup of the patient must be undertaken to confirm and identify the immune defect.

Laboratory Investigation

To evaluate a patient one can construct a flow chart with the different branches of the immune system

Adaptive Immunity		Innate Immunity	
Humoral Immunity	Cell-Mediated Immunity	NK Cells/ Phagocytes	Complement

During the development of humoral immunity, the major effector cell, the B cell, synthesizes its product, immunoglobulin (antibody), in response to antigen associated with pathogenic organisms, particularly encapsulated bacteria. In contrast, during the development of cell-mediated immunity, the T cell is the major effector cell, either as a $CD4^+$ T cell (acting through the release of cytokines or via cell–cell interactions) or as a $CD8^+$ cytotoxic T cell that will lyse virally infected target cells. However, it is important to remember that both types of immune responses depend on T helper cells and antigen-presenting cells such as macrophages or dendritic cells for the generation of the effector cells. Even complement components, which act as chemoattractants, opsonins, and as part of the antibody-mediated lytic process, impact the humoral and cell-mediated immune responses. In practice, therefore, one starts the evaluation of the patient with quantitating the final product or cell type in each arm of the immune system, evaluating them functionally and then, if necessary, working backward in the activation and developmental scheme until the block or deficiency is identified. In patients with combined immunodeficiencies (both humoral and cell mediated), the block could occur in a mechanism early in development and be common to both T and B cells or it could simply be present in T cells and interfere with help in both antibody production and cytotoxic T-cell maturation.

Quantitative Assays. The simplest initial test is the quantitation of products and cells that are present in the peripheral blood. Even when the clinical presentation points to a specific arm of the immune system, it is common to perform the simplest quantitative tests to establish that those parameters are normal in the patient. We can assign each quantitative test to an arm of the immune system as follows:

Adaptive Immunity		Innate Immunity	
Humoral Immunity	Cell-Mediated Immunity	NK Cells/ Phagocytes	Complement
B Cells	$CD4^+$ T Cells	NK Cells	C3, C4
Immunoglobulin isotypes	$CD8^+$ T Cells	Monocytes (macrophages)	C1esterase inhibitor
		Neutrophils/ Eosinophils/ Basophils	

Cellular Composition of Peripheral Blood. The first step in such quantitation is a **complete blood count (CBC)**, which results in the quantitation of the white blood cell types (differential count) present in the circulation; neutrophils, lymphocytes, monocytes, eosinophils, and basophils.

Further quantitation of immune cells in the blood involves analysis of the **lymphocyte subsets** by flow cytometry (see Unit V for assay descriptions) to determine the number and percentage of mature CD4$^+$ T cells, CD8$^+$ T cells, B cells, NK cells, and other cellular subsets in the circulation. This analysis is based on expression of characteristic cell surface markers (**CD: clusters of differentiation**) and is usually undertaken even if the number of lymphocytes in the peripheral blood is normal.

Immune-System Related Molecules in Peripheral Blood. Quantitation of the secreted protein products that are essential for immune function is also conducted on peripheral blood samples. For suspected B-cell deficiencies, assays are performed to determine the levels of total **serum immunoglobulins** along with individual isotype quantitation and analysis (IgM, IgG, IgA, and IgE). Levels of **complement components**, generally C3 and C4, are also part of a standard initial evaluation. Quantitation of protein molecules is generally performed by enzyme-linked immunosorbent assay (ELISA; see Unit V), which allows detection of low levels of specific proteins.

Analysis of Results of Quantitative Assays. Clearly, the absence of a specific cell type (such as mature B cells) or a molecule (such as an immunoglobulin isotype) will direct your further analysis. In particular, the absence of a mature cell population will now require analysis of the immature cells of that lineage, cells which may only be accessible from the primary lymphoid organs. Additional quantitative analysis may be undertaken subsequently as indicated by results of qualitative or functional assays. This might include further characterization of activation and memory markers on lymphocytes or adhesion molecules on granulocytes as examples. A number of immunodeficiency syndromes are characterized by defects in surface molecules that impair cell function but which do not result in altered cell numbers.

All laboratory results are compared with those from patients of similar age (as well as sex and sometimes ethnicity). In fact, immunoglobulin levels will be affected by both the patient's age as well as his or her prior exposure to antigen (vaccination history). In a young child, levels of some immunoglobulin isotypes are normally quite low and, as such, an inability to produce an effective immune response may not be apparent from these quantitative studies but will require a specific challenge.

Functional Assays and Further Quantitative Assays. Even the presence of normal numbers of mature circulating cells does not guarantee their functional capability. Depending on which arm of the immune system one suspects has a deficiency, several functional assays may be undertaken *in vitro* (in the test tube) and/or *in vivo* (in the patient).

B-Cell Functional Assays
PROLIFERATION ASSAYS. The ability of the cell to proliferate (divide) *in vitro* in response to nonspecific stimuli (or mitogens) is a cross between a functional assay and quantitative assay and in humans is usually performed using peripheral blood cells. This test does not evaluate the cell's ability to perform its differentiated function; rather, it measures a preliminary step that is necessary for most lymphocytes, T cells, and B cells to go through in the course of activation. B cells may be incubated with pokeweed mitogen (PWM), *Staphylococcus aureus* Cowen's I, and/or stimuli directed at the B-cell receptor (BCR). In the latter case, the assay is designed to evaluate the functionality of pathways normally taken to stimulate the division of B cells during an immune response. These include use of anti-μ antibody (the μ heavy chain is part of the BCR for antigen) and anti-CD40, a molecule crucial to the activation of the B cell. Thus, the selective proliferation of the B cell in response to some but not other signals is an important determinant of the ability of the B cell to respond to stimulation specific for a variety of pathways.

SPECIFIC ANTIBODY PRODUCTION *IN VITRO*
Retrospective Study (Prior Immunization). Antibody titer that exists as the result of prior exposure, whether to common antigens in the environment or to vaccination, is a simple way to assess B-cell function. However, the usefulness of these studies depends on the age and history of the patient. For instance, positive titers would be expected to antigens in vaccines administered during childhood and thus antibody levels may be measured for specific antigens, such as measles, mumps, rubella, tetanus, and diphtheria. One expects low levels of specific IgM and IgG antibodies to such antigens even in normal individuals unless they have received a recent challenge. In addition to these organism-specific antibodies, all individuals are expected to have **isohemagglutinins**, "natural" IgM antibodies to blood group antigens not expressed in the patient. These are also believed to be stimulated by organisms and appear to be the result of environmental exposure to organisms expressing antigens cross-reactive to human blood group antigens. Therefore, levels of isohemagglutinins are expected to be low in children less than one year of age.

Prospective Study (Active Immunization). For a more definitive assessment of B-cell function, one can administer a vaccine and then perform sequential measurements of specific antibody titers. However, because patients with immunodeficiency may develop active infections if given live attenuated viral vaccines, only nonliving antigens can be used to evaluate such patients. Evaluation for titer and immunoglobulin isotype at two and four weeks following immunization will provide information on the ability to respond to antigen and to switch immunoglobulin isotypes (see Case 4). Pneumococcus and *Haemophilus influenzae* vaccinations are commonly used as polysaccharide antigens and tetanus and diphtheria as protein antigens. The latter type will be more dependent on T-cell help to generate an effective response.

SPECIFIC ANTIBODY PRODUCTION *IN VITRO*
The B Cells on Their Own. Many of the nonspecific mitogens used to stimulate a proliferative response will result in the production of immunoglobulin by the B cells. These products may be measured in the culture media and quantitated by ELISA according to the isotype produced: IgM, IgG, and IgA.

T–B Collaboration. B cells may also be stimulated to produce immunoglobulin by coculture with T cells activated with anti-CD3/anti-CD28. Depending on the combination of patient versus control T cells, patient versus control B cells, or both, the function of each cell type and their ability to cooperate with one another can be measured. The assay also allows the evaluation of the function of T helper cells of the T_H2 subset. This parallels the natural situation of antibody response to T-dependent antigens.

T-Cell Functional Assays
PROLIFERATION ASSAYS. As with the B cell, nonspecific mitogens, in this case phytohemagglutinin (PHA) and concanavalin A (Con A), are used *in vitro* to test the ability of T cells to respond with cell division. A more physiologically relevant stimulation test employs cross-linking anti-CD3 antibody or anti-CD3 plus the cytokine interleukin-2 (IL-2), a T-cell growth factor, to stimulate the T cells.

T-CELL FUNCTIONAL ASSAYS *IN VITRO.* T helper cell function for antibody production was discussed above.

Cytokine Assays. The ability of T cells to produce and secrete their cytokine products after stimulation can be measured by harvesting the culture media and quantitating the specific cytokines in ELISAs. The cytokine products are characteristic of specific T helper cell subsets.

Mixed Lymphocyte Culture (MLC) and Cell-Mediated Lysis (CML) Assays. As will be discussed in some of the case studies, T cells recognize foreign molecules in the context of the individual's major histocompatibility complex (MHC) antigens and also recognize foreign MHC itself.

The recognition of foreign MHC *in vitro* can be used as a means of determining the ability to generate cytotoxic T cells and the ability to provide the help necessary for that generation, in this instance the T helper 1 subset. In the MLC assay, T cells are incubated with fixed cells (so that they do not divide) from an unrelated individual and the proliferation or cytokine production by these T cells is measured after several days. For the cytotoxicity assay, the responding cells are transferred from the first culture and incubated with labeled target cells that originate from the individual used for stimulatory cells in the first culture. The killing of those target cells is then a measure of the function of the cytotoxic T cells ($CD8^+$ T cells).

T-CELL FUNCTIONAL ASSAYS *IN VIVO*
Delayed-Type Hypersensitivity. This assay is commonly referred to as an assay of cell-mediated immunity. However, as will become apparent from its description, it actually measures the ability of T helper cells (and not T cytotoxic cells) and antigen presenting cells (APCs, e.g. macrophages) to collaborate. The reaction is dependent on the presentation of antigen in the context of MHC by the APCs in addition to the interaction of surface molecules and their receptors on the two cell types. An antigen to which the individual should have been previously exposed, such as antigen from *Candida*, a common environmental fungus, is injected intradermally in the forearm. The development of redness and swelling is evaluated 48–72 h later. The requirement for APCs to present antigen to the T cell and produce chemokines attracting additional cell types to the region illustrates the interaction between the innate and adaptive immune systems in both the afferent and efferent phases of this specific immune response. In fact, the results of this test are also dependent on vascular changes at the site, demonstrating both the potential difficulty of interpreting *in vivo* testing and the complexity of responses as they occur naturally in the body.

Allogeneic Skin Graft Rejection. Although used in the past, the ability to reject a skin graft from an unrelated donor is no longer a test employed in humans (although still acceptable in animal models). This assay would be the *in vivo* equivalent of the MHC–CML assay.

Phagocytic Cell Functional Assays
PHAGOCYTOSIS. The ability of cells to phagocytize (ingest or engulf particle through the formation of a vacuole) may be measured using a variety of small, usually labeled particles. Their ingestion can be detected by either flow cytometry (see Unit V) or microscopy. Killed bacteria, yeast, or synthetic particles may be labeled and used as the targets for phagocytosis.

ROLLING, ADHESION, AND MIGRATION. These are evaluated by flow cytometric detection of the surface molecules required for each function.

OXIDATIVE BURST. Two assays are employed to measure the oxidative burst of phagocytic cells.

Nitroblue Tetrazolium (NBT) Assay. This assay tests the oxidative burst capacity of neutrophils by measuring their ability to convert NBT, which is yellow, to formazan, which is blue/violet and detectable by microscopy.

Dihydrorhodamine Assay. Stimulated neutrophils loaded with dihydrorhodamine will oxidize the dye with H_2O_2 and demonstrate increased fluorescence, which is detectable by flow cytometry.

Evaluation of NK Cell Function. Although the function of NK cells can be evaluated by an *in vitro* test similar to the T-cell cytotoxicity assay, using susceptible targets and without presensitization, in actuality the functioning of these cells is rarely measured in the clinical situation. Deficiencies in NK cells may be part of a larger deficiency in the T-cell lineage and will be reflected in the peripheral blood NK cell numbers. The rarity of an NK cell defect as an isolated abnormality suggests that the NK cell's individual capabilities are compensated for, that these patients have yet to be described, or both.

Complement Function Assay. The CH50 assay is a functional assay for complement that generates a kinetics curve for the rate of lysis of antibody-coated sheep red blood cells and is reported at the 50% point. The assay measures the presence and function of C1–C9.

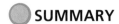 **SUMMARY**

Given identification of a quantitative or functional defect, the specific disorder may need to be further defined. For the quantitative tests, such as finding the absence of a surface molecule on neutrophils, the results of the assays and identification of the immunodeficiency disorder will be straightforward; one only needs to think to look for the specific defect. In analyzing of the results of functional studies, particularly those involving lymphocytes, the multitude of interactions among the components of the adaptive as well as the innate immune systems must be considered. Figure UI.1 attempts to illustrate these interwoven parts by placing arrows between the components of the branches and arms of the immune system that we described at the start of this chapter (Fig. UI.1). From this figure it is easy to appreciate how a defect in one cell may affect many functions or how a defect in one cell may be compensated for in the individual by the intact components of their immune system.

Once a quantitative or functional defect is identified, the underlying pathophysiology must be elucidated. For some of the immunodeficiency diseases, familiarity with the development and differentiation of the immune cells will be required. Figure UI.2 is a flow chart of the development and interaction of T and B lymphocytes and the positions of the blocks in differentiation and function that are seen in a variety of immunodeficiency disorders; use of such a chart is a good approach to the problem if the adaptive immune system is deficient. The diagnosis of the specific disorder (Table U1.1), whether it requires further functional studies

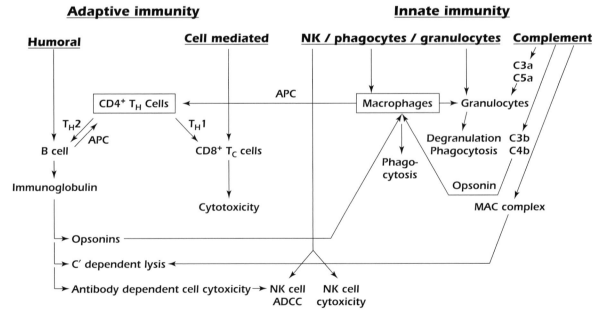

Figure UI.1. Flow chart depicting interactions between arms of immune system.

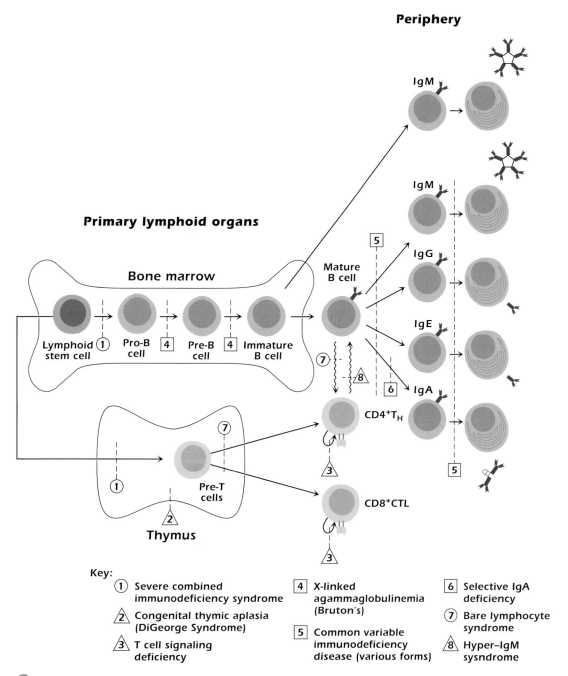

Periphery

IgM

Primary lymphoid organs

Bone marrow

Mature
B cell

Lymphoid ① Pro-B ④ Pre-B ④ Immature
stem cell   cell   cell   B cell

⑦

⑧

IgM

IgG

IgE

IgA

5

6

CD4⁺T_H

③

Pre-T
cells

⑦

①

△2

Thymus

CD8⁺CTL

③

5

Key:
① Severe combined
   immunodeficiency syndrome

△2 Congenital thymic aplasia
   (DiGeorge Syndrome)

△3 T cell signaling
   deficiency

④ X-linked
   agammaglobulinemia
   (Bruton's)

5 Common variable
   immunodeficiency
   disease (various forms)

6 Selective IgA
   deficiency

⑦ Bare lymphocyte
   syndrome

△8 Hyper–IgM
   sysndrome

⬤ Figure UI.2. Flow chart depicting B- and T-cell development with locations of immunodeficiency diseases. Circles denote diseases with severe combined immunodeficiency presentation; triangles are for diseases with predominantly T cell deficiencies and squares are for B cell defecent disorders.

and flow cytometric analysis of surface molecules, enzymatic studies as in adenine deaminase (ADA) deficiency, or even gene sequence analysis, is discussed in the individual

cases presented in this unit. It is apparent that we are lucky to have the footprints of investigators who came before us to follow in unraveling this complex set of diseases.

1

X-LINKED AGAMMAGLOBULINEMIA (BRUTON'S AGAMMAGLOBULINEMIA)

SUSAN R. S. GOTTESMAN

 ## CASE REPORT

"Sam always gets sick; now he has a bad earache and fever."

Day 1

Sam is a four-year-old boy who is brought to you in the emergency room (ER) by his distraught parents because he has a fever, has been vomiting in the last few hours, and seems slightly disoriented (confused). His mother relates that initially Sam complained of a right-sided earache that was only transiently relieved with acetaminophen. Over the next few days, he developed a fever and became less active and more irritable and did not want to eat. Yesterday he began complaining of a headache "all over his head" and this morning he began vomiting. His mother states that Sam has a history of frequent ear infections (otitis media) with effusion but is concerned that this time it is more than just an earache.

Sam has a generally normal appearance and size but that he has an acute illness marked by fever, withdrawal from his surroundings, and extreme irritability, that is,

crying spells unabated by his mother's attempts to calm him down. He has a temperature of 40°C, his skin is hot to the touch, and he appears to be mildly dehydrated (as evidenced by dryness around his mouth and eyes). His throat is injected (red) but without *exudate* (pus) and his right ear has an opacified tympanic membrane with a loss of the light reflex; his left ear is normal. He has *nuchal rigidity* (neck stiffness when his head is flexed). You evaluate him for other signs of meningeal irritation and find that he has a positive *Kernig's sign* (pain when lower leg is extended with his hip flexed at 90°) and a positive *Brudzinski's sign* (involuntary flexion of the knees and hips when you flex his neck).

His lungs are clear to auscultation and his abdomen has normal bowel sounds, is nondistended, and is nontender. His joints are nontender and mobile.

You are alarmed at the evolution of Sam's initial complaint and his neurologic signs. Suspecting that he has an infectious meningitis you immediately perform a lumbar puncture (after checking his eyes for papilledema with an ophthalmoscope) to confirm the diagnosis and to attempt to identify the organism. The cerebrospinal fluid (CSF) is obtained and blood and CSF samples are sent for emergency analysis and to the microbiology lab for culture.

Immunology: Clinical Case Studies and Disease Pathophysiology, By Warren Strober and Susan R. S. Gottesman
Copyright © 2009 John Wiley & Sons, Inc.

Results obtained quickly are as follows:

Cerebrospinal fluid:	Result	Reference Range
Opening pressure	180 mm Hg	50–80 mm Hg
Appearance	Cloudy	Clear
White blood cells (WBC)	1078/μL	<5/μL
Neutrophils	75%	<25%
Red blood cells (RBC)	0	0
Protein	300 mg/dL	20–45 mg/dL
Glucose	3 mg/dL	>50 mg/dL

Peripheral WBC count and differential:	Absolute Count	Reference Range
Total WBC	24,000/μL	5500–15,000
Neutrophils 75%	18,000/μL	1500–8500
Lymphocytes 19%	4,560/μL	2000–8000
Monocytes 5%	1,200/μL	300–650
Eosinophils 1%	240/μL	100–500

In view of the above history and laboratory findings, what is your initial diagnosis and treatment plan?

> *Sam shows all the typical signs and symptoms of meningitis. These include headache, vomiting, and disorientation as well as physical evidence of meningeal irritation (e.g., nuchal rigidity). These clinical findings and the elevated opening pressure on entry into the meningeal space, along with the presence of a cloudy CSF containing WBC, point unmistakably to infection of the meninges. Moreover, the predominance of neutrophils in the CSF, along with a low glucose, strongly suggests a bacterial meningitis, a type of meningitis that must be treated urgently to prevent permanent neurologic defects or even death.*
>
> *Recurrent otitis media is fairly common in young children and may occasionally lead to meningitis, as it apparently did in Sam's case. Viral meningitis is the more common form, although bacterial meningitis does sometimes occur in normal children as well.*
>
> *Sam's peripheral blood cell count is high due to a granulocytosis. **Granulocytosis** is an increase in cells of the granulocytic series, of which the neutrophils are by far the most prominent. This again suggests a bacterial infection and one that has spread to the peripheral blood. Given this likelihood, you start Sam on intravenous ceftazidine, an antibiotic that provides good broad-spectrum coverage.*

Day 2

The next morning, after almost 24 h of intravenous ceftazidine, you walk into Sam's hospital room to find that he is calm, smiling faintly, and beginning to eat. His parents are much relieved and are already asking when Sam can be taken home. The laboratory reports that *Streptococcus pneumoniae* was isolated from both his blood and CSF but antibiotic sensitivities are not yet available; you therefore continue the ceftazidine therapy. When they become available, you may elect to change the antibiotic on the basis of the sensitivities of the isolated streptococcal organism.

Now that the urgent problem of bacterial meningitis is resolving, you obtain a more complete history from the parents. The mother mentions again that Sam seems to get sick quite often, definitely more often than his playmates. She relates that Sam had skin abscesses at 9 and 10 months of age, three episodes of pneumonia documented by X-ray findings, multiple episodes of diarrhea, and one episode of left knee swelling. His parents take him to the pediatrician on a regular basis.

This history of multiple, severe, and in some cases unusual infections is disturbing and you decide that further investigation is needed. You consider the possibility that Sam has a primary immunodeficiency disorder and refer the family to an allergist/immunologist for more definitive workup once he has recovered from the acute infection.

Subsequent Workup Three Weeks Later

Three weeks later, Sam has fully recovered from the meningitis and has completed the recommended antibiotic treatment (the streptococcus was sensitive to ceftazidine). At this point he is seen by an allergist/immunologist who confirms that Sam is within the expected range for height and weight and has a normal appearance. On examination, however, he notices that Sam lacks tonsillar tissue, quite an abnormal finding in a 4-year-old child. There is no **lymphadenopathy** (enlargement of lymph nodes) or **hepatosplenomegaly** (enlargement of liver and spleen). He also checks Sam's blood count and finds that it has returned to normal.

From questioning the parents, the allergist/immunologist learns that Sam is an only child and that both parents are healthy. The pregnancy was uneventful and Sam was a full-term baby of normal size. The parents do not remember any fevers or infections during the first 6–8 months of his life. In relating the family history, Sam's mother states that her two sisters are healthy but that she had a brother who died at age 18. She recalls that the brother was always sick and had repeated pneumonias resulting in chronic lung disease. Her male cousin died of polio after receiving an oral polio vaccine during childhood. Sam's father's family history is negative for family members with multiple infections.

The allergist/immunologist concludes that Sam's history and the family history are sufficiently suggestive to warrant an immunodeficiency workup.

What information does one seek in such a workup?

*The initial goal of an immunodeficiency workup is to determine if the patient (a child in this case) has a B-cell deficiency, a T-cell deficiency, a combined T- and B-cell deficiency, a phagocytic cell deficiency, or a complement deficiency. By **deficiency** we mean a decrease in the amount or function of these immunologic elements. If a defect is detected, one would then attempt to define the specific underlying molecular abnormality. Sam's age suggests that a congenital deficiency needs to be considered; his maternal family history raises suspicion of an inherited disorder.*

Tests may be organized to investigate each arm of the immune system (see the introduction to this unit and below). In addition, specific assays either provide quantitative information or measure functional activity. In general, the results of quantitative assays are more quickly available. Given the fact that Sam has a sufficiently strong personal and family history to justify this workup, most of these tests are initiated at the outset. As the results are collected and evaluated, it will become obvious that some give predictable results. For learning purposes, we will present the results of this evaluation arranged according to the immune system being probed.

Humoral Immunity Studies (Mainly Involving B Cells)

Serum Immunoglobulin Levels: Quantitative Assay. Blood is drawn from Sam for determination of serum immunoglobulin levels. These are measured by a spectrometric assay called nephelometry, with the exception of IgE, which, because of its normally low level, requires a more sensitive method: radioimmunoassay (RIA) or enzyme linked immunosorbent assay ELISA (see unit V for detailed assay descriptions).

Result

		Reference Range
IgG	140 mg/dL	923 ± 256 mg/dL
IgM	32 mg/dL	65 ± 25 mg/dL
IgA	48 mg/dL	124 ± 45 mg/dL
IgE	1.5 μg/dL	2.0–10 μg/dL

What information do you obtain from overall immunoglobulin levels?

Overall immunoglobulin levels are used as a gross indication of the individual's ability to respond to antigenic exposure with a humoral response and to be capable of a secondary response (IgG) and as an indicator of allergic reactions (IgE). As the levels are the result of prior exposure, it is not unexpected that immunoglobulin levels increase with age. They generally reach adult levels at puberty. Thus, Sam's levels are compared with those of other four-year-olds.

Sam shows abnormally low levels of all the immunoglobulin subclasses.

Specific Antibody Responses to Antigenic Challenge: Functional Assays

RETROSPECTIVE. Studies of response to previous challenge. Blood is drawn for the determination of measles, mumps, rubella, and varicella serum antibody titers with the knowledge that Sam had been administered vaccines for these organisms at approximately 12 months of age. These antibodies are measured by ELISA using the specific antigens. This allows detection of low levels of antibody, as one would expect in response to a specific antigen, and allows titers to be obtained.

Result. Titers to all four organisms come back as "undetectable" or at the lowest limit of detection.

PROSPECTIVE. Response to a new challenge. In a more definitive test of ability to mount an antibody response, Sam is administered a standard dose of diphtheria and tetanus (DT) antigens as well as pneumococcal antigens to test his capacity to mount an antibody response to protein (DT) or to polysaccharide (pneumococcal) antigens [see Case 24 and Coico and Sunshine (Chapter 10) for description of T-dependent and T-independent antigens]. Blood is drawn just prior to antigen administration and again at two and four weeks after immunization. Serum antibody titers to each specific antigen are measured at the three time points. Although Sam would already have been given three doses of DT as part of the routine vaccination schedule, a normal individual will exhibit at least a 5- to 10-fold rise in titer to DT following this immunization protocol and a 4- to 5-fold rise in titer to one or more of the pneumococcal subtypes. The data are obtained about two weeks after the submission of the sera.

Result. Sam is unable to mount a significant antibody response to either DT or pneumococcal antigens.

Conclusion of Humoral Immunity Studies. The low "across-the-board" Ig levels and poor antibody responses point to a severe deficiency in B-cell function. However, from this information one cannot state definitively that this is the only immune defect present or that the B cells are the culprits.

T- and B-Cell Studies

Analysis of Lymphocyte Subsets in the Peripheral Blood: Quantitative Studies by Flow Cytometry. Sam's peripheral blood cells are stained with fluorochrome-bound antibodies recognizing CD markers characteristic of particular lymphocyte subsets. The number of cells staining with each antibody is quantitated using a flow cytometer (see Unit V).

Result.

		Reference Range	Absolute Count
CD3 (pan T-cell marker)	85%	55–82%	1755/μL
CD4 (marker of helper T cell)	55%	33–57%	1053/μL
CD8 (marker of cytotoxic T cell)	31%	8–34%	725/μL
CD19 (B-cell marker)	0%	6–22%	0
CD16/56 (NK cell markers)	15%	6–31%	350/μL

Combining the Data. *The lymphocyte subset quantification studies suggest that Sam's inability to mount an antibody response is due to the absence of mature B cells.*

In Vitro Proliferation Studies: Nonspecific Functional Assays. Sam's cells are cultured with various stimulators for three days, after which their level of proliferation is quantitated by their ability to incorporate tritium-labeled thymidine. Agents that stimulate T-cell proliferation include the mitogens phytohemagglutinin (PHA) and concanavalin A (ConA) and the T-cell-specific antibody combination anti-CD3 and anti-CD28. B cells are stimulated to proliferate by incubation with pokeweed mitogen (PWM), *Staphylococcus aureus* Cowen type I, and the B-cell specific antibodies anti-μ heavy chain or anti-CD40.

Sam's cells are cultured with the anti-CD3/anti-CD28, which is designed to mimic the manner in which T cells are normally stimulated, and with anti-CD40, which is designed to mimic the normal interaction between T helper cells and B cells.

Result.

> Anti-CD3/anti-CD28 stimulation: the proliferation response of Sam's T cells is normal as compared to simultaneously run control cells.
> Anti-CD40 stimulation: the proliferation of Sam's cells is significantly decreased as compared to simultaneously run control cells.

These phenotyping and proliferation studies reveal the presence of a B-cell defect, corroborating the humoral immunity studies which focused on B cells. Given the fact that Sam has no detectable levels of B cells in the peripheral blood, stimulation with B-cell specific mitogens or anti-CD40 was expected to be undetectable. It is also not surprising that Sam is unable to mount an antibody response given the absence of mature B cells (and tonsillar tissue). The results

additionally demonstrate that Sam has normal T- and NK cell numbers and that Sam's T cells can mount a normal proliferative response to stimulation via the specific receptors that would normally be involved in a T–B collaboration. Thus, his T cells appear to be normal.

Cell-Mediated Immunity Studies (Mainly Involving T Cells)

Delayed-Type Hypersensitivity (DTH) Test: In Vivo T-Cell Functional Assay. An antigen to which Sam has been previously exposed is injected intracutaneously on the forearm and development of redness and induration (swelling) is evaluated at 48 h. Since Sam has been immunized with tetanus toxoid in the past, tetanus toxoid is injected intracutaneously in the forearm area.

Result. At 48 h, a 1 cm area of redness and swelling is noted.

DTH is a classic test for cell-mediated immunity but in fact only measures the interaction between T helper cells and APCs (along with nonspecific vascular changes, etc.). Additional tests of cell-mediated immunity include studies of cytotoxic T-cell function; however since all evidence, both clinical and laboratory, suggests that this arm of Sam's immune system is intact, they will not be performed in this case (see differential diagnosis section below and Unit V).

Nonspecific Immunity and Complement Studies.
For completeness, Sam's blood is also sent to the laboratory for the determination of complement levels and the ability of his white cells to generate reactive oxygen species or hydrogen peroxide. The latter is a function of phagocytes and is impaired in chronic granulomatous disease.

Complement Studies: Quantitative Assay of Complement Components.

Result.

		Reference Range
CH50	180 μg/ml	150–310 μg/ml
C3	95 mg/dL	85–201 mg/dL
C4	30 mg/dL	16–47 mg/dL

Phagocytic Cells: Functional Assays of Neutrophils.

NITROBLUE TETRAZOLIUM (NBT) TEST.   Yellow NBT is converted to blue/violet formazan within normal neutrophils due to reduction of NBT by O_2^-, thus measuring their ability to generate reactive oxygen species.

Result. Sam's cells exhibit blue/violet crystals following incubation with NBT.

FLOW CYTOMETRIC ANALYSIS OF PMA-STIMULATED NEUTROPHILS LOADED WITH DIHYDRORHODAMINE. When dye is oxidized by H_2O_2, it exhibits increased fluorescence, demonstrating the neutrophils' ability to generate H_2O_2 when stimulated.

Result. Sam's cells exhibit normal flow patterns.

Complement levels and neutrophil functions are normal.

Based on the above results, what is your overall conclusion concerning the functioning of Sam's immune system and location of possible defect?

Overall, the above results show that, despite Sam's normal peripheral white blood cell and normal lymphocyte counts, he has low to undetectable numbers of B cells and has reduced or absent B-cell function. The fact that the B-cell defect was not reflected in the white count is not unexpected given the fact that B cells normally account for only a minority of peripheral lymphocytes. The absence of mature B cells goes along with the absence of tonsils since the latter is a secondary lymphoid organ in which the majority of cells are B cells. Finally, T-cell numbers and function, both in vitro and in vivo, are normal, strongly suggesting the B-cell defect is not secondary to a T-cell defect. The fact that the B cells are not just nonfunctional but are absent in the periphery points to an intrinsic inability of the B-cell precursors to differentiate or to a block in the differentiation of mature B cells from precursors.

Why was Sam healthy until the age of six months?

Neonates are protected against infection by the presence of maternal antibodies obtained during gestation and nursing. IgG crosses the placenta and IgG and IgA especially are components of breast milk (Case 4; see also Coico and Sunshine, Chapter 4 for function of different isotypes.). This is essentially a natural form of passive immunity and protects the infant until its immune system is developed enough to generate its own immune response. These principles also underlie the vaccination schedule in infants (Coico and Sunshine, Chapter 20).

Follow-Up Visit

Based on the laboratory results, the allergist/immunologist concludes that Sam has a B-cell disorder. Since this has led to an inability to produce normal levels of immunoglobulins and mount normal antibody responses, he starts Sam on intravenous immunoglobulin (IVIG) therapy administered every four weeks as a replacement for his own inability to produce immunoglobulins. After a single IVIG administration Sam's trough IgG level (the level obtained four weeks after the initial dose and just prior to the second dose) is 400 mg/dL. His trough level after six months of therapy is 550 mg/dL. Since studies have shown that no additional protection is achieved with trough IgG levels higher than 400 mg/dL, the six-month result indicates that optimal

therapy has been achieved. IgM and IgA levels remain low because the IVIG preparation does not contain significant amounts of these immunoglobulins. One year later, Sam shows definite clinical improvement; he has been without infections since IVIG therapy was started.

DIFFERENTIAL DIAGNOSIS OF SAM'S IMMUNODEFICIENCY

The differential diagnosis of Sam's immunodeficiency starts with the immunologic studies conducted above that show the presence of a B-cell defect. However, even before such data are obtained, certain features of Sam's clinical course allow informed speculation concerning his diagnosis. What are these features?

As discussed in the introduction to this unit, when considering the history of a patient with possible immunodeficiency, it is useful to take note of the infectious agents and whether they are most consistent with the presence of a defect of the humoral response (antibody) as opposed to a defect of cell-mediated immunity or phagocytic cell immunity. Thus one needs to consider if the organisms involved are bacterial (extracellular) as opposed to viral or fungal (intracellular).

It was mentioned above that, although Sam had a history of infections early in life, his first several months were infection free. This points to a primary immunodeficiency rather than a secondary immunodeficiency, but one which may have been masked by immune elements such as maternal immunoglobulins that Sam received from his mother in utero. Second, Sam's infections appeared, at least by history, to be due mainly to extracellular "high grade" bacterial pathogens that could cause infections in both normal and immunocompromised individuals, rather than "low grade" intracellular pathogens such as certain viruses, fungi, and parasites. This suggests the presence of a humoral abnormality rather than a cell-mediated immune defect, since the former is usually associated with infections with highly virulent, high grade bacteria. However, this infectious history does not rule out a complement disorder, which is also marked by infections with such pathogens. Finally, Sam's infection history is inconsistent with a disorder of the innate immune system such as a neutrophil or NK cell disorder, since these disorders would also be expected to give rise to infection with low grade pathogens. A deficiency in humoral immunity may be due to a defect in B cells. Alternatively, T helper cells or the interaction between T and B cells may be at fault.

In evaluating where Sam's defect lies, it is helpful to look at a scheme of B-cell development and function and consider where the block may occur (Fig. 1.1).

How does Sam's workup allow one to pinpoint the problem?

Sam's immunologic workup revealed a reduction in all the serum immunoglobulins and an absence of response to

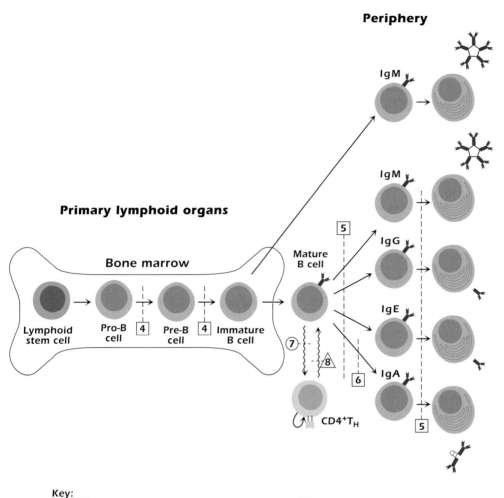

Periphery

Primary lymphoid organs

Bone marrow

Key:

4	X-linked agammaglobulinemia; μ heavy-chain deficiency; λ₅ (λ-like) deficiency
6	Selective IgA deficiency
7	Bare lymphocyte syndrome
5	Common variable immunodeficiency
8	X-linked hyper-IgM syndrome

Figure 1.1. Scheme of B-cell development and function and locations of blocks in development with various immunodeficiency disorders.

immunization. The absence of all immunoglobulin isotypes suggests that the block occurs at a stage prior to the development of isotype-specific plasma cells. Specifically, this eliminates a selective IgA deficiency and hyper-IgM syndrome. The latter is unlikely because Sam's IgM levels are low and because some forms of hyper-IgM syndrome result from T-cell abnormalities (see Case 4).

Working our way to the left in Figure 1.1, we encounter common variable immunodeficiency (CVID) and bare lymphocyte syndromes. Bare lymphocyte syndrome, in which the cells lack the expression of one of the human leukocyte antigen (HLA) classes, would lead to a defect in DTH and humoral immunity combined, since both depend on class II MHC expression. Lack of class I MHC antigen expression would affect T cytotoxic activity and spare T helper cell stimulation.

It is somewhat more difficult to clinically distinguish between CVID and X-linked agammaglobulinemia (XLA), which might both be part of your differential diagnoses. Like XLA, CVID is dominated by a humoral immune defect

manifested by the inability to mount normal antibody responses, and the two have similar infectious histories. However, CVID usually manifests later than XLA and indeed was initially called "acquired agammaglobulinemia" because it has its onset in adulthood more often than in childhood (see Case 5). Four years of age would be particularly young for CVID. In addition, patients with CVID not infrequently manifest various types of autoimmune manifestations leading to chronic gastrointestinal (GI) disorders, hematopoietic abnormalities, and liver abnormalities that are never seen in XLA. Importantly, in CVID, mature B cells are present, although the activation and differentiation to antibody-producing cells are blocked. In Sam, the defect is earlier and prevents the development of mature B cells. As you will note, we have worked our way back to the earliest stages of B-cell development to localize the point of Sam's block (Fig. 1.2).

A final differential must be made among the various types of B-cell abnormalities that result in a block in early B-cell development at the pro-B cell stage and thus lead to the

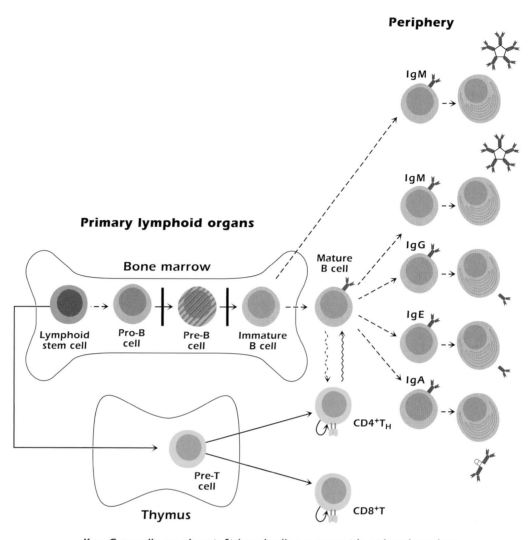

Figure 1.2. Remaining developing and mature lymphoid populations in XLA. Gray cells are populations missing in XLA patients. Bars indicate positions of developmental blocks.

Key: Grey cells are absent. Stripped cells are present in reduced numbers.

absence of mature B cells in the periphery: XLA, μ heavy chain deficiency, and λ5 deficiency (see the section on normal B-cell development below for events leading to B-cell maturation). The distinction among these diseases on clinical or even on immunologic grounds can be quite difficult. However, both μ heavy chain deficiency and λ5 chain deficiency show autosomal recessive patterns of inheritance and are quite rare. The family history of healthy females and affected male relatives on Sam's mother's side is classic for an X-linked Mendelian genetic disease and is thus more consistent with XLA. Another difference is that μ heavy chain deficient patients generally display even lower levels of IgG than XLA patients and have undetectable peripheral B cells. Both XLA and λ5 deficiency patients generally have very small numbers of circulating B cells, but in XLA the B cells have an immature phenotype, and in λ5 deficiency they have a mature phenotype.

In the end, distinction among these early B-cell defects requires confirmation by molecular analysis. This is usually done by analysis of patient monocytes, another cell that ordinarily expresses Bruton's tyrosine kinase (Btk) (see

below). Identification of the mutation may be necessary for screening of future pregnancies for the occurrence of affected fetuses.

CLINICAL ASPECTS OF X-LINKED AGAMMAGLOBULINEMIA

XLA is characterized by susceptibility to infection with pyogenic bacterial organisms, particularly encapsulated Gram-positive and Gram-negative organisms such as *Haemophilus influenzae*, *S. pneumoniae*, *S. aureus*, and *Pseudomonas* species. It thus results in severe recurrent acute infections starting at approximately six months of age when maternal antibodies transmitted to the child via the placenta *in utero* are no longer present in sufficient amount. Upper and lower respiratory infections are especially common, but life-threatening sepsis and meningitis (as in the present case) also occur. A particularly serious and long-term problem is recurrent pneumonia because it can lead to bronchiectasis, pulmonary fibrosis, and pulmonary failure. As previously noted, a clue to the early diagnosis and treatment of XLA (and a clinical pearl) is the absence of lymph node enlargement and underdeveloped tonsils in a young child who presents with what seem to be normal childhood infections.

Organisms that enter the bloodstream through the GI tract are a particular problem for patients with B-cell deficiencies. Thus, immunization with live poliovirus may lead to infection rather than protection. This was the probable scenario in Sam's mother's cousin who died of poliomyelitis following "vaccination." A particularly ominous type of infection that can occur in XLA (as well as in CVID) is enteroviral infection of the central nervous system (CNS). This infection can lead to a poorly understood type of autoimmune encephalomyelitis that results in progressive loss of CNS function characterized by motor and intellectual deterioriation and culminating in death. It is refractory to treatment since it is usually recognized when the infectious phase is over and the CNS is sterile. In some cases XLA is associated with a dermatomyositis-type disorder. As previously mentioned, in sharp contrast to CVID patients, XLA patients do not manifest the array of autoimmune disorders mentioned above. Other viral and fungal infections are well handled by XLA patients.

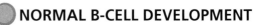 NORMAL B-CELL DEVELOPMENT

In the fetus, B-cell development first begins, along with all hematopoiesis, in the liver and then transfers to the bone marrow, the major site of development at birth. The orderly process of hematopoiesis is dependent on the interaction of precursor cells with their microenvironment, such as, bone marrow stromal cells and osteoblasts, in ways which are still being elucidated. In order to produce mature B cells, the first decision point is at the level of a pleuripotential hematopoietic stem cell in the bone marrow which commits to the lymphoid lineage. The next decision point is the determination as to whether differentiation will progress along the T/NK pathway or the B-cell pathway. We will pick up the story of B-cell development at the level of the progenitor B cell (pro-B), as illustrated in Figure 1.3. Note that most of the experimental data have been obtained on mice, and there are differences between human and mouse B-cell development. The nomenclature also varies (even from investigator to investigator) within one species. We will focus on human data where available.

During normal B-cell development, the pro-B cell initiates immunoglobulin synthesis with the rearrangement and transcription of the μ heavy-chain gene. This occurs first with the joining of the $D_H J_H$ segments, followed

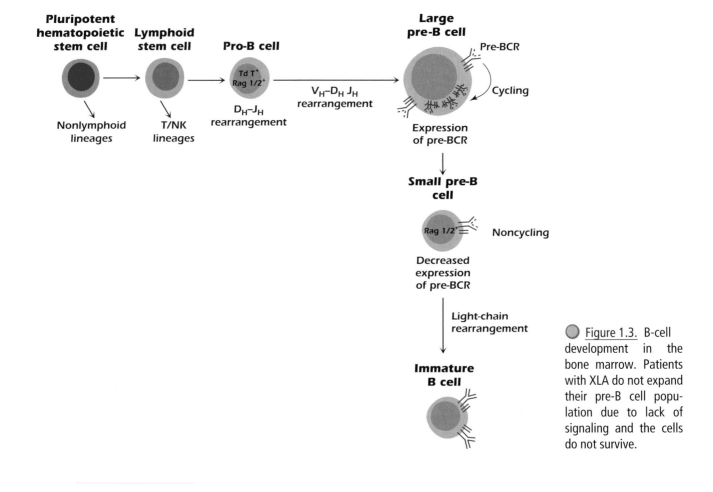

Figure 1.3. B-cell development in the bone marrow. Patients with XLA do not expand their pre-B cell population due to lack of signaling and the cells do not survive.

by the joining of V_H segments. Accomplishing this task requires the expression of a variety of transcription factors and recombination enzymes (Rag 1 and 2), endonucleases, and TdT (terminal deoxynucleotidyl transferase) similar to those operating in the developing T cell (see Case 2). The productive rearrangement of the μ heavy-chain gene culminates in the expression of μ protein on the cell surface plasma membrane and/or in the internal cytoplasmic membranes in association with a "surrogate" light chain. The surrogate light chain is the product of two genes, *VpreB* and λ5 (also called λ-like in humans). The heavy chains and surrogate light chains assemble into an Ig-like complex and become associated with two transmembrane signal-transducing molecules, Igα and Igβ (CD79a and CD79b). The molecular complex thus formed is called the pre-B-cell receptor (pre-BCR) and the cell is now termed a precursor (pre)-B cell. The down-regulation of the recombination enzymes, further differentiation, continued survival, and, in humans, the proliferation of the pre-B cell requires stimulation via the pre-BCR and the activation of a pre-BCR-dependent signaling cascade. This includes the activation of a key cytosolic tyrosine kinase enzyme known as Bruton's tyrosine kinase, which is a Tec family protein tyrosine kinase (PTK) (Fig. 1.4).

The activation of Btk and its role in B-cell development is illustrated in Figure 1.5. A description of this biochemical pathway is as follows:

Activation, possibly by cross-linking, of the pre-BCR causes phosphorylation of the cytoplasmic tails of Igα and Igβ on their ITAM domain (immunoreceptor tyrosine-based activation motif).These then activate the Src family kinases, particularly Lyn and then Syk and Blk. This allows the formation of a docking station for Syk, which then recruits and phosphorylates SLP-65 and Btk at its PH (Pleckstrin homology) domain. The adaptor protein SLP-65 (also known as BLNK or BASH) functions as a scaffold, bringing Btk to the membrane. This activated SLP-65 molecule further

recruits Btk and phospholipase Cγ2 (PLC-γ2). Btk activates PLC-γ2, which then hydrolyzes PIP_2 (phophatidylinositol bisphosphate) to IP_3 (inositol triphosphate) and DAG (diacylglycerol). This opens calcium channels and activates protein kinase C. In humans, SLP-65 and Btk control both differentiation and proliferation of the pre-B cell, whereas in mice, although differentiation appears dependent on these molecules, proliferation involves different pathways and appears dependent on IL-7 signaling. Proliferation involves the activation of the RAS and MAPK (mitogen-activated protein kinase) pathways. Thus in humans, mutations in Btk and the much more rare mutations in SLP-65 or λ5 result in a severe phenotype; mice with mutations in these molecules or "knockouts" demonstrate milder and "leakier" B-cell deficiency (see Unit V for description of knockout mice). Recent evidence suggests that, after activation, Btk and SLP-65 down-regulate the pre-BCR, thereby limiting pre-B-cell proliferation and possibly functioning as tumor suppressor molecules.

Activated Btk again functions in the mature B cell and may integrate pathways important for its survival, proliferative response, and modulation of the signal threshold necessary for B-cell activation via the BCR. In addition, Btk is expressed in mast cells and may play a role in their ability to degranulate in response to surface receptor cross-linking. Btk expression is restricted to the B-cell lineage, myeloid (granulocytic) cells, and erythroid cells.

The pre-B cell has now gone from a larger proliferating cell to a small pre-B cell. It has exited the cell cycle and down-regulated pre-BCR expression and is no longer synthesizing surrogate light chain molecules. Re-expression of the enzymes required for immunoglobulin gene rearrangement, Rag 1 and 2, initiates light chain gene rearrangement and protein synthesis. This light chain must be able to associate with the μ heavy chain on the surface for the cell to escape apoptosis. The cell is now the immature B cell and is subject to negative selection for elimination of autoreactive cells.

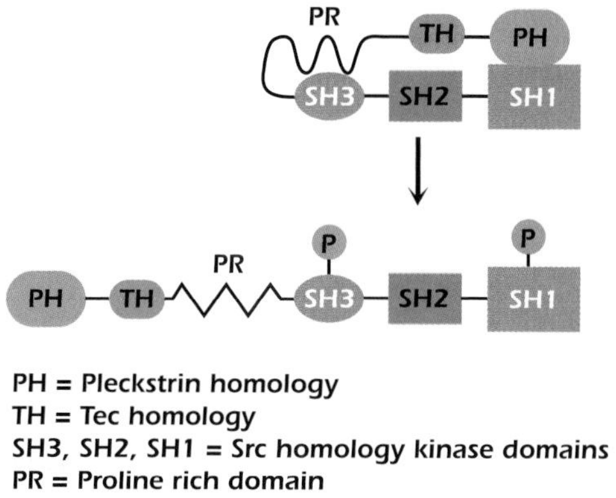

PATHOGENESIS OF XLA AND RELATED DISORDERS

X-linked agammaglobulinemia, or Bruton's agammaglobulinemia, was described by Ogden Bruton in 1952 and, indeed, was the first description of an immunodeficiency disorder. Dr. Bruton, a colonel in the U.S. army at Walter Reed Hospital in Washington DC, identified the first case when he noticed that a patient with recurrent infections had a very low gamma globulin band in the recently developed protein electrophoresis test. The disease has a frequency of 3–6 per million. It was not until 1993 that the responsible protein was identified and its gene mapped to the long arm of the X chromosome at Xq21.2–22. It was subsequently named for Dr. Bruton, Bruton's tyrosine kinase.

PH = Pleckstrin homology
TH = Tec homology
SH3, SH2, SH1 = Src homology kinase domains
PR = Proline rich domain

Figure 1.4. Structure of Bruton's tyrosine kinase, a Tec family protein tyrosine kinase. Upon activation by phosphorylation molecule unwinds into a linear strand.

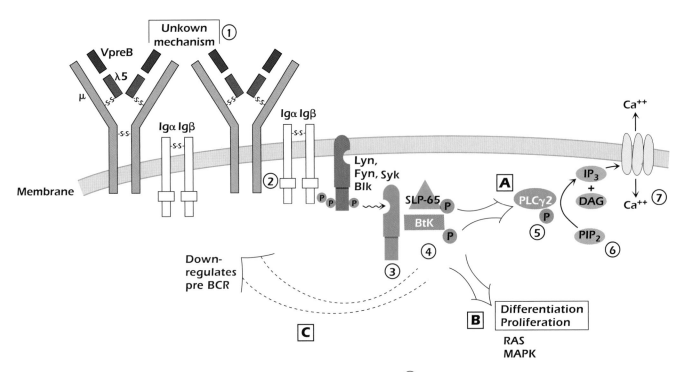

🔘 Figure 1.5. The activation of Btk and its role in B-cell development ① Activation of pre-BCR by unknown mechanism (? crosslinking by ligand) brings ② Src family kinases, Lyn, Fyn and Blk to the ITAMS on Igα and Igβ as a result of their phosphorylation on their ITAMS. This results in ③ a docking site for Syk which ④ recruits and phosphorylates SLP-65 and Btk. ⑤ BtK in turn associates with and activates PLC$_\gamma$. ⑥ Activated PLC$_\gamma$2 hydrolyzes PIP$_2$ to DAG + IP$_3$ ⑦ which opens Ca^{++} channels in the membrane. SLP-65 and BtK also activate differentiation and proliferation, the latter through RAS and MAPK pathways and then down-regulate the pre-BCR. Ⓐ, Ⓑ, and Ⓒ denote the three pathways affected by SLP-65 - Btk activation.

In the presence of a mutated Btk and the consequent absence of signaling of the pre-B cell via the pre-BCR, the pre-B cell undergoes apoptosis or fails to mature. The B lineage cells thus accumulate in the marrow at the pro-B cell stage with few pre-B cells identifiable. Instead of the larger cycling cells normally seen at the beginning of the pre-B cell stage, those pre-B cells which are present are small. This block in proliferation and differentiation leads to an absence of mature B cells in the periphery; no or few circulating immature B cells; tonsils and lymph nodes that lack germinal centers; and the absence of plasma cells. Recently it has been shown that bone marrow B cells in XLA patients do produce antibodies, but these antibodies have altered reactivity, leading in some cases to autoantibody activity. Thus, intact Btk function may also be necessary for deletion of B cells that react to autoantigens.

Over 300 different mutations that give rise to XLA have been identified in the *BTK* gene. These range from point mutations with single amino acid substitutions to deletions and stop codons. It should be noted that XLA is one of several immunodeficiency disorders caused by a mutation in a tyrosine kinase enzyme. The other two thus far identified are mutations in *JAK3*, which causes a form of

SCID, and mutations in *ZAP70*, which results in a type of T-cell deficiency.

Several other genetic abnormalities, μ chain deficiency, λ5 (also called λ-like in humans) deficiency, and Igα deficiency are similar to XLA in that they also lead to a defect in BCR expression at the pro/pre-B-cell stage of B-cell development. This emphasizes the fact that expression of the pre-BCR and its signaling are necessary for maturation of the B cell beyond the pro/pre-B-cell stage. These autosomal recessive abnormalities, which have been described in only a handful of patients, are clinically similar to XLA, although μ chain deficiency is a somewhat more severe disease with an earlier onset and a more profound lack of Ig. The exclusive accumulation of pro/pre-B cells in the bone marrow of patients with these genetic abnormalities allows definition of its phenotype as CD19$^+$CD34$^+$ B cells, defines the bone marrow as the site of B-cell maturation in nonavian species (birds have the bursa of Fabricius for maturation of B cells), and suggests the existence of little or no extramedullary B-cell maturation. Recall that the mouse model for XLA (the xid mouse), which is also due to a Btk mutation, is characterized by much less severe symptomatology, suggesting that in murine B cells, non-Btk signaling can partially compensate for Btk signaling or that Btk functions are more restricted in mice.

Bonus Question. What would you observe in a female carrier of XLA who is heterozygous for glucose-6-phosphate dehydrogenase (G6PD) isozyme?

The B cells of a female carrier of XLA would express only a single isozyme of G6PD, whereas her T cells, red blood cells, fibroblasts, and all other non-B cells would express a mixture of the two G6PD isozymes. G6PD is an enzyme that, like Btk, is encoded by a gene on the X chromosome. All those pre-B cells whose active X chromosome had the defective BTK gene would die in the marrow or fail to mature past the pro-B-cell stage, leaving only those B cells with the normal BTK gene to fully mature. Consequently the mature B cells would express only one G6PD isozyme, the one encoded by the X chromosome not bearing the defective BTK gene. In contrast, cells that do not depend on Btk for survival (non-B cells) would randomly inactivate one X chromosome (lyonization principle) and thus give rise to a non-B-cell population with a mixture of G6PD isozymes.

TREATMENT OF X-LINKED AGAMMAGLOBULINEMIA

XLA and related B-cell deficiencies are logically and effectively treated by the administration of IVIG. Such treatment usually prevents serious lower respiratory infection and thus prevents the development of bronchiectasis and other chronic pulmonary problems. IVIG therapy has supplanted intramuscular IG therapy because it results in higher levels of serum IgG and because it avoids the local skin and muscle problems associated with the injection of intramuscular injection of IG. IVIG contains only low amounts of IgM and IgA, and thus IVIG therapy does not restore the levels of these immunoglobulins. In addition, IgA normally functions at the mucosal surface and would not be effectively if replaced in this manner. If infection occurs in spite of IVIG therapy, it is important to treat the patient early with appropriate antibiotics. As with any genetic disorder resulting from the absence of a single protein, gene replacement therapy is the hope of the future.

As these patients live longer, the possibility of an increased incidence of malignancies, particularly hematologic malignancies, arises. Interestingly, gastric carcinoma, also frequent in CVID patients, is reported at a higher than expected rate in XLA patients.

REFERENCES

Espeli M, Rossi B, Mancini SJC, Roche P, Gaunthier L, Schiff C (2006): Initiation of pre-B cell receptor signaling: Common and distinctive features in human and mouse. *Sem Immunol* 18:56–66.

Geier JK, Schlissel MS (2006): Pre-BCR signals and the control of Ig gene rearrangements. *Sem Immunol* 18:31–39.

Kawakami Y, Kitaura J, Hata D, Yao L, Kawakami T (1999): Functions of Bruton's tyrosine kinase in mast and B cells. *J Leukocyte Biol* 65:286–290.

Nomura K, Kanegane H, Karasuyama H, Tsukada S, Agematsu K, Murakami G, Sakazume S, Sako M, Tanaka R, Kuniya Y, Komeno T, Ishihara S, Hayashi K, Kishimoto T, Miyawaki T (2000): Genetic defect in human X-linked agammaglobulinemia impedes a maturational evolution of pro-B cells into a later stage of pre-B cells in the B-cell differentiation pathway. *Blood* 96:610–617.

Yang WC, Collette Y, Nunès JA, Olive D (2000): Tec kinases: A family with multiple roles in immunity. *Immunity* 12:373–382.

2

SEVERE COMBINED IMMUNODEFICIENCY DISEASE

FABIO CANDOTTI and LUIGI D. NOTARANGELO*

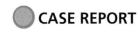

CASE REPORT

"My baby does not gain weight."

Case History

A mother brings her two-month-old child Joseph to you, his pediatrician, earlier than his scheduled check-up because she is distraught about his seemingly unending health problems. Joseph has not gained more than an ounce or two since birth and vomits at least once a day. On physical examination you note that the infant has white plaques in his oral cavity indicative of thrush (*Candida* infection) and has diaper area candidiasis as well. You eliminate the possibility of a tracheoesophageal fistula based on the timing and frequency of Joseph's vomiting and assume that the problem is due to reflux, perhaps the result of a gastric-emptying problem. You prescribe antacids, an agent that promotes gastric emptying, and oral anti-fungal agents for the thrush. Over the next few months you see Joseph repeatedly and note continued failure to thrive. At four months of age he develops persistent diarrhea as well as a chronic, nonproductive cough; at this point you decide he has an infectious syndrome and begin antibiotics. When he does not respond to the antibiotics after one week of treatment, you begin to

*With contributions from Warren Strober and Susan R. S. Gottesman

suspect that he may have an immunodeficiency disease and refer Joseph and his mother to a specialist.

Two days later he is seen by an immunologist who notes the above history and elicits a detailed family history.

Family History

The immunologist learns that Joseph was born to nonconsanguineous (unrelated) healthy parents after an uncomplicated full-term pregnancy. He has a three-year-old sister in good health. The maternal side of the family consists of two aunts and one uncle, also in good health; however, another uncle died in early infancy from unknown causes. Maternal grandparents are now deceased from natural causes. The paternal side of the family consists of one uncle in good health and paternal grandparents who are deceased due to prostate cancer and heart failure.

What "red flags" are raised by the patient and family histories?

A history in an infant or young child of recurrent or chronic infections, failure to thrive and a positive family history for similar conditions (or unexplained death at less than two years of age) raises the suspicion of a congenital or inherited host defense defect. In addition, although the family tree is small, it suggests an X-linked defect inherited from his unaffected mother.

Immunology: Clinical Case Studies and Disease Pathophysiology, By Warren Strober and Susan R. S. Gottesman
Copyright © 2009 John Wiley & Sons, Inc.

Physical Examination

Upon physical examination, the immunologist notes that Joseph has a severely dystrophic appearance and is below the third percentile in height and weight for his age (Fig. 2.1). He notes obvious oral thrush and, upon auscultation of Joseph's chest, detects bilateral rales (crackling lung sounds on inspiration). Finally, despite this evidence of infection, Joseph has no tonsillar tissue in his pharynx and no palpable cervical, axillary, or inguinal lymph nodes.

Based on the history and physical examination, the immunologist presumes that Joseph has an immunodeficiency syndrome and arranges hospitalization for a more definitive evaluation.

Initial Hospital Workup

In the hospital, Joseph is placed in a single-crib room with reverse precautions to protect him from hospital infection. A chest X ray shows absence of a thymic shadow and the presence of bilateral interstitial pneumonia. The severity of the latter is indicated by transcutaneous pulse oxymetry that shows 91% oxygen saturation on room air (normal: 98–100%). A complete blood count (CBC) shows lymphopenia (600 cells/mm^3; normal: 1500–5200 cells/mm^3) with normal neutrophil counts and normal red blood cell (RBC).

What do the significant features of the physical examination, history, and preliminary laboratory results suggest?

Failure to thrive is a serious but nonspecific finding in infants. The additional presenting symptom of widespread infection with Candida, *a fungal organism, may signify a problem with the cell-mediated immune system. Alternatively, it may be a consequence of the infant's generalized debilitated state combined with the normally immature immune system of a four-month-old. However, the absence of a thymic shadow, underdeveloped peripheral lymphoid tissues (tonsils and lymph nodes), and lymphopenia point to an immunologic deficiency. This deficiency would seem to involve at least the T cells and possibly the B cells as well, either primarily or secondary to a T-cell deficiency. The class of the causative organism of Joseph's pneumonia has not been determined (see introduction to this unit).*

Immunologic Workup

The immunologist recognizes the urgency of the condition, which requires immediate therapy to prevent death from a severe infection. He initiates an immunologic workup to define the specific defect.

Many of the tests ordered are the same as those ordered in the case study on X-linked agammaglobulinemia (XLA

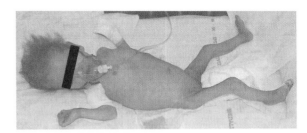

Figure 2.1. Dystrophy is marked in this SCID patient at presentation.

Case 1); however both the differential diagnosis and sense of urgency differ. First, this infant, Joseph, is only four months old and has failure to thrive; and this is in contrast to the child with XLA, who came to the specialist's attention at four years of age and was of normal height and weight despite a history of multiple infections. Second, whereas the XLA patient presented with bacterial infections of high virulence, Joseph presents with fungal infections that are normally of low or no virulence, in addition to possible bacterial infections.

Although immunologic workups may be divided into the arm of the immune system under investigation (see introduction to this unit and Case 1), quantitative lymphocyte subset analysis by immunophenotyping of peripheral blood lymphocytes is an obvious first step. In addition, immunoglobulin levels should be measured as an indication of overall B-cell function, and *in vitro* studies of the patient's lymphocyte proliferative responses to mitogenic stimulation should be conducted to evaluate both T- and B-cell function.

Quantitation of Peripheral Blood Lymphocyte Cell Type by Immunophenotyping

	Results	Reference Range
CD3$^+$ cells	<1%	55–82%
CD4$^+$ & CD8$^+$ subsets	undetectable	
CD19$^+$ cells	98%	6–22%
CD16/56$^+$ cells	<1%	6–31%

Joseph's lymphocytes consist of a severely reduced proportion of T cells (CD3$^+$), an increased percentage of B lymphocytes (CD19$^+$), and virtually undetectable levels of natural killer (NK) cells (CD16/56$^+$). Since Joseph has an absolute lymphopenia, his absolute peripheral blood B-cell number is actually at the upper limit of normal, rather than truly increased.

Serum Immunoglobulin Levels.

	Result	Reference Range
IgG	132 mg/dL	196–558 mg/dL
IgM	18 mg/dL	27–101 mg/dL
IgA	undetectable	4.4–73 mg/dL
IgE	< 1 μg/dL	0–5 μg/dL

Result. All immunoglobulin classes are severely reduced.

In Vitro Proliferation Studies. The proliferative responses of purified mononuclear cells following stimulation with phytohemoagglutinin (PHA, a T-cell mitogen), pokeweed mitogen (PWM, a B-cell mitogen), concanavalin A (Con A, a T-cell mitogen), anti-CD3 and anti-CD3 + IL-2 were virtually absent.

What is the interpretation of the preliminary immunologic studies?

*These laboratory data show that Joseph has an immunologic defect characterized by decreased number and (presumably) function of T cells. The B cells, although present in the peripheral blood, are likely to be decreased in total number in the periphery. The evidence for this conclusion is based on the decrease in peripheral lymphoid tissues, particularly the tonsils, in which B cells normally predominate. Evidence of decreased B-cell function is also shown by the lack of proliferation to the B-cell-specific mitogen and the paucity of serum immunoglobulins. The profound reduction in IgM, in particular, suggests that B-cell function is affected intrinsically, rather than simply as a result of lack of T-cell help. These observations establish the diagnosis of **severe combined immunodeficiency (SCID)**.*

Initial Management of Joseph's Case

Regardless of the underlying genetic defect, the extreme susceptibility of SCID patients to overwhelming infections from opportunistic pathogens requires strict protective measures such as reverse isolation and administration of prophylactic antibiotics, anti-virals and anti-fungals when indicated. Thus, placing Joseph in strict isolation was a necessary step. In addition, live vaccines must be avoided and blood products may be transfused only after irradiation and screening for cytomegalovirus (CMV)–negative units. However, such measures do not represent a realistic long-term management option. In the absence of successful reconstitution of the immune system, most patients succumb to infectious complications by two years of age.

Further Analysis to Identify Subtype of SCID in Joseph

SCID is not a single disease entity, but rather a large group of diseases that are related only by the fact that they affect both T- and B-cell immune function. The combined frequency of SCID is nevertheless low (frequency ~1 : 50,000). In recent years the genetic causes have been determined in approximately 70% of cases, and new defects are still being identified. Overall SCID may be organized into subgroups according to the lymphocyte subsets present in the peripheral blood; this can direct investigation into the underlying molecular cause of the patient's disease. The causes and pertinent characteristics of SCID are listed in Table 2.1 and will be reviewed below.

The lymphocyte immunophenotyping data demonstrate that Joseph lacks both T and NK cells but has a normal number of peripheral blood B cells. These findings suggest that his disease falls into the $T^-B^+NK^-$ variety of SCID, which is generally caused by mutations in the genes encoding the γc-cytokine receptor chain or Janus-associated kinase 3 (JAK3). Mutations affecting expression and/or function of γc, the **common γ chain** of several important cytokine receptors, are the most common cause of SCID, comprising almost 50% of cases and are X-linked (X-SCID). A related defect, **JAK3 deficiency**, is due to disrupted intracellular signaling from this receptor component and will also result in a $T^-B^+NK^-$ phenotype and an identical clinical picture. In the absence of specific molecular studies, the former defect is more likely, due to both its frequency and X-linked inheritance. Our patient, Joseph, is male with a family history of an uncle from the maternal side who died early in life.

Adenosine deaminase (ADA) deficiency is the second most common cause of SCID. Both ADA and ***purine nucleoside phosphorylase (PNP) deficiency*** are inherited in an autosomal recessive fashion and will result in a $T^-B^-NK^-$ type of SCID. Joseph's ADA and PNP enzymatic activity are tested for completeness and are found to be within normal limits.

Flow cytometric analysis of Joseph's cells is performed and reveals lack of the γc receptor component on the surface of his T cells; a preliminary diagnosis of X-SCID is thus established. This diagnosis is confirmed by molecular analysis of DNA extracted from his lymphocytes, which reveals a 660C-to-T mutation in exon 5 of the *IL2RG* gene resulting in a codon 216 that specifies premature termination. Analysis of DNA from the patient's mother indicates that she has the same molecular defect on one of her X chromosomes and is therefore a carrier of the disease.

TABLE 2.1. Severe Combined Immunodeficiency Diseases

Specific Disorder	Underlying Deficiency	Mode of Inheritance[a]
T^-B^+ *Subgroup*		
X-linked SCID	Mutated γ chain of cytokine receptors	X-linked
Autosomal recessive SCID	Mutated JAK3 tyrosine kinase	AR
T^-B^- *Subgroup*		
Adenosine deaminase deficiency	ADA enzyme	AR
Purine nucleoside phosphorylase deficiency	PNP enzyme	AR
Recombinase deficiency	Rag 1 or Rag 2 enzyme	AR
T^+B^- *Subgroup*		
Omenn's syndrome	Partial Rag deficiency	AR
T^+B^+ *Subgroup*		
Bare lymphocyte syndrome	MHC class II transcription activator (4 proteins)	AR
	MHC class I TAP defect	AR
ZAP-70 deficiency	Kinase domain of the TCR–associated protein tyrosine kinase, ZAP-70	AR
Multisystem disorders		
Wiskott–Aldrich syndrome	Wiskott–Aldrich syndrome protein (WASP)	X-linked
Ataxia telangectasia	ATM[b] protein for DNA repair	AR

[a] AR: autosomal recessive.
[b] ATM: ataxia telangectasia mutated

Treatment: Long and Short Term

As mentioned above, while the detailed workup is being completed, Joseph is placed in strict isolation and the parents are counseled on the severity of the disease and its mode of inheritance. With the final results, plans are made for Joseph to undergo allogeneic hematopoietic stem cell (HSC) transplantation. Although lacking T cells and therefore unlikely to reject the transplant, histocompatibility typing of family members is conducted to try to find a related matched donor (see below). As expected, each parent is found to be haploidentical, while Joseph's sister is a histocompatibility locus antigen (HLA)–identical match and plans are therefore made to harvest cells from this sibling (see Case 20 for discussion of transplantation).

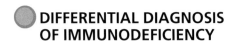 **DIFFERENTIAL DIAGNOSIS OF IMMUNODEFICIENCY**

As discussed in the introductory chapter and in the case study on XLA (Case 1) the initial evaluation of immunodeficiency often focuses on the types of infections with which the patient presents. In Joseph's case, the presentation of significant infection with fungal organisms of low virulence, occurring as early as the neonatal period, suggests a defect in cell-mediated immunity. Humoral immunity is still at least partially supplied by maternal antibodies at that time. In viewing a flow chart of lymphopoietic development (Fig. 2.2), there are several points

at which T-cell function can be disrupted, many affecting B-cell function as well, either as an intrinsic defect in B cells or as a secondary consequence of lack of T-cell help. From this flow table, you can appreciate how some types of SCID result in total lack of peripheral lymphocytes (T^-B^-); others allow the development of nonfunctioning B cells, and yet a third group of mutations allows for the development of both types of mature lymphocytes. Although DiGeorge syndrome (congenital thymic aplasia) may be a consideration given the absence of a thymic shadow and peripheral blood T cells, the lack of associated abnormalities (i.e., aparathyroidism), nonfunctional B-cell status (as demonstrated by the mitogen response), and tonsillar underdevelopment help rule out this entity (see Case 3). As will be discussed in detail below and has been proven by the results given above, Joseph has a mutation in the common γ chain of cytokine receptors, resulting in a total lack of mature T-cell development, impaired B-cell development, and lack of function of both cell types.

THE MOLECULAR BIOLOGY OF SCID AND NORMAL LYMPHOCYTE DEVELOPMENT

There are approximately 10 different subtypes of SCID. Delineation of the mutations underlying each subtype teaches us about the disease as well as the requirements for normal lymphocyte development and function. Thus,

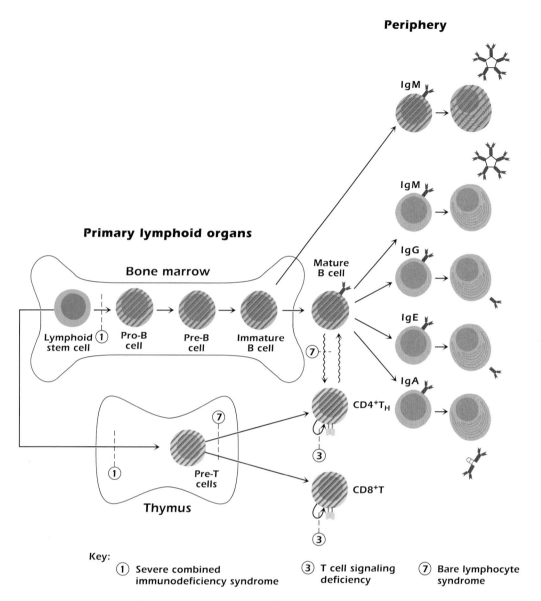

Figure 2.2. Sites of defective lymphopoietic development associated with various forms of severe combined immunodeficiency phenotype. Gray cells denote those which would not exist in any of the subtypes of SCID.

the discussion of each SCID subtype below is interwoven with the normal biology of T- and B-cell differentiation and function.

T⁻B⁻ Subgroup

The T⁻B⁻ subgroup of SCID would presumably result from a mutation in a component necessary to the development of the common lymphoid stem cell or a component involved in the maturation of both the T- and B-cell lineages. These include the housekeeping genes

ADA and *PNP*, and genes encoding enzymes required for V(D)J rearrangement of the T- and B-cell antigen receptors.

Mutations in ADA and PNP Housekeeping Enzymes. Adenosine deaminase is a ubiquitous enzyme that catalyzes the conversion of adenosine to inosine or 2′-deoxyadenosine to 2′-deoxyinosine. These metabolites are then converted to hypoxanthine, which can be utilized by the cell to synthesize new deoxynucleotides; thus, ADA is a key part of the purine "salvage" pathway. The main reason that ADA deficiency results in SCID is that its absence leads, first, to the accumulation of deoxyadenosine and its downstream product deoxyadenosine triphosphate (deoxyATP) and, second, to the inhibition of ribonucleotide reductase by deoxyATP. Since ribonucleotide reductase is a critical enzyme in the conversion of nucleotide monophosphates to nucleotide triphosphates (the basic building blocks of DNA), its inhibition blocks DNA synthesis. Thus, ADA deficiency results in "poisoning" of the cell with deoxyATP. While ADA is expressed in many cells, its dysfunction is most detrimental to cells undergoing rapid division, for example, developing T and B lymphocytes. Thus, these patients will lack both T and B cells and even NK cells in the periphery. Although the immunologic deficits of ADA deficiency are similar to other forms of SCID, these patients frequently also exhibit skeletal abnormalities such as flaring of the costochondral junctions and neurologic manifestations such as blindness. Patients with partial ADA deficiency will have less accumulation of toxic metabolites and may have a late onset of SCID associated with milder lymphopenia.

Like ADA deficiency, a deficiency in purine nucleoside phosphorylase, another enzyme in the purine salvage pathway, leads to a SCID phenotype with neurologic problems due to the buildup of toxic products. Both ADA and PNP deficiencies are inherited in an autosomal recessive pattern. ADA deficiency accounts for approximately 20% of the cases of SCID.

Mutations in Enzymes Involved in Rearrangement of DNA. Defects in genes involved in antigen receptor [V(D)J] gene rearrangements, the process that accounts for clonal diversity of T and B cells, also lead to SCID. Such defects account for approximately 20% of cases and, like ADA and PNP deficiency, are inherited in an autosomal recessive pattern. T- and B-cell precursors require signaling through their antigen receptors, which are the products of rearranged receptor genes, in order to develop and expand. This requirement was discussed in detail in the description of B-cell development in the XLA case study (Case 1). In XLA, rearrangement of the B-cell receptor (BCR) genes begins but no BCR or pre-BCR signaling takes place in the immature B cell to allow maturation to continue. A defect in a molecule (Btk) specific for pre-B cells, but not in pre-T cells, is to blame in XLA. In the types of SCID due to rearrangement defects, enzymes common to both T- and B-cell receptor gene rearrangement are the culprits. Thus, neither T nor B cells differentiate; however, cells that do not utilize antigen-specific receptors, such as NK cells, develop normally in the face of this deficiency.

How is antigen receptor gene rearrangement accomplished?

The variable or antigen recognizing region of an unrearranged receptor gene consists of a string of multiple V

(D) and J gene segments (Fig. 2.3). Normal rearrangement consists of the production of random but targeted breaks at two points in this string. One break occurs in one gene segment, and a second occurs in a different gene segment type. The breaks are followed by excision of the intervening DNA and ligation of the broken ends. In effect, this leads to the random juxtaposition of V and D segments and D and J segments, resulting in a newly formed (combined) VDJ or VJ segment that encodes a unique antigen-combining site (Fig. 2.3). A series of enzymes are involved in this process. First, the enzymes recombination-activating gene (Rag) 1 and Rag 2 initiate rearrangements by performing double-stranded DNA breaks. Both enzymes are necessary for rearrangement to proceed. Following the action of the Rag proteins, terminal deoxynucleotidyl transferase (TdT) randomly adds nucleotides to the broken ends without a primer, thus contributing further to the diversity of the rearranged receptor gene. Lastly, the DNA ends have to be religated, which is accomplished by the common DNA repair enzymes.

In about 50% of patients with SCID due to defects in rearrangement, the latter process is disrupted by mutations in the ***RAG1*** or ***RAG2 genes***. As expected, since the action of these genes is restricted to lymphocyte precursors, immunologic deficiencies are their only (although not minor) problem. The other 50% of patients with presumed rearrangement defect SCID manifest repair defects in other cell types, so the mutation is inferred to be a problem in DNA break repair. One group of patients has been found to be particularly sensitive to irradiation damage of their fibroblasts. Repair of irradiation damage, which causes double-stranded DNA breaks, uses the same common repair enzymes as VDJ recombination. The protein mutated in ***radiosensitivity-SCID (RS-SCID)*** has been recently identified and the gene cloned. The protein, called Artemis, is involved in V(D)J recombination and DNA repair following double-stranded breaks, as described in the legend for Figure 2.3.

In either situation, without functional antigen receptors, neither T nor B cells can expand and differentiate, resulting in a T⁻B⁻NK⁺ SCID.

Multisystem Disorders. Several multisystem disorders resulting from DNA repair defects are also associated with a SCID-like clinical picture of varying degrees of severity. These include ***ataxia telangiectasia, Bloom syndrome***, and ***Fanconi anemia***.

In addition to multisystem disorders that affect DNA repair, ***Wiskott–Aldrich syndrome*** causes a SCID-like clinical picture, although peripheral lymphocyte numbers are variable. Wiskott–Aldrich syndrome is due to a mutation in the gene for Wiskott-Aldrich syndrome protein (WASP) located on the X chromosome. This protein normally interacts with the cell's cytoskeleton, presumably affecting the cell's ability to respond to stimuli. The patients show a classic triad of recurrent infections (particularly bacterial) due to functional abnormality in the T and B cells,

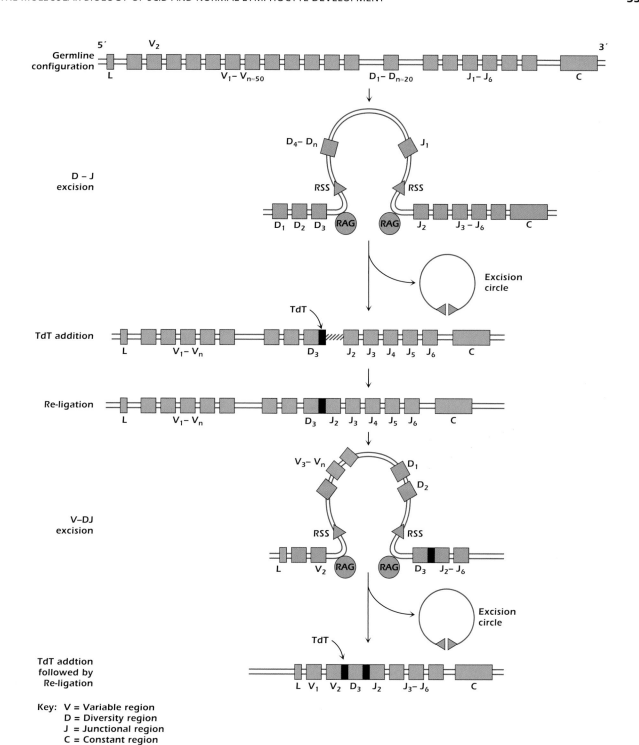

Key: V = Variable region
D = Diversity region
J = Junctional region
C = Constant region
L = Leader sequence

Figure 2.3. The first step in gene rearrangement for the TCR or BCR genes involves recognition of the recombination signal sequences (RSSs) by Rag 1 and Rag 2 proteins. RSSs are conserved sequences that flank each V, D, and J segment and that combine in a specific manner. With recognition of these sequences, the Rag endonuclease proteins introduce double-stranded DNA breaks. Diversity of these antigen-specific receptors is accomplished through the use of different V-region families (germline-encoded diversity) and the random association of different V, D, and J segments (combinatorial diversity). In addition, the enzyme TdT may randomly add (and delete) up to nine nucleotides to the broken ends without a template (junctional diversity). The broken DNA ends then have to be religated through a process known as nonhomologous DNA end joining (NHEJ). Although the latter uses enzymes ubiquitously expressed, NHEJ is not employed in all instances of DNA repair in nonlymphoid cells; it is most often used in repair of radiation damage. Patients deficient in Rag proteins would fail to rearrange their TCRs and BCRs resulting in SCID phenotype with neither mature T nor mature B cells.

bleeding tendencies due to low platelet numbers and small size of platelets, and, paradoxically, allergic reactions with elevated IgE.

T⁻B⁺ Subgroup

X-SCID (γc) and JAK3 and IL-7Rα Mutations.
X-SCID and JAK3 deficiency account for approximately 60% of SCID cases. The molecular basis of X-SCID was identified in 1993, when the gene encoding for the common γ chain (γc) of cytokine receptors (named *IL2RG*) was mapped to Xq13, where the X-SCID locus had also been assigned, and was mutated in X-SCID patients. γc was found to be an integral component of multiple cytokine receptors (those for IL-4, IL-7, IL-9, IL-15, and IL-21 as well as IL-2; Fig. 2.4).

X-SCID therefore may be regarded as a failure of multiple cytokine-mediated signaling pathways. Observations in mice and humans have provided insights into the role of the specific cytokine signaling pathways that are affected by mutations of γc, in contrast to mutations in individual cytokines and/or unique cytokine receptor chains.

Conceptually, if one knocks out (in an animal model) a gene for a particular cytokine or there is a mutation in a cytokine gene, the resulting deficiency will be limited to that specific cytokine's function. Similar results may

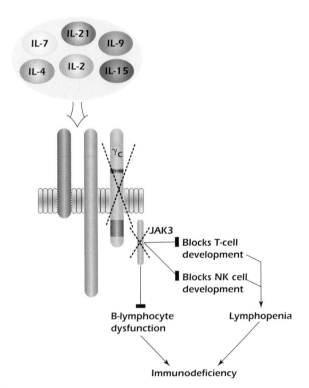

🔘 Figure 2.4. Molecular basis of X-SCID. Absence of γc chain (or JAK3) results in a SCID phenotype lacking mature T cells and NK cells while having mature but dysfunctional B cells.

be obtained by eliminating, through knockout experiments or mutation, a unique chain of a receptor specific for a single cytokine. Mutation of the γ-chain gene has broad effects because it codes for a chain crucial to the functioning of at least six different cytokine receptors (Fig. 2.4). Although the γ chain was first identified as a component of the high-affinity IL-2 receptor, elimination of IL-2 did not replicate the deficiency; that is, impaired IL-2 signaling alone did not lead to the profound lymphoid developmental block seen in X-SCID. This has been demonstrated by experiments targeting the IL-2 gene in mice, which resulted in disturbed peripheral T-cell homeostasis and autoimmunity but did not prevent T-cell development. In humans, defective IL-2 production has been reported in an immunodeficient patient who has detectable circulating T cells; in addition, mutations of the *IL2RA* gene, which encodes the α chain of the IL-2 receptor (IL2Rα), have been identified in another individual with immune deficiency and lymphoid proliferation. Both of these cases indicate that signaling through the IL-2R is important for peripheral T-cell homeostasis but less important for intrathymic differentiation.

The pronounced defect in T-cell development in X-SCID patients appears to be due primarily to impaired IL-7 signaling, which uses the same γ chain as IL-2 signaling. IL-7- and IL7Rα-deficient mice demonstrate a SCID-type picture; similarly, patients with T⁻B⁺ SCID due to *mutations of the IL7RA gene* that encodes the α chain of the IL7R have been identified. In humans, IL-7 signaling appears to be crucial to T-cell development and function and B-cell function (but not development), resulting in the T⁻B⁺ SCID phenotype. The development of B cells in humans proceeds in spite of the lack of IL7R signaling, correlating with the lack of dependence of human B-cell maturation on IL-7 (see Case 1).

Immunophenotypic analysis of X-SCID and IL7Rα SCID patients reveals subtle but important differences. The lack of circulating NK cells is a common feature of X-SCID, whereas NK cell differentiation is unaffected in IL7Rα SCID. This difference likely reflects impaired γc-mediated signaling by IL-15 in X-SCID, a hypothesis confirmed by the profound block in NK cell development seen in *IL15RA* gene knockout mice. Experiments using IL-4 and IL-21R knockout mice have demonstrated that IL-21 has a significant influence on regulation of B-cell function *in vivo*, which suggests that inactivation of these cytokines, which use receptors bearing γc chains, may bear primary responsibility for the B-cell defect in X-SCID. Notice from Figure 2.4 that, whereas one would expect absence of T and NK cells due to the block in their development, B cells will be present but nonfunctional, therefore resulting in the T⁻B⁺ phenotype.

As previously mentioned, a *JAK3* mutation would result in an identical patient presentation as a γc-chain mutation, although with autosomal recessive inheritance. This is because JAK3 tyrosine kinase is the intracellular molecule transmitting the signal from the γc chain of all the above-mentioned cytokine receptors to the interior of the cell (see below).

How do different cell types respond uniquely to individual cytokines if these cytokines act through a common receptor chain (γc) and a common intracellular signaling molecule (JAK3)?

The biological effects of cytokines are mediated through phosphorylation of intracellular proteins. The chains of the receptors do not have intrinsic kinase activity but recruit intracellular protein kinases following the receptors' interaction with their ligands and dimerization. These tyrosine kinases are members of the JAK family. Of the four JAK family members identified to date (JAK1, JAK2, JAK3, and Tyk2), JAK1 and JAK3 are the only kinases involved in γc-mediated cytokine signaling. The observation that distinct cytokines signal through the same set of kinases indicates that JAKs are not directly controlling the specificity of the response to the signal. Following cytokine/cytokine receptor interaction and dimerization of the cytoplasmic tails of the cytokine receptor chains, the JAKs are brought in close proximity, cross-phosphorylate, and phosphorylate the membrane distal region of the cytokine receptor chains, thus generating docking sites for SH2(Src homology2)–containing proteins.

One group of SH2-containing proteins is the STAT class of transcription factors (signal transducers and activators of transcription): STAT1, STAT2, STAT3, STAT4, STAT5a, STAT5b, and STAT6. Following interaction with phosphotyrosine residues of the cytokine receptor chain, STATs themselves are phosphorylated, which allows them to form STAT homo- or heterodimers. STAT dimers then translocate to the nucleus, where they bind to consensus sequences in the enhancer elements of the promoter regions of target genes, favoring gene transcription. The specificity of the cytokine response depends largely on the particular combination of STATs recruited by the signal-transducing chains of the cytokine receptor. As an example, STAT6 is recruited following activation by IL-4 of IL-4R, whereas STAT-3 and STAT-5 are recruited to the IL-2R upon IL-2-mediated signaling. Gene accessibility to STAT binding is another mechanism through which specific responses to distinct cytokines are obtained.

Finishing the story: A number of mechanisms terminate the activity initiated by cytokine signals. SH2 domain-containing protein tyrosine phosphatases SHP-1 and SHP-2 are important inhibitors of signaling events and are thought to dephosphorylate receptor chains and JAK molecules through SH2–phosphotyrosine interaction. Other mechanisms for attenuation involve the suppressor of cytokine signaling (SOCS) family of eight known proteins (CIS, SOCS1–7). These proteins are induced by cytokine stimulation following a classic feedback loop. Although their function is incompletely understood, SOCS proteins appear to inhibit cytokine signaling by a variety of mechanisms, including competition with STATs for the phosphorylated docking sites on receptor chains and inhibition of kinase activities.

Even Rarer Cases of Signaling Defects. Patients with mutations in *CD45* [CD45 is also known as leukocyte common antigen (LCA)] fall into the T⁻B⁺NK⁻ category, although CD45 normally functions in both the T- and B-cell lineages. CD45 is a tyrosine phosphatase present on the surface of all white blood cells that regulates the Src kinases involved in TCR and BCR signaling (see Case 1).

Lastly, patients with mutations in one of the ***CD3 chains***, γ or ζ, may be considered under T⁻B⁺NK⁺ SCID since these patients, although having a pure T-cell defect, often show a SCID-like clinical phenotype. CD3 is a group of five invariant polypeptide chains noncovalently linked to the TCR which serve to transmit the signal into the cell following stimulation of the TCR. ZAP-70 is the next molecule involved in the signaling cascade (see below).

T⁺B⁺ Subgroup: Immunodeficiencies Due to Defective T-Cell Function

A number of other immunodeficiencies are clinically similar to T⁻B⁻ and T⁻B⁺ SCID but are caused by abnormalities that primarily affect T-cell function while resulting in normal or near-normal T-cell numbers. These qualitative T-cell defects are rare but are of great theoretical interest because of the insights they provide into normal human immunology.

As in the other types of SCID, qualitative T-cell defects lead to frequent infection but also to autoimmunity and, in some cases, allergy. However, these clinical manifestations present a few years after birth rather than within the first several months of life. Respiratory infections leading to bronchiectasis and GI infections resulting in chronic diarrhea and malabsorption are common and are frequently due to opportunistic organisms. Autoimmune manifestations such as hemolytic anemia and thrombocytopenia (caused by antibodies against the patient's own RBC and platelets, respectively) are also common and can be quite severe. The underlying mechanism of the autoimmune disorders is not understood and could have a central (i.e., thymic) or peripheral origin; one interesting possibility is that the patients lack regulatory T cells. The presence of a qualitative T-cell defect should be suspected when a patient presents with normal or only mildly reduced T-cell numbers but exhibits poor T-cell function either *in vivo* or *in vitro*. In addition, B cells are usually present and respond normally to stimuli; however, B-cell function may be impaired by lack of T-cell help.

Bare Lymphocyte Syndrome. One immunodeficiency in this category is ***bare lymphocyte syndrome (BLS) type II***, in which there is defective expression of MHC class II molecules. Although in reality it is a defect of antigen presentation rather than T cells, it can be operationally considered a T-cell abnormality because, in the absence of normal antigen presentation, T-cell function is manifestly defective. The molecular basis of BLS type II is a mutation in a gene encoding one of the four interactive transcription factors that are necessary for MHC class II gene transcription rather than in the MHC class II gene itself. Three of these factors, called RFX (regulatory factor X) factors, form a complex that binds to the promoter of the MHC class II gene; the fourth factor, CIITA (class II transactivator), is a protein that interacts with and stabilizes the RFX complex but does not bind to the MHC class II gene promoter itself.

Bare lymphocyte syndrome type I involving MHC class I, which is less common than the class II abnormality, is due to mutations in genes encoding the transporter of peptides (TAP) 1 or TAP2. TAP1 and TAP2 are molecules involved in the transport of peptides from the cytosol to the endoplasmic reticulum so that they can be loaded into the class I molecule. Without such loading, the MHC class I molecule is not expressed on the cell surface. Diagnosis is made by flow cytometry (see Unit V) showing absence of class I expression on cells and reduced numbers of CD8$^+$ T cells.

The reduction in T subset numbers in class I and class II deficiencies is due to the lack of positive selection in the thymus of CD8$^+$ and CD4$^+$ T cells, respectively. Thus the defect is later in the differentiation of T cells in the thymus than the previously described mutations. The T-cell precursor has already rearranged its T-cell antigen-specific receptor genes and expressed them. It has also benefited from cytokine stimulation, particularly IL-7, which has promoted its expansion and differentiation. The block in further development occurs at the point of positive selection, a necessary step for the continued survival and expansion of the CD4 or CD8 single positive T cells (see Case 3 on DiGeorge syndrome for description of thymic education and T cell differentiation).

The clinical presentation of MHC class II immunodeficiency is much like that of other immunodeficiencies described above, except that it has its onset in the first few months of life. Although patients usually die in childhood of opportunistic infections, there have been some long-term survivors. Diagnosis is made by flow cytometry showing lack of MHC class II antigens on cells ordinarily expressing these molecules, particularly antigen-presenting cells and B cells. CD4$^+$ T cells are reduced in number and antigen-specific responses *in vivo* and *in vitro* are profoundly impaired. The patients also manifest hypogammaglobulinemia, which primarily affects IgG and IgA. For these immunoglobulins to be produced, the B cells must express MHC class II to interact with and receive the help from T cells that is essential for Ig class switching (see Case 4). Interestingly, some MHC class II expression can be found in the thymus, suggesting that, at least in some cases, the mutation is "leaky." This can account for the fact that patients' CD4$^+$ T cells do have

the capacity to distinguish between self and nonself and for the development of limited numbers of CD4$^+$ T cells.

In evaluating a patient with BLS type I or type II, what results would you expect from the panel of immunologic tests, both quantitative and functional, used to diagnose immunodeficiency diseases (see introduction to this unit)?

Although there will be a quantitative decrease in T cells (or one subset of T cells), with normal numbers of B and NK cells, the in vitro "functional" assays may give surprisingly normal results. Proliferative responses of both T and B cells may be normal on a per-cell basis. This is because there is no intrinsic T-cell defect, and these in vitro assays using mitogens or anti-CD3 stimulation do not rely on T cell receptor (TCR) stimulation, which requires an antigen presented in the context of MHC. In these assays, you are not testing the ability of the antigen-presenting cell to stimulate, which is where the defect lies. In vivo, delayed-type hypersensitivity (DTH) responses will be absent in class II deficiencies since DTH relies on macrophage stimulation of T cells (see introduction to this unit and Case 1). Secondary antibody responses in vivo will be diminished in class II defects. Certainly, a challenging diagnosis unless one is thinking of it!

ZAP-70 Deficiency. ZAP-70 (ζ-chain-associated protein) is a tyrosine kinase that transduces the signal from the TCR–CD3 complex into the cell. Stimulation through this complex then activates ZAP-70. Two points should be noted here. First, in contrast to a defect in a CD3 chain, which will result in a pure T-cell deficiency, **a mutation in *ZAP-70*** results in a more truly SCID-like clinical presentation. This suggests that ZAP-70 has a broader role, affecting B cells as well as T cells. Second, patients with the ZAP-70 defect are completely missing CD8$^+$ T cells, suggesting that ZAP-70 has a role in CD8$^+$ T-cell differentiation in the thymus. ZAP-70 is the third tyrosine kinase joining Btk (see Case 1) and JAK3, which when mutated, results in immunodeficiency disease.

Brief Review of Normal T-Cell Differentiation in the Thymus

We have used the information obtained from the SCID patients and experimental models to construct a scheme of lymphocyte (particularly T-cell) differentiation and to understand the disease presentation in each patient. We will continue this discussion of T-cell differentiation in the description of DiGeorge syndrome (see Case 3). To review, first, if early progenitor cells are being progressively poisoned by the buildup of toxic metabolites (i.e., by mutations in enzymes of the purine salvage pathway), there will be no maturation of T cells, B cells, or even NK cells. Next, assuming survival of the early progenitors, the pro-T cell and pro-B cell must undergo rearrangement and expression of their antigen-specific receptor genes to receive signals for continued differentiation and survival. Disruption in productive rearrangement will lead to an absence of T and B cells but allow for the generation of NK cells. Disruption of further T-cell development in the thymus will affect both cell-mediated and humoral immunity and thus may produce a SCID clinical picture, whereas disruption of B-cell development will only impact humoral immunity, as was seen in Case 1 on XLA.

The goal of differentiation in the thymus is to generate two subsets of T cells (at least in the $TCR\alpha\beta^+$ T cells): $CD4^+$ T cells and $CD8^+$ T cells, which recognize antigen in the context of self-MHC antigens (Class II and Class I, respectively) while having minimal or no reactivity to unadulterated self-antigens. This education process in the thymus is the result of positive and negative selection. Positive selection requires signals for survival, differentiation, and proliferation (expansion), whereas negative selection results in cell death (as does the absence of positive selection). One can presume that defects or "holes" in negative selection, if they could be identified, would result in autoimmune disease (see Introduction to Unit III), while a lack of positive selection will result in immune deficiencies. Thus, the lack of proliferation and signaling for differentiation (i.e., the inability to respond to cytokines) will result in deficient T-cell numbers and function (and B and NK cell, if they use common cytokines); an inability to signal through the T-cell receptor (CD3 chain deficiencies) will result in deficient T-cell numbers and function only; while the lack of an MHC molecule will prevent positive selection of one T-cell subset, in addition to the inability to stimulate in the periphery any mature T cells which manage to develop ("leaky" phenotype). Indeed, proof of concept that positive selection is needed to expand the T-cell subsets came partially from analysis of the lymphocytes of patients with BLS and those of animals where MHC antigen display is prevented.

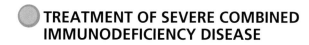

TREATMENT OF SEVERE COMBINED IMMUNODEFICIENCY DISEASE

Hematopoietic Stem Cell Transplantation

In 1968, a five-month-old boy with X-SCID became the first human to be successfully treated with allogeneic hematopoietic stem cell transplantation (SCT). The stem cells were harvested from the donor's bone marrow although now peripheral blood stem cells would be the first choice. Successful engraftment of normal donor hematopoietic stem cells has been achieved for more than 30 years in X-SCID patients with excellent results in terms of restoration of immune function and survival. Two unique features of SCID make this procedure particularly effective for the disease: (1) the lack of T-cell immunity in SCID patients prevents graft rejection even in the

absence of pretransplant treatment with myeloablative therapy (therapy to eliminate recipient bone marrow cells) and (2) the selective growth and survival advantage of normal cells over recipient cells which favors development and function of donor cells in the host environment. For these reasons, SCT for X-SCID is commonly performed without prior myeloablation of recipients, allowing X-SCID patients to avoid the serious risks of irradiation and/or chemotherapy. If an HLA-identical related donor is available, survival and immune reconstitution are excellent, making SCT the treatment of choice for X-SCID. The overall survival of SCID patients after SCT from HLA-nonidentical or haploidentical donors is lower than that from HLA-matched donors, ranging between 40 and 80%. One reason is the risk of graft-versus-host disease (GvHD), which may be severe and even fatal in some cases. Because GvHD occurs when immunocompetent donor T lymphocytes react against "foreign" HLA or minor histocompatibility antigens of skin, liver, and GI tract tissue cells of the recipient, it is less common and less severe in HLA-identical SCT compared to HLA-nonidentical transplants.

Although restoration of adequate T-cell number and function can be achieved by SCT in the absence of myeloablation, B-cell restoration is usually not achieved under these conditions. This may be due to the fact that X-SCID patients have normal numbers of host B cells, which can successfully compete with donor B cells for survival. Whatever the reason, a considerable fraction of transplanted X-SCID patients still require IVIG replacement therapy because of poor B-cell immunity even when normal T-cell function is reconstituted. Some transplant groups have resorted to transplantation preceded by myeloablation to remedy this situation, but this approach poses unacceptable risks to severely immunoincompetent patients.

Gene Therapy

The development of viral vectors as efficient tools for gene transfer into mammalian cells has made possible a new approach to the treatment of genetic disorders of the immune system that avoids problems arising from histoincompatibility inherent in SCT. In 1990, gene therapy given to patients with ADA-deficient SCID led to at least partial genetic reconstitution; in 2000, gene therapy was applied to patients with X-SCID with excellent reconstitution.

Gene therapy for X-SCID is currently performed by the transfer of a functional copy of normal γc complementary DNA (cDNA) to autologous hematopoietic stem cells (HSCs) obtained from the patient. HSCs are characterized by expression of CD34 and are purified from patient bone marrow aspirates by flow cytometry (see Unit V). Gene transfection is accomplished *in vitro* by the exposure of patient HSCs to modified murine retroviruses carrying stable γc cDNA inserts and the transfected cells are then returned to the patient.

The first clinical gene transfer protocol for X-SCID consisted of the transfer of the γc gene to X-SCID patients who lacked HLA-identical stem cell donors. As early as 60–90 days after the infusion of gene-corrected cells, mature T cells expressing γc appeared in the circulation; within 4–6 months normal values were attained in most cases. Importantly, these T lymphocytes were polyclonal and functionally competent as demonstrated by normal responses to stimulation with mitogens and specific antigens. In addition, at this time point, close to normal serum levels of IgM and IgG and the ability to mount antibody responses were demonstrated in three patients despite low numbers of B cells with the transferred gene. Based on the predicted lack of selective advantage in myeloid lineages, it is not surprising that only 0.01–1% of the patients' monocytes and granulocytes showed evidence of genetic correction. Overall, this first series of patients clearly demonstrated that γc gene therapy was sufficient to provide protective immunity and to allow the patients to lead normal lives.

Unfortunately, a serious adverse effect, the development of lymphoid neoplasia, developed about three years after initiation of gene therapy in several of the treated patients. They presented with a T-cell disorder characterized by uncontrolled clonal proliferation of T cells, which is characteristic of T-cell acute lymphoblastic leukemia. These neoplastic events were most likely caused by the insertion of the retroviral vector near the *LMO2* (LIM-domain-only 2) oncogene. The *LMO2* oncogene is known to cause acute T-cell leukemias when activated by chromosomal translocation. It appears plausible that the retroviral insertion led to activation of the *LMO2* gene via juxtaposition of the retroviral promoter; this, in concert with the selective proliferation of the gene-corrected cells due to expression of the γc, led to a "second hit" that resulted in overt malignancy. In any case, this serious side effect of gene transfer has had major repercussions in the field of gene therapy in general. It is clear that the benefits of this therapy must be weighed against the possibility of the development of neoplasia in making the decision to subject patients to gene therapy with currently available vectors of gene delivery. Meanwhile, the search for safer vectors (i.e., ones that do not insert near known oncogenes) continues.

REFERENCES

Anderson WF (1992): Human gene therapy. *Science* 256:808–813.

Antoine C, Muller S, Cant A, Cavazzana-Calvo M, Veys P, Vossen J, Fasth A, Heilmann C, Wulffraat N, Seger R, Blanche S,

Friedrich W, Abinun M, Davies G, Bredius R, Schulz A, Landais P, Fischer A (2003): Long-term survival and transplantation of haemopoietic stem cells for immunodeficiencies: Report of the European experience 1968–99. *Lancet* 361:553–560.

Blaese RM, Culver KW, Miller AD, Carter CS, Fleisher T, Clerici M, Shearer G, Chang L, Chiang Y, Tolstoshev P, Greenblatt JJ, Rosenberg SA, Klein H, Berger M, Mullen CA, Ramsey WJ, Muul L, Morgan RA, Anderson WF (1995): T lymphocyte-directed gene therapy for ADA-SCID: Initial trial results after 4 years. *Science* 270:475–480.

Buckley RH (2004): Molecular defects in human severe combined immunodeficiency and approaches to immune reconstitution. *Annu Rev Immunol* 22:625–655.

Buckley RH, Schiff SE, Schiff RI, Markert L, Williams LW, Roberts JL, Myers LA, Ward FE (1999): Hematopoietic stem-cell transplantation for the treatment of severe combined immunodeficiency. *N Engl J Med* 340:508–516.

Candotti F, Johnston JA, Puck JM, Sugamura K, O'Shea JJ, Blaese RM (1996): Retroviral-mediated gene correction for X-linked severe combined immunodeficiency. *Blood* 87:3097–3102.

Cavazzana-Calvo M, Hacein-Bay S, de Saint Basile G, De Coene F, Selz F, Le Deist F, Fischer A (1996): Role of interleukin-2 (IL-2), IL-7, and IL-15 in natural killer cell differentiation from cord blood hematopoietic progenitor cells and from γc transduced severe combined immunodeficiency X1 bone marrow cells. *Blood* 88:3901–3909.

Cunningham-Rundles C, Ponda, PP (2005): Molecular defects in T- and B-cell primary immunodeficiency diseases. *Nature Rev Immunol* 5:880–892.

de la Salle H, Zimmer J, Fricker D, Angenieux C, Cazenave JP, Okubo M, Maeda H, Plebani A, Tongio MM, Dormoy A, Hanau D (1999): HLA class I deficiencies due to mutations in subunit 1 of the peptide transporter TAP1. *J Clin Invest* 103:9–13.

Endo TA, Masuhara M, Yokouchi M, Suzuki R, Sakamoto H, Mitsui K, Matsumoto A, Tanimura S, Ohtsubo M, Misawa H, Miyazaki T, Leonor N, Taniguchi T, Fujita T, Kanakura Y, Komiya S, Yoshimura A (1997): A new protein containing an SH2 domain that inhibits JAK kinases. *Nature* 387:921–924.

Foxwell BM, Beadling C, Guschin D, Kerr I, Cantrell D (1995): Interleukin-7 can induce the activation of Jak 1, Jak 3 and STAT 5 proteins in murine T cells. *Eur J Immunol* 25:3041–3046.

Gatti RA, Meuwissen HJ, Allen HD, Hong R, Good RA (1968): Immunological reconstitution of sex-linked lymphopenic immunological deficiency. *Lancet* 2:1366–1369.

Giri JG, Ahdieh M, Eisenman J, Shanebeck K, Grabstein K, Kumaki S, Namen A, Park LS, Cosman D, Anderson D (1994): Utilization of the beta and gamma chains of the IL-2 receptor by the novel cytokine IL-15. *EMBO J* 13:2822–2830.

Hacein-Bey-Abina S, Von Kalle C, Schmidt M, McCormack MP, Wulffraat N, Leboulch P, Lim A, Osborne CS, Pawliuk R, Morillon E, Sorensen R, Forster A, Fraser P, Cohen JI, de Saint Basile G, Alexander I, Wintergerst U, Frebourg T, Aurias A, Stoppa-Lyonnet D, Romana S, Radford-Weiss I, Gross F, Valensi F, Delabesse E, Macintyre E, Sigaux F, Soulier J, Leiva LE, Wissler M, Prinz C, Rabbitts TH, Le Deist F, Fischer A, Cavazzana-Calvo M (2003): LMO2-associated clonal T cell proliferation in two patients after gene therapy for SCID-X1. *Science* 302:415–419.

Haddad E, Le Deist F, Aucouturier P, Cavazzana-Calvo M, Blanche S, De Saint Basile G, Fischer A (1999): Long-term chimerism and B-cell function after bone marrow transplantation in patients with severe combined immunodeficiency with B cells: A single-center study of 22 patients. *Blood* 94:2923–2930.

Johnston JA, Kawamura M, Kirken RA, Chen YQ, Blake TB, Shibuya K, Ortaldo JR, McVicar DW, O'Shea JJ (1994): Phosphorylation and activation of the Jak-3 Janus kinase in response to interleukin-2. *Nature* 370:151–153.

Jung D, Giallourakis C, Mostoslavsky R, Alt FW (2006): Mechanism and control of V(D)J recombination at the immunoglobulin heavy chain locus. *Annu Rev Immunol* 24:541–570.

Kondo M, Takeshita T, Ishii N, Nakamura M, Watanabe S, Arai K, Sugamura K (1993): Sharing of the interleukin-2 (IL-2) receptor gamma chain between receptors for IL-2 and IL-4. *Science* 262:874–1877.

Leonard WJ, O'Shea JJ (1998): Jaks and STATs: Biological implications. *Annu Rev Immunol* 16:293–322.

Miyazaki T, Kawahara A, Fujii H, Nakagawa Y, Minami Y, Liu ZJ, Oishi I, Silvennoinen O, Witthuhn BA, Ihle JN, Taniguchi T (1994): Functional activation of Jak1 and Jak3 by selective association with IL-2 receptor subunits. *Science* 266:1045–1047.

Moshous D, Callebaut I, de Chasseval R, Corneo B, Cavazzana-Calvo M, Le Deist F, Tezcan I, Sanal O, Bertrand Y, Phillippe N, Fischer A, de Villartay JP (2001): Artemis, a novel DNA double-strand break repair/V(D)J recombination protein, is mutated in human severe combined immune deficiency. *Cell* 105:177–186.

Noguchi M, Yi H, Rosenblatt HM, Filipovich AH, Adelstein S, Modi WS, McBride OW, Leonard WJ (1993): Interleukin-2 receptor gamma chain mutation results in X-linked severe combined immunodeficiency in humans. *Cell* 73:147–157.

Peschon JJ, Morrissey PJ, Grabstein KH, Ramsdell FJ, Maraskovsky E, Gliniak BC, Park LS, Ziegler SF, Williams DE, Ware CB (1994): Early lymphocyte expansion is severely impaired in interleukin 7 receptor-deficient mice. *J Exp Med* 180:1955–1960.

Puck JM, Deschenes SM, Porter JC, Dutra AS, Brown CJ, Willard HF, Henthorn PS (1993): The interleukin-2 receptor gamma chain maps to Xq13.1 and is mutated in X-linked severe combined immunodeficiency, SCIDX1. *Hum Mol Genet* 2:1099–1104.

Puel A, Ziegler SF, Buckley RH, Leonard WJ (1998): Defective IL7R expression in T(−)B(+)NK(+) severe combined immunodeficiency. *Nature Genet* 20:394–397.

Reith W, Mach B (2001): The bare lymphocyte syndrome and the regulation of MHC expression. *Annu Rev Immunol* 19:331–373.

Roifman CM, Zhang J, Chitayat D, Sharfe N (2000): A partial deficiency of interleukin-7R alpha is sufficient to abrogate T-cell development and cause severe combined immunodeficiency. *Blood* 96:2803–2807.

Russell SM, Johnston JA, Noguchi M, Kawamura M, Bacon CM, Friedmann M, Berg M, McVicar DW, Witthuhn BA, Silvennoinen O, Goldman AS, Schmalstieg FC, Ihle JN, O'Shea JJ, Leonard WJ (1994): Interaction of IL-2R beta and gamma c chains with Jak1 and Jak3: Implications for XSCID and XCID. *Science* 266:1042–1045.

Schorle H, Holtsche T, Hunig T, Schimpl A, Horak I (1991): Development and function of T cells in mice rendered interleukin-2 deficient by gene targeting. *Nature* 352:621–623.

Sun JY, Pacheco-Castro A, Borroto A, Alarcon B, Alvarez-Zapata D, Regueiro JR (1997): Construction of retroviral vectors carrying human CD3 gamma cDNA and reconstitution of CD3 gamma expression and T cell receptor surface expression and function in a CD3 gamma-deficient mutant T cell line. *Hum Gene Ther* 8:1041–1048.

Tonegawa S (1983): Somatic generation of antibody diversity. *Nature* 302:575–581.

Weinberg K, Parkman R (1990): Severe combined immunodeficiency due to a specific defect in the production of interleukin-2. *N Engl J Med* 322:1718–1723.

3

DiGEORGE SYNDROME (CONGENITAL THYMIC APLASIA)

SUSAN R. S. GOTTESMAN

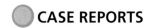 CASE REPORTS

A History of Discovery

The following is a story of discovery, the discovery of DiGeorge syndrome (congenital thymic aplasia) as related in published and personal communications by Dr. Angelo DiGeorge himself. The brilliance of Dr. DiGeorge's observations may be appreciated by considering the general understanding of the immune system at that time.

The Power of Observation

The year was 1963 and Dr. DiGeorge was a pediatric endocrinologist. He was caring for an infant with congenital hypoparathyroidism who also had mild diarrhea and a mucopurulent nasal discharge (mucus, dead white blood cells, and bacteria), indicating an infection. Upon the infant's sudden death, an autopsy was performed in an attempt to understand the cause. At autopsy, no evidence of thymic tissue was found. Dr. DiGeorge relates that he was particularly intrigued by this structure, having just reread a report of an infant with congenital absence of the parathyroid glands, absence of the thymus, aortic arch anomaly, and a history of diarrhea, pneumonia, and mucopurulent nasal discharge.

During the next six months, two more infants with hypoparathyroidism came to his institution; however, because they had normal peripheral blood lymphocyte counts and serum immunoglobulin levels, Dr. DiGeorge assumed that they probably had a thymus. Both these infants also succumbed to infection and, on autopsy, neither had thymic tissue and both had cardiovascular structural abnormalities. This brought to three the number of infants Dr. DiGeorge had observed with absence of the thymus and hypoparathyroidism (one had minimal parathyroid tissue). Dr. DiGeorge knew that both the parathyroid and thymus glands originate from the third and fourth pharyngeal pouches during embryonic development; he thus reasoned that the associated congenital abnormalities in the children represented a disorder in the development of these structures during embryonic life. As a treating physician, what frustrated him was the death of these infants despite control of their calcium levels; now we know that the deaths were of course due to infection. What excited him was the realization that the thymus might be linked to the development of the immune system and the possibility of studying these patients to uncover the then unknown function of the thymus.

From Endocrinologist to Immunologist

In 1965, when the next infant with hypoparathyroidism arrived at his door, Dr. DiGeorge was prepared. A chest X

Immunology: Clinical Case Studies and Disease Pathophysiology, By Warren Strober and Susan R. S. Gottesman
Copyright © 2009 John Wiley & Sons, Inc.

ray confirmed the lack of thymic shadow and he initiated studies of the infant's immune capabilities.

Workup

Lymphocytes. Absolute lymphocyte counts and morphology of lymphocytes were normal. Bone marrow examinations showed no abnormality.

Immunoglobulins. Levels of IgG, IgM, and IgA were all as expected for age. Evaluation of the immunoglobulin allotype was undertaken to exclude measurement of passively transferred maternal antibodies.

Lymph Node Morphology. Repeated biopsies of axillary and inguinal lymph nodes disclosed a disrupted architecture. Plasma cells were normal in quantity in early biopsies obtained soon after the baby presented but were decreased later in postmortem samples. In the earlier biopsies, acid-fast organisms were seen, but without necrosis (cell death) of the lymphocytes. The organism was found to be a type of mycobacterium, which is usually innocuous in immunocompetent hosts.

Delayed-Type Hypersensitivity Responses. Skin testing for commonly encountered antigens elicited no response at 48–72 h to any antigen tested. The antigens used included *Candida*, streptokinase–streptodornase, blood group substances, mycobacterial antigens, and the chemical antigen 1-chloro-2,4-dinitrobenzene. Response to chlorodinitrobenzene was measured following three applications to induce sensitization.

Homograft Response. A skin graft from an unrelated female donor was placed when the child was 8 months of age; a second graft from the same donor was applied at 11 months of age. Neither graft was rejected.

Specific Antibody Response. Immunization with diphtheria, pertussis, and tetanus toxoid (DPT) five times, oral poliomyelitis vaccine twice, Salk vaccine twice, and inactivated measles vaccine twice gave no antibody responses except to polio at nine months. In addition, there were no antibody responses to two organisms isolated from the child, *Staphylococcus aureus* and *Pseudomonas aeruginosa*.

Natural Antibodies. Isohemagglutinins (IgM) to blood groups A and B were detected at 8 months, although these were decreased at 16 months (1 month prior to death).

Lymphocyte Proliferation Studies. Culture of lymphocytes with phytohemagglutinin, a T-cell mitogen (polyclonal activator of proliferation), failed to generate a proliferative response.

In summary, Dr. DiGeorge found normal lymphocyte counts in the circulation, normal plasma cells in the lymph nodes, and normal immunoglobulin levels. In contrast, the infant had "runting" (failure to thrive), oral fungal infection with absent skin tests (delayed hypersensitivity) to fungal antigens and to a synthetic chemical, and absent allogeneic (unrelated individual of the same species) skin graft rejection. In spite of normal immunoglobulin levels, he failed to generate antibodies following vaccination protocols.

How do these results fit with what we now know about the divisions of the immune system?

If we consider the results of the immunologic studies on this infant, we can recognize that the defect is in his **cell-mediated immunity** *arm: absent response to fungal infection, absent delayed-type hypersensitivity, absent response to a haptenating chemical, and absent graft rejection. [A haptenating agent, in this case 1-chloro-2,4-dinitrobenzene, is a substance that introduces a* **hapten** *(low-molecular-weight chemical group) onto normal body self-proteins and converts them into antigens that induce T-cell responses. Individuals with normally functioning T cells demonstrate a positive response on reexposure to the haptenating agent.] The baby's* **humoral immunity** *was relatively intact; as evidenced by the presence of immunoglobulin and plasma cells; however he lacked the ability to generate specific antibody responses to challenge. This division of the immune system into two distinct but interacting parts was at that time only suspected, and the role of the thymus was unclear.*

Although he was not yet ready to report on these data, Dr. DiGeorge relates that he found himself compelled to do so during a discussion at the meeting of the Society of Pediatric Research in May 1965.

State of the Art, Circa 1965

At that meeting, Max Cooper, Raymond Peterson, and Robert Good presented a concept of the lymphoid system based on their findings in chickens, with parallel evidence in mammals. They had previously published a report demonstrating that the chicken has two distinct lymphoid structures; the bursa of Fabricius and the thymus. In hatchlings, ablation of the bursa plus total body irradiation resulted in a lack of plasma cells, a lack of follicular cells and germinal centers in the spleen, and the absence of gammaglobulins. In contrast, thymectomy and irradiation reduced the number of small lymphocytes in the blood and spleen and impaired delayed-type hypersensitivity, graft-versus-host reactivity, and graft rejection. However, the capability to produce immunoglobulins, albeit less specific ones for antigens, remained. Thus, the major impairment following thymectomy and irradiation was in what we now know as cell-mediated immunity.

Cooper et al. proposed that the immune system was similarly compartmentalized in mammals but that the tonsils were the mammalian analogue of the bursa of Fabricius and the site of maturation of plasma cells. Other investigators at the meeting objected to making too direct a comparison between these species and argue I against the tonsils as the primordial site for plasma cell (in that they were correct).

Based on the knowledge we have today, the difficulty these investigators were having is understandable. Mammals have no equivalent to the bursa of Fabricius in that they do not have a separate organ solely for the development of B cells; maturation instead occurs in the bone marrow, the site of all hematopoiesis, which is not easily ablated without causing death. The second area of confusion arose from the comparison of experimental animal studies with observations on patients. At that time, two groups of patients had been described: those with Bruton's agammaglobulinemia and those, more severely ill patients, with "Swiss-type agammaglobulinemia," then also known as thymic alymphoplasia. Swiss-type agammaglobulinemia encompasses many of the entities that we now recognize as severe combined immunodeficiency (SCID). In an attempt to mimic these "experiments of nature," the investigators eliminated both the structure (via thymectomy or bursectomy) and the cells (via irradiation) in experimental animals. They met with more immediate success in chickens than in mammals.

At this point in the meeting, during the arguments over the comparison between chickens and mammals and humans and experimental animal models, Dr. DiGeorge describes how he could no longer sit quietly but felt compelled to describe his patient series. He therefore made the following statement: "A group of patients that has not, to my knowledge, come to the attention of investigators interested in the immunologic function of the thymus in man are the infants born with congenital absence of the thymus. Such infants are not to be confused with patients who have the Swiss type of agammaglobulinemia or the ataxia telangiectasia syndrome."

Dr. DiGeorge was invited to present his experiences and patient series at the First Immunologic Conference: Immunologic Deficiency Diseases in Man in 1967. The publication of the proceedings followed in February 1968. His experimental report on the fourth infant, the child on whom the immunologic studies described above were conducted, was published in *Nature* in May 1967 (following rejection by the first journal to which the manuscript was submitted). By that time the infant had died, and an autopsy had confirmed the lack of thymic tissue. In the *Nature* article, Dr. DiGeorge separated the consequences due to absence of thymic structure from those due to absence or disorder of stem cell differentiation and proposed thymic transplants as treatment for the former. In calling attention to the thymus as the locus of T-cell development, he thus

added a vital piece of evidence to the growing understanding of the bipartite nature of the immune system.

Footnote on History

A remarkable and eerie coincidence is recorded in a communication by Dr. Ogden Bruton in 1948, almost 20 years before Dr. DiGeorge's publication described above. At that time, Dr. Bruton was inspecting the pediatric care at Army hospitals in post–World War II Germany and Austria as part of his military service. He describes meeting and evaluating a promising young doctor who had become Chief of medical services in the army hospital in Linz, Austria, after only one year of general training. This doctor's stated goal was to become a pediatric endocrinologist; his name was Lieutenant Angelo DiGeorge. Dr Bruton himself was to publish his description of X-linked (Bruton's) agammaglobulinemia in 1952.

DIFFERENTIAL DIAGNOSIS TODAY

DiGeorge syndrome, a rare, usually sporadically occuring congenital disease, needs to be considered in a differential diagnosis of any infant with failure to thrive and recurrent infection. The classical triad of cardiac structural anomalies, hypocalcemia, and immune deficiencies, along with abnormal facies, easily distinguishes this entity from other immunodeficiencies and makes the diagnosis, or at least suspicion of the diagnosis, obvious. Patients may demonstrate less severe and more variable presentations, and it is often difficult to distinguish DiGeorge syndrome from other congenital syndromes with cardiac and facial structural abnormalities. We will concern ourselves here with the differential diagnosis with respect to congenital immunodeficiency disorders only.

Infants with DiGeorge syndrome are unusually susceptible to fungal and viral infections as well as opportunistic infections by organisms that do not cause disease in normal individuals. This clinical profile, plus the presence of a normal or elevated number of peripheral B cells and normal isohemagglutinins, places the syndrome in the category of a T-cell defect (Fig. 3.1) and makes it easily distinguishable from X-linked (Bruton's) agammaglobulinemia. Patients with DiGeorge syndrome may be similar to those with hyper-IgM syndrome with respect to peripheral B-cell numbers and isohemagglutinins. However, full-blown DiGeorge syndrome patients may have reduced numbers of T cells in the peripheral blood; in contrast, T-cell levels are normal in those with hyper-IgM syndrome (see Case 4). Children who present with partial DiGeorge syndrome (see Clinical Features below) may require functional studies of lymphocyte populations to distinguish their illness from hyper-IgM syndrome.

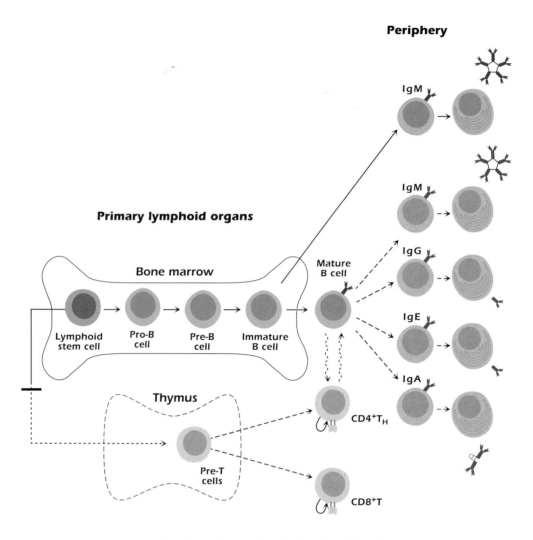

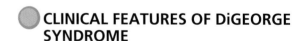
Figure 3.1. Lymphopoietic development remaining in athymic patient. Thymic structure is missing.

The distinction between DiGeorge syndrome and SCID is more problematic. Referring again to our flow chart of lymphopoietic development (Fig. 3.1), the DiGeorge abnormality prevents development at the same level of T-cell maturation as in SCID. Although there is no corresponding disruption of B-cell development in DiGeorge syndrome, the humoral response will be at least partially disrupted because of the lack of required T-cell help for specific antibody production. In addition, some SCID subgroups have normal or near-normal B-cell numbers (see Case 2), necessitating further analysis to distinguish the two entities. Clinically, both may present with failure to thrive, but hypoparathyroidism and lack of a thymic shadow on radiographic studies are unique to DiGeorge syndrome. Patients with SCID will have tonsillar underdevelopment and absent responses to B-cell mitogens in spite of the presence of peripheral blood B cells. Those with DiGeorge syndrome will have B cells that are functionally normal if properly stimulated.

Workup today is therefore likely to include immunophenotypic studies of peripheral blood lymphocytes by flow cytometry, mitogen proliferation studies employing both T- and B-cell mitogens (PHA and PWM, respectively), and studies of T–B-cell collaboration in the generation of antibody responses, pairing patient cells of one lineage with normal cells of the other lineage (see Cases 1 and 2).

CLINICAL FEATURES OF DiGEORGE SYNDROME

General

Since infants with DiGeorge syndrome have congenital abnormalities that involve multiple organ systems, their overall clinical presentations include cardiac, endocrine, and often neurologic complications as well as infectious problems resulting from the thymic aplasia. The abnormal development of the palate and facial structures results in dysmorphic features and severe feeding difficulties. The hypocalcemia, as a consequence of hypoparathyroidism, is often the most urgent clinical problem. Cardiac complications are of varying severity, depending on the degree and the specific anomaly seen in the individual patient. In fact, all of the clinical features show a range of expression in individual patients (variable phenotype), suggesting that this congenital disease is the result of disruption of complex tissue interactions during fetal development.

Immune Dysfunction

As discussed above, the immune deficiency is related to the decreased production of mature T cells. Although at the time the disease was described by Dr. DiGeorge the patients succumbed to infectious complications, most of these children have only mild and transient immunodeficiency. Similar to the variability seen in the other involved organs, many of the children have small rests of thymic tissue, enough to produce some mature T cells that increase over time. In addition, there is the hypothetical possibility of extrathymic T-cell maturation, a thesis supported by some data from animal studies.

In general, DiGeorge syndrome patients may be subdivided based on their degree of immunodeficiency into those with complete DiGeorge syndrome and those with partial DiGeorge syndrome. This difference is reflected in the severity of the T-cell deficit, which, for unknown reasons, is more severe in the $CD8^+$ T-cell compartment, rendering DiGeorge patients particularly susceptible to viral infections. As expected, those with severe T-cell defects are susceptible to opportunistic infections as well (infections due to organisms that do not cause disease in immunocompetent individuals).

In children who survive until a later age, there is also an earlier and increased incidence of autoimmune diseases, which is understandable based on the need for the thymus to eliminate autoreactive T-cell clones (central tolerance, see below) and to generate regulatory T cells (peripheral tolerance). Juvenile rheumatoid arthritis is the most common type of autoimmune disease observed, but organ-specific autoimmune diseases have been reported as well.

Those patients with minimal hypoparathyroidism and/or cardiac problems may not be recognized as having DiGeorge syndrome until a later age. This is particularly understandable since the disease would not be expected in the family given that it is most often the result of a sporadic rather than an inherited mutation (see below).

⬤ NORMAL THYMIC FUNCTION

The Thymus as a Black Box

In the 1950s and early 1960s, a time when the functions of virtually all the body's organs had been known (if not understood) for decades, the basic role of the thymus remained a mystery. In fact, in the 1950s children found to have a large thymus on chest X rays performed for other reasons were sometimes irradiated to decrease its size, a stunning example of pre-evidence-based medicine! It was not until 1961 that Miller published studies comparing the immune status of mice thymectomized within the first day of life and those thymectomized at five days of age with sham thymectomized animals. His findings that thymectomized animals had significant immune defects but only if the procedure was done within a few hours of birth put to rest any doubts that the thymus was involved in the immune competence of the animal. However, as late as 1964, it was uncertain as to whether thymic lymphocytes were derived from an outside source (which we now know is the bone marrow) or were derived from thymic epithelial cells as stem cells! Certainly, it was erroneously but commonly believed at the time that thymic lymphocytes were the precursors of plasma cells, although they were not thought to become plasma cells within the thymus themselves. Thus, Max Cooper's presentation in 1965 of the two arms of the immune system in chickens met with great resistance.

Thymectomy in the neonatal period in mice resulted in a decrease in lymphocytes in the blood and lymphoid organs (but not the bone marrow), a decreased ability to make specific antibodies to some (but not all) antigens, no effect on serum immunoglobulin levels, marked impairment in delayed-type hypersensitivity reactions, and impaired ability to reject foreign skin grafts. Histologic examination of the lymph nodes and spleens showed a marked decrease in germinal centers and few plasma cells. Indeed, these animals died at several months of age from a type of wasting syndrome. You will recognize that these findings on neonatally thymectomized mice are virtually identical to those found by Dr. DiGeorge in the workup of his fourth patient. In 1964, Miller reported evidence that stem cells from the bone marrow had to experience the thymic environment, or at least humoral factors from the thymus, in order to mature. Upon leaving the thymus, they homed and recirculated among all the other lymphoid tissues in the body (but not back into the thymus). Given the long life span of those lymphocytes which had matured in the thymus, he believed it likely that the animal could then retain immune competence and did not ordinarily need a functioning thymus after the first few days of life. Miller's results explained why it was so difficult to prove the requirement for the thymus in immune competence; the general approach of "cutting out" an organ (usually an endocrine organ) in animals and seeing what disease emerged or what functions were missing had not initially worked for the thymus because the experiments were done in adult or young animals. Even five-day-old mice were too old to show the effect. The innovation of using neonatal animals before mature T cells had well seeded the periphery exposed the function of the thymus as the site required for the maturation of at least some lymphocytes.

Thus, the thymus was recognized to be the place that immature lymphocytes enter and from which mature "thymus-derived" or T lymphocytes emerge. T lymphocytes occupy the interfollicular area of the lymph nodes and are important for defense against fungi, viruses, and some bacteria. The avian counterpart in the humoral immune system is the bursa of Fabricius. Immature lymphocytes enter this organ and emerge as "bursa-derived" or B lymphocytes, the cells responsible for germinal center formation and antibody production. The mammalian equivalent of the bursa of Fabricius is the bone marrow (which, conveniently, also begins with a "B").

At this point, the thymus was a black box and for decades there was little or no understanding of what occurred in the thymus even once we understood the characteristics of mature T lymphocytes.

What must the T cell accomplish during its sojourn in the thymus?

During the precursor T lymphocytes' tenure in the thymus, teleologically speaking, the cells have to accomplish the following tasks:

1. *They have to productively rearrange their **T-cell receptor (TCR) genes** in order to express a receptor, either αβ or γδ.*

2. *If they express the αβ TCR, they have to commit to either the **CD4** or **CD8 lineage**.*

3. *They must be expanded if their receptor recognizes self-MHC (major histocompatibility complex) antigen with low avidity, assuming that they will then recognize modified self. This process is known as **positive selection**.*

4. *They must be eliminated if their receptor recognizes self-MHC antigen with too high an avidity (autoreactive), a process known as **negative selection**.*

Some of these tasks obviously require the participation of other cell types, such as epithelial cells or dendritic cells as well as growth factors and cytokines to interact with the thymocytes in negative and positive selection. In fact, the commitment to single positive cells (CD4 vs. CD8) also depends on these cells (as will become clear below). Presumably, even gene rearrangement cannot occur without cytokine stimulation from other cells. Thus, DiGeorge syndrome, in which progenitor T cells exist but the epithelial structure of the thymus is absent, results in an absence, or near absence, of mature T lymphocytes.

Fast Forward to the 21st Century: The Black Box Partially Illuminated

Commitment to T-cell Lineage. Since T cells derive from the same ***common lymphoid progenitor (CLP)*** as B cells, NK cells, and some dendritic cells and use many of the same lymphocyte-specific enzymes as B cells to accomplish their maturation (see Case 1), signals must necessarily be received by the progenitor cells to commit them to the T-cell lineage. These signals derive from the thymic stromal cells. The fetal liver is the source of the CLP during fetal life; the bone marrow takes over at birth.

Traveling through the Thymus and Accomplishing Their Four Tasks. The thymus, an epithelial structure populated by immature lymphocytes and located in the anterior mediastinum, can be divided into two regions, cortex and medulla, each made up of three predominant types of stromal cells (Fig. 3.2). Thymic epithelial cells have abundant cytoplasm with long processes that form a meshwork within the cortex. They are also present in the medulla where, upon degeneration, it is believed that they comprise the whorls of Hassall's corpuscles. During embryogenesis, the thymus develops from an endodermal epithelial cell bud, which is encapsulated by mesenchyme contributed by the neural crest. The thymic epithelial cells (those cells missing in DiGeorge syndrome) differentiate into cortical and medullary thymic epithelial cells. The other two cell types comprising the thymic stroma are derived from bone marrow. These are dendritic cells that are present mostly at the corticomedullary junction and in the medulla and macrophages, which reside mostly in the medulla.

The progenitor cells enter the cortical region or corticomedullary junction of the thymus and traffic through the cortex, then into the medulla, and eventually out through the rich vasculature and efferent lymphatics (Fig 3.3). That is if they survive! Greater than 90% of the thymocytes die within the thymus as the result of lack of stimulation and negative selection.

1. TCR Gene Rearrangement. Early T-cell progenitors depend on IL-7 signaling for proliferation (see Case 2). Similar to B-cell development, a precursor receptor called the pre-TCR is expressed. The cell requires signaling through this receptor for continued survival and proliferation; however, a ligand has not been identified and none may in fact be needed. The pre-TCR in those cells destined to express αβ TCR consists of a pre-Tα chain and a β chain.

Since the progenitor cells use the same set of enzymes (and same mechanisms) to achieve rearrangement of the TCR genes as are used in B-cell receptor (BCR) or immunoglobulin gene rearrangement, how is the gene target of these enzymes determined? A corollary question is when and where does lineage commitment take place?

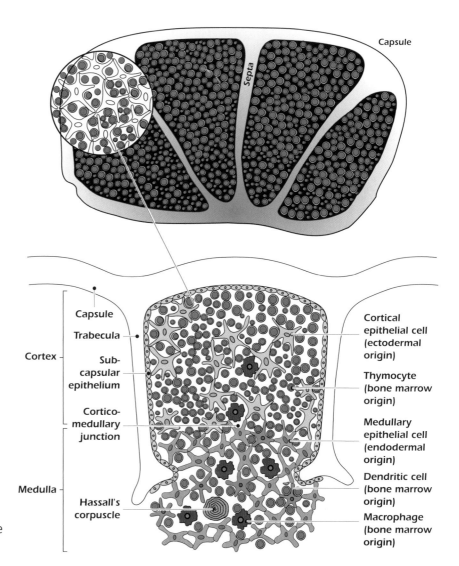

Capsule

Cortex
- Capsule
- Trabecula
- Sub-capsular epithelium
- Cortico-medullary junction

Medulla
- Hassall's corpuscle

Cortical epithelial cell (ectodermal origin)

Thymocyte (bone marrow origin)

Medullary epithelial cell (endodermal origin)

Dendritic cell (bone marrow origin)

Macrophage (bone marrow origin)

Septa

Figure 3.2. Cellular organization of the thymus.

The answer to the second question is in fact still being hotly debated. There is experimental data in mice supporting both concepts; that T cell lineage commitment occurs before and after arrival of the progenitors to the thymus.

More is known about what determines how T-cell-specific genes are turned on in thymocyte progenitors. The key molecule is a Notch 1 protein. The Notch family of cell surface proteins interacts with ligands on stromal cells in their environment to initiate proteolytic cleavage of the Notch molecules. The intracellular portion of the Notch protein then migrates to the nucleus. The cleaved portion of Notch 1 will collaborate with the transcription factor GATA 3 to turn on the T-cell lineage-specific genes (perhaps at that point committing the CLP to the T-cell lineage) and initiate recombination of the pre-TCR (Fig. 3.4).

The mechanisms of TCR gene rearrangement are then identical to BCR gene rearrangement (see Case 2). More is understood about the differentiation of thymocytes, specifically $\alpha\beta$ T cells, than about B-cell precursors but there are common themes.

As the maturation of the thymocyte progresses, it moves through the thymus from the cortex to the medulla, interacting with different stromal cells in each region. It is proposed that the stromal cells create a series of microenvironments in the thymus that result in the differentiation and education of the thymocytes. In the adult thymus, the CLP enters mostly through the blood vessels in the corticomedullary junction and then travels through the cortex and back down again (Fig. 3.3). These movements are at least partially governed by CCR7 and its recognition of CCL21 and CCL19 differentially expressed on the stromal cells. The pro-thymocyte in the cortex first expresses c-kit (CD117), the receptor for stem cell factor (SCF) made by stromal cells, as well as CD44 and CD25, the α chain of the IL-2 receptor. There is no expression of TCR, CD3, or the ξ chain. At this juncture, it is believed that cells with productively rearranged γ and δ genes will express the TCR $\gamma\delta$ on their surfaces, split off as the separate lineage of $\gamma\delta$ T cells, and exit the thymus. This population remains negative for both CD4 and CD8 and forms a minor population in the periphery. For the remainder of the prothymocytes (and perhaps in some of those cells that become γδ T cells), the genes for the β chain of the TCR are rearranging. In the prothymocyte, the genes for the β chain have been successfully rearranged and TCR β is synthesized. The TCR β is placed on the membrane with the pre-Tα, CD3, and ξ protein; signaling, which is perhaps ligand independent, initiates recombination of the TCR α-chain genes and inhibition of further TCR β-chain gene recombination. The δ-chain genes are in the midst of the α-chain locus; thus recombination of α-chain genes deletes them and eliminates any possibility of γδ TCR development in that cell. The cell goes from being "double negative" (DN; CD4⁻CD8⁻) to "double positive" (DP; CD4⁺CD8⁺) with numerous intervening stages.

The DN stage has been characterized further and divided into four substages: DN1, DN2, DN3, and DN4. The progression of the thymocyte through these stages is governed by signals produced by the thymic stromal cells as the thymocyte migrates through the different microenvironments created by the stromal cells of the cortex (Fig. 3.4). The different DN subpopulations may be distinguished by their differential expression of CD44 and CD25. In progressing from DN1 (CD44⁺CD25⁻) through DN2 (CD44⁺CD25⁺), the cells become specified and committed to the T-cell lineage, receiving the Notch signaling discussed above as well as other signals. TCR β-chain rearrangement begins in the DN2 stage and continues through DN3; these are both CD25⁺ stages. When the cell progresses from DN2 to DN3 (CD44⁻ CD25⁺), it is signaled through its pre-TCR, which continues until the DP stage. This process is partially stimulated by signaling from the protein sonic hedgehog (SHH), which is produced and secreted by the epithelial cells and may facilitate β-chain rearrangement. SHH protein is one of a family of secreted molecules that is important for body pattern development during embryogenesis and has other, organ-specific functions later in maturation. The SHH receptor PTCH1 on the developing thymocyte surface sets into motion a signaling cascade that turns on genetic programs via activation of transcription factors. PTCH1 interacts with smoothened (SMO) in the thymocyte; this molecule is the actual transducer of the signal. The expression of SMO is highest in the DN2 stage and is then down-regulated. Thus the progressive maturation of the thymocyte is the result of complex interactions between these developing cells and stromal cells in which the thymocyte travels through different microenvironments and partially controls its own responsiveness by expressing molecules to receive and transduce the signals from the thymic epithelial cells. Between the DN4 stage (CD44⁻ CD25⁻) and the DP stage is a brief single-positive stage in which CD8 is first expressed (ISP).

2. Commitment to CD4 or CD8 Lineage. The maturation from a CD4⁺ CD8⁺ double-positive thymocyte to a single-positive cell, either CD4⁺ or CD8⁺, requires interaction of the TCR with the MHC, which is expressed with a bound peptide on the surface of nonlymphoid cells of the thymus. It is part of the same series of interactions that results in positive and negative selection (see below) and can almost be considered a byproduct of those interactions. CD4 binds to the nonpolymorphic β₂ domain of the MHC class II molecule, functioning as a coreceptor that increases the signal transduction and the affinity of binding between the T cell and the epithelial cell. CD8 similarly functions as a coreceptor, interacting with the α₃ portion of the MHC class I molecule on the surface of the presenting cell.

As a result of the costimulation by either CD4 or CD8 when the TCR interacts with the MHC and peptide, the reciprocal molecule is down-regulated on the thymocyte surface and a single-positive T cell results. This interaction also results in proliferation and positive selection if the avidity of binding is at the appropriate level. Several properties of mature T cells can be understood as a consequence of this developmental process. This includes (1) the specific recognition by mature CD4⁺ T cells of antigen presented in the context of MHC class II versus the specific recognition by mature CD8⁺ T cells of antigen presented in the context of MHC class I (MHC class II vs. class I restriction) and (2) the failure to generate CD8 single-positive T cells and CD4 single-positive T cells in the absence of class I or class II MHC expression, respectively, as occurs in diseases known as bare lymphocyte syndromes (see Case 2). This is due to the lack of positive selection of the single-positive T cells (see below).

The Specter of Death: Recall that more than 95% of thymocytes do not survive to exit the thymus. The developing T cell has many paths to take to cell death. At many stages, lymphocytes need survival signals to prevent apoptosis (see Cases 1 and 25). In the thymus, the survival signal is provided by stimulation through the TCR and coreceptors, without which the thymocyte undergoes death by neglect (Fig. 3.5). Approximately 90% of the DP cells will die by neglect. That is, their mature TCR does not engage a ligand. The remainder will bind a peptide–MHC complex, which serves as a signal for the cells to proliferate, survive, and expand. The thymus is also the site of purposeful cell death, called negative selection (see below). The end result is the production of a mature T-cell population that will recognize infected or altered self (and outright foreign cells) but will not react with self-peptides (autoimmunity). There is debate as to whether this is achieved through events which are temporally and/or spatially distinct requiring separate thymic microenvironments.

3. Positive Selection. Hand in hand with the commitment to single-positive mature T cells is the process of positive selection, which will result in expansion of a

Trafficking of Developing Thymocytes through Thymus

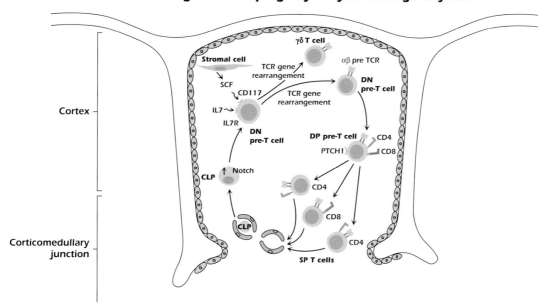

Figure 3.3. Trafficking pattern and maturation of developing thymocytes. Within the thymus thymocytes migrate from corticomedullary junction to cortex and back again falling under the influence of different micro environments.

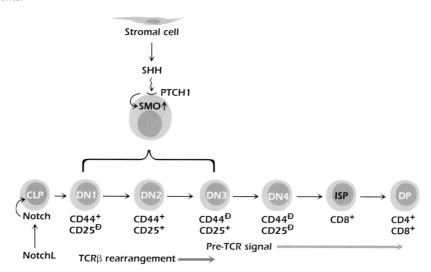

Figure 3.4. External signaling and surface antigen changes during thymocyte maturation from CLP to double-positive (CD4+ CD8+) thymocyte stage. Cell passes through four DN stages, receiving signals from stromal cells. TCR gene rearrangement takes place during these stages.

population of T cells responding to foreign antigen in the context of self-MHC. It is primarily the cortical epithelial cells of the thymus that "educate" the developing T cell, with some contribution from the dendritic cells of the cortex. These cells express MHC class I and class II associated with peptide. If the thymocyte recognizes the MHC molecule and peptide with low avidity, it survives and proliferates (Fig. 3.5). The TCR and its coreceptor or T-cell subset marker (CD8 or CD4) recognize the MHC (class I or II, respectively) with bound peptide, preventing cell death and reinforcing the expression of the TCR, CD3, and the coreceptor CD8 or CD4. The epithelial cells must therefore express the MHC molecules and must be able to process and display peptides in those molecules. The peptides are believed to serve as space holders, without which the MHC cannot be expressed on the cell surface.

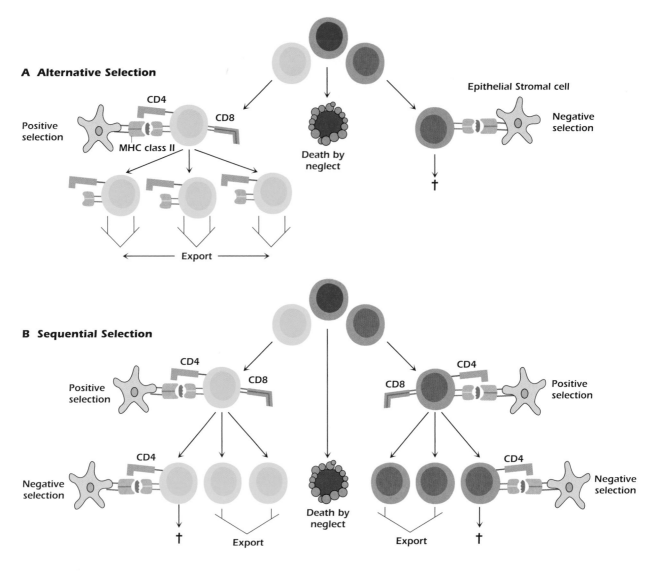

A Alternative Selection

Positive selection

CD4

CD8

MHC class II

Death by neglect

Epithelial Stromal cell

Negative selection

Export

B Sequential Selection

CD4

Positive selection

CD8

CD4

CD8

Positive selection

CD4

Negative selection

CD4

Negative selection

Death by neglect

Export

Export

C Positive Selection + Lineage Committment to CD4⁺ subset

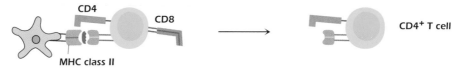

CD4

CD8

MHC class II

CD4⁺ T cell

🔘 <u>Figure 3.5.</u> Fate of developing thymocyte and emergence of selected, single-positive (CD4⁺ or CD8⁺) T cells (CD4⁺ T cell emergence shown as example) Whether the thymocytes are alternatively positively or negatively selected (as in **A**) or sequentially selected (as in **B**) is still under investigation. **C**. Following positive selection, the DP cell undergoes lineage committment to CD4 cell (shown here) or CD8 cell. This requires stimulation of the T cell through the TCR.

4. Negative Selection. The last decade has witnessed an explosion in our understanding of negative selection in the thymus. Negative selection occurs predominantly in the medulla of the thymus, the medullary epithelial cells having the major instructive role and dendritic cells serving a secondary function (Fig. 3.5). The existence of negative selection in the cortex is a point of debate.

The objective is to eliminate developing autoreactive T cells and prevent them from entering the periphery, a process resulting in ***central tolerance***. In the thymus, central tolerance is accomplished mostly by clonal deletion of autoreactive cells. The fate of those T cells that react strongly to their own MHC is cell death, but the mechanism behind the thymic deletion of T cells reactive to molecules expressed in the periphery and not encountered in the thymus was unexplained. Or are these antigens expressed in the thymus? The emerging story is that negative selection is in fact based on the expression of specific **peripheral tissue antigens (PTA)** on thymic medullary epithelial cells and dendritic cells. These PTAs are ectopically expressed on the medullary epithelial cells and include insulin, a salivary gland protein, myelin basic protein, thyroglobulin, and C-reactive protein, among others, for a total of at least 500 antigens.

What governs the expression of organ-specific self-peptides in this "aberrant" or unexpected location?

A rare inherited polyendocrine autoimmune disorder called autoimmune polyendocrinopathy–candidiasis–ectodermal dystrophy (APECED) helped provide the answer to this question. These patients suffer an assortment of autoimmune diseases, including type I diabetes, autoimmune hepatitis, and ovarian failure. Although manifestation is affected by environment and the patient's MHC, the mutated region of DNA contains a gene that codes for a transcription factor named AIRE (autoimmune regulator). In mouse model studies, this protein was found to be expressed mainly in the thymus, specifically in the medullary epithelial cells; its function is the regulation of the transcription of many, but not all, of the PTA genes. Normally there is deletion in the thymus of those T-cell clones reactive to self-peptides expressed on peripheral organs. Without AIRE, PTAs are not expressed on these antigen-presenting epithelial cells and the autoreactive thymocytes are not eliminated. Mutation or elimination of AIRE in thymic medullary epithelial cells, resulting in autoimmune disease, is therefore evidence that expression of organ-specific antigens by these thymic stromal cells underlies the mechanism of central tolerance.

The dendritic cells of the thymic medulla may also serve as inducers of central tolerance by using their "skills" as professional antigen presenters to display antigen captured from the medullary epithelial cells. In that way, the dendritic cells may more effectively eliminate T cells with lower affinity receptors for self-antigens without having to turn on the genes to ectopically produce those proteins themselves. In addition, there are peripheral tolerance mechanisms that help maintain the state of tolerance or anergy, result in B-cell tolerance, and establish tolerance to antigens not encountered in the thymus.

While negative selection results in clonal deletion of autoreactive T cells, these same self-antigen expressing epithelial cells may be responsible for the generation of another subset of T cells called T regulatory (T_{reg}) cells. Following thymic education, T_{reg} cells recognize self-antigens and exert a negative regulatory effect on other immune cells in the periphery, preventing autoimmune disease and playing a role in the mechanism of peripheral tolerance. The function of T_{reg} cells and major mechanisms achieving and maintaining tolerance to self will be examined in more detail in Unit III.

The thymus is therefore much more than simply an inert physical structure in which progenitor T cells mature. It is even more than a provider of a milieu of soluble mediators simply supporting cell growth. The thymic epithelial cells serve as the "teachers" of self and nonself to the maturing thymocytes and the gatekeepers for preventing autoimmune attack.

What difficulties might theoretically be encountered in attempting to restore complete immune competence in DiGeorge syndrome patients with thymic transplants?

Investigations using mouse models have elucidated much of what we know about thymic education and mature T-cell function. In addition to those systems specifically devised by investigators using thymectomy and irradiation with reconstitution, there is a naturally occurring mouse model for DiGeorge syndrome, the nude mouse. In nude mice, neither the thymus nor hair follicles develop (hence the mouse is "nude"). This is the result of a single point mutation in the gene for a forkhead box transcription factor Foxn1, located on chromosome 11. Experimental attempts to reconstitute the T-cell immune responses of these mice met with only partial success. Thymic transplants that did not strictly match the recipient MHC resulted in the generation of mature T cells of recipient origin, which were not capable of the vigorous immune response expected. In fact, these observations led to the concept of antigen recognition in the context of self-MHC. In subsequent studies, it was shown that, if the thymic epithelial cell utilizes a foreign MHC to present peptide to the developing thymocyte (as in a transplanted thymus) and it is recognized with low avidity, the thymocyte will survive and expand. After this positive selection and maturation, the T cell leaves the thymus having been educated to "self" but it is the self-MHC of the donor thymic epithelium. In the periphery, where the job of the T cell is to respond to altered self, the mature T cell will respond most effectively to antigen-presenting cells displaying the MHC that matches the donor thymus. In actuality, the mature T cell encounters antigen-presenting cells displaying the recipient's own MHC, not the MHC to which it has been positively selected or educated. Thus, the overall interaction in the periphery will not be as effective after maturation in a foreign thymic structure.

Luckily, thymic transplantation is often unnecessary in DiGeorge syndrome patients.

⬤ PATHOPHYSIOLOGY OF CONGENITAL THYMIC APLASIA

As noted previously, the pathophysiology of this syndrome is the result of the impaired development of several organ structures in the fetus; the urgent problems of the patients may be a consequence of the cardiac, endocrine, and/or neurologic anomalies. From an immunologic standpoint, the pathophysiology of DiGeorge syndrome, also called congenital thymic aplasia, is a consequence of the lack of the thymic structure during fetal development and the absence of its function. Specifically, absence of the thymic epithelial cells results in a T-cell deficiency caused by an inability of the T cells to mature. In this respect, the patients overlap with many SCID patients; recall that we began this chapter by recounting how these two groups of patients could not be distinguished because of the state of knowledge at that time.

In many patients with DiGeorge syndrome, there are reduced numbers of mature T cells, perhaps due to their development in small rests of thymic tissue. In patients surviving longer with DiGeorge syndrome, the incidence of autoimmune disease is increased. As one might surmise from the discussion of normal thymic function, this may be the result of improperly educated T cells. Maturation of T cells in disrupted thymic tissue may allow the escape of autoreactive T-cell clones due to inadequate central tolerance. In addition, peripheral tolerance mechanisms that control autoreactive B cells as well depend on one or more populations of regulatory T cells which are also normally products of thymic education. Without T-cell control, B cells expand in number, including those that are autoreactive.

Cytogenetic studies have linked DiGeorge syndrome to disruption of chromosome 22q11 with patients showing deletions, translocations, and microdeletions in that region. Deletion of region 22q11.2 is the most common deletion syndrome, with an incidence of 1 in 4000 live births. Genes in the area affect organ development during embryogenesis, resulting in a variety of cardiac malformations, craniofacial anomalies, and neurologic abnormalities, in addition to hypoplasia (decreased size) of the parathyroids and thymus. Patients with complete DiGeorge syndrome account for only a minor fraction ($<0.5\%$) of cases, although most patients with 22q11.2 deletion syndrome show some degree of immunodeficiency and dysregulation. Neither the severity of the disease nor its variability neatly correlates with the extent of the genetic material disrupted. Thus, genetic analysis including prenatal screening cannot predict phenotype.

TREATMENT OF DiGEORGE SYNDROME

Treatment of DiGeorge syndrome depends on the severity of the immunodeficiency. In less severe cases, the immunodeficiency is managed by supportive therapy and careful observation. This may include prophylaxis against *Pneumocystis jiroveci* pneumonia and, of course, will include the avoidance of live viral vaccines.

For those with more severe immunodeficiency, treatment may be similar to that of SCID patients, including isolation and the possibility of reconstitution of the immune defect, in this case with both bone marrow and thymic transplantation. Given that the immune capability of these patients may improve over time, particularly during the first year of life, it is often advisable to wait before undertaking these measures.

REFERENCES

Cooper MD, Peterson RDA, Good RA (1965a): A new concept of the cellular basis of immunity. With discussions by P. Fireman and A. DiGeorge. *J Pediatr* 67:907–908.

Cooper MD, Peterson RDA, Good RA. (1965b): Delineation of the thymic and bursal lymphoid systems in the chicken. *Nature (Lond)* 205:143–146.

Crompton T, Outram SV, Hager-Theodorides AL (2007): Sonic hedgehog signaling in T-cell development and activation. *Nature Rev Immunol* 7:726–735.

DiGeorge A. Personal communication, 2006.

DiGeorge A. (1968): Congenital absence of the thymus and its immunologic consequences: Concurrence with congenital hypoparathyroidism. Birth Defects Original Article Series. National Foundation March of Dimes N.Y. ed. Bergoma, D. Scientific ed. Robert A. Good Immunologic Deficiency Diseases in Man, vol. 4, pp. 116–123.

Gallegos AM, Bevan MJ (2006): Central tolerance: Good but imperfect. *Immunol Rev* 209:290–296.

Hemming VG (1996): Ogden Bruton and Angelo DiGeorge: 1948. *Pediatrics* 88:A36.

Lischner HW, Punnett HH, DiGeorge AM (1967): Lymphocytes in congenital absence of the thymus. *Nature (Lond)* 214:580–582.

Mathis D, Benoist C (2007): A decade of AIRE. *Nature Rev Immunol* 7:645–650.

McLean-Tooke A, Spickett GP, Gennery AR (2007): Immunodeficiency and autoimmunity in 22q11.2 deletion syndrome. *Scand J Immunol* 66:1–7.

Miller JFAP (1961): Immunological function of the thymus. *Lancet* ii:748–749.

Miller JFAP (1964): The thymus and the development of immunologic responsiveness. *Science* 144:1544–1551.

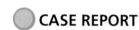

HYPER-IgM SYNDROME

WARREN STROBER

⬤ CASE REPORT

"My baby has a high fever and a bad cough."

Clinical History and Initial Evaluation

Lee, a six-month-old infant, is brought to the pediatric emergency room (ER) by his mother at about 8 AM on a Saturday. She tells you that Lee was well until two days ago, when he developed a cough and seemed lethargic. At that time, she called her family physician. He advised her that it was probably a cold, to keep him well hydrated, and to administer one baby acetaminophen every 6 h if Lee develops a fever. Lee slept poorly that night and the next day was noted to have a low-grade fever of about 38°C. Since he seemed to be getting worse, the family physician was called again, but he continued to think Lee merely had a cold and should be treated symptomatically. Over the course of the day Lee's cough became more frequent, and by the evening he was breathing more rapidly than usual (tachypneic). These symptoms became more intense during the night and prompted the mother's visit to the ER with the baby.

Your physical examination of Lee discloses a child of appropriate length and weight (normal growth) who has a normal overall appearance, that is, no dysmorphic facial

features or bone abnormalities. He has an elevated temperature of 38.5°C and obvious respiratory symptoms (coughing and rapid breathing) but no meningeal signs such as neck rigidity or inconsolable irritability. Auscultation of his chest reveals coarse breath sounds but no bronchospasm or evidence of pulmonary consolidation. Examination of the pharynx reveals no evidence of pharyngitis or tonsillitis (inflammation of the phyarynx and tonsils); in fact, the tonsils seem reduced in size.

You surmise that the patient has a pulmonary infection (probably a bacterial pneumonia) and have him admitted to the pediatric ICU (PICU). You also order a chest X ray, blood cultures, and a complete blood count (CBC).

Course in Hospital and Initial Diagnosis

The chest X-ray result is available shortly after admission to the PICU and reveals the presence of bilateral perihilar infiltration. A complete blood count shows an increased white blood cell (WBC) count (15,500 cells/μL, reference range <12,000 cells/μL) comprised of 72% neutrophils, 7% monocytes, and 20% lymphocytes. Although this differential is compatible with the presence of an infection, you note that the total white count is lower than you expected for a bacterial pneumonia. In any case, you start the patient on IV cefotaxine, a broad-spectrum third-generation cephalosporine antibiotic to treat what

Immunology: Clinical Case Studies and Disease Pathophysiology, By Warren Strober and Susan R. S. Gottesman
Copyright © 2009 John Wiley & Sons, Inc.

you consider is the likely cause of his pneumonia, a bacterial pathogen. You also order a lung computer-aided tomography (CAT) scan to obtain an objective baseline for the extent of the infection.

Over the next several days you return frequently to the PICU to check on Lee's condition. Over this period Lee's respiratory status remains stable but does not improve despite the antibiotic therapy. He continues to be febrile and to be tachypneic. Pulse oxymeter readings show periodic episodes of oxygen desaturation (<92%) that require treatment with an oxygen mask. The blood cultures have proved negative, so you know neither the identity of the organism nor its sensitivity to antibiotics. Thus, you cannot be sure his infection is being adequately treated and, in fact, his lack of more rapid clinical improvement suggests otherwise. On the morning of the fourth day after admission, Lee's status seems to have deteriorated; his breathing is more labored and oxygen desaturation episodes are more prolonged and frequent. Indeed, a repeat CAT scan shows more extensive lung involvement. After consultation with a pulmonologist, a bronchoscopy is performed to obtain bronchial lavage fluid and brushings for microscopic examination and culture. This is done without incident. The next morning the laboratory report is returned; to your surprise, Lee has an infection with *Pneumocystis jiroveci* (formerly called *Pneumocystis carinii*) a protozoal organism that ordinarily causes infection only in immunocompromised hosts. You immediately change the antibiotic to IV trimethoprim-sulfamethoxazole (Bactrim), a specific and effective therapy for this organism.

The results of this treatment are dramatic. Within 24 h Lee shows noticeable improvement. Over the next several days he defervesces and his pulmonary status returns to normal. After four days of IV Bactrim therapy you switch to oral therapy and two days later Lee is discharged to home with the proviso that he continue on oral Bactrim therapy for another two weeks.

What is unusual about a pneumonia due to *Pneumocystis jiroveci (carinii)*?

As discussed in Case 1 on X-linked agammaglobulinemia (XLA), neonates are protected against infections, particularly bacterial infections, by maternal antibodies that have crossed the placenta (IgG) or been obtained through the mother's milk (IgM and IgA) until the infant's own immune system is more mature and the infant can mount his or her own antibody responses. Protection by placentally transmitted antibodies has almost completely dissipated by six months after birth; thus the occurrence of a pneumonia at this age, even a bacterial pneumonia, is unusual but not rare. It is the particular organism causing Lee's pneumonia, Pneumocystis jiroveci, *which is unusual and which raises a red flag that an underlying immune problem may exist.* Pneumocystis *belongs to a category of organisms known as "opportunistic pathogens" because they do not cause disease in healthy individuals, but do so in those with a compromised immune system that allow them the opportunity*

to act as pathogens. Although infants with their incompletely mature immune systems may be partially immunodeficient relative to the general population, the occurrence of an infection due to an opportunistic pathogen in a young child should still alert one to the possibility that an underlying immunologic defect is present. In particular, it suggests the presence of an immunodeficiency disease characterized by an abnormal T-cell-mediated immunologic response, since T-cell immunity provides the main host defense against opportunistic pathogens. DiGeorge syndrome and the various forms of severe combined immunodeficiency disease (SCID) are among the immunodeficiency diseases characterized by defective T-cell-mediated immunity (see introduction to this unit as well as Cases 2 and 3). More commonly, however, an acquired immunodeficiency such as that associated with human immunodeficiency virus (HIV) infection accounts for the presence of an infection with an opportunistic organism (see Case 9).

Immunologic Workup and Diagnosis

Initial Approach. Recognizing that Lee may have an immunologic disorder, you refer him to an immunologist for further workup. The immunologist starts the workup with a second look at the facts already in hand.

History. First, the history of normal development and lack of disease during Lee's first six months of life speak against SCID, an immunodeficiency that generally declares itself early and is associated with a failure to thrive (see Case 2). This tentative conclusion is corroborated by the CBC, which did not show the presence of a lymphopenia (reduced lymphocyte count). It should be noted, however, that Lee was observed to have a reduced tonsillar mass, possibly indicating some loss of ability to populate peripheral lymphoid compartments.

Re-review of the chest X-ray and CAT scans confirms the presence of a thymic shadow, with a size appropriate for age. Combined with the lack of evidence of hypoparathyroidism, dysmorphic facial features, and cardiac anomalies, the presence of a thymic shadow on radiologic examination eliminates consideration of thymic aplasia (DiGeorge syndrome).

Another major consideration in the differential diagnosis is the presence of a neonatal HIV infection (HIV transmitted to Lee from his mother during birth). This is unlikely because an HIV diagnostic test performed on Lee's mother during childbirth (as required by your state's law) was negative. Nevertheless, to be absolutely certain, Lee is tested for the presence of HIV using a Western blot–based technique to detect HIV protein, in case he lacks the ability to mount an antibody response to this organism (see Case 9 and Unit V for test descriptions). The results of this test are likewise negative, and HIV infection is definitively ruled out.

The immunologist also elicits a family history from the mother. He learns that Lee has a maternal uncle (his mother's brother) who died mysteriously at an early age due to pneumonia. This suggests that Lee may have an X-linked disease.

The conclusions drawn from the above review and family history are very valuable but do not identify a specific immunodeficiency state. A more extensive workup is therefore initiated. Although the *Pneumocystis* infection is drawing attention to the T cells or cell-mediated arm of the immune response, the status of his humoral immunity is also investigated.

Testing and Interpretations. As described in Cases 2 and 1 on SCID and XLA, respectively, and the introduction to this unit, an orderly approach to the investigation of the capability of the immune system must be pursued, keeping in mind the stages of development of mature immune cells and the interactions that must take place among them to mount an effective immune response.

LYMPHOCYTE SUBSET ANALYSIS. Quantitation of peripheral lymphoid subsets by an initial flow cytometry study reveal normal percentages and absolute numbers of $CD4^+$ T cells, $CD8^+$ T cells, B cells, and natural killer (NK) cells. Additional studies are performed in a specialty laboratory that does a more extensive panel of CD markers. Analysis of the $CD4^+$ cell subsets reveals that the percentage of $CD4^+$ cells in the $CD4^+/CD45RA^+$ (naive) CD4 T-cell subset is high and, correspondingly, the percentage in the $CD4^+/CD45RO^+$ (mature) CD4 T-cell subset is low even if one considers the fact that the ratio of $CD45RA^+$ cells to $CD45RO^+$ cells is high in young children as compared to adults. In addition, while Lee has a normal number of B cells, virtually none bear surface IgG or IgA.

These findings suggest a defect in T- and B-cell maturation at a point governed by antigen exposure.

IMMUNOGLOBULIN LEVELS

	Results	Reference Range
IgM	407 mg/dL	65 ± 25 mg/dL
IgG	<50 mg/dL	923 ± 256 mg/dL
IgA	<5 mg/dL	124 ± 45 mg/dL

How do the results obtained thus far differ from what would be found in studies of patients with XLA, SCID, and common variable immunodeficiency disease (CVID; see Case 5)?

In XLA, a primary B-cell defect leads to absence of circulating B cells and lack of production of all Ig classes by circulating cell populations. In SCID syndromes, a primary

defect affecting T cells is usually present that reduces the capacity of T cells to elaborate the helper cytokines necessary for B-cell maturation and Ig production; in addition, this primary defect may also have a direct effect on B cells. The result is that the number of T cells in the circulation is usually reduced as are B cells and serum immunoglobulin levels. Finally, in CVID, B-cell function is also usually impaired by a primary B-cell defect, and production of all immunoglobulin classes, including IgM, is correspondingly decreased, although not to the level seen in either XLA or SCID. In CVID the levels of both T and B cells in the circulation are normal or only mildly decreased. Lee's immunoglobulin profile differs from that of all of these diseases in that his IgM level is normal or even elevated, whereas the other immunoglobulins are decreased. Lee has normal numbers and distribution of lymphocyte subsets, unlike patients with XLA, who exhibit selective absence of B cells, and most patients with SCID, who exhibit absence of T cells associated, in many cases, with absence of B cells as well. Finally, while some SCID patients do have normal numbers of circulating lymphocytes such as those with a T^+B^+ phenotype, Lee's capacity to produce IgM makes it unlikely that he fits into this category of immunodeficiency disease.

PROLIFERATION STUDIES. Culture of Lee's cells with nonspecific mitogens, which induce proliferation of T cells (phytohemmaglutinin and concanavalin A) and B cells (pokeweed mitogen) show normal proliferative ability (see Case 1).

IN VITRO IMMUNOGLOBULIN PRODUCTION. The ability of each cell type to function in the steps required to produce immunoglobulin is next tested.

The B Cells on Their Own. Lee's peripheral blood (circulating) B cells are isolated and cultured *in vitro* with a CD40L trimer (plus IL-4 and IL-10) to produce antibody in conditions circumventing T-cell dependence. CD40L (CD154) is a molecule appearing on activated T cells that interacts with CD40 on B cells and induces B-cell maturation and class switching; thus, soluble CD40L trimer mimics or replaces the stimulatory activity of T cells. The culture fluid is then assayed for the presence of secreted immunoglobulins.

Result. Lee's B cells, stimulated under these culture conditions, produced normal amounts of IgM as well as normal amounts of IgG and IgA.

This provided solid evidence that his B-cell responses were intrinsically normal and that the serum Ig levels did not reflect an intrinsic B-cell abnormality.

T–B Cell Interaction. In concomitant studies, Lee's T cells are cultured with control B cells and his B cells are cultured with control T cells under conditions to induce polyclonal T-cell stimulation (surface-bound anti-CD3 and soluble anti-CD28). T-cell stimulation leads to the expression of CD40L and cytokine production, and the activated T cell should be capable of inducing B-cell stimulation and isotype switching to IgG and IgA production.

Result. Lee's T cells, stimulated by anti-CD3/anti-CD28, fail to induce normal B cells to produce IgG or IgA, whereas control T cells demonstrate this capacity; on the other hand, control T cells, stimulated by anti-CD3/anti-CD28, induce Lee's B cells to produce IgG and IgA.

These results suggest that Lee's T cells have reduced "helper T-cell activity", that is he has basic T-cell defects, whereas his B cells are normal. Thus his T cells are unable to interact with B cells to induce isotype class switching. This may be the result of a defect in CD40L expression and/or function or a defect in cytokine production.

Further Diagnostic Studies

Cell-Mediated Immunity Studies. Lee's clinical presentation (infection with an opportunistic pathogen) and immunologic workup thus far suggest an underlying T-cell abnormality in spite of the fact that Lee appears to have a B-cell deficiency as manifested by low IgG and IgA levels. The immunologist places particular importance on the T–B-cell interaction studies described above which, given that Lee's B cells are capable of producing immunoglobulin, point to a T-cell defect rather than a B-cell defect. One type of immunodeficiency that fits this pattern is hyper-IgM syndrome, an immunodeficiency that may be caused by failure to express CD40L (CD154) on the surface of activated T cells.

CD40L–CD40 also mediates interactions between T cells and antigen-presenting cells (APCs; monocytes or dendritic cells) to produce cytokines. The absence of effective interaction between T cells and macrophages would be expected to manifest in defective cell-mediated immune responses. To investigate this possibility, the immunologist conducts further T-cell studies that evaluate both *in vivo* and *in vitro* T-cell function and T-cell/APC interactions.

DELAYED-TYPE HYPERSENSITIVITY TEST. These "*in vivo*" studies consist of intradermal skin tests with tetanus toxoid and diphtheria antigens. Both are antigens to which Lee has already been exposed as part of his normal vaccination schedule. The skin test sites are "read" at 48 h for the presence of induration and erythema to determine if Lee can mount a delayed-type hypersensitivity (DTH) response.

Result. The test proves negative in that neither of these antigens elicits a significant inflammatory response.

Since the DTH reaction depends on T-cell stimulation of APCs via CD40L to produce cytokines (normally resulting in induration and erythrema), the absence of response in

these studies is compatible with a CD40L defect. This test of in vivo T-cell immunity also predicts that Lee will unfortunately have further difficulties with opportunistic infections.

IN VITRO ACTIVATION AND MONOCYTE CYTOKINE PRODUCTION: AN INVESTIGATION OF CELL COMMUNICATION. Lee's peripheral blood mononuclear cells are cultured either with anti-CD3 (an antibody that acts as a T-cell mitogen as noted above) or *Staphylococcus aureus* Cowan strain 1 (SAC) plus interferon-γ (IFN-γ). The latter combination acts as a direct stimulant of APCs, which, in peripheral blood, consists mainly of monocytes. This time the culture fluid is assayed for the cellular production of secreted cytokines (see Unit V). T cells, when activated by the anti-CD3, normally express CD40L (CD154), which then interacts with CD40 on the monocyte membrane, inducing the monocytes to produce inflammatory cytokines such as interleukin-12 (IL-12) and tumor necrosis factor (TNF)-α. On the other hand, SAC plus IFN-γ stimulates monocytes directly and results in production of IL-12 and TNF-α in the absence of T cells.

Result. Lee's peripheral monocytes produce greatly reduced amounts of IL-12 and TNF-α when they are stimulated by his T cells (cultured with anti-CD3). In contrast, his monocytes produce normal amounts of these cytokines when they are directly stimulated with SAC plus IFN-γ.

Lee's T cells do not stimulate monocytes to produce cytokines, but his monocytes are intrinsically intact. This is likely the result of defective CD40L expression on the T cells. However, a defect in IFN-γ production by the T cells could also be the culprit; therefore that possibility is tested next.

IFN-γ PRODUCTION. Lee's mononuclear cells are cultured with anti-CD3, but this time CD40L stimulation of the monocytes is "artificially" provided by addition of CD40L trimer, the soluble form of CD40L that can stimulate monocytes via CD40 in the absence of T cells. The CD40L trimer was used for a similar purpose in B-cell cultures (see above). T cells in cultures with anti-CD3 and activated monocytes should produce a cytokine such as IFN-γ as a result of stimulation by the anti-CD3 and the helper cytokines produced by the CD40L-stimulated monocytes.

Result. Whereas Lee's T cells produced greatly decreased amounts of IFN-γ in the absence of CD40L trimer, they produced normal amounts in its presence. The control T cells, on the other hand, produced IFN-γ in the presence and absence of CD40L trimer.

These data thus offer excellent functional evidence that Lee's T cells are functionally deficient either because they do not express CD40L or because they express an inactive CD40L, rather being unable to produce IFN-γ.

Definitive Diagnosis and Classification

Detection of the Molecule. At this point the immunologist closes in on the diagnosis of X-linked hyper-IgM syndrome (XHIGM; HIGM-I) by performing flow cytometry studies using fluorochrome-labeled anti-CD40L. These studies indeed demonstrate that Lee's cells do not express CD40L. The immunologist also sends a sample of Lee's DNA to a sequencing facility for sequencing of the CD40L gene. The results show that Lee's CD40L gene has a mutation in the extracellular domain of the gene that results in a truncation of this domain and thus low expression of CD40L on the T-cell surface. The diagnosis of XHIGM is now secure. Given the family history of a maternal uncle with an illness that could have been caused by HIGM, Lee is assumed to have inherited this mutated X-linked gene rather than to have a new mutation. This was subsequently verified by sequencing of Lee's mother's DNA, which showed that the mother carries the mutated gene on one X chromosome.

What is the explanation for the initial observations that Lee's tonsils are underdeveloped and that his peripheral helper T cells are skewed toward the naive (CD45RA) subset rather than the memory (CD45RO) subset?

As will be discussed in more detail later in the chapter, germinal center formation is dependent on interactions between T cells and dendritic cells and T cells and B cells. Both interactions occur in a CD40L–CD40-dependent fashion. The underdevelopment of germinal centers and predominance of only small primary follicles in the tonsils and even in the lymph nodes result in the reduced size of these structures. The change in the T-cell subset distribution is similarly the result of the inability of the T cells to express CD40L. Without CD40L, they are unable to stimulate the dendritic cells to express B7, which in turn is required to induce the T cell to mature. Thus Lee's peripheral T cells are skewed to the naive T-cell subset (CD45RA$^+$), with corresponding decrease of the memory T-cell compartment (CD45RO$^+$).

Lee is placed on monthly intravenous immunoglobulin (IVIG) infusions of 20 mg/kg to bring his "trough" (low-point) IgG level above 500 mg/dL, the target IgG level for immunodeficiency patients who cannot produce normal amounts of IgG. In addition, he is placed on prophylactic Bactrim therapy to prevent recurrence of *Pneumocystis* infection.

Lee's Subsequent Medical Course

At the age of three years, Lee developed a neutropenia (2000 neutrophils/μL versus the reference level of 5000 neutrophils/μL), a known concomitant of XHIGM syndrome. At age six years, he was placed on granulocyte colony-stimulating factor (G-CSF) therapy and partial amelioration of the neutropenia was achieved. This neutropenia was associated with recurrent apthous mouth ulcers, which tended to improve when neutrophil levels increased. Extensive attempts to culture an organism from these ulcers were unsuccessful.

At age eight, Lee suddenly developed mild right-sided weakness. Unfortunately, this symptom was not investigated until three months later, when he had a grand mal seizure. At that point a magnetic resonance imaging (MRI) examination of the brain revealed multiple punched-out lesions with enhancement. This picture is typical of toxoplasmosis, a known complication of XHIGM. Lee was therefore put on long-term pyrimethamine-sulfadiazine therapy that had an immediate effect as evidenced by the decrease in the enhancement in the MRI and had the long-term effect of preventing progression of the toxoplasmosis.

CLINICAL FEATURES OF HYPER-IgM SYNDROME

As will be detailed in a later section, the clinical syndrome of hyper-IgM has several possible pathophysiologic bases. Here we will discuss the clinical features of XHIGM syndrome. Although the name "hyper-IgM" places the emphasis on the inability to isotype switch to IgG and IgA immunoglobulin production, the infectious complications of XHIGM remind one that this is a deficiency in an interaction (CD40–CD40L) important in both humoral and cell-mediated immune responses. Thus there is overlap in its clinical features with those of some forms of SCID and T-cell immunodeficiency in that these patients have infections not normally found in conditions such as CVID (see Case 5 and below), a disorder with usually intact cell-mediated immunity.

Pulmonary Problems

Since patients with all forms of HIGM syndrome have increased or normal amounts of IgM levels but decreased IgG and IgA levels, it is not surprising that they are susceptible to infection with extracellular pathogens, similar to patients with CVID (see Case 5). Indeed, upper and lower respiratory infections by extracellular pathogens are the most common problems of hyper-IgM patients. In the absence of IVIG replacement therapy, bronchiectasis is likely to result as a consequence of recurrences. However, respiratory infection in X-linked hyper-IgM syndrome is also not infrequently due to opportunistic organisms (unlike CVID), and in over 40% of patients in whom pneumonia marked the onset of disease in the first year of life, *Pneumocystis jiroveci* was the cause of infection. Other opportunistic organisms causing infection in XHIGM patients include cytomegalovirus (CMV), cryptococcus, and atypical mycobacterial infection. These are the consequence of the inadequate interaction between T cells and macrophages via CD40–CD40L.

Gastrointestinal Problems

XHIGM patients frequently have diarrhea, and in 20–30% of cases, this can have a chronic course, associated with malabsorption and failure to thrive (again similar to what occurs in CVID). At times, the diarrhea results from opportunistic infection, such as with cryptosporidia or giardia, but in other instances it appears to be noninfectious in nature. In these latter cases, the patients may have intestinal nodular lymphoid hyperplasia and villous atrophy, suggesting the presence of an autoimmune process involving the GI tract (also see Case 5).

Liver Problems

Severe liver problems occur in almost 20% of XHIGM patients. These can take the form of sclerosing cholangitis (frequently due to cryptosporidiosis) as well as infection with hepatitis B and hepatitis C or even CMV. The hepatic infections can lead to cirrhosis and liver decompensation, which may necessitate a liver transplant. Historically, hepatitis in hyper-IgM syndrome has been associated with exposure to contaminated blood products, thus, IVIG used for replacement therapy must come from an unimpeachable source. Another complication of chronic hepatitis in XHIGM patients is hepatocellular carcinoma, which usually has a fatal outcome.

Hematologic Manifestations

The main hematologic problems in XHIGM patients are anemia and neutropenia. The former occurs in about one-third of patients and is usually due to iron deficiency; however, the anemia can occasionally be due to bone marrow failure (aplastic anemia) or peripheral lysis of the red cells (hemolytic anemia). Neutropenia, the more common hematologic abnormality, occurs in almost 70% of patients. It takes the form of a block in myeloid cell development, occurring at the promyelocytic–myelocytic stage. In some cases, the neutropenia is chronic and in other cases it is cyclic. It is frequently associated with gingivitis and perioral ulceration.

Neoplasia in XHIGM patients

Visceral neoplasms involving the gall bladder, liver, and pancreas have been reported, but this is not a frequent phenomenon. Lymphomas, often increased in other immunodeficiency states, are not associated with XHIGM, possibly because patients do not live long enough to develop this complication.

Miscellaneous Problems

A degenerative encephalopathy is not infrequently seen in XHIGM patients and is usually due to infection with any of several opportunistic pathogens, including *Cryptococcus*, toxoplasmosis, CMV, Echo virus, and *Mycobacterium bovis*. Because some of these infections are treatable, vigorous search for a causative agent should be done at the onset of CNS symptoms. Once degenerative changes occur, they can rarely be completely reversed.

Finally, secondary arthritis occurs in a small group of patients. This is usually associated with neutropenia and is presumably due to infection, but in most cases a causative agent cannot be identified.

NORMAL B-CELL STIMULATION AND FUNCTION

The maturation of B cells occurs in two phases. The first is an antigen-independent phase occurring in the fetal liver and bone marrow and the second is an antigen-dependent phase that occurs in lymphoid peripheral tissues such as the Peyer's patches, the spleen, and the lymph nodes. The steps necessary to advance the B cell from the progenitor stage to a naive mature B cell leaving the bone marrow were reviewed in Case 1 on XLA. In that first phase, the "germline" B-cell repertoire is established in individual B cells by rearrangement of both the heavy- and light-chain immunoglobulin genes. These rearrangements result in the formation of a VDJ segment from the variable segments, diversity segments, and joining segments (V, D, and J segments, respectively) as a consequence of a random recombination process. At the conclusion of these molecular events, the Ig heavy-chain gene consists of a "recombined" VDJ segment that determines antigen specificity. This segment sits upstream of a string of heavy-chain constant-region segments, the first of which are the Cμ and Cδ segments. The cell is now able to produce IgM and IgD antibodies.

In the second (antigen-dependent) stage of development, which occurs in the periphery, B cells undergo proliferation. At the same time, their Ig genes may undergo further changes, that of somatic hypermutation in the variable region (resulting in affinity maturation) and that of isotype class switch rearrangement. Somatic hypermutation is the result of point mutations in the VDJ segments, which lead to subtle changes in the affinity of the immunoglobulin for antigen. This process allows for the generation of cells producing high-affinity antibodies. Isotype class switch rearrangement results in a substitution of the constant-region portion of the heavy-chain molecule. Thus, the VDJ becomes associated with various downstream "C-region" heavy-chain genes such as γ, α, or ε C regions. In this way cells producing the various classes and subclasses of immunoglobulins are formed and combined with the hypermutated variable portion; these antibodies thus produced have a generally higher affinity for antigen than IgM.

In patients with hyper-IgM syndrome, the first phase of B-cell maturation, the antigen-independent phase in the bone marrow, is intact. It is in the second, antigen-dependent stage in the periphery that progression is halted (Fig. 4.1).

The Structural Basis of Class Switching

What is the molecular basis of the process by which B cells switch from the production of IgM to IgG or IgA; in other words how do they undergo Ig class switch differentiation?

A switch region (S) sits in the intron 5′ of each heavy-chain constant region with the exception of δ (Fig. 4.2). These switch regions are repetitive, conserved base sequences of

1–10 kilobases. When the cell receives the signal to switch (see below), two switch regions line up with the intervening DNA looping out. Recombination then takes place between these repetitive (and somewhat homologous) sequences and the DNA between them is cleaved. "Fingerprints" of this event are evident from the small loops of this cleaved DNA, which can be transiently detected before degradation. Switching may occur in an adjacent constant region or a constant region further downstream or sequential switching events may occur, with the cell progressing first to IgG and then to IgA. Isotype switching requires transcription and is initiated by promoters. Transcription is presumed to be required so that the DNA of the switch region can be opened up and accessed by the enzymes needed to accomplish the feat. Activation-induced cytidine deaminase (AID), an enzyme expressed exclusively in B cells and integral to the mechanism of somatic hypermutation, is also involved in isotype switching. It functions in both of these processes by deaminating cytidine directly on DNA. AID is a member of a

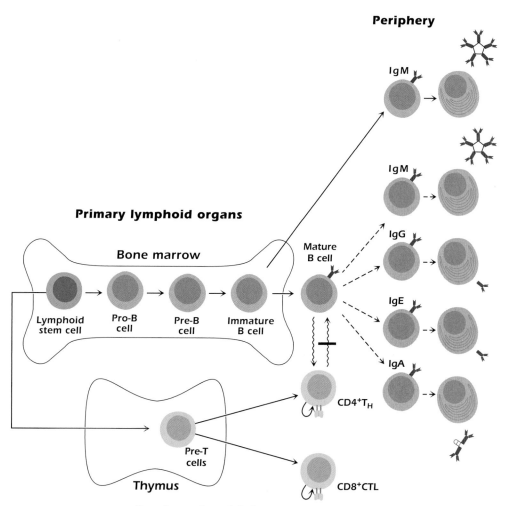

Key: Grey cells and their products are absent.

Figure 4.1. Sites of defective lymphopoietic development associated with primary immunodeficiency syndromes. Developing and mature lymphoid populations remaining in patients with hyper-IgM syndrome. Gray cells denote absent populations. Bar denotes block in interaction.

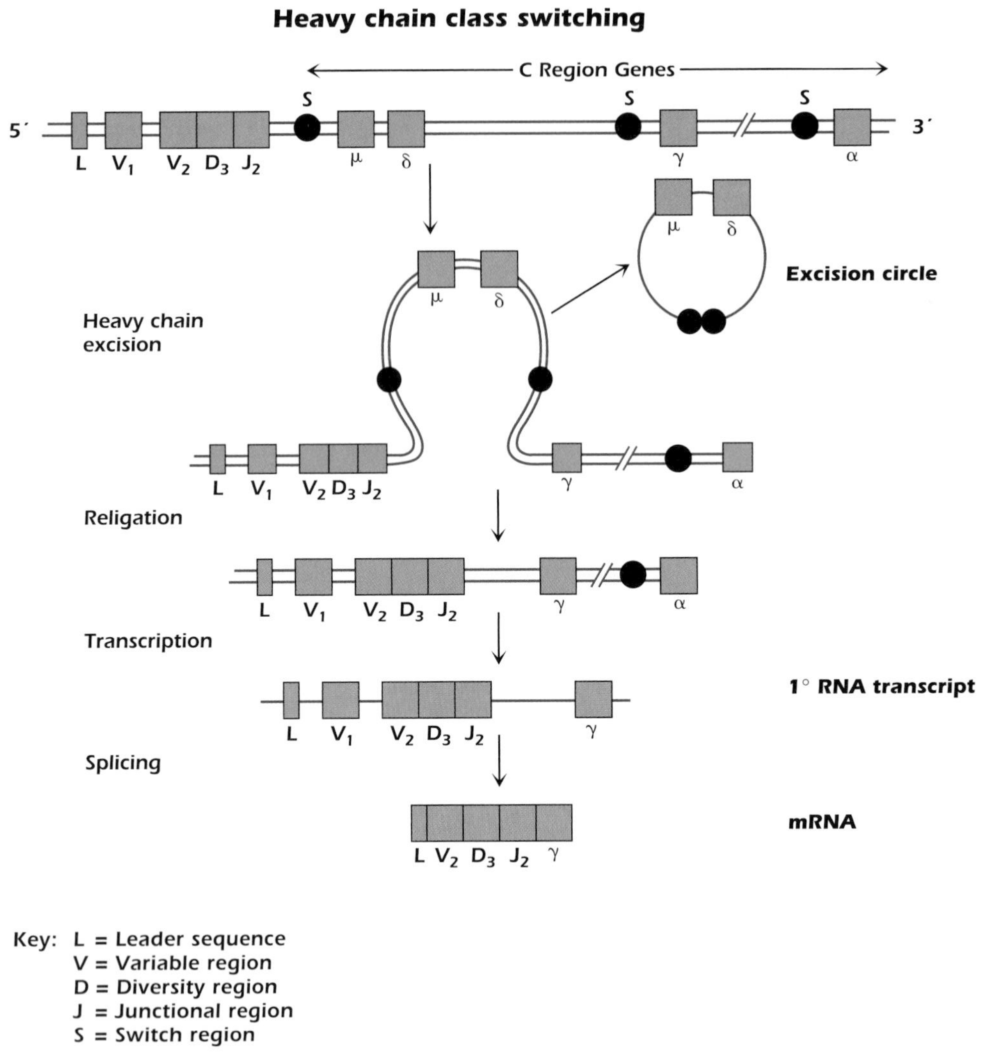

Heavy chain class switching

Key: L = Leader sequence
      V = Variable region
      D = Diversity region
      J = Junctional region
      S = Switch region

Figure 4.2. Mechanism of class switching in Ig synthesis; S = switch region, upstream of each heavy-chain constant region. Switching requires T cell interaction.

class of molecules capable of "RNA editing"; it may be essential to class switching because it is necessary to edit the RNA of a key switch molecule. Obviously the breaking and ligation of DNA involve a host of coordinated enzyme activities and enzymes, including an endonuclease necessary for genetic DNA breaks and DNA repair enzymes necessary to anneal such breaks. Interestingly, as opposed to the V-region genes, in which rearrangements not infrequently cause disruption of the gene and are therefore nonproductive, all isotype switch recombinations are successful, resulting in a productive immunoglobulin gene. This preserves the ongoing and effective immune response.

What signals the B cell to undergo isotype switching?

The T cells are the prime players providing the signals for isotype switching to the B cells. CD40 engagement on the surface of the B cell and signaling from T-cell-derived cytokines are required. The helper T cell, in response to its specific antigen and to costimulatory molecules presented by the B cell, up-regulates CD40L (CD154) on its surface and secretes cytokines (see the pathogenesis section below). Additional adhesion is achieved through LFA-1–ICAM-1, ICOS–B7, and CD30–CD30L interactions, the first molecule listed in the pair being on the T cells and the second on the B cells. This cognate interaction between the T and B cells ensures the specificity of the immune interaction by being antigen driven and by focusing the signals to the area of contact between the two cells. It is the specific cytokines received by the B cell which govern the heavy-chain isotype that is produced and these cytokines differ depending on the T helper subset responding. Viruses and many bacteria will activate T_H1 cells to secrete IFN-γ, stimulating isotype switching to IgG_{2a} and IgG_{2b} subclasses; helminths will stimulate T_H2 cells to produce IL-4, the main cytokine resulting in IgE, as well as IgG_1 production. T_H2 cells also *secrete transforming growth factor (TGF) β (resulting in IgG₂ᵦ and IgA switching) and IL-5 (causing IgA secretion). Thus the T cell has a central role in controlling the character of the antibody response.*

The "Purpose" of the Different Immunoglobulin Constant Regions

Whereas the variable region governs the antigen-binding properties of the immunoglobulin molecule, the constant region determines its biologic properties. This region is required for recruiting other cells via their Fc receptors, binding complement, and specifically transporting the immunoglobulin molecule via active transport mechanisms to other sites. Macrophages and neutrophils, the body's phagocytic cells, have Fc receptors for IgG_1 and IgG_3, whereas high-affinity FcRε are found on mast cells, basophils, and eosinophils, the cells containing mediators needed for response to parasitic infections. Complement, which may directly destroy pathogens or activate phagocytes, is bound most efficiently by IgM, IgG_3, and IgG_1. IgG_1 and IgG_3 cross the placenta and make their way into the fetal circulation. IgA is specifically and actively transported across the epithelial cell into mucous secretions, tears, and milk (Table 4.1).

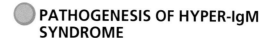

PATHOGENESIS OF HYPER-IgM SYNDROME

As its name implies, HIGM syndrome is defined by the fact that patients have B cells that produce IgM but not IgG, IgA, or IgE. Thus, they have a defect in class switch recombination. As is evident from the discussion above, class switch recombination is a multistep process and thus the HIGM syndrome could result from molecular defects affecting any of these steps. As shown in Figure 4.3, five distinct defects leading to the HIGM syndrome have so far been identified. Three of these defects (designated HIGM-I, III, and IV) affect the function of B cells, T cells, and APCs; two of these defects, HIGM-II and V, affect the function of B cells only. The most common form is X-linked HIGM, described in our patient, Lee.

Molecular Basis of XHIGM, HIGM-I Syndrome

An important clue to the molecular origin of the most prevalent form of hyper-IgM syndrome came from the discovery that class switch rearrangement is an antigen-driven process that occurs in germinal centers of lymphoid follicles. Thus, when it was discovered that interaction between CD40 on APCs and CD40L on T cells was necessary for

TABLE 4.1. Most Important Features of Immunoglobulin Isotopes

Characteristic	Isotype				
	IgG	IgA	IgM	IgD	IgE
Placental passage	++	—	—	—	—
Presence in secretion	—	++	—	—	—
Presence in milk	+	+	0 to trace	—	—
Activation of complement	+	—	+++	—	—
Binding to Fc receptors on macrophages, polymorphonuclear cells, and NK[a] cells	++	—	—	—	—
Relative agglutinating capacity	+	++	+++	—	—
Antiviral activity	+++	+++	+	—	—
Antibacterial activity (Gram negative)	+++	++ (with lysozyme)	+++ (with complement)	—	—
Antioxin activity	+++	—	—	—	—
Allergic activity	—	—	—	—	++

	IgG_1	IgG_2	IgG_3	IgG_4
Complement binding	+	+	+++	—
Placental passage	++	±	++	++
Binding of monocytes	+++	+	+++	±

[a] Natural killer.

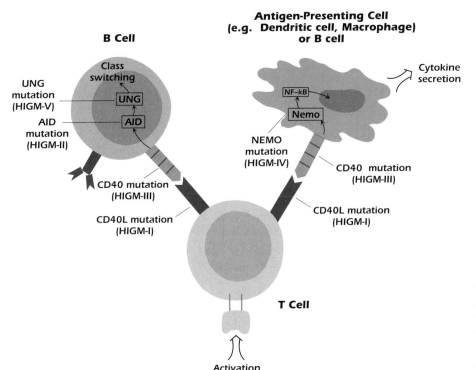

Figure 4.3. Defects in hyper-IgM syndromes. Some defects interfer with T-macrophage interaction as well as T-B interaction. Others interfere with mechanisms of class switching within the B cells.

germinal center formation, investigators considered the possibility that this interaction was important for class switch rearrangement and by extension was somehow involved in hyper-IgM syndrome. This suspicion was heightened by the fact that most patients with HIGM syndrome have lymphoid organs characterized by poorly developed germinal centers. It was ultimately shown that an X-linked form of hyper-IgM syndrome (XHIGM or HIGM-1), representing about 50% of all cases, is due to a mutation of the CD40L gene, resulting in nonexpression of CD40L or expression of a defective CD40L that cannot exert signaling function. Figure 4.4 shows a diagram of the CD40L molecule and the approximate locations in the molecule of mutations associated with XHIGM. Most of the mutations occur in the gene segment encoding the extracellular domain of the molecule and result in stop codons or base substitutions that cause loss of expression of CD40L on the cell surface or a CD40L molecule that cannot signal via CD40.

The CD40L molecule is a member of the TNF-α receptor family of molecules; its interaction with CD40 results in activation of important signaling pathways that affect the function of the CD40-expressing cells, B cells, and APCs, particularly dendritic cells. As noted above, CD40 signaling in the B cell is necessary for B-cell proliferation, germinal center formation, and class switch rearrangement. In dendritic cells, CD40 signaling is important in the production of key cytokines such as IL-12 and in the expression of costimulatory molecules such as CD80 and CD86. Thus, as shown in Figure 4.5, the consequences of a mutation of CD40L include not only the functional abnormalities in B cells that

are the hallmark of the disease, but also T-cell abnormalities due to defective interactions with APCs. The latter is illustrated in Figure 4.5C, which shows the sequential activation of T cells leading to expression of CD40L and the signaling of dendritic cells to produce IL-12. Both the B-cell and APC "defects" are actually secondary to the absence of signal from the real culprit, the T cell that lacks functional CD40L. The main immunologic consequence of the inadequate APC–T cell interaction is decreased IL-12 production, leading in turn to decreased production of IFN-γ by T cells. This explains why hyper-IgM patients with CD40L mutations (XHIGM patients) have increased susceptibility to infection with opportunistic organisms. With the advent of Ig replacement therapy, this defect in XHIGM patients is now the most significant clinical abnormality remaining and is one that explains their clinical course.

Interestingly, XHIGM patients with mutations in CD40L have IgM+/IgD+ B cells (unswitched B cells) that express CD27 (a maturation marker) and that exhibit evidence of some somatic hypermutation. These cells may have been generated in non–germinal center areas (e.g., marginal zones) as a result of other interactions, such as those involving OX40/OX40L, another TNF receptor family member. They can probably react with thymic independent (polysaccharide) antigens and thus provide patients some protection against disease. Along these lines, it also has been noted that a substantial fraction of patients produce IgA but not IgG. This may arise from class switching in certain types of B cells that does not require CD40L.

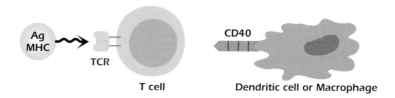

**CD40L Gene
Points of Mutation**

Exons or
Exon segments

Intracellular coding region

Transmembrane coding region

Extracellular coding region

Introns

Figure 4.4. Structure of CD40L (CD154) gene. Arrows denote positions of mutations.

A. T-cell activation

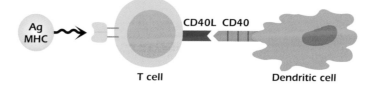

Ag
MHC

TCR

T cell

CD40

Dendritic cell or Macrophage

B. Expression of CD40L and interaction with CD40

Ag
MHC

CD40L   CD40

T cell

Dendritic cell

C. Induction of costimulation and cytokine secretion

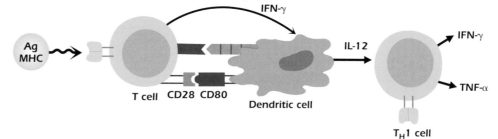

Ag
MHC

IFN-γ

IL-12

IFN-γ

TNF-α

T cell   CD28 CD80

Dendritic cell

T_H1 cell

Figure 4.5. Sequence of events in T cell-APC interaction through CD40-CD40L following antigen stimulation.

Other Forms of Hyper-IgM Syndrome

In recent years several other forms of hyper-IgM syndrome have been described; they are not due to a CD40L mutation, but like XHIGM they present as a defect in class switch recombination. As discussed below, some of these syndromes are characterized by considerably different clinical patterns than that found in XHIGM.

Hyper-IgM Syndrome due to CD40 Mutations: HIGM-III. Several patients with hyper-IgM syndrome

have been reported to have an autosomal recessive form of the disease in which various mutations in the CD40 gene lead to failure to express CD40 on the cell surface. Inasmuch as this abnormality leads to the same immunologic defects as seen in XHIGM (absence of CD40–CD40L interaction), it is not surprising that the clinical pattern found in these patients closely resembles that of XHIGM. This form of hyper-IgM syndrome which has been found in females (and can potentially occur in males as well) is classified as *HIGM-III*.

Hyper-IgM Syndrome Due to NEMO Mutations: HIGM-IV. Another form of HIGM syndrome is X linked but has a different molecular defect than XHIGM (HIGM-I). This is known as XHIGM-ED or HIGM-IV. It occurs in association with hypohydrotic ectodermal dysplasia (ED) and has been shown to be due to mutation in nuclear factor κB (NF-κB) essential modulator (NEMO). NF-κB is a master transcription factor controlling expression of numerous gene programs and functioning in different cell types. NEMO is a docking molecule for Iκκα and Iκκβ, two phosphorylases involved in the phosphorylation and degradation of IκBα and thus in the activation of NF-κB components; it is also involved in the translocation of these components to the nucleus. As shown in Figure 4.6, interaction of CD40L with CD40 leads to the activation of second messengers that interact with NEMO and initiate the activation and nuclear translocation of NF-κB components. Thus, a mutation in NEMO that results in impairment of its function leads to a defect in CD40L signaling and another form of the HIGM syndrome. It should be noted, however, that intact NEMO function is also necessary for the activation of NF-κB by numerous other cell stimulants, such as Toll-like receptors; this explains the fact that cells of patients with this form of HIGM display abnormal responses to these stimulants as well as CD40L.

The clinical features of this form of hyper-IgM syndrome are thus similar to those with XHIGM due to CD40L deficiency. However, given the ubiquitous nature of NF-κB and its interacting molecules, it is not unexpected that these patients have additional abnormalities. XHIGM-ED is associated with ectodermal dysplasia because the development and function of ectodermal tissue depend on another TNF family receptor that also depends on NEMO for signaling (the DL or ED receptor). The ectodermal abnormalities include inability to sweat (hypohydrosis), teeth malformations (hypodontia), and hairlessness. Susceptibility to infection is confined to high-grade extracellular pathogens rather than including opportunistic pathogens as well but is aggravated by the fact that the patients have thick secretions that impede elimination of organisms from the airways.

Hyper-IgM Due to Activation-Induced Cytidine Deaminase (AID) Mutations: HIGM-II. This fourth form of hyper-IgM syndrome, HIGM-II, which is inherited

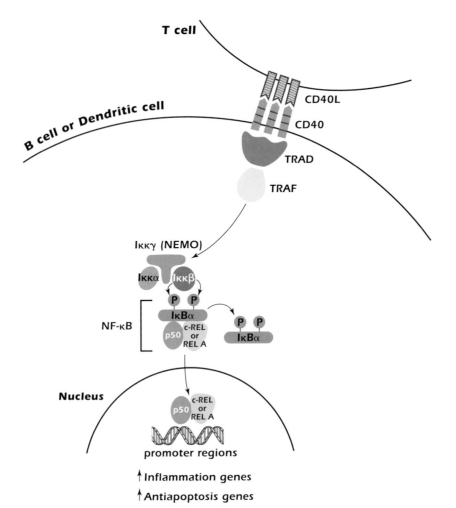

Figure 4.6. CD40L signaling at the cell surface leads to activation of NF-κB with subsequent translocation of its components to the nucleus. The initial step of NF-κB activation involves the interaction of TRAF with NEMO.

in an autosomal recessive manner, is caused by a mutation in the gene encoding AID, a molecule essential for both somatic hypermutation and class switching in B cells. As in the case of XHIGM-ED, these patients have normal CD40L and CD40 expression. Because somatic hypermutation is severely impaired in the absence of AID, the B cells of patients with HIGM–AID elaborate only low-affinity IgM antibodies.

Patients with this form of hyper-IgM syndrome differ from patients with other hyper-IgM syndromes in that they have a defect exclusive to their B cells. The CD40–CD40L interactions between T cells and macrophages and T cells and dendritic cells are intact; therefore these patients are not subject to opportunistic infection or other problems related to cell-mediated immunity. In this form of the syndrome, patients do manifest lymphoid hyperplasia and various autoimmune manifestations.

Hyper-IgM Syndrome Due to Uracil–DNA Glycosylase Mutations: HIGM-V. Yet another form of hyper-IgM syndrome has been identified and this one (HIGM-V) is due to mutations in a gene known as uracil–DNA glucosylase (UNG) This enzyme is expressed in activated B cells and operates downstream of AID during the class switch recombination: AID deaminates cytosine to form uracil and then the uracil is removed by UNG. The clinical picture in this hyper-IgM syndrome is similar to that seen due to AID deficiency.

TREATMENT OF HYPER-IgM SYNDROME

Replacement of IgG by IVIG administration is the main thrust of therapy and, indeed, has resulted in a marked decrease in infection in these patients. In some (but certainly not all) cases, this leads to normalization of elevated IgM levels and even correction of the neutropenia. Adjunctive therapy consists of treatment of the neutropenia with G-CSF, and prophylactic Bactrim therapy for the prevention of *Pneumocystis* pneumonia in XHIGM patients. Despite these therapies, many patients with XHIGM continue to experience opportunistic infections. Because of this, survival of these patients beyond the second decade has been less than 20%.

On a more fundamental level, several patients have been treated successfully with bone marrow transplantation, usually from a human leukocyte antigen (HLA)–matched sibling. In view of the poor prognosis of XHIGM patients, this therapy should probably be considered more frequently, especially when a matched donor is available.

REFERENCES

DiSanto JP, Bonnefoy JY, Gauchat JF, Fischer A, de Sain Basile G (1993): CD40 ligand mutations in x-linked immunodeficiency with hyper-IgM. *Nature* 11:41–43.

Ferrari S, Gillani S, Insalaco A, Al-Ghonalum A, Soresina AR, Loubser M, Avanzini MA, Marconi M, Badolato R, Ugazio AG, Levy Y, Catalan N, Durandy A, Tbakhi A, Notarangelo LD, Plebani A (2001): Mutations of CD40 gene cause an autosomal recessive form of immunodeficiency with hyper IgM. *Proc Natl Acad Sci USA* 98:12614–12619.

Imai K, Slupphaug G, Lee WI, Revy P, Nonoyama S, Catalan N, Yel L, Forvelle M, Kavil B, Krokan ME, Ochs HD, Fischer A, Durandy A (2003): Human uracil-DNA glycosylase deficiency associated with profoundly impaired immunoglobulin class-switch recombination. *Nature Immunol* 4:945–946.

Jain A, Atkinson TP, Lipsky PE, Slater JE, Nelson DL, Strober W (1999): Defects of T-cell effector function and post-thymic maturation in X-linked hyper-IgM syndrome. *J Clin Invest* 103:1151–1158.

Jain A, Ma CA, Liu S, Brown M, Cohen J, Strober W (2000): Specific missense mutations in NEMO result in hyper-IgM syndrome with hypohydrotic ectodermal dysplasia. *Nature Immunol* 2:223–228.

Muramatsu M, Kinosita K, Fagarasan S, Yamada S, Shinkai Y, Honjo T (2000): Class switch recombination and hypermutation require activation-induced cytidine deaminase (AID), a potential RNA editing enzyme. *Cell* 102:553–563.

Prasad ML, Velickovic M, Weston SA, Benson EM (2005): Mutational screening of the CD40 ligand (CD40L) gene in patients with X linked hyper-IgM syndrome (XHMI) and determination of carrier status in female relatives. *J Clin Pathol* 58:90–92.

Quartier P, Bustamamente J, Sanai O, Plebani A, Debre M, Deville A, Litzman J, Levy J, Fermand JP, Lane P, Horneff G, Aksu G, Yakin I, Davies G, Texcan I, Ersoy F, Catalan N, Imai K, Fischer A, Durandy A (2004): Clinical immunologic and genetic analysis of 29 patients with autosomal recessive hyper-IgM syndrome due to activation-induced cytidine deaminase deficiency. *Clin Immunol* 110:22–29.

Stavnezer J (1996): Immunoglobulin class switching. *Curr Opin Immunol* 8:199–205.

Tomizawa D, Imai K, Ito S, Kajiwara M, Minegishi Y, Nagasawa M, Morio T, Nonoyama S, Mizutani S (2004): Allogeneic hematopoietic stem cell transplantation for seven children with X-linked hyper-IgM syndrome: A single center experience. *Am J Hematol* 76:33–39.

Winkelstein JA, Marino MC, Ochs H, Fuleihan R, Scholl Pr, Geha R, Stiehm ER, Conley ME (2003): The X-linked hyper-IgM syndrome: Clinical and immunologic features of 79 patients. *Medicine* 82:373–384.

Zhu Y, Nonoyama S, Morio T, Muramatsu M, Honjo T, Mizutani S (2003): Type two hyper-IgM syndrome caused by mutation in activation-induced cytidine deaminase. *J Med Dent Sci* 50:41–46.

5

COMMON VARIABLE IMMUNODEFICIENCY DISEASE

WARREN STROBER

 CASE REPORT

" I have had low gammaglobulin levels since I was a child and now I have diarrhea all the time."

Clinical History and Initial Evaluation

Sandy is a 26-year-old woman who has been sent to you, an allergist/immunologist, by her internist because of steadily worsening gastrointestinal (GI) symptomatology. A pale, asthenic person, Sandy is obviously intelligent and articulate and is a lawyer with a large law firm. She carries a diagnosis of common variable immunodeficiency disease (CVID), and although her physicians have handled the immunodeficiency aspects of Sandy's illness well enough, both she and they seem confused about her steadily worsening GI symptoms over the last several years. You start with a detailed medical history and quickly peruse the extensive medical records she provides.

Sandy was the product of a normal pregnancy and delivery and was healthy until the age of two when she began experiencing recurrent episodes of lower respiratory infections that on several occasions proved to be X-ray-documented pneumonias. By age six, she had a chronic cough and sputum production that eventually led to a bronchoscopic exam and the diagnosis of **bronchiectasis** (destruction and widening of the large airways often caused by

recurrent inflammation or obstruction). This diagnosis and the recurrent pulmonary infections triggered evaluations for malformations of the bronchial tree, cystic fibrosis, α_1-antitrypsin deficiency, and asthma. These all proved negative or inconclusive. Over the next two years, Sandy's pulmonary symptoms gradually intensified. At age eight, she underwent a lobectomy of the right middle lobe to remove the most severely affected area; however, because bronchiectasis was present in other regions of the lung as well (albeit less severe), her pulmonary problems persisted. At about this time, Sandy's doctor thought her pulmonary problems might be due to an immunodeficiency state and he obtained serum immunoglobulin levels. These were as follows:

	Results	Reference Range
IgG	750 mg/dL	800–1800 mg/dL
IgM	100 mg/dL	70–280 mg/dL
IgA	36 mg/dL	90–450 mg/dL
IgE	<0.5 μg/dL	2.0–10.0 μg/dL

What are the abnormalities seen in the above results and how do these differ from what is expected in patients with X-linked agammaglobulinemia (XLA) and hyper-IgM (HIGM) syndrome (see Cases 1 and 4, respectively)?

Immunology: Clinical Case Studies and Disease Pathophysiology, By Warren Strober and Susan R. S. Gottesman

First, Sandy is now considerably older (eight–nine years) than when a workup was initiated in the patients with XLA or HIGM syndrome. Even though Sandy's workup was delayed for several years after she first came to medical attention, her presentation at age two was older than the usual age of presentation for the other two humoral immunodeficiency diseases. The onset of recurrent infections at age two, in contrast to earlier (six months to one year), suggests an immunodeficiency disorder acquired after birth rather than a congenital immunodeficiency, although at this young age the latter cannot be ruled out by history alone.

Second, with regard to the immunoglobulin levels, in XLA, there would be an absence of all immunoglobulin isotypes, documenting a global failure of immunoglobulin production including "natural antibodies" (IgM). In a patient with HIGM, the secondary isotypes would be missing (IgG and IgA). Although we will see that eventually Sandy's immunoglobulin profile will partially overlap with that seen in HIGM in that IgG will be decreased as well as IgA, in HIGM, IgM levels would likely be increased over normal. Both isolated IgA deficiency and common variable immunodeficiency affecting all immunoglobulin classes (IgG, IgA, and sometimes IgM) are "prime suspects" when a patient presents with a late-onset, seemingly acquired immunodeficiency state; Sandy's profile suggests one of these possibilities.

On the basis of this information, Sandy's doctor assumed she had either IgA deficiency (IgAD), the most common immunodeficiency state, or mild CVID and started her on intramuscular immunoglobulin (Ig) replacement therapy, the only form of replacement therapy available at that time. The pulmonary symptoms abated but did not disappear.

Why might you expect a deficiency in IgA to be associated with respiratory infections? At what other sites might infections occur?

IgA is the main immunoglobulin in mucosal secretions. It is actively transported across the epithelial surface from mucosal associated lymphoid tissue and plasma cells in the lamina propria. IgA is found in the lung, GI tract, urogenital tract, salivary and lacrimal glands, and the breast during lactation (see Table 4.1 for description of individual Ig isotypes). It is secreted as a dimer; the two monomeric units (each consisting of two heavy chains and two light chains) are joined to each other and to the J chain by disulfide bonds end to end (Fig. 5.1). The J chain is a 15-kDa polypeptide chain that also functions to polymerize IgM molecules. IgA picks up a secretory component in the epithelial cell as it is actively transported across the cell to its luminal surface. On the surface, IgA prevents bacteria and toxins from gaining access to the epithelial cells. Thus, without IgA, one would expect infections in the respiratory tract and other mucosal sites. In reality, as discussed below, most patients with isolated IgAD are asymptomatic. The redundancy of our protective systems, both nonspecific barrier mechanisms

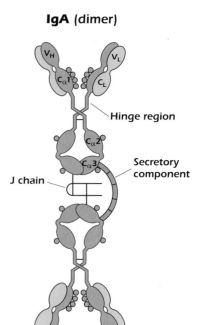

IgA (dimer)

🔵 Figure 5.1. Structure of IgA. Light chains are shown in green; heavy chains are shown in blue. Orange circles denote areas of glycosylation. The dimeric IgA molecule contains a polypeptide known as the J chain. Its secretory component is shown in red.

such as mucous secretion and ciliated epithelium and the compensatory presence of other immunoglobulins such as IgM and IgG, may explain the lack of symptoms.

On the other hand, Sandy is and has been symptomatic. Her unfortunate history is the result of the long delay in diagnosing her immunodeficiency in spite of severe recurrent infections, leading to the delay in initiating effective Ig replacement therapy. Recurrent lower respiratory infections (pneumonia) in a child are never normal and always require a search for a possible immunodeficiency, although most patients with CVID do not present as young as Sandy (see below). In Sandy's case, the low IgA level was accompanied by a borderline low IgG level, which lent credence to the presence of an immunodeficiency disorder. Isolated IgAD is sometimes associated with a decrease in one of the IgG subclasses (especially IgG$_2$), which could lead to a mildly decreased, but not frankly abnormal, overall IgG level. Alternatively, the low IgG level could presage the development of frank IgG deficiency involving all IgG subclasses and resulting in the presence of panhypogammaglobulinemia characteristic of CVID. Most cases of CVID present initially with panhypogammaglobulinemia rather than an initial deficiency involving mainly IgA.

Why does Ig replacement therapy replace IgG and not IgA? Did the discovery of isolated IgA deficiency associated with only a borderline low IgG level justify placing Sandy on Ig replacement therapy?

Ig replacement therapy would not provide enough IgA to even partially correct the deficiency and, if given, the IgA would not arrive at the effective location, the mucosal surface. In addition, the IgA could even elicit an allergic reaction in the patient, since it might be recognized by the immune system as a foreign antigen. Treatment of isolated IgAD is therefore limited to treatment of infections after they occur. For Sandy, Ig replacement therapy was advisable because her IgG level was borderline low and she was experiencing destructive pulmonary infections. In this situation this therapy was worth trying based on the chance that the low IgG levels were a significant factor in causing the disease. Nevertheless, it would have been useful to test Sandy's capacity to produce antibodies to both protein and polysaccharide antigens and thus try to verify that a humoral immune defect in the IgG response existed, even though her overall IgG level was at that time relatively normal. This could have been accomplished by subcutaneous administration of polyvalent pneumococcal vaccine and diphtheria toxoid followed by measurement of IgG antibody responses to these antigens at two and four weeks.

You read on through her history to learn that about one year after Sandy was started on intramuscular gammaglobulin replacement her doctor repeated her serum Ig studies. He conducted these tests just before administering the next dose when the level of exogenous (administered) gammaglobulin would be at its lowest (trough level). The results were as follows:

	Results	Reference Range
IgG	352 mg/dL	800–1800 mg/dL
IgM	90 mg/dL	70–250 mg/dL
IgA	11 mg/dL	90–450 mg/dL

Sandy's IgG level was now clearly below reference range and indicated that her condition had evolved into full-blown hypogammaglobulinemia. Thus Sandy probably had CVID rather than just isolated IgAD. At about that time, preparations of gammaglobulin became available that could be given by intravenous infusion. Intravenous immunoglobulin (IVIG) replacement therapy is easier to administer than intramuscular therapy and, more importantly, achieves a higher concentration of circulating IgG. Sandy's therapy was changed to monthly infusions of IVIG, which she has been on ever since.

After this therapeutic change, Sandy had milder pulmonary symptoms and felt generally better. Nevertheless, chronic sputum production continued, reflecting ongoing damage to her bronchi. A pulmonologist recommended a strict regimen of twice-daily postural drainage to clear out as much of the pulmonary secretions as possible. Sandy has followed this regimen to the letter and has been able to avoid further episodes of pneumonia and prevent green (pus-like) sputum production, which is indicative of low-grade chronic bronchial infection.

During her teenage years Sandy experienced normal pubertal changes and was moderately active. Perhaps her biggest complaint during this period was that she had some difficulty maintaining an ideal weight. In her final year of college, at the age of 21, she noted increased frequency of bowel movements, which consisted of soft or poorly formed stools. Sandy's doctor assumed that this was due to an infection. He had her stools cultured on a number of occasions and examined for ova and parasites; however, all studies proved negative.

Over the last two years, Sandy's GI symptoms have intensified so that she currently has multiple bowel movements each day and her stools are abnormally greasy and foul smelling. This has been associated with a mild (5 lb) weight loss despite a conscious effort to eat a sufficient amount to maintain weight. It is this complex of symptoms that has led to her visit to you.

Workup for Confirmation of Diagnosis

As an initial step in her workup you perform a series of immunologic tests to verify the diagnosis of CVID and to better define the type and severity of the immunologic abnormality, since CVID, as its name implies, is a highly variable disease. Ordinarily some of these tests would have been performed earlier, perhaps at the time of initial diagnosis.

What is CVID and how does one arrive at this diagnosis?

*CVID and the closely related disease, isolated IgAD, was originally a "catch-all" immunodeficiency category for a large group of patients that had in common a humoral defect of the immune system characterized by a reduced ability to produce immunoglobulins. It was alternatively referred to as **acquired agammaglobulinemia** because in virtually all cases the disease was not evident at birth and became apparent (was "acquired") later, most often in the second to third decade, usually in the absence of a known precipitating factor. For years it was suspected that CVID was not a single disease entity, but rather a group of genetically diverse diseases with different pathophysiologies that had a common clinical and immunologic profile. Recently, this suspicion has been validated by the discovery of a number of genetic defects that have defined different groups of patients.*

CVID and IgAD together account for the majority of patients with primary immunodeficiency. The incidence of IgAD is actually much higher than CVID; IgAD occurs in 1 in 300–1,300 people in various populations, and the incidence of CVID is 1 in 50,000–200,000. Most patients with IgAD are totally asymptomatic, and thus the incidence of symptomatic patients in the two syndromes is similar and equal to that of CVID (which is almost always symptomatic). Given that CVID patients sometimes have relatives with IgAD and that IgAD sometimes evolves into CVID, it is best to consider these diseases as genetically and mechanistically related; IgAD can be thought of as an incomplete form of CVID.

The diagnosis of CVID can be established in any individual over one year of age in whom the total IgG level is more than two standard deviations below the mean level in the normal population (or below 250 mg/dL). Decreases of similar magnitude in IgM and IgA levels should also be present; if not, other diseases must be considered. In IgAD, only the IgA level is similarly decreased. In patients who show lesser decreases in IgG (in the 300–600-mg/dL range), CVID can be suspected but not proven. When this occurs, one is likely to be dealing with an IgG subclass deficiency that frequently occurs in association with IgA deficiency. The clinical significance of an IgG subclass deficiency in the absence of IgA deficiency is not always clear, because lack of antibody responses in one subclass can be compensated for by responses in another subclass. In this situation one must test the patient's ability to mount responses to standard antigens such as tetanus toxoid or pneumococcal polysaccharide to determine if an immunodeficiency is present.

Sandy's previous immunoglobulin profile at age eight to nine years fulfilled the criteria for CVID. Identification of her specific defect requires further study, since an inability to produce immunoglobulin may be caused by different underlying pathologies.

Lymphocyte Phenotype Profile. A lymphocyte profile was obtained by flow cytometric analysis of peripheral cells stained with antibodies that delineate cell subsets (see Unit V for assay description).

Result

T cells. mildly reduced numbers of T cells associated with a normal CD4/CD8 T-cell ratio.

B cells. normal numbers of B cells but greatly reduced numbers of $CD27^+/IgD^-$ B cells.

How do these results correlate with Sandy's serum immunoglobulin levels? What is the significance of the reduced number of $CD27^+/IgD^-$ B cells?

Sandy was previously noted to have a defect in IgA and IgG levels, immunoglobulin isotypes produced by $CD27^+/IgD^-$ B cells. This is the expected phenotype of memory B cells, cells that have undergone maturation and been exposed to

antigen. CD27 is a cell surface molecule expressed on B cells after antigen contact, presumably in the germinal center, in a T-dependent fashion. Its ligand, CD70, is a tumor necrosis factor (TNF) receptor (R) family molecule expressed on T cells. In the germinal center, the stimulated B cells undergo somatic mutation of their immunoglobulin V region genes and some isotype switch to IgG or IgA (see Case 4). The progeny become plasma cells or memory cells, both of which leave the germinal center. One therefore expects the $CD27^+$ B cells in the peripheral blood to have mutated V-region genes, which in fact they do.

While most patients with CVID have normal numbers of B cells, some may have mildly or greatly reduced numbers. Only rarely does one find a patient with absent B cells, as occurs in XLA. Since Sandy maintains some ability to produce at least IgM, you would not expect absence of B cells in her. CVID B cells, even when normal in number, may contain reduced numbers of $CD27^+$ cells (i.e., increased numbers of $CD27^-/IgD^+$ cells). In humans, peripheral blood B cells are normally comprised of approximately 60% $IgM^+IgD^+/CD27^-$ (naive with unmutated V genes), 15% IgG^+ or $IgA^+/CD27^+$, and 25% $IgM^+/CD27^+$ cells. The latter two groups of cells have mutated V-region genes and, upon reexposure to antigen in vitro, will respond rapidly with immunoglobulin production but will not undergo further isotype switching. The absence or decreased number of B cells with a memory phenotype, particularly of the IgM^-IgD^- phenotype, correlates with the low level of production of IgG and IgA. This indicates that the cells have not undergone normal Ig class switching (see section on normal B cell stimulation and function in Case 4). A decrease of all memory B cells is not unexpected in patients who are panhypogammaglobulinemic.

Normal T-cell numbers and ratios are found in the majority of CVID patients, although there are subgroups with numerical T-cell alterations, one with high CD8 levels and low CD4/CD8 T-cell ratios and another with CD4 lymphopenia, particularly affecting the $CD45RA^+$ (naive) T-cell subset. Finally, the subset of patients with GI disease, such as Sandy, have somewhat reduced numbers of T cells, affecting both the CD4 and CD8 subsets, and reduced numbers of $CD18/CD56^+$ natural killer (NK) cells.

In Vitro T- and B-Cell Responses. Sandy's peripheral mononuclear cells were separated into T- and B-cell subsets and stimulated *in vitro* to determine their capacity to produce cytokines and Ig, respectively.

T-Cell Response. When stimulated with the T-cell mitogen concanavalin A or anti-CD3/anti-CD28, Sandy's T cells exhibited normal proliferative responses and produced normal amounts of interleukin-2 (IL-2) and interferon-γ (IFN-γ) in comparison to control T cells.

B-Cell Response. While her B cells exhibited normal proliferative responses to the B-cell mitogen *Staphylococcus aureus* Cowen's I and to another B-cell mitogen (anti-IgM), they produced greatly reduced amounts of IgG and IgA and somewhat reduced amounts of IgM when stimulated with these mitogens, again as compared to control cells. Furthermore, Sandy's B cells failed to produce normal amounts of IgG when cultured with normal T cells stimulated with anti-CD3/anti-CD28; control B cells did produce normal amounts of IgG when cultured with Sandy's T cells under these conditions.

These results suggest that the abnormality lies in Sandy's B cells.

As indicated earlier, CVID is actually a group of diseases having in common a reduced ability to produce Ig. It is not surprising, therefore, that their *in vitro* T- and B-cell responses are variable and that classification of patients with CVID is still in flux, reflecting the heterogeneous nature of this disease category. In most patients with CVID, the B cells fail to produce IgG and IgA, even when cocultured with normal T cells. (IgM responses are usually reduced as well, but not to the same extent as IgG and IgA responses.) This is usually due to a true B-cell abnormality rather than a failure of T cells to act as effective helper cells and was shown to be the case in the study of Sandy's cells. T cells from normal individuals do not facilitate Ig production by Sandy's B cells, but Sandy's T cells do facilitate Ig production from normal B cells.

While most patients exhibit normal T-cell proliferative and cytokine responses, some do manifest decreased T-cell responses. This is particularly true of patients who have granulomatous nodules in various tissues (a sarcoid-like picture). In addition, some CVID patients have T cells with increased suppressor function, which is demonstrated in *in vitro* studies by their capacity to suppress Ig production by normal cells. A subset of patients with CVID have autoimmune syndromes such as autoimmune cytopenias (decreased peripheral blood counts). Even in most of the cases with T-cell abnormalities, the CVID patient's B cells still manifest an intrinsic defect in Ig production when they are separated from their T cells. The primary defect thus still resides in the B cells.

How do these studies of Sandy's cells help you define her immunodeficiency?

The major outcome of the studies of Sandy's cells is that while she has adequate numbers of B cells, her B cells do not function normally to produce Ig. The fact that B cells are present rules strongly against the diagnosis of XLA [Bruton's agammaglobulinemia (BTK) deficiency], a disease characterized by a profound absence of B cells. Those CVID patients who manifest numerical B-cell deficiency must be distinguished from XLA by sequencing studies of the BTK gene and by family history demonstrating a lack of X-linked inheritance. The immunologic studies also show that Sandy's B cells are defective in IgM production and that her T cells "help" normal B cells produce Ig in vitro. These findings rule against a diagnosis of HIGM syndrome (usually X-linked HIGM syndrome), in which IgM

production is normal or increased and the T cells cannot help normal B cells because they do not express normal amounts of CD40L. The possibility of HIGM syndrome based on a CD40 defect (a non-X-linked HIGM III) must be considered as the results of in vitro functional studies for the latter would be similar to CVID. This is easily done by staining for CD40 on the B-cell surface using anti-CD40 antibody and flow cytometric analysis.

Dealing with Sandy's Clinical Manifestations of CVID

Having defined Sandy's immunologic defect and confirmed that she really does have CVID, you now initiate an investigation of her GI function in consultation with a gastroenterologist so that you can better manage her disease. GI symptomatology is her major current clinical problem, her pulmonary complications being well controlled.

Initial studies reveal that Sandy has a mild microcytic anemia (**microcytic:** small cells; **anemia:** decreased hemoglobin- or oxygen-carrying capacity). This is probably due to iron deficiency, as suggested by her reduced serum iron level. Her albumin level is moderately reduced to 3.0 gm/dL, but her liver function tests are within normal limits (the liver produces albumin). Sandy's serum calcium is at the lower limit of normal and a bone density study shows mildly decreased density.

GI workup discloses reduced D-xylose absorption and moderately increased fat excretion in the stools, conclusive evidence that Sandy has malabsorption. This probably explains the low serum iron and mild iron deficiency anemia as well as the calcium/bone problem. An α_1-antitrypsin excretion test reveals mild loss of albumin into the stool, confirming the presence of protein-losing enteropathy as the cause of the low serum albumin. However, a breath hydrogen excretion test is normal, indicating absence of small bowel bacterial overgrowth. In addition, comprehensive cultures of stools for pathogenic bacteria or parasites are negative. These results prompt the performance of a small bowel biopsy of the duodenum via upper GI endoscopy. The duodenum shows partial villous atrophy (villous blunting) and intestinal nodular lymphoid hyperplasia. The lamina propria is infiltrated with lymphoid cells and has increased numbers of intraepithelial lymphocytes. These findings are reminiscent of the changes found in celiac disease; however, it differs from the latter in that there is no B-cell infiltrate and the intestinal epithelium is hypoplastic rather than hyperplastic. This is, in fact, the typical histologic picture found in CVID patients with a complicating autoimmune syndrome affecting the GI tract.

Unfortunately, this CVID-associated GI syndrome is not easily treated and can progress to a point where the patient requires parenteral nutrition to maintain body weight. High-dose steroid therapy can be effective but is risky in a patient who already has immunodeficiency. Ultimately, agents that block the proinflammatory cytokines underlying this inflammation may become available, but for now the patient can only be given supportive medications.

After a frank discussion with Sandy, you elect to treat her conservatively with measures that address the malabsorption (the iron and calcium deficiencies) and with close follow-up to make certain she maintains adequate nutrition. She of course continues her program of monthly IVIG and postural drainage to prevent pulmonary complications and leaves your office optimistic that she can likewise deal with her GI symptoms now that the underlying cause is understood.

 ## CLINICAL ASPECTS OF CVID

Infections

The major clinical feature of CVID is recurrent infections, particularly of the upper and lower airways. For the most part, these are due to "high-grade" pathogens, pathogens that are capable of causing infections in immunocompetent hosts such as the extracellular bacterial organisms *Haemophilus influenza* and *Streptococcus pneumoniae*. These are to be distinguished from the low-grade or opportunistic pathogens, which are usually intracellular, that cause disease only in hosts with severe T-cell defects. This is not surprising, since CVID is characterized mainly by loss of humoral immunity, the arm of the immune response responsible for the clearance and killing of extracellular invaders via complement-mediated lysis (IgM), opsonization and phagocytosis (IgG), or prevention of binding to epithelial cells (IgA).

Of the types of infections to which patients with CVID are prone, those involving the lower airways are usually the most important. Initially, they take the form of recurrent discrete episodes of pneumonia but later manifest as chronic colonization of the large airways and bronchiectasis. Such infections result in pulmonary insufficiency and its sequelae, including right heart failure. Patients in this advanced state are now susceptible to infection with a larger group of organisms, such as *Pseudomonas aeruginosa*, and have structural lung disease that cannot be reversed. Early treatment with IVIG replacement therapy can prevent this outcome and provides a strong argument for institution of this therapy in cases of newly diagnosed CVID prior to lung damage.

Now that IVIG therapy has provided some control of infection with high-grade pathogens, it has become apparent that some CVID patients are also subject to infection with opportunistic organisms. This reflects the fact that CVID is associated with defects in T-cell function, a concept discussed in greater detail below. Infections of this type

include those due to protozoal organisms such as *Pneumocystis jiroveci* and *Giardia lamblia;* fungal organisms such as *Candida albicans*, cryptococci, and nocardia; bacteria such as mycoplasma and mycobacteria; and, finally, various viral organisms. A particularly unfortunate example of the latter is enteroviral infection of the central nervous system (CNS), usually by echovirus type II. This infection leads to chronic meningoencephalitis resulting in progressive loss of mental and neurologic function and, not infrequently, death. It may also be accompanied by a dermatomyositis-like skin disease and hepatitis. This syndrome also occurs in XLA and appears to result from the fact that, in the absence of circulating antibodies, viral organisms usually confined to the GI tract may gain access to the circulation and the CNS.

Infection of the GI tract, the second most common site in CVID, takes several forms. Perhaps the most common is infection with *G. lamblia*, an organism that can infect and cause self-limited disease in normal individuals, usually following exposure to an infected water supply. In CVID patients, it manifests as a spontaneously occurring and then persistent and/or recurrent diarrheal disease. Treatment of this infection in CVID may require various combination antibiotic therapies. Other GI infections include those due to "conventional" GI pathogens, such as *Salmonella* and *Shigella* organisms, as well as unusual organisms such as "dysgonic fermentor-3," a gram-negative bacterium. Although IVIG therapy has decreased GI infections in CVID, these infections, particularly those due to *G. lamblia*, still occur at a higher than normal frequency. This may again reflect the presence of T-cell abnormalities that cannot be corrected by IVIG therapy.

Autoimmunity

CVID is almost as much a disease of immune dysregulation as it is a disease of immunodeficiency. Several pathophysiologic factors probably contribute to this. First, for reasons that are as yet unknown, because CVID and IgAD are strongly associated with a histocompatibility locus antigen (HLA) haplotype frequently found in patients with frank autoimmune disease, genes that predispose to CVID also predispose to autoimmunity (see the introduction to Unit III, Autoimmune Disorders). Second, both CVID and IgAD patients lack a competent mucosal immune system and therefore would fail to exclude many environmental antigens from the body that may cross-react with self-antigens and thus induce autoimmunity. Third, as already discussed, CVID is associated with T-cell abnormalities, which may include loss of suppressor mechanisms that normally prevent autoimmunity.

In addition to autoimmunity involving the GI tract (discussed below), the most common forms of autoimmunity in CVID are autoimmune hemolytic anemia, autoimmune neutropenia, and idiopathic thrombocytopenia, collectively referred to as autoimmune cytopenias. As in patients without CVID, these are due to autoantibodies to the blood elements. Although it seems paradoxical that a severe defect in the ability to mount antibody responses is associated in some instances with production of pathologic autoantibodies, recall that CVID patients invariably retain the ability to produce low but significant amounts of IgG antibodies (100–300 mg/dL). Thus, in some patients, the retained capacity to differentiate B cells may be subverted to the production of pathologic antibodies. As mentioned previously, the usual therapy for these forms of autoimmunity is steroids. In CVID patients, however, steroid therapy can exacerbate the immunodeficiency and lead to overwhelming infection.

The GI syndrome in CVID (and in IgAD) is marked by severe, persistent diarrhea, malabsorption leading to progressive weight loss and vitamin deficiency, and protein-losing enteropathy resulting in hypoalbuminemia, edema, and inability to maintain adequate Ig levels following IVIG administration. The latter is due to loss of administered Ig into the GI tract. Pathologically, this syndrome is associated with and/or due to moderate to severe intestinal villi blunting, increased numbers of intraepithelial lymphocytes, and epithelial cell apoptosis. In addition, many patients exhibit a pathology that is more or less unique to CVID among the immunodeficiency states, known as *intestinal nodular lymphoid hyperplasia*. These are collections of lymphocytes throughout the GI tract large enough to be appreciated both on radiographic examinations and endoscopy. These collections are comprised of surface IgM-bearing B cells surrounded by T cells, most of which are CD8$^+$ T cells.

In a recent study GI mucosal inflammation was shown to be present in many CVID patients without GI symptoms, although it was less severe than the degree of inflammation seen in those with frank malabsorption. In symptomatic patients, inflammation extends to the colon as well as involving the small bowel. Thus, GI disease emerges as a major complication of CVID.

Superficially, the villous atrophy of CVID resembles celiac disease or gluten-sensitive enteropathy (GSE) and for a period was thought to be due to gluten sensitivity. These patients do not respond to a gluten-free diet or any other elimination diet, and closer examination of the GI lesion reveals subtle differences from GSE, such as the presence of a hypoplastic rather than a hyperplastic crypt epithelium. In CVID, this GI syndrome was thought to be due to either bacterial overgrowth of the normal intestinal flora or to cryptic infection with an as-yet unidentified organism. Several factors suggest otherwise. First, a similar syndrome does not occur in XLA, an immunodeficiency characterized by an equally if not more severe antibody deficiency, but one lacking T-cell abnormalities; thus, the GI disease is associated with and probably due to a T-cell defect of some kind. Second, the GI abnormalities usually

occur in association with other evidence of T-cell dysfunction. Third, and most importantly, the GI abnormalities have not been tied to any particular infection, and bacterial overgrowth, when present, is very mild; in fact, patients without structural changes to the intestinal mucosa do respond to steroid therapy, a treatment that could worsen an infection. Taken together, these factors suggest that the GI syndrome in CVID results from an autoimmune attack on the villous epithelial cells, one most likely mediated by autoreactive T cells. This is consonant with a recent study of T cells in CVID, in which it was shown that the T cells of the lamina propria secrete IFN-γ, a cytokine known to cause epithelial cell death when produced in excess. On the other hand, these T cells do not produce IL-23, a proinflammatory cytokine produced by T cells in Crohn's disease (see Case 18).

In addition to the characteristic malabsorption syndrome, patients with CVID may manifest other GI abnormalities, including gastric atrophy and pernicious anemia, and, very occasionally, bowel syndromes resembling ulcerative colitis or Crohn's disease. Whether these are also forms of autoimmune GI disease in CVID remains unknown.

Lymphoproliferative Disorders, Lymphoma, and Carcinoma

CVID is similar to other immunodeficiency states in that patients are at increased risk for the development of tumors, particularly B-cell lymphomas and carcinomas. One possible explanation is that the patients have T-cell abnormalities that lead to faulty "immune surveillance" and thus defective immune elimination of malignant cells. Another possibility is that the chronic infections increase the chance of sequential gene mutations necessary for the development of neoplasia. This latter hypothesis is suggested by the fact that about 30% of patients manifest nonmalignant lymphoproliferation leading to splenomegaly, diffuse lymphadenopathy, or both. The clinical observation that the lymphoproliferation is sometimes transient suggests that it may be due to viral infection. Also relevant to the issue of chronic infection in CVID is that patients frequently exhibit diffuse infiltration of organs with persistent noncaseating (sarcoid-like) granulomata of undefined origin.

● NORMAL MEMORY B-CELL FORMATION

In the preceding chapters, we have been able to correlate the clinical presentation and laboratory results of the deficiency we are studying with one or a few molecular defects and therefore identify a specific block in the development, differentiation, or function of B cells. These have provided insight into the requirements for normal functioning of the humoral immune system. CVID is more difficult to use as a model for learning the mechanisms of normal function for several reasons. First, CVID is not a single disease entity; second, for many patients, the particular underlying defect is unknown, and, third, for some, environmental factors may also influence the onset and progression of the disease. Keeping in mind that the universal defect in CVID patients is a reduced capability to produce Ig (particularly of the secondary isotypes), any discussion of the pathogenesis of CVID will necessitate a review of the steps required to induce a B cell to produce antibody and form memory cells. On careful analysis of patients and with the information gathered from mouse models, the mechanism of memory B-cell formation is gradually being elucidated and will serve as our basis for understanding the pathogenesis and even the variability of this disease.

Immature (IgM$^+$IgD$^+$) B cells released from the bone marrow that undergo maturation to mature naive (naive with respect to antigen exposure) B cells change from CD19$^+$CD21$^-$CD27$^-$ cells to CD19$^+$CD21$^+$CD27$^-$/IgM$^+$ IgD$^+$ cells. In addition, these naive B cells [as well as antigen-presenting cells (APCs)] constitutively express a surface molecule, ***inducible costimulator molecule–ligand*** **(ICOS-L)**. ICOS-L serves as a ligand for a costimulatory molecule, ***ICOS***, whose expression is induced on the surface of activated T cells (Fig. 5.2). Thus, when T cells are stimulated by APCs with antigen via the T-cell antigen receptors (TCRs) and several costimulatory molecules to become effector T cells, they are also costimulated via the ICOS-L–ICOS interaction. This is relevant to the B-cell defect in CVID because costimulation via ICOS has the effect of inducing T$_H$2 T cells, a subset of T helper cells that is critical to the support of the humoral immune response. In particular, ICOS signaling turns on transcription of cytokines, IL-4, IL-5, IL-6, IFN-γ, and, most importantly, IL-10, all of which are necessary for

the terminal differentiation of B cells to memory cells and plasma cells (Fig. 5.2). As would be predicted, ICOS expression can be detected on T helper cells located in the apical light zone of the germinal center (follicular helper T cells), the site of T-cell dependent antibody production.

The naive B cell must transverse several steps to become a memory cell or plasma cell. Receiving cytokine signals from the T$_H$2 cell as described above is just one of the requirements and is in fact a late occurrence. First, the naive B cell in the circulation traffics through the lymph nodes and the lymph node follicles in search of its specific antigen. It is attracted there by chemokines secreted from activated follicular dendritic cells, which also attract T cells. In the follicle, the B cell will survive for only a limited time unless stimulated by antigen. When the naive B cell enters the follicle, a survival signal is also provided by ***B-cell activation factor of TNF family (BAFF)*** through its specific receptor on the B cell, BAFF-R, a TNF receptor superfamily member (Fig. 5.3). BAFF-R signaling is required for mature follicular B-cell survival and for the differentiation of marginal zone B cells in mice, but it may have a less stringent role in humans (also see Cases 24 and 25).

Upon finding its specific antigen, the B cell receives a signal via its antigen-specific receptor (BCR), with the invariant Ig chains Igα and Igβ transmitting the intracellular signal (see Case 1). A coreceptor complex consisting of CD19, CD21, CD81, and CD225 on the B-cell membrane is brought into close proximity to the BCR when CD21 binds to complement component C3d (Fig. 5.4). This can occur when C3d is bound to the antigen (e.g., a microbe). CD21 binding initiates signaling into the cell via CD19, a molecule with a long intracytoplasmic tail. CD19 increases the phosphorylation of the Ig-invariant chains, enhancing their signaling.

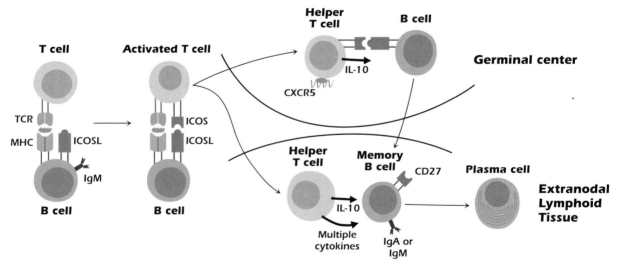

Figure 5.2.   Interaction of T cells and naive B cells leading to B-cell terminal differentiation.

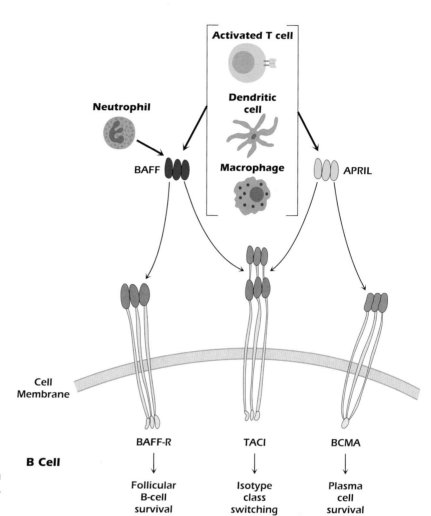

Figure 5.3. Signaling of B cells through specific surface receptors activate differentiation and survival pathways.

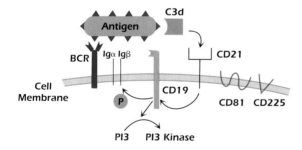

Figure 5.4. B-cell receptor signaling complex.

This enhancement of signal by the coreceptor complex also serves to link the innate immune system (direct complement component binding to organisms) with the adaptive humoral immune system. Of particular importance is the role of CD19 in the activation of phosphatidylinositol-3 (PI3) kinase, a signaling component that is essential, at least in mice, for germinal center B-cell development that also plays a role in human follicular center cell antibody response.

BAFF and an additional chemokine, *a proliferation-inducing ligand (APRIL)*, also signal the B cell through two other TNF-R family members, *transmembrane activator and calcium-modulating cyclophilin ligand interactor (TACI)* and *B-cell maturation antigen (BCMA)*. TACI and BCMA function in later stages of B-cell differentiation and activation (Fig. 5.3). BAFF is produced by neutrophils, and BAFF and APRIL are both produced by activated T cells, dendritic cells, and macrophages in the follicle and bone marrow. TACI signaling of the B cell is required for isotype class switching [along with IL-10 or transforming growth factor β (TGF-β)], to IgA and IgG isotypes and may help induce expression of activation-induced cytidine deaminase (AID), an enzyme required for somatic hypermutation that also plays a role in class switching (see Case 4). BCMA signaling is required for survival of long-lived plasma cells.

Thus the B cell, in the environment of the germinal center, receives numerous coordinated signals/cytokines from antigen, complement components, dendritic cells, T cells, macrophages, and even myeloid cells. Some are unique, but many have redundancy. As a consequence, the B cell survives, undergoes somatic hypermutation of its immunoglobulin V-region genes, may isotype class switch, and form a memory or plasma cell before finally leaving the germinal center.

 ## PATHOGENESIS OF CVID AND IgAD

Although the diagnosis of CVID is based on serum Ig levels, the reality is that different underlying pathophysiologies can result in the "CVID phenotype" and its variants. Classification schemes of CVID patients have been proposed based on the peripheral blood lymphocyte subsets; these groupings have correlated loosely with some of the clinical presentations detailed above and the results of the immunologic studies (see below). A closer look allows the detection of additional functional abnormalities and identification of the cellular abnormalities represented in a portion of these patients.

In recent years, molecular analysis has identified several genetic mutations in receptor molecules as the underlying cause of disease in individual families with CVID. In some instances these may be correlated with the cellular abnormalities which have been elucidated and which correspond to what we know about the role of these molecules in the generation of the memory B-cell response and Ig production. The variability in the severity of the disease and in its temporal and clinical manifestations may stem from the fact that some of the mutations occur in costimulatory molecules and thus in stimuli whose importance to the B cell response is not absolute. Coreceptors serve to lower the threshold for activation and may be functionally redundant. Alternatively they may modify only a particular type of response such as the IgA or IgE response. Finally their effects may occur only under certain circumstances such as differing environmental conditions. Thus one can assume that a mutation in one costimulatory receptor may diminish and/or modify an immune response, rather than eliminating it entirely. This may account for the relatively late clinical appearance of CVID.

Cellular Abnormalities

If we return to our flow chart of T- and B-cell development (Fig. 5.5), you will see that CVID affects more terminal events leading to Ig production. These events depend on interactions among several cell types, and thus it is not surprising that there are several possible scenarios that may result in the CVID phenotype.

B-Cell Abnormalities. One consistent finding in CVID and IgAD is that these diseases are associated with B-cell dysfunction. Within the CVID patient population as a whole, this abnormality exists as a spectrum, ranging

from patients with severely reduced circulating B-cell numbers (about 10%) to those with moderately reduced or normal B-cell numbers. Regardless of the quantitative findings, in most patients these cells are qualitatively abnormal. This is documented by their surface phenotype with a reduced percentage exhibiting markers of maturity or memory (CD27) or evidence of having undergone heavy-chain class switch differentiation (into IgG and IgA B cells) and instead remain as $IgD^+/CD27^-$ B cells (see above).

The abnormalities of B-cell subset distribution correlate to some extent with the capacity of the patient's B cells to produce Ig when stimulated *in vitro* with a T-cell-independent, B-cell stimulant such as *S. aureus* Cowan's I plus IL-2. In general, regardless of whether they have normal overall B-cell numbers, patients with reduced numbers of $CD27^+$ cells manifest decreased IgG production *in vitro*. Production of IgM *in vitro*, on the other hand, is not highly correlated with markers of B-cell maturation; patients may produce substantial amounts of this Ig *in vitro* despite low circulating IgM levels. Finally, in keeping with the evidence described above that CVID B cells exhibit reduced B-cell maturation, CVID B cells display decreased somatic hypermutation of Ig variable-region genes, leading to reduced affinity maturation of the antibodies that are produced. This abnormality applies even to IgM antibodies and to those that recognize polysaccharide antigens. It may be that the *in vitro* stimulation conditions push naive B cells from the peripheral blood to produce Ig. However, these B cells would be expected to lack evidence of somatic hypermutation and thus have low overall affinity because they have not previously trafficked through the germinal center.

Initial activation events following B-cell stimulation in CVID are normal, at least in the majority of patients that display normal B-cell proliferation. This suggests a defect downstream from initial activation. Along these lines, persistent stimulation of B cells via CD40, which mimics the stimulation of B cells by activated T cells expressing CD40L, has been shown to result in nearly normal Ig production. This again occurs in a hierarchical fashion wherein IgM production is more nearly normalized than IgG production, and IgA production is hardly affected at all. Thus, to some extent, defect(s) in CVID B cells can be bypassed by accessory pathways. Alternatively, the defect may be quantitative so that the defective synthesis of certain key differentiation components can be increased and the defect overcome by strong *in vitro* stimuli. Although evidence of somatic hypermutation has not been examined, one would predict its absence in this *in vitro* stimulation model.

The B-cell responses generated *in vitro* also correlate with the *in vivo* immune capability and clinical status of patients. Patients with IgM^+ B cells expressing CD27

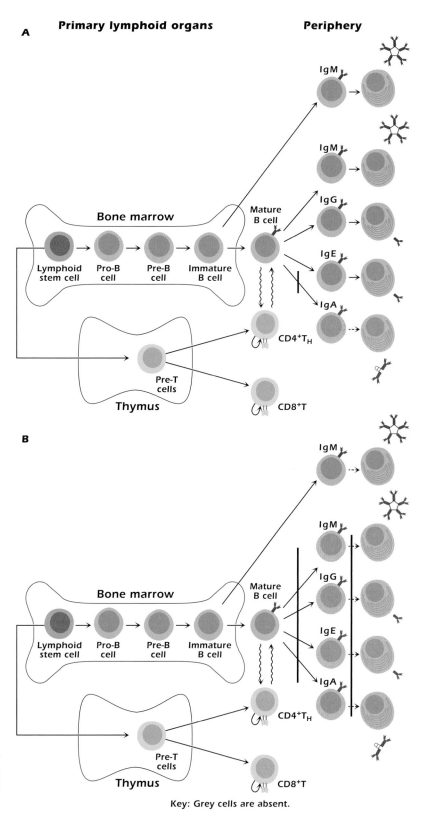

A **Primary lymphoid organs**

Periphery

B

Key: Grey cells are absent.

Figure 5.5. Scheme of T- and B-cell differentiation with indication of position of block in differentiation in (A) selective IgA deficiency and (B) CVID.

could sometimes produce antibodies against pneumococcal antigens whereas patients without these cells could not. Similarly, patients with class-switched memory B cells that produce some IgG and IgA *in vitro* are capable of mounting responses to both polysaccharide and protein antigens. On this basis, it can be argued that some patients can be successfully vaccinated. The presence or absence of memory B cells also tends to predict which patients are subject to the development of bronchiectasis, splenomegaly, and granulomatous disease: Those with absence of memory B cells are more likely to develop these abnormalities. On the other hand, low numbers of memory B cells are not predictive of autoimmunity in that even CVID patients with normal memory B-cell numbers are subject to this complication.

T-Cell Abnormalities.   Studies of T cells in CVID over the past two decades have uncovered patient groups with reduced CD40L expression, defects of cell activation, and cytokine production defects, including reduced production of IL-2, IL-4, and IFN-γ. However, these abnormalities are not a general feature of CVID and thus their significance to its pathogenesis is poorly understood. A more consistent set of abnormalities was found in a recent study of a large cohort of CVID patients. This study disclosed that, on average, patients have low numbers of CD4$^+$ T cells and, in the naive (CD45RA$^+$) T-cell population, both CD4$^+$ and CD8$^+$ naive T cells are reduced. These patients tend to have high numbers of memory T cells (CD45RO$^+$) and T cells that display markers of previous activation such as CD25 (IL-2Rα) and HLA-DR. Thus, it is not surprising that when cells of patients with low levels of naive T cells were subjected to microarray analysis for mRNA expression, they expressed many genes associated with cell activation. Other characteristics of CVID T cells in patients with decreased numbers of naive T cells were evidence of reduced thymic T-cell output, increased T-cell turnover and apoptosis, and the presence of T cells producing increased amounts of IFN-γ and decreased amounts of IL-10 (but normal amounts of IL-4 and IL-2). Patients with low numbers of naive CD4$^+$ T cells tended to be the same patients with low numbers of memory B cells, suggesting a similar pathophysiology leading to both abnormalities. However, the correlation is far from perfect.

Another T-cell abnormality in CVID is the occurrence of high numbers of CD8$^+$ T cells and reversed CD4/CD8 ratios. This is seen in about 20–25% of patients who are not otherwise different from other CVID patients. The CD8$^+$ T cells are mature T cells that produce low amounts of IL-2 and elevated amounts of IFN-γ and other cytokines. In addition, they exhibit increased capacity to mediate cytotoxic T-cell function. Whereas most patients in this group have (CD8$^+$) T cells with the capacity to suppress Ig synthesis by normal B cells, these patients' B cells still fail to produce normal amounts of Ig when their T cells are removed. Thus, the presence of suppressor T cells is not the cause of the hypogammaglobulinemia in this subset of patients. In fact, while patients with CVID due only to the presence of suppressor T cells do occur, they are quite rare.

Consideration of T-cell abnormalities is particularly relevant in patients with autoimmune parameters. The possible association of villous atrophy of the GI tract with autoreactive T cells secreting IFN-γ in the lamina propria has already been discussed.

Dendritic Cell Abnormalities.   Recent reports demonstrate an association of CVID with defective dendritic cell function. They show that CVID dendritic cells fail to express markers of differentiation and maturation, produce reduced amounts of IL-12, and have poor antigen-presenting function. It should be noted, however, that stimulation of dendritic cells in lamina propria cell populations from patients with villous atrophy and malabsorption reveals that these cells produce increased amount of IL-12. Thus, it is still not clear that dendritic cells in CVID are truly defective.

Genetic Factors in CVID

A number of genetic factors have been discovered that are associated with CVID and that account for at least some of the T- and B-cell abnormalities described above.

Major Histocompatibility Complex (MHC). The first documented genetic association is that between CVID/IgAD and MHC region genes on chromosome 6. The MHC codes for class I and class II antigens; the latter influences the level of immune response to protein antigens and is associated with many autoimmune diseases (see Unit III). CVID is associated not with a particular MHC gene, but rather with one of two "extended" MHC gene haplotypes. An extended haplotype is a group of genes in a cluster (in this case in the highly polymorphic MHC gene complex) that tend to be inherited together and thus are said to be in "linkage dysequilibrium." The reason for such dysequilibrium is most likely due to the fact that, when inherited together, the specific alleles in that cluster provide a selective survival advantage. The extended haplotypes associated with CVID and IgAD occur in 70–80% of patients and are similar to those seen with many autoimmune diseases, including celiac disease and systemic lupus erythematosus. However, as noted below, the particular genes in the MHC haplotype associated with CVID and IgAD are probably different from those associated with autoimmune syndromes.

A study of a large family with multiple members having CVID has allowed more precise localization of the susceptibility gene(s) within the extended haplotypes to an area in the MHC class III region (a region between the class I and class II regions). In contrast, the regions associated with autoimmune diseases tend to localize to the class

II region. The class III region contains 21 known genes, including those encoding TNF-α and lymphotoxins α and β. How the genes in this area actually act as susceptibility genes awaits more precise identification of the genes involved.

ICOS Gene Defects.

As discussed earlier in the case, ICOS is a costimulatory molecule on the surface of T cells that, upon interaction with B-cell ICOS-L, causes the T cell to increase its production of cytokines, including IL-4 and IL-10 that are involved in B-cell maturation. Mice lacking either ICOS or ICOS-L exhibit germinal center defects and impaired Ig production.

Based on this mouse data, ICOS deficiency was sought in CVID patients and found in two Austrian families, each of which contained multiple members who manifested disease typical of CVID associated with panhypogammaglobulinemia. Genetic analysis of these individuals disclosed homozygous ICOS gene mutations leading to total absence of ICOS expression. Large groups of CVID patients in both the United States and Europe were then tested, but no additional patients with ICOS mutation were found. This, plus the fact that the two families in Austria were distantly related, led to the conclusion that CVID due to the ICOS mutations arose as a spontaneous mutation in a single family (occurring several hundred years ago) and that such mutations are not a general cause of CVID. Nevertheless, the identification of an ICOS defect as one cause of CVID did establish that this disease could arise from this single gene defect. Patients with ICOS defects have a fairly typical form of CVID characterized by decreased numbers of memory B cells that exhibit evidence of class switching and T cells that lack the subpopulations that produce IL-10 and that are involved in germinal center formation.

CD19 Deficiency.

CD19-deficient mice have poor primary and secondary (high-affinity) antibody responses, as would be expected from a deficiency in a molecule that is part of the B-cell costimulatory complex. In humans, a mutation in the gene encoding CD19 has been found in four CVID patients from two unrelated families. As in the case of ICOS, the gene encoding CD19 is autosomal, and homozygous mutations in this molecule give rise to affected patients. CVID patients with CD19 mutations exhibit absent or greatly reduced CD19 expression on the B cells and this is associated with decreased expression of CD21, another member of the BCR costimulatory complex. While B-cell numbers are normal, the subset of memory B cells expressing CD27 is reduced. In contrast to mice with CD19 deficiency, patients have normal germinal center formation; nevertheless, peripheral B cells manifest poor proliferative responses in response to BCR stimulation with anti-IgM or a B-cell mitogen. This translates to poor antibody formation upon *in vivo* antigen stimulation.

TNF Superfamily Receptor Defects: TACI and BAFF-R Mutations.

Mutation in the B-cell receptors TACI and BAFF-R have been found in some patients with CVID. As discussed earlier, B-cell survival and isotype switching depend on signaling of TACI, BAFF-R, and a third TNF receptor superfamily member BCMA by their ligands—BAFF (for all three receptors) and APRIL (for TACI and BCMA). Like other TNF receptor superfamily members, such as CD40, these ligand–receptor signaling cascades involve interactions between trimolecular complexes that result in activation of nuclear factor κB (NF-κB) and certain mitogen-activated protein kinases (MAPKs). The interaction of BAFF and APRIL with several of these receptors suggests that the receptors have overlapping functions. However, studies of mice in which only one receptor has been deleted establish that they also have some unique functions. Thus, whereas BAFF-R signaling is important for the survival of certain B-cell subsets, TACI signaling appears to also negatively regulate B cells and one sees autoimmune manifestations and lymphoma development occur in its absence. In addition, APRIL signaling via TACI appears to be important in IgA isotype induction, perhaps as a result of APRIL's stimulation of TGF-β production. Finally, TACI signaling, but not BAFF-R, is important in supporting T-cell-independent B-cell responses in mice.

Mutations in TACI have been identified in two separate cohorts of patients. Within one family, a single TACI mutation has been found in one individual with CVID and another with IgA deficiency, underscoring the genetic relationship between these immunodeficiencies. Patients with mutations in one allele and in both alleles have been identified, suggesting that some patients have an autosomal dominant abnormality whereas others have an autosomal recessive abnormality. The dominance may actually result from the fact that, as mentioned above, signaling requires the formation of a trimolecular receptor and the latter may be disrupted by some mutated molecular forms. While most mutations occur in gene segments encoding the extracellular portion of the molecule, mutations in the intracellular portion (that presumably permit ligand binding but nevertheless fail to generate a signal) have also been observed.

Overall, TACI mutations have been found in about 8–10% of the large multicentered CVID cohort studied. Most of the affected patients exhibit heterozygous mutations which are also found in normal populations, albeit at a lower frequency. This suggests that, at least as far as the heterozygous mutation is concerned, TACI mutations are best considered *susceptibility factors* in CVID, that is, factors that require the presence of other genetic factors to produce disease. While TACI mutations in mice are associated with increased B-cell numbers, they are not associated with a similar phenomenon in CVID patients; furthermore, TACI mutations are not correlated with a particular CVID phenotype. In this regard, it was recently found that, while some CVID patients have high levels of circulating BAFF, APRIL, and TACI, there was no correlation between these levels and patient clinical findings or with the presence of TACI mutations. Finally, one individual with a BAFF-R mutation consisting of large deletions in exon 2 of the gene has been identified; this patient exhibits an as-yet poorly characterized abnormality of B-cell survival.

The discovery of various genetic defects in CVID signals the opening of a new era in the study of this complex group of abnormalities that result in hypogammaglobulinemia and poor antibody responses. Clearly, much remains to be learned, with respect to both the discovery of new genetic abnormalities and the clearer definition of how these abnormalities contribute to the immunologic phenotype found in the individual patient. Given the probability that this disease is likely to be a multigenic rather than a monogenic disease, this task may prove quite difficult.

PROGNOSIS AND TREATMENT OF CVID DISEASE

CVID is a life-long disease that does not spontaneously remit, except in very rare cases. In the absence of treatment with gammaglobulin replacement, patients will usually develop chronic lung infection leading to irreversible pulmonary insufficiency and death. Initial attempts to treat patients with intramuscular Ig slowed the progress of pulmonary disease but did not eliminate it. The picture changed with the introduction of IVIG therapy; here it was found that initiation of therapy prior to lung damage could prevent the development of irreversible disease. On this basis, there is now consensus that IVIG therapy should be initiated as soon as possible and certainly after the first episode of pneumonia. The rule of thumb is to administer sufficient IVIG to maintain "trough levels" of 500 mg/dL of IgG.

Although IVIG therapy has dramatically influenced the course of CVID, patients still have difficulties with autoimmune manifestations, neoplasia, and opportunistic infections. Each of these problems is believed to be due to T-cell abnormalities, which are beyond the reach of IVIG therapy. These problems have a significant impact on the overall well-being of CVID patients and their survival is

significantly reduced when compared to normal individuals or even to XLA patients who have only a B-cell defect.

IgAD is usually a silent condition, although there is evidence that the disease is a risk factor for the development of certain autoimmune diseases such as lupus erythematosus. The occasional patient with IgAD with chronic respiratory symptoms is not treated with IVIG unless there is concomitant IgG subclass deficiency since IVIG preparations do not contain IgA. These patients are handled with antibiotics and other conventional measures.

REFERENCES

Agematsu K, Nagumo H, Yang FC, Nakazawa T, Fukushima K, Ito S, Sugita K, Mori T, Kobata T, Morimoto C, Komiyama A (1997): B cell subpopulations separated by CD27 and crucial collaboration of CD27$^+$ B cells and helper T cells in immunoglobulin production. *Eur J Immunol* 27:2073–2079.

Bacchelli C, Buckridge S, Thrasher AJ, Gaspar HB (2007): Translational minireview series on immunodeficiency: Molecular defects in common variable immunodeficiency. *Clin Exp Immunol* 149:401–409.

Klein U, Rajewsky K, Küppers R (1998): Human immunoglobulin (Ig)M$^+$ IgD$^+$ peripheral blood B cells expressing the CD27 cell surface antigen carry somatically mutated variable region genes: CD27 as a general marker for somatically mutated (memory) B cells. *J Exp Med* 188:1679–1689.

Klein U, Rüppers R, Rajewsky K (1997): Evidence for a large component of IgM-expressing memory B cells in humans. *Blood* 89:288–1298.

Litinskiy MB, Nardelli B, Hilbert DM, He B, Schaffer A, Casali P, Cerutti A (2002): DCs induce CD40-independent immunoglobulin class switching through BLys and APRIL. *Nature Immunol* 3:822–829.

Maurer D, Fischer GF, Fae I, Majdic O, Stuhlmeier K, von Jeney N, Holter W, Knapp W (1992): IgM and IgG but not cytokine secretion is restricted to the CD27$^+$ B lymphocyte subset. *J Immunol* 148:3700–3705.

Wamatz K, Denz A, Dräger R, Braun M, Groth C, Wolff-Vorbeck G, Eibel H, Schlesier M, Peter HH (2002): Severe deficiency of switched memory B cells (CD27$^+$ IgM$^-$ IgD$^-$) in subgroups of patients with common variable immunodeficiency: A new approach to classify a heterogeneous disease. *Blood* 99:1544–1551.

6

AUTOIMMUNE LYMPHOPROLIFERATIVE SYNDROME (ALPS)

KONETI RAO and THOMAS A. FLEISHER*

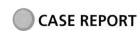 ## CASE REPORT

"I found a lump on my child's neck."

History and Physical Examination

Emily is a three-year-old girl whose mother notices a soft, painless lump on the left side of her neck, distorting the outline of her jaw. Disturbed by this discovery, the mother brings her to you at the pediatric clinic.

The mother states that Emily has been a healthy child except for several episodes of sore throat and upper respiratory infection in the last two years. She does recall being told that Emily's spleen was large during a well-baby clinic visit at age 18 months; however, this was not further evaluated. She also says that Emily has not been febrile, has a good appetite, and has not lost weight; in addition, she is up to date with her immunizations.

On physical examination you note that Emily has considerable, nontender lymphadenopathy. This includes a visible left anterior cervical node measuring approximately 2 cm in diameter as well as enlarged right cervical lymph nodes and enlarged right and left axillary and inguinal nodes. The latter node measures approximately 1 cm in diameter. In addition, she has an enlarged spleen, palpable to 5 cm below the left costal margin.

*With contributions from Warren Strober and Susan R. S. Gottesman

Differential Diagnosis and Initial Workup

At this point, you ask yourself what is the differential diagnosis of peripheral lymphadenopathy and splenomegaly in a three-year-old child?

As for adults, the differential diagnosis of lymphadenopathy includes malignancy, particularly lymphoma, and infection (see Case 25). Lymphadenopathy, defined as enlarged lymph node tissue measuring more than 1 cm in diameter, is a frequent presenting symptom in children. In most cases this is due to the presence of one of the bacterial or viral infections that commonly occur in childhood and that resolve either spontaneously or after appropriate antibiotic therapy. These "reactive" lymph node enlargements are typically tender, painful masses that are confined to one region, suggesting that the node is draining a localized site of infection. Regional lymphadenopathy can also occur in association with more serious infections. Thus, mycobacterial infections produced by Mucobacteria tuberculosis or nontuberculous Mycobacteria species need to be considered.

Generalized lymphadenopathy may also be due to an infection; however, under these circumstances, it would be systemic rather than localized. Persistent viral infection due to organisms such as Epstein–Barr virus (EBV), human immunodeficiency virus (HIV), hepatitis, or coxsackie virus is part of the differential diagnosis. EBV infection would also explain the splenomegaly, although infectious mononucleosis (caused by EBV) is more common in a slightly older age group; teenagers and young adults.

If the child has an infection as a result of an organism which does not normally cause disease, an opportunistic infection, or repeated severe or unusual infections, an underlying immunodeficiency disease needs to be considered. A cardinal feature of immunodeficiency particularly that due to T-cell abnormalities, is the occurrence of opportunistic infection with ordinarily benign infectious agents. Examples of immunodeficiencies of this type include X-linked severe combined immunodeficiency due to a mutation in the common gamma chain of the IL-2 receptor (and other cytokine receptors) and acquired immunodeficiency syndrome (AIDS) due to HIV infection (see Cases 2 and 9).

A final category of disease giving rise to lymphadenopathy is hematologic malignancy. This is usually due to lymphoma but can occasionally be the result of childhood-onset myelodysplastic syndrome (chronic myelomonocytic leukemia) characterized by peripheral monocytosis and a dysplastic bone marrow. These diseases present with generalized lymphadenopathy, usually associated with splenomegaly.

To summarize the above, the differential diagnosis of peripheral lymphadenopathy of childhood usually falls into one of three categories: (1) reactive lymphadenopathy associated with local or generalized infection; (2) lymphadenopathy associated with immunodeficiency (which is also reactive to infection; in association with immunodeficiency, the infection is often opportunistic); and (3) hematologic malignancy. As we shall see, however, our patient, Emily, falls into "none of the above."

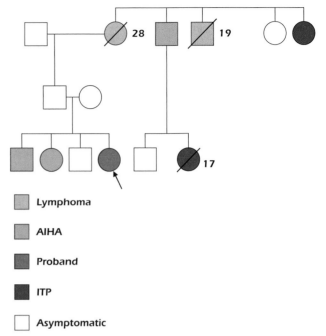

Figure 6.1. Pedigree of Emily's family. Several family members have ALPS-related conditions, including autoimmunity (ITP) or lymphoma. These individuals are all related through the paternal side of the family. Other family members, including Emily's father, bear mutations associated with ALPS but are asymptomatic.

To help distinguish among the above-listed possibilities, you draw blood samples for a complete blood count (CBC), erythrocyte sedimentation rate (ESR—a nonspecific screen for the presence of infection, inflammation, or neoplasm), serum immunoglobulin levels, and specific antibody and antigen tests for EBV, HIV, and hepatitis viruses. These are reported back as normal with the exception of an elevated ESR of 35 mm/h (reference range 0–25 mm/h) and an overall IgG level of 2,020 mg/L (age-specific reference range 441–1135 mg/L). No evidence of recent viral infection is found. You also order a computerized tomography (CT) scan, which corroborates the clinical findings of generalized lymphadenopathy; the scan shows enlarged nodes in the mediastinum, mesenteric, and para-aortic regions and splenomegaly.

Diagnosis of ALPS

Based on these abnormalities you assume that Emily has a malignancy and you refer the family to a pediatric hematologist for further study. She reviews your findings and also elicits a family history of diseases involving the hematopoietic system. As shown in Emily's pedigree chart depicted in Figure 6.1, two adult first-degree relatives (one male, one female) have had illnesses similar to Emily's,

characterized by lymphadenopathy and complicated by **autoimmune hemolytic anemia** (**AIHA**; destruction of red blood cells by autoantibody); in both cases the latter ultimately necessitated splenectomies. In addition, several second- and third-degree relatives on Emily's paternal side died at relatively young ages following the diagnosis and unsuccessful treatment of lymphoma in the 1960s. Additional relatives had autoimmune hemolytic anemia and autoimmune thrombocytopenia (ITP). In one instance death was caused by sepsis, a complication of splenectomy for ITP.

The hematologist, now suspecting a genetically determined lymphoproliferative disorder, continues her evaluation by arranging for a biopsy of one of Emily's peripheral lymph nodes as well as immunophenotyping of her peripheral blood cells. The biopsy procedure subsequently performed is an excisional biopsy of the 1 cm inguinal node identified in Emily's initial examination. The tissue is examined by the pathologist, who uses both conventional hematoxylin–eosin (H&E) staining and immunohistochemical stains for evaluation of the tissue. The latter employ labeled antibodies to allow one to detect the presence of specific cell types (see Unit V for assay descriptions).

The pathology report based on conventional histologic examination is as follows: Reactive follicular hyperplasia, marked paracortical hyperplasia, and interfollicular expansion with focal progressive transformation of germinal centers. The overall architecture of the node is preserved. Increased numbers of immunoblasts (large reactive lymphocytes) and plasma cells are evident with no cells displaying characteristics of malignant cells (Figs. 6.2A–C).

Thus, on conventional staining, the node provides evidence of abnormally increased lymphoid proliferation but no evidence of malignancy. Additional studies to detect various lymphoid subpopulations with labeled antibodies are more diagnostic. These reveal that the node contains greatly increased numbers of T cells [CD3$^+$ cells, bearing the αβ T-cell receptor (TCR)] that bear neither CD4 nor CD8 subset marker; these are therefore "double-negative" (DN) T cells (Figs. 6.2D,F).

Immunophenotyping by flow cytometry (see Unit V) of the peripheral blood lymphocytes corroborates and expands on the above biopsy findings. This reveals increased levels of circulating B lymphocytes and more importantly, as shown in Figure 6.3, a marked expansion in T cells expressing the αβ TCR that do not bear CD4 or CD8, as was also seen in the biopsy.

These clinical and laboratory findings point strongly to the diagnosis of **autoimmune lymphoproliferative syndrome (ALPS)**, a disorder of lymphocyte apoptosis inherited in an autosomal dominant fashion. This is based on the presence of two of the three criteria necessary for the diagnosis: (1) nonmalignant lymphadenopathy with or without splenomegaly and (2) an elevated percentage (>1%) and/or number (>20) of double-negative (CD3$^+$CD4$^-$CD8$^-$) T cells that express the αβ TCR. A third and critical criterion is the demonstration that the patient does in fact have a disorder of lymphocyte apoptosis.

What is apoptosis?

Apoptosis is programmed cell death. Cells which die in this manner undergo chromosome breakage and are noted histologically to first have nuclear condensation, followed by fractionation of the nucleus. The plasma membrane starts to change its orientation of phospholipids and demonstrates blebbing. The cell is then phagocytosed. This process of cell death is caused by caspases, enzymes normally present in the cytoplasm in inactive form. Signals to initiate caspase activation come from either a mitochondrial based pathway (passive apoptosis) or signaling through "death receptors" on the cell surface (activation-induced apoptosis). This is discussed in more detail below.

A test for activation-induced apoptosis is ordered. In this assay, peripheral blood lymphocytes from the patient and a control individual are first activated with mitogen (nonspecific stimulator of cell proliferation) and then cultured in IL-2-containing media to up-regulate the expression of cell surface Fas (CD95). Apoptosis is then induced in the Fas$^+$ lymphocytes by the addition of anti-Fas monoclonal antibody that cross-links Fas. This initiates activation of caspases 10 and 8, which starts the process leading to DNA fragmentation. The degree of cell death can be measured by the TUNEL assay, which detects the broken ends of DNA, or by flow cytometry, which detects apoptotic cells by their uptake of annexin V, a labeled reagent that binds to newly exposed phospholipids on cells undergoing apoptosis (Fig. 6.4).

Emily's lymphocytes display a moderately severe decrease in apoptotic capacity compared to the control sample and the diagnosis is now established. Emily's parents are then also tested and her father is found to have a defect

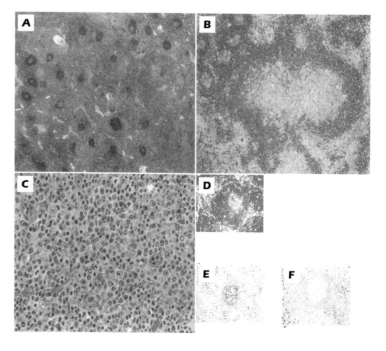

Figure 6.2. Histopathologic findings in lymph node in ALPS. (**A, B, C**) Stained by H&E. (**A**) Paracortical region of lymph node at low power showing marked expansion of interfollicular cells; original magnification: ×100. (**B**) Progressively transformed (and greatly enlarged) germinal center (in center of picture); this finding is a focal but relatively frequent finding; original magnification: ×200. (**C**) Paracortical region of patient's lymph node at high power showing presence of lymphocytes, plasma cells, and immunoblasts; original magnification: ×600. (**D**) Immunoperoxidase stain for CD3 demonstrating expansion of interfollicular regions by CD3$^+$ T cells. (**E, F**) Immunoperoxidase stain of same area as in D to detect CD4 and CD8 showing that the CD3$^+$ T cells are largely CD4$^-$ (**E**) and CD8$^-$ (**F**); most of the CD4$^+$ cells are within germinal center (**E**). [Modified from Lim MS et al. (1998): *Am J Path* 153:541–550.]

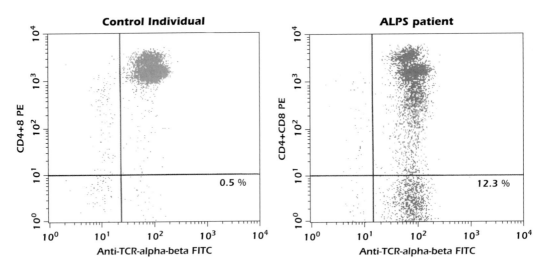

Figure 6.3. Two-Color flow cytometric study of lymphocytes of patient with ALPS. Vertical axis captures cells stained with anti-CD4– and anti-CD8–phycoerythrin and horizontal axis captures cells stained with anti-αβ TCR–fluoroscein isothiocyanate (FITC) dye (CD4/CD8-positive cells are above the horizontal line). Note that a control individual (left panel) has only 0. 5% double-negative cells whereas an ALPS patient (right panel) has over 12.3% double-negative T cells.

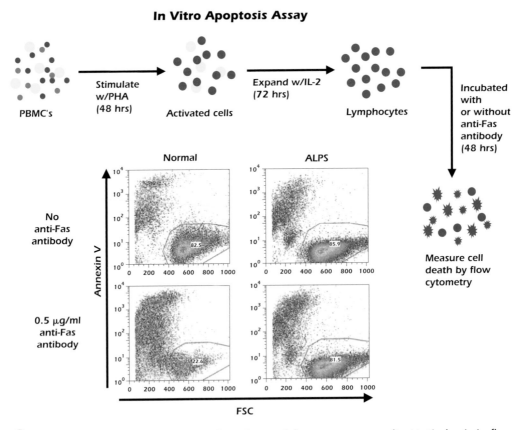

Figure 6.4. *In vitro* apoptosis assay. Procedure and flow cytometry results. Vertical axis in flow cytometry study captures dying cells that take up a dye (annexin V) that binds to proteins in dying cells; horizontal axis captures living cells that exhibit forward light scatter (FSC). ALPS patient study shows decreased number of dying cells and therefore decreased Fas-mediated apoptosis.

in apoptosis, although he lacks clinical evidence of the disease.

What do these results disclose about the pattern of inheritance?

These findings, combined with the pedigree already obtained, document an autosomal dominant pattern of inheritance with a second gene defect or environmental factor required to trigger disease.

The family is counseled as to the significance of these findings, but no specific treatment is advised at this point. Emily is referred back to her pediatrician for observation by regular clinic visits every six months.

Emily's Subsequent Clinical Course

In the years following the initial diagnosis of ALPS, Emily remains relatively well. Although her lymphadenopathy and splenomegaly progressed somewhat, the increase in size was not great enough to interfere with everyday life, even though it was noticeable and slightly disfiguring. However, this benign course changes at age seven when she has the onset of an illness that initially appears to be a seasonal viral flu-like process but soon becomes more serious with the development of jaundice, pallor, and petechiae (minute hemorrhages). Emily's mother brings her in on an urgent basis. On physical examination at this time, Emily has persistent lymphadenopathy that, as noted above, is some-what increased over that at age 3. In addition, she exhibits markedly increased splenomegaly, with a spleen that now measures 10 cm below the costal margin.

To investigate these changes, you obtain a CBC, ESR, and immunoglobulin levels.

Results.

	Results	Reference Range
Selected Blood Counts		
Hemoglobin	6.5 g/dL	11.5–15.5 g/dL
WBC	1800/μL	4800–10,800/μL
Neutrophils	700/μL	1900–8000/μL
Platelets	13,000/μL	130,000–400,000/μL
Reticulocyte %	15.0%	0.3–2.1%
Inflammatory Marker		
ESR	105 mm/h	3–13 mm/h
Immunoglobulin Levels		
IgG	3040 mg/dL	633–1280 mg/dL
IgM	112 mg/dL	48–207 mg/dL
IgA	172 mg/dL	33–202 mg/dL

Interpretation. The results of these studies reveal marked anemia, marked thrombocytopenia (low platelet count) and leukopenia (low white blood cell count) with neutropenia, and an elevated reticulocyte percentage. Thus, she has marked pancytopenia (reduced levels of all blood cell elements). Her ESR is now markedly increased and she has a further elevation of her IgG level; however, the latter is associated with normal IgA and IgM levels. Based on the marked pancytopenia and the presence of jaundice, hemolysis is suspected. This is confirmed by serum chemistries and a direct Coomb's test which proves to be strongly positive.

What do the elevated reticulocyte percentage and jaundice signify?

Reticulocytes are young red blood cells recently released from the bone marrow into the circulation. They are detected by their content of remnant RNA still in the cytoplasm. Their presence signifies intact bone marrow function and helps distinguish between bone marrow failure versus peripheral loss or destruction of red blood cells as the cause of anemia. With peripheral destruction, one expects a high percentage of reticulocytes, both because the denominator is low (total red blood cell count) and because the marrow tries to compensate for the anemia by increased red cell production and release. Also suggesting peripheral destruction is the observation of jaundice. Jaundice, as evidenced by the yellow discoloration of eyes and palms, is due to an increase in indirect bilirubin and is an indication of extravascular hemolysis.

What is a Coomb's test?

A direct Coomb's test detects the presence of antibodies coating the patient's red blood cells. The cells are incubated with an anti-human IgG (Coomb's reagent) and a positive reaction is detected by agglutination of the red cells. When the patient has antibodies in their plasma not bound to their red cells, they are detected by incubating patient plasma with test red blood cells, followed by addition of the Coomb's reagent. This is an indirect Coomb's test.

Knowing that ALPS can lead to autoimmunity, you now draw the tentative conclusion that Emily has developed autoimmune hemolytic anemia associated with immune cytopenia involving other blood elements ("Evan's syndrome" or autoimmune cytopenia) and again refer Emily to the hematologist. The hematologist admits her to the hospital for treatment of her cytopenias and decides to perform a bone marrow biopsy to confirm the diagnosis of an autoimmune cause of the pancytopenia rather than bone marrow failure.

Results of bone marrow biopsy. The biopsy exhibits increased cellularity with megaloblastoid dyserythropoietic changes and absent iron stores, increased myeloid cells with a left shift in maturation, and increased numbers of megakaryocytes. In addition, there is plasmacytosis.

What do these bone marrow findings signify?

The findings confirm what the hematologist suspected based on the reticulocyte count; that the bone marrow is producing red blood cells. Importantly it also demonstrates that the bone marrow is still producing myeloid cells and platelets. Evidence for this comes from the findings of increased myeloid cells and megakaryocytes (the producers of platelets). The changes in maturation such as megaloblastoid changes and myeloid left shift, are not uncommon when the marrow is stressed to rapidly produce and release cells. The increased plasma cells in the marrow are also not unexpected given Emily's inflammatory and autoimmune state.

Why has the spleen size increased so dramatically?

The initial splenomegaly and lymphadenopathy were due to ALPS itself with hyperplasia of the lymphoid tissue. The spleen is further increased in size with this current episode of autoimmune hemolytic anemia because it is the site of phagocytosis and destruction of the antibody-coated red blood cells. This same phenomenon of phagocytosis of coated platelets, and a degree of hypersplenism, are the causes of the extremely low platelet count.

These findings support the diagnosis of autoimmune cytopenia and Emily is promptly placed on high-dose corticosteroids (intravenous methylprednisone). When this therapy proves ineffective, she is given several courses of high-dose intravenous γ-globulin (IVIG) therapy. In addition, she is given G-CSF (granulocyte colony-stimulating factor) to support her neutrophil levels and blood transfusions to support her red blood cell levels. Nevertheless, her hemogloblin level continues to deteriorate, reaching a nadir of 4.5 g/L. At this point, the hematologist, in concert with her colleagues, considers splenectomy to stop the destruction of the antibody-coated red blood cells by the spleen. This step is not taken lightly because the spleen is an important organ of host defense and its removal will cause Emily to be more prone to sepsis. However, the continued presence of unsustainable hemoglobin and platelet levels tips the scales toward splenectomy. After obtaining consent from Emily's parents, the procedure is performed. Not long after splenectomy, Emily's blood parameters exhibit progressive improvement. After several weeks, her hemoglobin and platelet levels increase to levels just below the lower limit of normal. To counter the possibility of sepsis, Emily is placed on an antibiotic regimen that she will have to follow for life.

Since the time of Emily's episode of immune cytopenia, other therapeutic modalities have become available that may have averted splenectomy. These include the use of mycophenolate mofetil and anti-CD20 (Rituximab) as immunosuppressive agents. CD20 is a surface antigen specific for mature B cells.

Emily does reasonably well over the next 10 years. Then, at 17 years of age, she presents with sudden enlargement of a right posterior cervical lymph node and the appearance of an abdominal lump associated with fever, malaise, and weight loss. She is again referred to the hematologist, who arranges for a biopsy of the enlarged node. This reveals the presence of lymphoma and Emily is immediately begun on a chemotherapy regimen that fortunately leads to successful clearing of the lymphoma. Emily remains in remission during the ensuing 8 years of observation and is currently 25 years old and a recent law school graduate.

CLINICAL FEATURES AND COURSE OF ALPS

ALPS typically announces itself by the early appearance of lymphoid enlargement. This is characterized by prominent lymphadenopathy, particularly in the neck and axillary regions, where it can be massive and distort anatomic landmarks. The adenopathy is actually generalized and enlargement of the abdominal and thoracic lymph nodes is usually noted on CT scans. Regardless of its extent, the lymphadenopathy is persistent, lasting for two or more years in virtually all patients. Splenomegaly is also a constant feature of the lymphoid enlargement and is often massive in proportion; it too can persist for many years.

A second early feature of ALPS (one not initially seen in Emily's case but occurring later on) is the development of autoimmunity. Thus, in 20–25% of patients, the lymphadenopathy described above is accompanied by chronic, refractory hemolytic anemia, thrombocytopenia, and/or neutropenia. These are B-cell-mediated autoimmune states and thus they are characterized by circulating autoantibodies to the target cells, such as RBC and platelets. These autoimmune cytopenias are frequently refractory to more benign forms of treatment, so approximately 50% of patients undergo splenectomy and are thus rendered susceptible to postsplenectomy sepsis. Other non-hematologic autoimmune diseases have been reported in association with ALPS, including Guillain-Barré syndrome, glomerulonephritis, uveitis, and autoimmune liver disease. The frequency of these autoimmune manifestations is substantially lower than the autoimmune cytopenias. Eosinophilia is an additional hematologic finding in ALPS patients, but its cause is unknown.

A third feature of ALPS is the increased incidence of lymphomas, both Hodgkin and non-Hodgkin. The reasons underlying this phenomenon are discussed below.

THE MOLECULAR BASIS OF ALPS

ALPS was first recognized in a child with severe lymphadenopathy who was found to have greatly increased numbers of double-negative T cells upon immunophenotyping of her peripheral blood. This suggested to her doctors that her syndrome resembled that seen in mice carrying the *lpr* mutation. The MRL mouse strain with *lpr* mutations (standing for lymphoproliferation) was originally thought to be a model for systemic lupus erythematosus (SLE). Similar to people with ALPS, these mice develop autoimmune phenomena which resemble SLE. The *lpr* mutation was later shown to be due to a molecular abnormality in the expression of the *Fas* gene, a gene that encodes a key molecule initiating lymphocyte apoptosis. Later molecular studies of this and similar patients confirmed the supposition that abnormalities of apoptosis underlying the main form of this disorder were due to mutations in *Fas*. Other molecular defects were subsequently identified that led to the same syndrome; in these cases, different molecules in the apoptosis pathway malfunctioned and led to similar or identical apoptosis syndromes, also called ALPS.

To understand how these defects present in the various forms of ALPS impact the immune system, one must first be aware of the fact that lymphocyte stimulation could lead to excessive cellular expansion were it not for the presence of built-in homeostatic mechanisms that ultimately limit such expansion. Perhaps the most important mechanism of this kind, known as activation-induced cell death (AICD), is set in motion when T cells, having been stimulated via their antigen receptor to produce IL-2 and undergo proliferation, are restimulated under certain conditions to undergo a second round of IL-2 production and signaling that activates the Fas-mediated apoptotic death pathway. This was demonstrated in culture using T-cell clones. The conditions just described that lead to apoptosis by this pathway, rather than further T-cell proliferation and expansion, are still poorly understood. One factor is probably the type of costimulation delivered to the cell, since certain forms of costimulation lead to proliferation and others to apoptosis. Another factor is the type of cytokines produced by the cell since it has been shown that interferon-γ (IFN-γ) production favors the apoptotic pathway. In any case, in the absence of an intact Fas-mediated apoptotic pathway, the relatively unchecked lymphocyte proliferation and resulting accumulation of lymphoid cells give rise to the key feature of ALPS, lymphadenopathy and splenomegaly. In addition, the failure to eliminate cells by apoptosis also affects B-cell homeostasis by a similar mechanism, causing the accretion of B cells as well as T cells. Finally, the Fas-mediated apoptotic mechanism is also important in the regulation of autoreactive cells; in the absence of this mechanism, such cells accumulate and autoimmunity

ensues. This tendency may be abetted by the fact that the Fas pathway normally inhibits innate T_H1 responses stimulated via Toll-like receptors; its malfunction creates a bias toward T_H2 responses that tends to support B-cell autoimmunity rather than T-cell autoimmunity (see Unit III). The presence of elevated numbers of double-negative T cells remains unexplained, although there is suggestion that they originate from $CD8^+$ T cells which have lost that subset marker.

Fas is part of the tumor necrosis factor receptor (TNFR) family of molecules. When T cells or B cells are activated, they express Fas molecules on the cell surface in the form of disorganized complexes of monomers. However, as shown in Figure 6.5, upon engagement with trimeric Fas ligand (FasL), expressed mostly on T cells, these complexes of Fas monomers are organized into trimers that form a cytoplasmic tail. This tail can interact with intracellular components to form a "death-inducing signaling complex," or DISC. In the first step in the formation of DISC, part of the cytoplasmic tail of Fas known as the "death domain" interacts with a similar death domain on a second molecule, FADD (Fas-associated protein with death domain). In the second step in the formation of DISC, the trimeric FAS–FADD complex interacts with either caspase 8 or caspase 10 via "death effector domains" (DED domains) on FADD and the caspases. The DISC now formed causes clustering (oligomerization) of the caspases and their autoproteolytic cleavage into active caspase components. In T cells, caspases 8 and 10 thus activated are sufficient to cleave and activate downstream caspases (particularly caspase 3) that mediate the apoptotic program. In other cells, activated caspase 8 also acts through an amplification loop that involves cleavage of pro-apoptotic members of the Bcl family which, in turn, activates caspases through release of mitochondrial caspase activators (see Case 25).

The Fas-mediated apoptotic pathway is down-regulated by a number of mechanisms that prevent or abrogate Fas-mediated apoptosis. Perhaps the most important of these mechanisms is the production of c-FLIP, a molecule that is structurally similar to caspase 8, in that it contains DED domains that enable its binding to FADD. However, it lacks an enzymatic domain necessary for caspase activation; thus, insertion of c-FLIP into the nascent DISC instead of caspase 8 or caspase 10 interrupts the apoptotic program. In view of this function of c-FLIP, it is reasonable to suppose that IL-2 activates the Fas-mediated apoptotic pathway, at least in part by regulating c-FLIP production.

In most cases of ALPS, the Fas pathway malfunctions because of mutations of Fas, FasL, caspase 8, or caspase 10. By far the most common of these mutations, accounting for 75% of all ALPS, are mutations affecting the gene encoding Fas itself (*TNFRSF6*). This and other mutations affecting

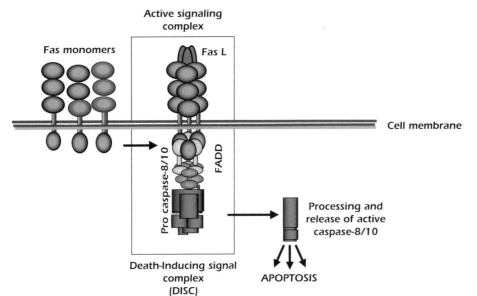

Figure 6.5. Mechanism of FasL–Fas–mediated apoptosis.

molecules of the Fas pathway are heterozygous mutations, meaning that they cause disease even though the mutation occurs in only one of the two autosomal genes. This is attributable to the fact that these various components of the Fas pathway function within the DISC as trimers; abnormal gene products from one gene are sufficient to disrupt the formation of the trimer and thus the function of the DISC. In spite of this dominance characteristic of the mutated protein, not everyone with the mutation manifests the disease clinically, although they do have demonstrable apoptotic deficiencies.

ALPS is classified as ALPS types Ia and Ib when it arises from a mutation in the genes encoding Fas and FasL, respectively, and as ALPS type II when it arises from mutations in genes encoding caspase 10 or caspase 8. Unlike other forms of ALPS, caspase 8 deficiency is associated with immunodeficiency. Finally, ALPS is classified as ALPS type III when the causative gene has not yet been identified. Patients falling into this category nevertheless have clinical and laboratory features of ALPS that are identical to those with identified mutations.

ALPS AND MALIGNANCY

ALPS type Ia patients with mutations in the intracellular death domain (Exon 9) of the gene encoding Fas (*TNFRSF6*) have been shown to be at a 14–51 times increased risk for the development of Hodgkin and non-Hodgkin lymphoma. These occur in all age groups and consist of lymphomas of diverse types. Importantly, the tumor cells retain the heterozygous *Fas* mutations found in the peripheral blood and manifest defective Fas-mediated killing; nevertheless, the lymphomas respond to conventional chemotherapy in the same manner as

non-ALPS-related lymphomas of similar histology. These data imply that Fas-mediated apoptosis plays a role in preventing B- and T-cell lymphomas; in addition, they suggest that defects in Fas-mediated lymphocyte apoptosis represent a risk factor for lymphoma development.

REFERENCES

Aspinall AI, Pinto A, Auer IA, Bridges P, Luider J, Dimnik L, Patel KD, Jorgenson K, Woodman RC (1999): Identification of new Fas mutations in a patient with autoimmune lymphoproliferative syndrome (ALPS) and eosinophilia. *Blood Cells Mol Dis* 25:227–238.

Avila NA, Dwyer AJ, Dale JK, Lopatin UA, Sneller MC, Jaffe ES, Puck JM, Straus SE (1999): Autoimmune lymphoproliferative syndrome: A syndrome associated with inherited genetic defects that impair lymphocytic apoptosis—CT and US features. *Radiology* 212:257–263.

Benkerrou M, Le Deist F, de Villartay JP, Caillat-Zucman S, Rieux-Laucat F, Jabado N, Cavazzana-Calvo M, Fischer A (1997): Correction of Fas (CD95) deficiency by haploidentical bone marrow transplantation. *Eur J Immunol* 27:2043–2047.

Canale VC, Smith CH (1967): Chronic lymphadenopathy simulating malignant lymphoma. *J Pediatr* 70:891–899.

Chun HJ, Zheng L, Ahmad M, Wang J, Speirs CK, Siegel RM, Dale JK, Puck J, Davis J, Hall CG, Skoda-Smith S, Atkinson TP, Straus SE, Lenardo MJ (2002): Pleiotropic defects in lymphocyte activation caused by caspase-8 mutations lead to human immunodeficiency. *Nature* 419:395–399.

Fisher GH, Rosenberg FJ, Straus SE, Dale JK, Middleton LA, Lin AY, Strober W, Lenardo MJ, Puck JM (1995): Dominant interfering Fas gene mutations impair apoptosis in a human autoimmune lymphoproliferative syndrome. *Cell* 81:935–946.

Fuss IJ, Strober W, Dale JK, Fritz S, Pearlstein GR, Puck JM, Lenardo MJ, Straus SE (1997): Characteristic T helper 2 T cell cytokine abnormalities in autoimmune lymphoproliferative syndrome, a syndrome marked by defective apoptosis and humoral autoimmunity. *J Immunol* 158:1912–1918.

Kroemer G, Zamzami N, Susin SA (1997): Mitochondrial control of apoptosis. *Immunol Today* 18:44–51.

Lim MS, Straus SE, Dale JK, Fleisher TA, Stetler-Stevenson M, Strober W, Sneller MC, Puck JM, Lenardom MJ, Elenitoba-Johnson KSJ, Lin AY, Raffeld M, Jaffe ES, et al. (1998): Pathological findings in human autoimmune lymphoproliferative syndrome. *Am J Pathol* 153:1541–1550.

Rieux-Laucat F, Fischer A, Deist FL (2003): Cell-death signaling and human disease. *Curr Opin Immunol* 15:325–331.

Sleight BJ, Prasad VS, DeLaat C, Steele P, Ballard E, Arceci RJ, Sidman CL (1998): Correction of autoimmune lymphoproliferative syndrome by bone marrow transplantation. *Bone Marrow Transplant* 22:375–380.

Sneller MC, Wang J, Dale JK, Strober W, Middelton LA, Choi Y, Fleisher TA, Lim MS, Jaffe ES, Puck JM, Lenardo MJ, Straus SE (1997): Clincial, immunologic, and genetic features of an autoimmune lymphoproliferative syndrome associated with abnormal lymphocyte apoptosis. *Blood* 89:1341–1348.

Straus SE, Jaffe ES, Puck JM, Dale JK, Elkon KB Rösen-Wolff A, Peters AM, Sneller MC, Hallahan CW, Wang J, Fischer RE, Jackson CM, Lin AY, Bäumler C, Siegert E, Marx A, Vaishnaw AK, Grodzicky T, Fleisher TA, Lenardo MJ (2001): The development of lymphomas in families with Autoimmune Lymphoproliferative Syndrome (ALPS) with germline Fas mutations and defective lymphocyte apoptosis. *Blood* 98:194–200.

Straus SE, Sneller M, Lenardo MJ, Puck JM, Strober W (1999): An inherited disorder of lymphocyte apoptosis: The autoimmune lymphoproliferative syndrome. *Ann Intern Med* 130:591–601.

Vaishnaw AK, Orlinick JR, Chu JL, Krammer PH, Chao MV, Elkon KB (1999): The molecular basis for apoptotic defects in patients with CD95 (Fas/Apo-1) mutations. *J Clin Invest* 103:355–363.

van der Werff ten Bosch J (2003): Autoimmune lymphoproliferative syndrome: Etiology, diagnosis, and management. *Paediatr Drugs* 5:185–193.

van der Werff ten Bosch JE, Otten J, Thielemans K (2001): Autoimmune lymphoproliferative syndrome type III: An indefinite disorder. *Leuk Lymphoma* 41:55–65.

7

X-LINKED LYMPHOPROLIFERATIVE SYNDROME

JEFFREY I. COHEN*

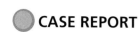 CASE REPORT

"Mark has had swollen glands and a fever for the last 24 hours."

History and Physical Examination

A couple brings their three-year-old son to you, his pediatrician, because of a high fever (104°F) and obviously swollen neck glands. They relate that he was playing and eating normally until the day before when they noticed that he was tired and listless, with poor appetite. Mark's parents are particularly concerned because their first son died of severe Epstein–Barr virus (EBV) infection several years ago, shortly before Mark was born.

The child is warm to the touch in spite of having had ibuprofen and still has a fever of 102°F. He is quiet and slightly irritable. You note a faint, macular rash (flat red spots) over much of his body, pharyngeal erythema (redness of the throat), and diffuse lymphadenopathy involving the anterior and posterior cervical chains, the axillae, and the supraclavicular regions. The neck is supple and there are no neurologic abnormalities. Lungs are clear to auscultation. On examination of the abdomen you note hepatomegaly

*With contributions from Warren Strober and Susan R. S. Gottesman

and splenomegaly (large liver and spleen). Extremities are normal with the exception of the rash.

Differential Diagnosis

Fever and swollen glands ordinarily would not be a cause for much concern, but the presence of hepatosplenomegaly suggests a more unusual and serious disease. You turn over in your mind the various diagnostic possibilities:

The differential diagnosis of diffuse lymphadenopathy associated with hepatosplenomegaly includes malignancy, immunologic diseases, lysosomal storage diseases, sarcoidosis, and infections of various types.

Malignancies associated with lymphadenopathy and splenomegaly include Hodgkin lymphoma, non-Hodgkin lymphoma, and acute or chronic lymphocytic leukemia. Hodgkin lymphoma and non-Hodgkin lymphoma often present with lymphadenopathy and systemic symptoms such as fever, weight loss, and night sweats. Hodgkin lymphoma presents with regional or unilateral lymphadenopathy whereas diffuse, symmetric lymphadenopathy is more characteristic of non-Hodgkin lymphoma. The non-Hodgkin lymphomas most frequent in young children are large B-cell lymphoma and Burkitt lymphoma. Burkitt lymphoma is distinctive in that it is often marked by the presence of

Immunology: Clinical Case Studies and Disease Pathophysiology, By Warren Strober and Susan R. S. Gottesman
Copyright © 2009 John Wiley & Sons, Inc.

masses in the abdomen or the jaw and other facial bones depending on the specific etiology of the disease. Acute lymphoblastic leukemia, the most common cancer in childhood, can also be a cause of diffuse lymphadenopathy, hepatosplenomegaly, and fever. The white blood cell (WBC) count can be elevated, reduced, or normal in acute lymphoblastic leukemia and may be nondiagnostic; however, tell-tale malignant lymphoblasts are usually present in the peripheral blood. This condition is usually associated with anemia and particularly thrombocytopenia (low platelet count), reflecting bone marrow involvement where it is seen more often than with lymph node involvement. Although chronic lymphocytic leukemia may present with similar symptoms, it is exceedingly rare in young children. While none of these diagnoses can be ruled out as the cause of Mark's illness on the basis of history and physical examination alone (and in the absence of hematologic studies), the acute nature of Mark's illness, along with the presence of a pharyngitis and rash, make these diseases unlikely causes of his symptoms. Juvenile myelomonocytic leukemia, although rare, is a consideration. It may be seen in children as young as one month of age; the majority present at three years of age or younger. The disease presents with leukemic infiltration of every organ, particularly liver and spleen and sometimes lymph nodes and skin, resulting in a rash. In addition, most present with malaise, fever, and infection with tonsillitis and bronchitis in almost half the affected children.

Immunologic diseases giving rise to systemic symptoms, lymphadenopathy, and/or hepatosplenomegaly include collagen-vascular diseases such as systemic lupus erythematosus (SLE) or juvenile rheumatoid arthritis (JRA) and immune-mediated drug reactions. In addition, some immunodeficiency syndromes could present in this manner because they cause susceptibility to infections that are the more immediate cause of these symptoms. SLE most often occurs in women of child-bearing age and is usually associated with arthralgias or myalgias. JRA may present abruptly with fevers, transient rash, and hepatosplenomegaly but most commonly includes musculoskeletal symptoms. Sarcoidosis, a disease of unknown etiology, frequently presents with generalized lymphadenopathy, including mediastinal and hilar adenopathy with pulmonary infiltrates; however, splenomegaly is uncommon and is rarely, if ever, a presenting feature. The drugs most often associated with lymphadenopathy are diphenylhydantoin (dilantin), hydralazine, and allopurinol. In this case, lymphadenopathy due to a drug is ruled out with a negative history of drug ingestion.

Lysosomal storage disorders such as Gaucher's disease or Niemann–Pick disease in a young child can present with lymphadenopathy and splenomegaly which develops gradually over time and is not commonly accompanied by fever.

Thus, for a variety of individual reasons, these immunologic diseases and storage diseases do not recommend themselves as the likely cause of Mark's illness.

Still to be considered, however, is the presence of an immunodeficiency that leads to an infection.

Infectious causes of lymphadenopathy and splenomegaly include organisms that can cause infectious mononucleosis (IM) or an IM-like syndrome, tuberculosis, histoplasmosis, rubella, and cat scratch disease. IM is caused by EBV, but cytomegalovirus, human herpesvirus-6, and acute human immunodeficiency virus (HIV) infection can produce similar symptoms. Tuberculosis usually presents with pulmonary symptoms in a young child, but if the infection is primarily extrapulmonary, it often presents as lymphadenitis (inflammation of the lymph node). In the latter case, most patients have symptoms confined to the cervical or supraclavicular lymph nodes and splenomegaly is uncommon. Disseminated (miliary) tuberculosis and acute disseminated histoplasmosis frequently present with fever, lymphadenopathy, and hepatosplenomegaly; however, pulmonary disease (especially later in the course of disease) and anemia also accompany these symptoms. Rubella has a classic clinical picture of fever and rash and can present with cervical lymphadenopathy, but diffuse lymphadenopathy and sore throat are uncommon. Cat scratch disease is usually associated with painful regional lymphadenopathy and fever is less common. Toxoplasmosis also needs to be considered in a patient with fever and lymphadenopathy, but it only infrequently causes pharyngitis and splenomegaly. Acute HIV infection (acute retroviral syndrome) can present with fever, pharyngitis, and lymphadenopathy, but splenomegaly and hepatomegaly do not usually accompany this disease (see Case 9). Other infections that present with fever, lymphadenopathy, and splenomegaly include leishmaniasis and trypanosomiasis; however, these two diseases are not seen in persons who have not lived outside the United States. Of all the diseases listed above, the most common causes of fever and generalized lymphadenopathy in children are IM, toxoplasmosis, HIV, cat scratch disease, and tuberculosis. IM is the disease that also accounts for the hepatosplenomegaly.

With this differential diagnosis in mind, you send routine laboratory tests that focus on Mark's hematologic and liver status. The following results are obtained:

Parameter	Results	Reference Range
Blood Counts		
Red blood cells (RBC)	$4.5 \times 10^6/\mu L$	4.5–$5.3 \times 10^6/\mu L$
Hemoglobin (Hgb)	13.2 g/dL	11.5–15.5 g/dL
Hematocrit (Hct)	41.2%	34–45%
WBC	20,000/μL	5000–15,000/μL
Platelets (PLT)	275,000/μL	130,000–400,000/μL

Parameter	Results	Reference Range
Neutrophils	25%	40–74%
Lymphocytes	40%	20–48%
Atypical lymphocytes[a]	20%	0–4%
Monocytes	4%	3.4–9%
Eosinophils	1%	0–7%
Basophils	0%	0–1.5%
Selected Chemistries[b]		
Alanine aminotransferases (ALT)	550 IU	7–55 IU
Aspartate aminotransferases (AST)	650 IU	8–60 IU

[a] Atypical lymphocytes seen are characterized by enlargement of the cytoplasm, indented edges, and cytoplasmic vacuoles.
[b] All other chemistry values were within reference range.

How do Mark's history and these findings narrow the differential diagnosis?

The presence of an elevated WBC count in the absence of anemia and thrombocytopenia points toward an infection rather than a malignancy. AST (previously known as SGOT) is an enzyme found in liver, muscle, kidney, and brain, while ALT (or SGPT) is mostly found in liver. Elevation of both enzymes indicates damage to liver cells, although not necessarily liver disease. Viral hepatitis (caused by a number of different types of viruses) is associated with high levels of AST and ALT, which revert to normal upon resolution of the infection.

Of the various infections in the differential diagnosis, EBV-associated infectious mononucleosis is strongly favored, since in this disease the most frequent presenting symptoms are fever, sore throat, and malaise and the physical examination usually discloses lymphadenopathy. Splenomegaly is present in about half of cases occurring in children and approximately 30% have hepatomegaly as well. This diagnosis is also favored by the presence of atypical lymphocytes in the circulation. This clinical constellation (including the atypical lymphocytes) can also be found in other infections, but in each case they do not fit Mark's situation as well. For example, cytomegalovirus infection can present with similar findings but usually occurs in adolescents and adults. In addition, lymphadenopathy and splenomegaly are less common than in EBV infection. Similarly, human herpesvirus-6 can be the cause of an IM-like illness; however, children with infection due to this organism present with roseola (exanthema subitum), in which the rash follows the fever. Finally, acute viral hepatitis, due to one of the hepatitis viruses themselves, and toxoplasmosis often present with fever and fatigue, but lymphadenopathy is unusual in the former disease, and in the latter case pharyngitis and splenomegaly are less frequent.

At this point you suspect that Mark has IM, probably due to EBV infection. In view of the fact that a sibling had a similar infectious illness that was fatal, you turn his care over to an infectious disease specialist who is also knowledgeable about immunodeficiency states. This physician sees the patient promptly and orders serologic tests to help him establish whether EBV infection (rather than infection with another virus) is in fact the cause of the child's illness. The specialist has Mark admitted to the hospital for IV antibiotic treatment and supportive care.

Initial Course, Treatment, and Further Diagnostic Tests

Upon admission, Mark is placed in reverse isolation (in view of the possibility that he has an immunodeficiency disorder) and is treated with intravenous acyclovir and intravenous immunoglobulin. However, over the ensuing 48 h he continues to have high fevers and his transaminases continue to rise, with the ALT now at 1200 IU and the AST at 1800 IU, signaling continued hepatic cell damage.

The results of serologic tests submitted at the time of admission now become available. While a monospot test is negative, tests for antibodies specific for EBV viral capsid antigen (VCA) reveal a titer of 1:160 for IgM and a titer of 1:80 for IgG. On the other hand, the IgM immunofluorescent antibody test (IgM IFA) for toxoplasmosis and the IgM antibody test for cytomegalovirus are negative. Similarly, hepatitis A IgM, anti–hepatitis B core antibody, and hepatitis B surface antigen are negative.

What is a monospot test and what is the significance of IgM versus IgG titers to these infectious organisms?

The monospot test is used to detect heterophil antibodies, which nonspecifically cause clumping or agglutination of sheep or horse RBC (see below). IgM antibodies to antigens of specific organisms provide evidence of an acute or current infection, while IgG antibodies are indicative of an acute or past infection with that organism. Some organisms, such as hepatitis B, produce acute and chronic disease that can be diagnosed by following the pattern of antigen expression and antibody response to the surface, core, and envelope proteins. Mark's results indicate response to an acute EBV infection.

The infectious disease specialist is fairly certain that Mark has an acute EBV infection. The negative monospot test does not carry much weight in this situation because, although it is usually positive in adolescents and young adults with IM, it is often negative in young children with EBV infection. This is why EBV-specific serologic tests are particularly useful for the diagnosis of this disease in young children.

Meanwhile, you investigate more of the family history with Mark's parents and discover that, in addition to a brother with fatal IM, two maternal uncles died from

Hodgkin lymphoma during childhood. In view of this family history and Mark's severe acute illness, a diagnosis of the genetic disorder **X-linked lymphoproliferative syndrome (XLPS)** is entertained.

XLPS is an immunodeficiency disease that occurs in young boys who are usually healthy until they become infected with EBV and then develop severe or even fatal IM frequently associated, as in Mark's case, with a fulminant EBV hepatitis. Severe and potentially fatal IM can also occur sporadically in the absence of a family history of severe EBV infection (see further discussion below).

The specialist orders a test to detect the presence of the **SLAM-Associated Protein (SAP)**, which has been shown to be absent in CD8$^+$ cytotoxic T cells of most patients with XLPS (see discussion below). This is a flow cytometry–based assay. Several days later, the results of this test are returned and show that the SAP protein is indeed absent in Mark's CD8$^+$ T cells.

Further Hospital Course and Rationale for Treatment

Recognizing the gravity of the situation, Mark's physician now provides maximal therapy for systemic EBV infection. Initially, Mark is treated with high-dose corticosteroids (methylprednisone in divided doses), along with the acyclovir and intravenous immunoglobulin (IVIG), but this does not stem the course of the inflammation. Mark's liver enzymes rise further over the next several days, and he has onset of gastrointestinal bleeding. Mark is now transferred to the pediatric intensive care unit where he is given supportive care; platelets, fresh frozen plasma, and packed RBC transfusions, and one dose of anti-CD20 antibody (rituximab). At this point, Mark's liver enzyme levels stabilize, his bleeding stops, and his condition gradually improves over the next few weeks. His fever, lymphadenopathy, and hepatosplenomegaly gradually abate. This allows his physician to slowly taper the steroids and switch Mark to oral acyclovir. After six weeks in the hospital, Mark is finally improved enough to be discharged home.

What is the rationale for Mark's various treatments?

Acyclovir is an agent which inhibits the replication of EBV. However, this treatment merely contains the infection, because it is effective only against replicating virus and therefore does not eliminate the nonreplicating latent EBV, which drives the proliferation of EBV-infected B cells. Mark is treated with IVIG because this is a source of neutralizing antibody to EBV. IVIG is derived from pooled donors, most of whom have been infected with EBV in the past. While anti-EBV antibodies may limit the spread of cell-free EBV, it does not have an effect on latently infected proliferating B cells and thus cannot completely clear the infection. Thus, its effectiveness in the severe EBV infection in Mark's case is limited. Immunosuppressive therapy with corticosteroids is given in an attempt to control the life-threatening hepatitis that is caused by the T-cell proliferation resulting from the

infection. However, corticosteroids were insufficient (as in most cases of EBV hepatitis) and anti-CD20 monoclonal antibody (rituximab) is added to Mark's regimen. Rituximab, directed against a surface marker on mature B cells, eliminates B cells, which are the main reservoir for EBV in the body. Treatment with rituximab markedly diminishes the number of virus-infected B cells and thereby likely limits the proliferation and activation of T cells in response to the EBV infection. Finally, Mark is given fresh frozen plasma containing clotting factors to stem the gastrointestinal bleeding resulting from the deterioration in his liver function and loss of the liver's ability to synthesize clotting factors. Platelet transfusions are also given because patients with bleeding disorders rapidly consume platelets.

Follow-Up Care

At a follow-up outpatient visit two weeks after discharge, Mark appears well. Recognizing that EBV infection associated with XLPS is frequently followed by the development of hypogammaglobulinemia, Mark's physician has blood drawn for determination of immunoglobulin levels. Indeed, the results of this test show that Mark has hypogammaglobulinemia. To prevent the occurrence of severe respiratory infections to which Mark is susceptible given his low immunoglobulin levels, Mark begins monthly infusions of IVIG.

Mark's parents are asked to visit a genetic counselor to obtain information on the inheritance of XLPS and the chances of having additional children with the disease.

THE BODY'S NATURAL RESPONSE TO EBV

EBV is a double-stranded DNA virus, a member of the Herpes family. It is ubiquitous throughout the world; however, exposure varies in different climates. The virus enters human B cells via its receptor CD21 on the cell surface. There, the linear viral DNA circularizes to form an episome within the nucleus. In the B cell, the virus may cause a productive infection—replicating in and lysing the host B cell, and thus releasing virions to infect additional cells.

In most B cells, the virus takes a latent form. B cells with latent virus will express the full complement of EBV latency-associated genes and are therefore positive for Epstein–Barr nuclear antigen (EBNA) 1 and 2 and latent membrane protein (LMP) 1 and 2. These B cells are normally eliminated by the body's immune system, specifically by cytotoxic cells, mainly CD8$^+$ T cells but natural killer (NK) cells as well. The reactive T cells proliferate in the lymph nodes and spleen, causing their enlargement, and circulate in the peripheral blood as "atypical" lymphocytes. They are anything but atypical; they are normal activated cytotoxic T cells required for the body to control the EBV infection. The infected B cells are capable of secreting antibodies and make immunoglobulins that nonspecifically agglutinate sheep or horse RBC. These properties of the antibodies form the basis for the heterophil antibody test or monospot used in the diagnosis of IM. The constellation of reactions just described, along with fever, muscle aches, and malaise as the result of cytokine production, are in fact recognizable as the clinical presentation of IM. Some patients present with a hepatitis picture due to the infiltration of the liver by lymphocytes and subsequent necrosis (death) of liver cells. In addition to the cytotoxic reaction, which is most important in controlling the infection, the infected individual will produce specific antibodies to EBV: "early" or IgM antibody against the viral capsid antigen and "late" or IgG antibody, which persists for the patient's lifetime. These are the footprints of recent and remote EBV infection, respectively.

A small population of resting B cells may retain the virus in latent form, expressing only EBNA1 and LMP2. However, the virus can at any time reactivate EBNA2 and LMP1, causing B-cell proliferation. EBNA2 stimulates transcription of several host genes, specifically cyclin D, which results in cell cycle progression from G_2 to S. LMP1 mimics B-cell activation by CD40 stimulation; in fact, an autostimulatory loop of CD40/CD40L expression and stimulation is established in the infected B cell. EBV is thus a polyclonal activator, or mitogen, for human B cells that actually acts from inside the cell.

This continuous proliferation or transformation of the B cell, unchecked by the individual's immune system, also creates a fertile soil for malignant transformation. Specifically, a translocation between c-*myc* and an immunoglobulin gene, usually the heavy-chain gene [t(8;14)], leads to the overexpression of MYC, contributing to the proliferative push. Those cells may undergo additional genetic mutations, most importantly mutations in *p53* or other tumor suppressor genes, resulting in malignant transformation of the B cell. Thus, although EBV by itself is neither necessary nor sufficient for the malignant transformation process, there is a strong association of the virus with Burkitt lymphoma, diffuse large B-cell lymphoma (DLBCL), nasopharyngeal carcinoma (there is some evidence that EBV can infect epithelial cells), and possibly Hodgkin lymphoma. Burkitt lymphoma cells no longer express the virally encoded membrane antigens that serve as cytotoxic T-cell targets. For endemic Burkitt lymphoma and nasopharyngeal carcinoma, the association with EBV is virtually 100%. For nonendemic Burkitt, DLBCL, and Hodgkin lymphoma, it is lower. As one might expect, a T-cell immunodeficiency, such as in AIDS patients or in iatrogenically immunosuppressed transplant patients, can allow first a polyclonal and oligoclonal B-cell proliferation followed by progression to a monoclonal B-cell tumor.

CLINICAL FEATURES OF XLPS

Mark's course mirrors the majority of cases of XLPS in that the most common presentation of this disease is fulminant IM in young boys (mean age three years) (Table 7.1). In the absence of effective treatment, EBV infection affecting the liver commonly leads to hepatic failure and, affecting the bone marrow, frequently leads to anemia, leukopenia, and thrombocytopenia. In such cases, death due to gastrointestinal or central nervous system hemorrhage, hepatic encephalopathy, or opportunistic infections due to impaired immune responses often ensues.

Another frequent manifestation of XLPS is hypogammaglobulinemia. While this is commonly noted in patients who survive EBV infection, it may also be present in patients with no history of such infection. Typically, the patients have low serum levels of IgG, associated with elevated levels of IgM and/or IgA; however, in some cases serum levels of all immunoglobulin classes are decreased.

The incidence of lymphomas is increased in XLPS patients, regardless of whether the patient has had an EBV infection. This is thought to result from the immunodeficiency and defective immune surveillance. Most of the lymphomas are B-cell lymphomas that occur outside the lymph nodes, notably in the intestine, central nervous system, and kidneys. The most frequent type of lymphoma in patients with XLPS is Burkitt lymphoma, usually involving the intestine, followed by DLBCL.

Less common complications of XLPS include aplastic anemia, vasculitis involving the central nervous system, or lymphomatoid granulomatosis that can cause severe damage to the lungs or brain.

The prognosis of XLPS is "guarded"; fewer than 10% of patients survive the fulminant IM that usually heralds the recognition of this disease. Hopefully, this percentage will increase with currently available therapy, such as that given to Mark. Patients who survive the EBV infection, however,

 TABLE 7.1. Clinical Manifestations of XLPS

Clinical Phenotype	Frequency (%)	Survival Rates (%)
Fulminant IM	58	4
Lymphoproliferative disorders[a]	30	35
Dysgammaglobulinemia[a]	31	55
Aplastic anemia	3	50
Vasculitis, lymphomatoid granulomatosis	3	29

[a]These phenotypes occur in some patients with XLPS and no exposure to EBV.

Source: Seemayer TA, et al. (1995): X-linked lymphoproliferative disease: Twenty-five years after the discovery. *Pediatric Res* 38:471–478.

almost always develop hypogammaglobulinemia and are at risk for B-cell lymphomas later in life.

PATHOLOGIC FEATURES OF XLPS

The liver is usually involved in EBV infection associated with XLPS, and liver failure is the most frequent cause of death (Fig. 7.1). Hepatomegaly is due to infiltration of the liver by T and B cells as well as due to increased amounts of fat and fluid. Staining of liver tissue for EBV-encoded RNAs (EBERs) is usually positive, indicating the presence of virus-infected B cells. If the inflammatory process does not resolve, hepatic necrosis can occur. In addition, even with lesser degrees of hepatic decompensation, the failure to produce hepatic clotting factors can result and lead to death due to hemorrhage.

The lymph nodes and spleen usually show proliferation of B and T cells as well as infiltration with macrophages, which can efface the normal architecture. If B- and T-cell proliferation is not controlled, necrosis of the lymph nodes can occur. EBER-positive B cells are frequently present as well as evidence of EBV-associated *erythrophagocytosis* or *leukophagocytosis*. This ingestion of RBCs or WBCs by macrophages is the result of their enhanced phagocytic activity in response to the T_H1 cytokines in the environment.

Early in the course of EBV infection associated with XLPS, the bone marrow contains an increased number of hematopoietic precursors. Then, as the disease progresses, the marrow becomes infiltrated with lymphocytes and phagocytic cells and there is loss of the normal cellular components. When severe, this infiltration is associated with bone marrow failure. Other organs, including the intestine, brain, and lung, are also often affected by the infectious process.

THE MAJOR GENETIC DEFECT IN XLPS: SAP MUTATIONS

XLPS is usually due to a mutation in a gene located on the X chromosome, the gene designated as *SH2D1A* that encodes SAP. The SAP gene mutations found in XLP are diverse, but in each case they lead to an absent, unstable, or nonfunctioning SAP protein in males. Female carriers are asymptomatic.

XLPS is a rare syndrome (one to three cases per million births) and is referred to as a syndrome rather than a disease because patients who lack SAP mutations have also been identified with a course identical to that described above for Mark. These cases are caused by one or more other genetic defects that are not necessarily X-linked; thus females as well as males can be affected.

SAP Function

The SAP gene is expressed in a wide variety of hematopoietic cells, including T cells, NK cells, NKT cells, B cells,

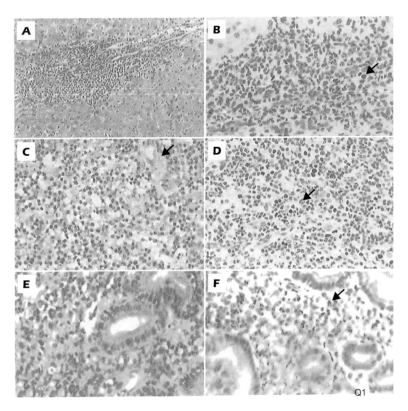

Figure 7.1. Pathology of acute EBV infection in a patient with XLPS. Hematoxylin and eosin stained sections of (**A**) liver, (**C**) lymph node, and (**E**) intestine show a predominant lymphocytic infiltrate in the liver and intestine and macrophage (arrow) infiltrate in the lymph node. In situ hybridization with an EBV encoded RNA EBER probe shows EBV-infected lymphocytes (arrows, brown staining) in (**B**) liver, (**D**) lymph node, and (**F**) intestine. [Reproduced with permission from Nichols KE (2000): X-linked lymphoproliferative disease: genetics and biochemistry. *Rev Immunogenet* 2:256–286.]

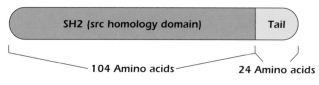

 Figure 7.2. Structure of the SAP protein.

eosinophils, and platelets. Thus, mutations in this gene have the potential to affect the functions of many cells. The SAP gene product, SAP protein, is an intracytoplasmic adaptor molecule that links surface receptor molecules with downstream effector molecules, thereby facilitating receptor signaling. It consists of a protein-binding domain, termed SH2 (src homology-2), attached to a short tail (Fig. 7.2). During cell activation and the formation of the complex of molecules on the cell surface comprising the "immunologic synapse," one region of the SH2 domain of SAP binds to the cytoplasmic tail of one or more of at least six surface receptor molecules known as the **SLAM (signaling lymphocyte activation molecule)** family of receptors (Table 7.2). These include the T-cell surface receptor SLAM (CD150) itself as well as the NK-cell receptors 2B4 and NTBA. Such binding is then followed (via a second SH2 site) by SAP interaction with and activation of the tyrosine kinase, FYN, and other tyrosine kinases that phosphorylate the cytoplasmic tails of SLAM, 2B4, and perhaps other surface molecules. Thus, docking sites for downstream molecules positively or negatively involved in cell-signaling programs are created.

The Impact of SAP Mutations on Immunologic Function

Insight into the function of SAP has come from SAP knockout mice that lack the SAP gene and thus cannot express the SAP protein. These mice are susceptible to infections with certain viruses, such as lymphocytic choriomeningitis virus. SAP knockout mice cannot become infected with EBV since mice lack the EBV receptor. SAP knockout mice exhibit exaggerated T_H1 responses characterized by the production of high amounts of interferon-γ (IFN-γ) upon stimulation, associated with a reciprocal defect in the ability to mount T_H2 responses (IL-4 and IL-10). Other

defects in SAP-deficient mice include defects in mounting T- or NK cell-mediated cytotoxic responses and the inability to generate memory B cells, probably due to lack of T-cell help. Thus, SAP deficiency leads to increases in some immune functions and decreases in others. This is to be expected, given the fact that SAP is involved in a number of different signaling pathways, some having positive effects and others having negative effects. In any case, the effect of SAP deficiency in mice is an increased susceptibility to viral infection with impaired ability to produce long-term antibody responses.

Patients with XLPS have defects in the functions of T cells, NK cells, and B cells that to some extent mimic those seen in the SAP-deficient mice (Table 7.3). However, these abnormalities are sufficiently subtle to escape detection until after the patient presents with EBV infection and is thus subjected to more intense immunologic study. The most prominent T-cell abnormality consists of a defect in cytotoxic function; this is most notably manifested by an impaired killing of autologous EBV-infected B cells. This decrease in cytotoxic function extends to NK cells as well, in this case involving both spontaneous and IFN-γ-induced cytotoxic function. In addition, following stimulation or in the presence of infection, the helper T cells display overexuberant T_H1 responses characterized by excessive production of IFN-γ and other T_H1 cytokines. Finally, B-cell function in patients with XLPS is impaired and includes a failure to switch from IgM to IgG after immunization, resulting

TABLE 7.3. Immunologic Abnormalities Associated with XLPS

Cell Type	Immune Defect
B cell	Hypogammaglobulinemia; impaired anti-EBNA IgG
NK cell	Decreased cytotoxicity against target cells; decreased IFN-γ-stimulated NK-cell activity
T cell	Defective killing of autologous EBV-infected B cells; reduced proliferation to mitogens; uncontrolled T_H1 responses; excessive production of IFN-γ
NKT cell	Reduced innate responses to infection

TABLE 7.2. Proteins That Bind to SAP and Their Activities

Protein	Location	Effect of SAP Interaction with Protein
SLAM	T cells, B cells, dendritic cells	Inhibits IFN-γ production when T cells are activated through T-cell receptor
2B4	NK cells, T cells	NK cell proliferation and cytotoxicity
NTB-A	NK cells, T cells, B cells	NK cell proliferation and cytotoxicity
Ly9	B cells, T cells	Not reported
CD84	B cells, myeloid cells	Not reported

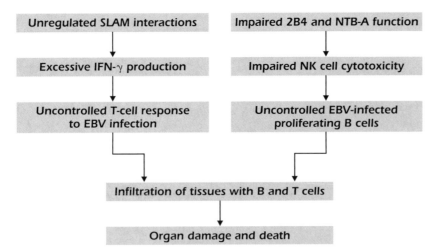

Figure 7.3. Model of SAP function relating to the control of the immune response to EBV.

in low levels of IgG. This process requires T helper cell help (see Case 4). This failure in switching is manifested by impaired antibody responses to EBV, including reduced or absent responses to EBNAs.

The absence of the SAP protein in humans may result in impaired NK-cell killing of EBV-infected B cells, allowing uncontrolled proliferation of the virus-infected cells (Fig. 7.3). The excessive T_H1 responses and IFN-γ levels may stimulate the overexuberant proliferation of T cells and macrophages that could then cause uncontrolled B- and T-cell infiltration of tissues or the severe inflammatory responses characteristic of patients with XLPS. This can lead to the severe hepatitis and bone marrow failure that occur during acute EBV infection in these patients. It is still unclear why patients with XLPS have severe and often fatal EBV infections but do not have severe infections with related viruses such as herpes varicella-zoster virus (chickenpox) or herpes simplex virus (cold sores).

TREATMENT AND PREVENTION OF XLPS

Specific facets of therapy of EBV infection occurring in XLPS have already been discussed in relation to Mark's treatment. Here we focus on general principles of therapy that are applicable to all patients.

Acyclovir and IVIG infusions have been used to limit virus replication and to neutralize cell-free virus, respectively. Unfortunately, much of the B-cell proliferation is driven by virus expressed in latently infected B cells that are beyond the reach of such therapy. Thus, at best, acyclovir or immunoglobulin therapy can do no more than limit the spread of virus.

Much of the immunopathology of XLPS is due to infiltrating T cells and the cytokines that they produce. Thus, despite the fact that it may seem counterintuitive to administer immunosuppressive therapy during an infection, such therapy has proven useful. Regimens targeting T cells

or macrophages, including corticosteroids, etoposide (VP-16), or cyclosporine, have been used with some benefit. However, recent experience has shown that T-cell proliferation may be better controlled with the use of monoclonal anti-B-cell antibody, anti-CD20 (rituximab), since this agent depletes B cells and thus eliminates the EBV-infected B cells stimulating the T-cell response.

Patients who survive infection with EBV and who develop hypogammaglobulinemia are treated with monthly infusions of IVIG. Patients with lymphomas are treated with cytotoxic chemotherapy.

At present a vaccine able to prevent EBV infection is not available. Even if one were available, it is not certain that patients with XLPS would be able to mount a protective anti-EBV response. IVIG is recommended for patients who have not yet been infected with EBV, since the product contains antibodies that can neutralize virus. Unfortunately, patients have developed fatal EBV infections despite the use of immunoglobulin therapy.

The only truly effective modality to prevent XLPS and its associated complications is stem cell transplantation. Patients who receive transplants at younger ages (<15 years old) have a more favorable outcome than older patients. Since the gene associated with XLPS has been identified, the disease may be amenable to gene therapy in the future.

REFERENCES

Cohen JI (2003): Benign and malignant Epstein-Barr virus-associated B-cell lymphoproliferative diseases. *Semin Hematol* 40:116–123.

Engel P, Eck MJ, Terhorst C (2003): The SAP and SLAM families in immune responses and X-linked lymphoproliferative disease. *Nature Rev Immunol* 3:813–821.

Gaspar HB, Sharifi R, Gilmour KC, Thrasher AJ (2002): X-linked lymphoproliferative disease: Clinical, diagnostic and molecular perspective. *Br J Haematol* 119:585–595.

Ma CS, Nichols KE, Tangye SG (2007): Regulation of cellular and humoral immune responses by the SLAM and SAP families of molecules. *Annu Rev Immunol* 25:337–379.

Milone MC, Tsai DE, Hodinka RL, Silverman LB, Malbran A, Wasik MA, Nichols KE (2005): Treatment of primary Epstein-Barr virus infection in patients with X-linked lymphoproliferative disease using B-cell-directed therapy. *Blood* 105:994–996.

Nichols KE (2000): X-linked lymphoproliferative disease: Genetics and biochemistry. *Rev Immunogenet* 2:256–286.

Seemayer TA, Gross TG, Egeler RM, Pirruccello SJ, Davis JR, Kelly CM, Okano M, Lanyi A, Sumegi J (1995): X-linked lymphoproliferative disease: Twenty-five years after the discovery. *Ped Res* 38:471–478.

8

HEREDITARY ANGIOEDEMA

MILAN BASTA*

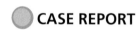

CASE REPORT

"My student's face swelled up."

Days 1–2: Clinical Presentation and Workup

Charlie, a 16-year-old high school junior, is brought to the emergency room of a small hospital by his school counselor where you see him as the emergency room physician on call; you are an allergist-immunologist in your regular practice. He has obvious massive swelling of his lower lip and face and is directed to you for urgent evaluation.

The swelling of his face is severe, but you immediately note that he is having no difficulty breathing. As you begin your preliminary examination, you ask him a few questions. He can speak with some difficulty.

Charlie relates that at the time the swelling started he was taking his semester final examination in physics and had encountered a problem that he could not answer. He is particularly anxious about physics, since he intends to apply for a special engineering scholarship. Charlie says that he is usually confident during tests and is an A student. He denies any allergies, eating new foods, or using new toiletries or drugs that morning. Charlie is athletic and has had no joint pain or swelling or muscle cramps. He does

recall one similar incident of facial swelling a few months ago when he and his girlfriend broke up, but he stayed alone in his room until the next day and did not tell anyone. When asked specifically about the current swelling, he says that, although it is uncomfortable and embarrassing, it is neither painful nor itchy.

Your initial examination reveals large, nonpitting, painless edema (swelling) of the lower lip and both sides of the face that has caused almost complete shutdown of his eyelids. He is breathing without difficulty and without stridor, which excludes edema of the air passages, the larynx specifically. The involved skin has normal temperature and there are no signs of urticaria (hives). His lungs are clear. The abdomen is not distended or tender to palpation.

What are the possible underlying causes of edema?

*Edema, an increase in fluid between cells, in this case is present in the deep dermis or subcutaneous or submucosal tissue. Specifically, this is a case of **angioedema**, caused by dilatation and increased permeability of the capillaries rather than edema secondary to systemic cardiovascular difficulties; the latter would be seen in dependent areas, usually the lower extremities. The separation of endothelial cells which allows fluid to escape may have several causes. It may be due to the release of vasoactive mediators in an allergic reaction (see Case 11); damage to the vessels*

---

*With contribution from Warren Strober and Susan R. S. Gottesman *resulting from immune complex deposition as is seen in autoimmune diseases (see Cases 22 and 13); infectious organisms; or abnormalities of the **complement system**, the cascade of enzymatically active proteins that participate in the body's innate and humoral immune responses (see discussion below).*

What is the significance of the absence of itching and urticaria?

Angioedema often accompanies urticaria in severe allergic reactions (see Case 11). The lack of itching or wheals and hives suggests that the underlying problem is not allergen related. This helps narrow the broad differential diagnosis but does not direct your immediate therapy.

Charlie's parents have arrived and you explain to all three of them that, even though there is no evidence that the airways are compromised, your goal is to maintain their patency. Since you do not yet have a diagnosis as to the underlying cause of the edema, you intend to treat with a combination of steroids (prednisone), subcutaneous epinephrine, and diphenhydramine (an antihistamine), since these cover the broad base of different conditions characterized by swelling. With his parents' permission, you proceed with the treatment and also send a series of blood tests including complete blood count (CBC), chemistries, immunoglobulin (Ig) levels, and complement component (C) levels in addition to a urine analysis.

You keep Charlie in the emergency room for treatment and observation. During that time you take a history from his parents. They relate that Charlie has always been healthy, with only the occasional seasonal colds and ear infections. No unusual or frequent infections have been noted in Charlie or in his two siblings. They also confirm the absence of a history of allergies and joint or muscle problems. Both parents report being healthy themselves, although on specific questioning his mother relates that she used to experience episodes of severe abdominal pain. One incident led to an appendectomy; however, the appendix was not inflamed and no underlying cause for the pain was ever found. The episodes became less frequent and she has not experienced one for years. Her parents attributed these to the "hysteria" of teenage and early adult years. She remembers that her father (Charlie's grandfather) said that he had episodes of facial swelling when stressed. He is now 73 years old and in good health.

What is suggested by this family history?

If the family history of facial swelling and abdominal pain are linked, the possibility of an inherited syndrome, or at least a familial tendency towards a disease, becomes likely. If this inherited syndrome is due to a single gene mutation, it would presumably be an autosomal dominant mutation since it affects both males and females and does not skip a generation.

Charlie's age at presentation, lack of frequent infections, and the current health of his mother and grandfather eliminate many of the immunodeficiency diseases which we have discussed in preceding chapters and which have full penetrance and severe clinical courses, such as hyper-IgM syndrome (see Case 4). Common variable immunodeficiency (see Case 5) is unlikely given the lack of infections in his history. As alluded to above, the differential diagnoses in this case include allergic states and autoimmune diseases rather than immunodeficiency disease.

After a few hours, the swelling has not gotten worse, although it has not significantly improved after treatment with prednisone and diphenhydramine as you would expect in an allergic reaction. This leads you to suspect that the cause of Charlie's swelling is not an allergic reaction and brings to the fore the possibility of a complement problem. Routine laboratory tests (CBC, chemistries, and urine analysis) are now available and are normal with the exception of an elevated hematocrit value. You assume that this is due to a shift of fluid from the intravascular space to the extravascular space during the acute episode. Since Charlie lives nearby, you decide to send him home with instructions to come back immediately if the swelling worsens or if he feels any shortness of breath or chest tightening. You set up an appointment to see him at your office the next day.

When you see Charlie the next day, you note that his upper lip swelling has completely resolved and the swelling of his face has subsided as well. You are satisfied with Charlie's progress, but you ask him to return to the office one more time the following day to make certain that the symptoms have cleared completely.

Day 3: Diagnosis

Charlie comes to your office once again, this time in the company of his parents. The facial swelling has now resolved completely, and it is clear that the swelling episode is over. The remaining test results are back, and you review them to determine if they provide you with a diagnosis.

As indicated above, routine CBC, chemistries, and urine analysis results were available earlier and were significant only for an increased hematocrit. Ig levels are normal, including the level of IgE (see Case 11). Complement component (C) measurements show normal levels of C1q, but concentrations of both C4 and C2 are decreased. In addition, the level of C1 esterase inhibitor (C1-INH) is decreased to 7.0 mg/dL (normal serum concentration is 10–25 mg/dL) as is the level of C1-INH determined in a functional assay for this component.

Circulating immune complex (CIC) levels are not increased and the serum histamine level is normal.

How do you interpret these results?

These results give no indication of an ongoing allergic reaction, which would usually be accompanied by an elevated IgE level, an abnormal white blood cell (WBC) differential with increased eosinophils, and/or an elevated serum histamine level. In addition, the normal WBC count does not support an infectious agent. On the other hand, studies related to the complement system do show abnormal findings. In particular, levels of both C2 and C4, components of the classical complement pathway (see below), are decreased. This could be due to decreased production on a genetic basis, but this is unlikely since two components are affected. A major cause of decreased production, infection, is not present. Alternatively, the decreased C2 and C4 levels could be due to increased consumption, as is seen in immune complex diseases or in uncontrolled activation of the complement cascade. Immune complex disease is unlikely in view of the normal CIC result. On the other hand, Charlie has an abnormally low concentration of C1-INH, an enzyme that normally inhibits the complement cascade by its inhibition of C1 esterase activity. Thus, C1-INH deficiency would result in uncontrolled activation of the complement system and low C2 and C4 levels due to excessive consumption of these components.

On the basis of these laboratory findings you conclude that the cause of the swelling episode is a C1-INH deficiency. Since Charlie has a positive family history, you conclude that this deficiency is due to one of the three forms of hereditary angioedema (see discussion below).

Proposed Treatment

You explain to Charlie and his parents that he has ***hereditary angioedema (HAE)*** and that this abnormality of the complement system led to uncontrolled complement activation. You explain further that complement activation results in leakage of fluid from small blood vessel walls and that this was the cause of Charlie's facial swelling (and his mother's episodes of abdominal pain). For some reason, stress can precipitate this complement reaction; in fact, HAE was originally called angioneurotic edema. Finally, you stress that swelling due to HAE can be dangerous if it occurs in an area of the body that threatens the airway, such as the larynx. Because of this potentially serious complication, you propose a plan of prophylactic therapy that will reduce the possibility of a serious swelling episode during this stressful school year. You prescribe danazol (an androgen) since, when taken every two to three days, this agent has been shown to reduce the frequency of HAE attacks. Furthermore, you emphasize that if Charlie is to have any type of surgery or dental procedure, events that could provoke an HAE attack, he will require prophylaxis on a daily basis for 10 days before the potential triggering event.

DIFFERENTIAL DIAGNOSIS OF HEREDITARY ANGIOEDEMA

HAE should be considered when one is faced with a patient who has a family and personal history of recurrent painless swelling of the extremities and face, compromised airways, or abdominal pain. In spite of its self-limiting course of three to four days, it is important to correctly diagnose and differentiate this condition from other edematous states due to its association with potentially fatal airway obstruction and its high rate of recurrence. HAE is often misdiagnosed because its symptoms mimic several common conditions such as allergic reactions, acute appendicitis, gallbladder attack, submucosal abdominal tumor, diverticulitis, and irritable bowel syndrome. When a family history is not available, initial misdiagnosis is common and leads to unnecessary and ineffective medical procedures, such as laparoscopy, administration of antihistamines and corticosteroids, and/or psychiatric referrals (due to "unexplained" recurrent abdominal pain).

Subcutaneous swelling due to HAE must be distinguished from subcutaneous swelling due to an allergic reaction (allergic angioedema). Several features of the latter usually allow one to distinguish between these two conditions. First, allergic angioedema is characterized by coincident urticaria (hives), an easily recognized manifestation marked by a wheal-and-flare reaction and considerable itchiness. Second, allergic angioedema is mast cell/histamine–mediated and thus responds to therapy with antihistamines and steroids. However, if allergic angioedema involves the face and throat, it can progress to involve swelling of the tongue and larynx, occlusion of the airways, and acute dyspnea (shortness of breath). Under these circumstances, differentiation between HAE and allergic reaction on clinical grounds alone may be more difficult and may require laboratory study. In either case, one should be prepared to perform a tracheotomy and then proceed with disease-specific treatment once the emergency has been taken care of and an accurate diagnosis has been established.

Drug-induced angioedema following exposure to multiple widely used agents can also mimic HAE. These agents include (but are not limited to) nonsteroidal anti-inflammatory drugs, angiotensin-converting enzyme (ACE) inhibitors, and estrogens. Patients with drug-induced angioedema are identified by careful history and lack of evidence of familial disease. In addition, this type of angioedema responds to cessation of drug administration.

Finally, hereditary angioedema has to be differentiated from acquired angioedema (AAE), a form of angioedema that results from increased destruction or consumption of C1-INH. There are two types of AAE. Type 1 occurs in patients with hematologic and lymphoproliferative disorders (including leukemia, multiple myeloma, macroglobulinemia, and essential cryoglobulinemia). These patients sometimes develop antibodies against specific immunoglobulins expressed on the surface of B cells, which results in the formation of immune complexes that lead to the activation of C1. This, in turn, leads to consumption of C1-INH, whose function it is to inactivate activated C1 by binding to it. If the amount of immune complex formation is sufficiently high, the consumption of C1-INH will exceed its synthetic rate and the level of C1-INH will decline. Type 2 AAE occurs in patients who develop IgG autoantibodies against the active site of C1-INH, leading to the blockade of its inhibitory function and its rapid catabolism. Patients with both types of AAE have significantly reduced levels of early classical complement components (see below), especially C1q, C4, and C2. Decreased C1q helps distinguish AAE from HAE, in which C1q levels are usually normal. Also, HAE presents in younger patients who have a family history of angioedema.

CLINICAL COURSE

The onset of HAE symptoms is usually in the first or second decade of life. Very few cases of perinatal angioedema have been reported. Some 40% of patients have their first HAE attack before the age of 5 years, while 75% experience it before age 15. HAE lasts a lifetime but appears to present with fewer symptoms as patients age. Five percent of adults carry the mutation for the C1-INH gene without symptoms and only become aware of it when their children present with symptoms of HAE.

Trauma, especially dental trauma, appears to be the most frequent event that precipitates HAE attacks. Other precipitating events include mental or physical stress, exercise, infection, alcohol consumption, anesthesia, menstruation, ovulation, and use of medications such as estrogen and ACE inhibitors.

All types of HAE present with similar symptoms characterized by edema involving major organ systems such as the skin, gastrointestinal tract, upper respiratory system, and occasionally the genitourinary tract. Edema is usually localized to a site in just one organ system, but combined involvement of two systems is not rare. In over 50% of cases attacks are localized to the skin, followed by localization to the gastrointestinal tract (~32%), gastrointestinal tract and skin (~7%), and larynx alone (~4%). Genitourinary involvement alone or a combination of genitourinary tract and skin accounts for the clinical presentation in about 5% of cases. The lifetime incidence of laryngeal attack is estimated at 70% and occurs at least once in over 95% of women with type III HAE. Mortality rates, resulting from laryngeal edema and subsequent asphyxiation, are estimated at 15–33%.

THE COMPLEMENT SYSTEM

As implied by its name, the major function of C1-INH is the prevention of autoactivation of the first component (C1) of the classical pathway complement system. To understand how C1-INH fits into the complement cascade as a whole, we need to briefly review the three complement pathways.

The *classical complement pathway* is initiated by C1, a complex pentameric molecule consisting of one C1q, two C1r, and two C1s molecules (Fig. 8.1A). The initiating event is the interaction of specific Ig with its target antigen and the binding of the C1q component of C1 to the constant domain of the Ig molecule; this is followed by the subsequent recruitment of C1r and C1s (see Fig. 11.1 for Ig structure). Incorporation of C1s into this complex allows the complex to acquire esterase activity and cleave the next complement component (C4) as well as the subsequent complement component C2, to create a complex (C4b/C2a) called C3 convertase that then activates and cleaves C3, the central and most abundant complement component.

The assembly of fragments from C2, C4, and C3 forms a complex (C4b/C2a/C3b) called C5 convertase, which then triggers a cascade of events in which complement components C5a to C9 activate each other in a "domino" fashion. They form a multimember complement complex called the membrane attack complex (MAC), which is responsible for the lysis of cells targeted by specific antibodies (Fig. 8.2). Activation of complement components refers to their cleavage into small fragments (C3a, C4a, C5a) that are released into the circulation where they exert potent biologic effects, while the remaining large fragments attach to the surface of the cell and to previously activated components, leading ultimately to the formation of MAC. The complement system can thus be somewhat arbitrarily divided into early components C1, C4, C2, and C3 and late components C5–C9.

Only some Ig isotypes "fix" complement to activate the classical pathway. These are IgM, IgG$_3$, IgG$_1$, and to a lesser extent IgG$_2$. In addition to the complement system's ability to cause direct killing of pathogens through its assembly of MAC, its various components function as opsonins (C3b), which promote phagocytosis by macrophages and neutrophils, and as anaphylatoxins (C3a, C4a, and C5a), which play a significant role in the development of systemic inflammatory reactions (Fig. 8.3A). Activated fragments of the C3 molecule (C3b and C3d) play roles in enhancing B-cell responses, in the removal of immune complexes and necrotic debris, and in the response to viruses (Fig. 8.3B).

The two other complement activation pathways—the lectin and alternative pathways (Fig. 8.1B, C and 8.4)—differ from each other and from the classical pathway in the recognition (initial) phase of activation and subsequent

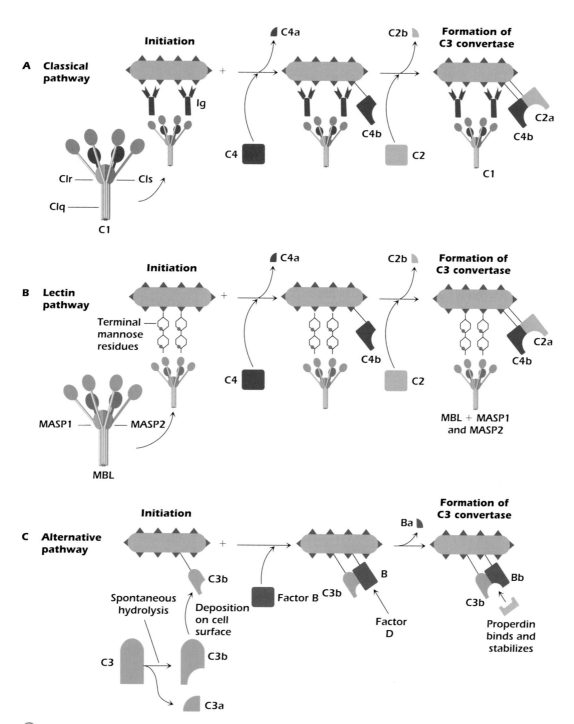

Figure 8.1. Activation of (**A**) classical, (**B**) lectin, and (**C**) alternative complement pathways, showing how each pathway is initiated and how C3 convertase is formed.

cleavage of C3. In the ***lectin pathway***, the initial component is mannose-binding lectin (MBL), a protein that recognizes pathogen-specific patterns of the simple sugar (mannan) residues expressed on an organism's cell surface. MBL is similar in structure to C1q; in conjunction with three associated serine proteases (MASP1–3) that are similar in function to C1r and C1s in the classical pathway, MBL can

activate C4 and C2. In this pathway, C1-INH inhibits the protease activity of MASP2.

The ***alternative pathway*** begins by direct spontaneous activation of C3 by water molecules in the fluid phase (so called C3 tick-over), without engaging early components of the classical pathway (Fig. 8.1C). C3 (H_2O) molecules are capable of reacting with Factor B to form C3bBb complexes

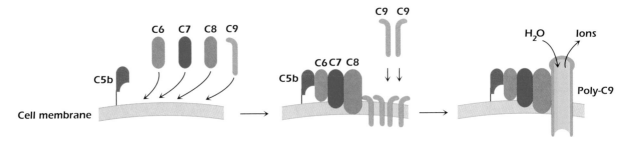

○ Figure 8.2. Formation of MAC. Late-stage complement components C5b–C9 bind sequentially to form a complex on the cell surface. Multiple C9 components bind to this complex and polymerize to form poly-C9, creating a channel that disrupts the cell membrane.

that, in turn, activate more C3 molecules, leading to assembly of C3b multimers and formation of (C3b)nBb. This process is tightly controlled by Factors H and I to prevent excessive and potentially autodestructive activation of the complement cascade. Amplification of the alternative pathway is initiated when cellular surfaces of pathogenic microorganisms provide a site where spontaneously activated molecules of C3 (C3b) are protected from regulatory actions of Factors H and I of the host. Multimers of C3b molecules then reach a point at which a critical mass of (C3b)nBb complexes is achieved and is sufficient to form the alternative pathway C5 convertase This convertase then triggers the assembly of the late complement components (C5–9) into the MAC (Fig. 8.4). It has been suggested that C1-INH might down-regulate the alternative pathway convertase and intercept the amplification loop by binding to C3b molecules, thus inhibiting binding of Factor B to C3b.

C1-INH Interaction with Non-Complement Proteases

In addition to inhibition of complement system-associated proteases, C1-INH is a major inhibitor of several proteases that play a key role in contact, coagulation, and fibrinolytic system activation. Those functions include inactivation of coagulation factors XIIa and XIIf and conversion of factor XIa to factor IX (thromboplastin); inhibition of activated kallikrein and subsequent formation of bradykinin; and inactivation of plasminogen and plasmin (preventing formation of fibrin split products).

Activation of the above systems results in generation of mediators that are capable of increasing vascular permeability (edema, swelling, and ascites), causing vasodilatation (congestion, erythema or redness, and hypotension) and causing contraction of vascular smooth muscles (cramps, spasm, and pain). The list of such mediators includes but is not restricted to C1s itself, C2 peptide, C3a, C4a, and C5a anaphylatoxins released during complement activation and bradykinin, plasminogen, and factors XIIa, XIIf, and IX liberated as a consequence of contact system activation.

● PATHOPHYSIOLOGY OF HAE

HAE is a congenital condition associated with a lack of or functional defect in C1-INH. C1-INH belongs to the family of serine protease inhibitors (SERPINs) that also includes α_1-antitrypsin and antithrombin. It is synthesized mainly by hepatocytes and peripheral blood monocytes. The gene for C1-INH has been cloned and has been mapped to chromosome 11 (11q11–q13.1). The C1-INH protein has 478 amino acids and a two-domain appearance on electron microscopy: an elongated, rodlike N-terminal domain and a globular C-terminal serpin domain. Two disulfide bridges connect the domains. The N-terminal domain contains 10 out of 13 glycosylation sites of the C1-INH molecule (all 7 O-linked and 3 out of 6 N-linked oligosaccharides). The reactive center loop (RCL) is a peptide on the surface of the molecule near the carboxy terminus. The inhibitory activity of C1-INH depends on the exposure of the reactive center within the RCL that consists of a peptide bond between residues P1 (Arg444) and P1′ (Thr445). This cleavable bond represents a specific substrate recognized by the target proteases. Upon breaking of the bond, the cleaved RCL moves to the opposites poles of the protein and traps the active protease. Subsequent conformational change leads to a covalent complex between C1-INH and the substrate. C1-INH is thus consumed in the process of performing its normal function.

The incidence of HAE varies from 1:10,000–1:150,000 individuals. There are three variants of HAE, the first two (type I and II) being related to levels of functional C1-INH. Type I (85% of cases) is defined by low antigenic levels of functional plasma C1-INH, while type II (15%) is characterized by normal or even elevated antigenic levels of nonfunctional mutant protein and reduced levels of normal C1-INH. Types I and II have been reported in all races with no bias in different ethnic groups. Men and women are equally affected with HAE types I and II, indicating that the defect has an autosomal mode of inheritance. Mutations in the C1-INH gene that result in substitutions of Arg444 with other amino acids are estimated to account for up to 70% of cases in type

II HAE. Approximately 150 different genetic mutations have been described in HAE; they include mutations both within the reactive loop and away from the reactive center. The spontaneous mutation rate in HAE has been estimated at 25%. Recently, a third type of HAE has been described that was first thought to occur exclusively in women, suggesting an X-linked dominant pattern of inheritance in which C1-INH is both quantitatively and qualitatively normal. Recent family studies show, however, that males can also have this form of HAE.

When C1-INH is deficient or nonfunctional, the activation of the complement cascade as well as the kallikrein–bradykinin pathway and coagulation–fibrinolytic systems may continue unchecked. Even though current consensus favors bradykinin as the major mediator of HAE attacks, it is likely that the multitude of activated components of the complement and contact systems act in conjunction to bring about the clinical picture of HAE.

Additional Complement-Associated Defect Conditions

Whereas C1-INH deficiency results in an overexuberant activation of the complement system, other deficiency states

A

Cell lysis

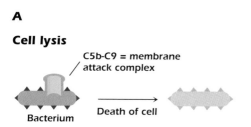

Opsonization

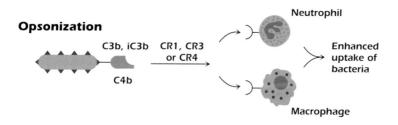

Anaphylatoxin production

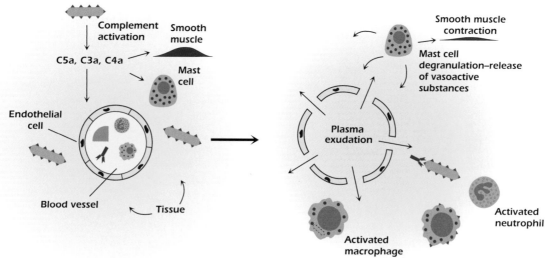

Figure 8.3. Functions of complement: (**A**) cell lysis, opsonization, and production of anaphylatoxins; (*Continued*)

B

Enhancement of B-cell responses

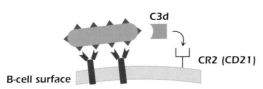

(a) B-cell activation

(b) Memory

Removal of immune complexes

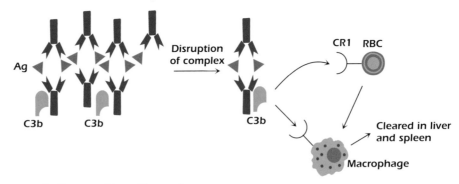

Removal of necrotic cells and subcellular membranes

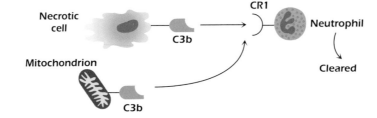

Responses to viruses

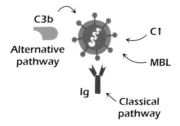

Figure 8.3. (**B**) enhancement of B-cell responses, removal of immune complexes, removal of necrotic cells and subcellular membranes, and responses to virus by C3 fragments.

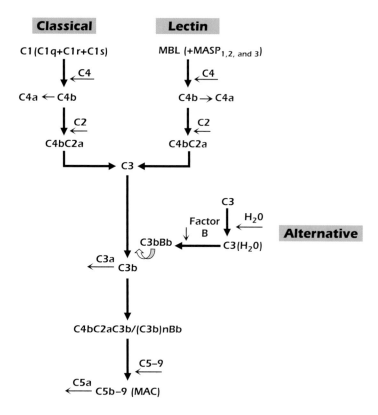

Figure 8.4. Complement activation pathways.

of the complement system present with increased incidence of infection and are associated with autoimmune symptomatology. Complement deficiency states are very rare, which indicates either a strong selective pressure favoring maintenance of a functional complement cascade or redundancy in this aspect of the immune system that keeps patients relatively symptom free and therefore undiagnosed. The estimated prevalence of complement deficiency is 0.03% in the general population, with the exception of MBL deficiency, which has an incidence as high as 3%. Complement protein alleles are codominant; therefore, heterozygotes for null alleles are usually phenotypically normal but contain half the normal levels of the affected complement component. Homozygotes are characterized mainly by infectious and autoimmune manifestations (Table 8.1).

Deficiencies of the early complement components (C1, C4, C2, or C3) result in increased infections with encapsulated organisms and increased autoimmune symptomatology, presumably from ineffective clearance of immune complexes (antigen-Ig). Similar features are seen with MBL deficiencies. Defects in late complement components are manifest by infection with Gram-negative bacteria, particularly *Neisseria*.

The body's cells are able to protect themselves from spontaneous activation of complement on their cell membrane. This is achieved by a family of proteins with glycosyl phosphatidyl inositol (GPI) anchors and includes CD55 (decay-activating factor) and CD59, among others. These prevent the progressive assembly of complement components leading to MAC formation on the body's normal cells (see Fig. 13.5 and related text discussion in Coico and Sunshine, 6th edition, Chapter 13). Additional proteins controlling the complement pathway are factors H and I, mentioned earlier. Defects in these proteins, as either an inherited or an acquired syndrome, result in spontaneous lysis of cells, particularly red blood cells, resulting in severe anemia, thrombosis, and chronic infection. An acquired form, with absence of all GPI-anchored proteins, is named paroxysmal nocturnal hemoglobinuria, reflecting the increased red blood cell lysis in the kidneys, particularly at night when the alternative complement pathway is activated by the acidic environment.

Clearly the complement system is very important in our defense against pathogens, but its potent activities must be tightly regulated.

TREATMENT OF HAE

Although the treatment of choice for acute HAE attacks is intravenous C1-INH, the current preparations are not yet available in the United States due to the limited number of controlled studies. Two plasma-derived preparations and one recombinant form are currently in clinical trials, each with an accompanying placebo. Study of one plasma preparation available in Europe demonstrated that approximately 69% of attacks treated with C1-INH subsided within

TABLE 8.1. Inherited Complement Deficiencies and Associated Clinical Correlates

Component	Pathway	Disease Association
C1, C4, C2	Classical	Systemic lupus erythematosus (SLE), infections caused by encapsulated bacteria
C3	Common to all three pathways	Recurrent pyogenic infections, glomerulonephritis
C5-C9	MAC	Recurrent *Neisseria* infections
MBL	Lectin	Pyogenic infections, sepsis, SLE
Factor H	Alternative	Membranoproliferative glomerulonephrititis, atypical hemolytic–uremic syndrome
Factor I	Alternative	Recurrent pyogenic infections

30 min and up to 95% of attacks responded within 4 h. It has been used both for on-demand (upon attack) basis and as continuous prophylaxis. If C1-INH concentrate is unavailable, fresh frozen plasma can be used as replacement therapy.

Several other experimental therapies are currently in clinical trials. Icatibant is a synthetic peptide that specifically and selectively acts as a bradykinin B_2 receptor antagonist. The safety and efficacy of Icatibant have been proven, and phase III studies have shown that the primary endpoint (significant reduction in the time to onset of symptom relief) had been reached. Dx-88 is a small recombinant peptide based on the reactive site of aprotinin (a broad-spectrum protease inhibitor). Dx-88 was found to inhibit the activity of human plasma kallikrein *in vitro* with specificity 300 times greater than that of C1-INH.

Current prophylactic treatments of HAE include attenuated androgens, such as danazol and stanazol, which are given to patients with frequent and severe episodes. Long-term administration of androgens may cause arterial hypertension and virilization in women, therefore keeping the dose to the lowest effective level is important. Contraindications include prostate cancer, pregnancy, childhood, and breastfeeding. Androgens are thought to exert their effect by stimulating the production of C1-INH by hepatocytes. Although antifibrinolytic agents such as ε-aminocaproic acid or tranexamic acid are less effective as prophylactic agents, they are the option of choice for pregnant women.

Intubation and/or tracheostomy may be required as life-saving procedures when laryngeal edema occurs.

Approval of the above-mentioned experimental therapies will provide more options for the management of acute attacks as well as prophylaxis of any future HAE episodes that may be experienced by Charlie and other patients suffering from this condition.

REFERENCES

Cicardi M, Zingale L, Zanichelli A, Deliliers DL (2007): Established and new treatments for hereditary angioedema: An update. *Mol Immunol* 44:3858–3861.

Davis AE (1998): C1 inhibitor gene and hereditary angioedema. In Volanakis JE, Frank MM (eds): *The Human Complement System in Health and Disease*, 1st ed., New York: Marcel Dekker, pp. 455–460.

Frank MM, Fries LL (1989): Complement. In Paul WE (ed): *Fundamental Immunology*, 2nd ed. New York: Raven, pp. 679–698.

Gal P, Ambrus G, Lorinez Z, Zavodszky P (2004): The initiation complexes of the classical and lectin pathways. In Szebeni J. (ed): *The Complement System. Novel Roles in Health and Disease*, 1st ed. Boston: Kluwer Academic, pp. 33–35.

Jiang H, Wagner E, Zhang H, Frank MM (2001): Complement 1 inhibitor is a regulator of the alternative complement pathway. *J Exp Med* 194:1609–1616.

Nzeako UC, Frigas E, Tremaine WJ (2001): Hereditary angioedema. A broad review for clinicians. *Arch Intern Med* 161:2417–2429.

Wen L, Atkinson JP, Gicias PC (2004): Clinical and laboratory evaluation of complement deficiency. *J Allergy Clin Immunol* 113:585–592.

9

ACQUIRED IMMUNODEFICIENCY SYNDROME

CARYN G. MORSE and FRANK MALDARELLI*

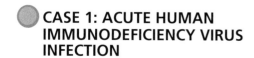
CASE 1: ACUTE HUMAN IMMUNODEFICIENCY VIRUS INFECTION

"I have a fever and I ache all over."

Clinical History and Initial Evaluation

Jack, a 20-year-old male, presents to your office in the early fall. You have been the family's doctor for many years and know Jack to be healthy and physically fit. Jack tells you that he was well until seven days ago when he began feeling fatigued and feverish with malaise and muscle aches. He also says that since about two days before these symptoms began he has had a red, raised rash on his trunk. He mentions that his parents are concerned about Rocky Mountain spotted fever (RMSF) and Lyme disease since he had recently been hunting in Texas and was also exposed to ticks while bathing the family dog during the week before the onset of these symptoms. Although he thinks that this is the "flu," the rash and his parents' concerns prompted him to come see you.

On review of symptoms, Jack reports temperatures to 100.5°F but denies chills, night sweats, weight loss, or appetite change. He also describes mild irritation of his

*With contributions from Warren Strober and Susan R. S. Gottesman

eyes, a sore throat, and swollen glands in his neck. Jack states that he has "never really been sick before," but because of these symptoms, in the last week he has even fallen behind in his schoolwork at the local community college.

On examination, Jack appears relatively well. His temperature is 101.0°F but his heart rate, respiratory rate, and blood pressure are normal. He has a reddish, papular rash on his neck, chest, back, and legs. His conjunctivae are slightly injected (reddish) bilaterally. He has a mildly erythematous posterior pharynx (red throat) which does not have exudates (pus); however, he has small ulcerations in the posterior pharynx. You find no meningismus (signs of meningeal irritation which are elicited by flexion of the neck) and his lungs are clear. Small (<1 cm) lymph nodes are palpable in the anterior and posterior cervical and inguinal (neck and groin) areas. Liver and spleen are nonpalpable.

On speaking with Jack, you elicit a history of social alcohol and tobacco use. He has been sexually active and is currently in a monogamous sexual relationship with his girlfriend of three months. He denies a history of sexually transmitted diseases. He has not traveled recently, other than the hunting trip, and has never been outside the United States. While hunting, he fords streams and is occasionally scratched by branches. He has a pet two-year-old Labrador retriever who has been healthy.

What is the differential diagnosis of fever, rash, and lymphadenopathy (enlarged lymph nodes)?

Fever, rash, and lymphadenopathy have numerous potential etiologies. Identifying the precise cause usually requires a stepwise approach, starting with the most likely possibilities arising from history and physical examination. Some key points emerging from Jack's history include an acute rather than gradual onset of symptoms, suggesting an infectious cause; generalized lymphadenopathy, suggesting a systemic problem; and a generalized nonpurpuric rash (one not characterized by extravasation of blood), suggesting the presence of an immune response or—more ominously—sepsis (systemic response to infection accompanied by a change in vital signs). Constitutional symptoms are significant but not extreme or unstable, indicating that sepsis is not present.

Based on your suspicion of infectious disease and history of likely exposures, you send a complete blood count (CBC), chemistries, and serologies for infectious mononucleosis, syphilis, RMSF, and Lyme disease and perform a rapid strep screen and throat culture. In a confidential counseling session with Jack, you discuss testing for human immunodeficiency virus (HIV) infection and he decides to be tested. You therefore send peripheral blood samples for an ELISA (enzyme-linked immunosorbent assay) screening test for HIV antibody and a quantitative NAT (nucleic acid testing) for HIV RNA.

Why were both tests sent for HIV?

*Jack's symptoms, which developed 7–10 days ago, suggest recent exposure to an infectious agent. Following infection with HIV, there is a "**window period**" of 5–10 weeks during which the individual will not yet have mounted an immune response to the virus. This window period is actually comprised of two phases: (1) the eclipse phase of approximately 2 weeks during which there is no circulating virus (the virus is still confined to tissue sites such as gastrointestinal and genital mucosa, lymph nodes, and liver) followed by (2) the viremic phase of approximately 22 days, during which there is circulating virus, usually at relatively high levels. The use of NAT technology to detect viral nucleic acid has decreased but not eliminated the effective window period (see testing for HIV below).*

Results. The rapid strep test, which was available immediately, and the throat culture, which was read the next day, are both negative. Jack's white blood cell count (WBC) is decreased at 3.0K/μL (reference range: 4.8–10.8K/μL) with 40% polymorphonuclear cells and 50% lymphocytes and no immature forms. His hemoglobin and platelet counts are normal. Chemistries are remarkable only for slight elevation in the liver enzymes, alanine aminotransferase (ALT) and aspartate aminotransferase (AST), which suggests the presence of inflammation in the liver.

The monospot [screening for heterophile antibodies to Epstein–Barr virus (EBV), the etiologic agent of infectious mononucleosis] and tests for syphilis, RMSF, and Lyme disease are negative. An HIV ELISA antibody test returns as nonreactive, but quantitative HIV viral RNA assay detects 750,000 copies/ml (viral load or titer).

How do you interpret these results?

The negative monospot test rule out infectious mononucleosis, which would have a similar presentation to HIV infection and might be associated with a hepatitis-like picture. As indicated in the discussion above, you are not surprised by the discrepancy between the negative ELISA test for HIV antibody and the positive HIV viral titer. The low WBC count and mildly elevated liver enzyme studies are also consistent with acute HIV infection, the phase of infection that you suspected from the history and clinical symptoms.

Follow-Up and Initiation of Therapy

You call Jack and ask to see him. In your office later that day, you explain to him that, based on his symptoms and the results of the tests, he is in the ***acute phase*** of HIV infection (Fig. 9.1). You take additional blood samples for a repeat HIV ELISA, a confirmatory Western blot (see below), and T-cell subset analysis by flow cytometry. You emphasize that, although he has HIV infection, he does not now have acquired immunodeficiency syndrome (AIDS), but he will need to be monitored and he will probably require antiviral

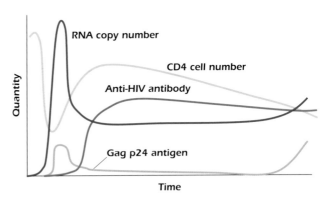

Figure 9.1. Schematic time course of HIV infection. After infection, a sharp rise in HIV viremia occurs followed by humoral and cellular immune response. There is a variable window period during which virus infection is present but not detectable by standard means. As chronic infection is established, a relatively stable HIV RNA level is achieved and a slow, inexorable decline in CD4 cell count occurs. In general, the rate of decline of CD4 cells is related to the degree of viremia, i.e., the higher the viral RNA level, the faster the CD4 decline.

medication sometime in the future. You indicate that the combined therapies now available are usually able to control the infection. While you suggest strongly that he tell his parents, you emphasize that you will maintain his confidentiality. You are most concerned that he communicate these results to his girlfriend and offer to take part in that discussion. You also ask again about any other sexual contact in the last several months.

Jack recalls that he went to a bachelor's party a few weeks ago and that party ended with unexpected sexual contact with the hired "entertainment." Since he did not think of this as a significant encounter, he did not recall the event when you initially asked him about his sexual activities. Jack agrees to tell his girlfriend about the HIV infection and events leading up to it but is not yet ready to tell his parents. He understands the necessity of close follow-up and has even done some reading on the subject in the time between his testing and the results. You set him up with a counseling service that you work closely with which will help monitor him and provide psychological support if needed.

After several additional weeks of monitoring, a repeat HIV-1/2 ELISA is reactive and an HIV-1 Western blot is positive with bands at gp160/120, p24, and p17 (Fig. 9.2). These indicate that Jack is now making antibody to the virus and that he has the HIV-1 serotype, as expected in this country. Repeat viral load testing shows a marked decline in viral titers. T-cell subset analysis, which initially showed a marked decrease from normal in CD4$^+$ T-cell numbers, now demonstrates a rise to values almost within reference range [range of values—mean ± 2SD—expected in healthy individuals of the same sex, age, and ethnicity]. This pattern of change is expected (Fig. 9.1).

CASE 2: CHRONIC HIV INFECTION

"I feel fine. Why do you think I should have an HIV test?"

Clinical History and Initial Evaluation

William, a 22-year-old sexually active student, has come to you for a routine physical exam required upon entry into medical school. He is entirely well and has had no recent illnesses. As you take his history, William discloses that he has had unprotected sex with both men and women for several years. He has had normal childhood diseases and several episodes of flulike illnesses and was diagnosed with infectious mononucleosis in college. His physical exam reveals normal vital signs and minimally enlarged, mobile, rubbery, nontender cervical lymph nodes (1 cm × 1 cm). The remainder of the exam is normal.

During the exam, you broach the subject of HIV testing with William, given his sexual history. He is at first startled by the suggestion because he feels well but then agrees that there is benefit in knowing. He does not, however, want the test administered through the school and arranges to call your private office for an appointment.

The next day William comes to your private office to be tested. You first have a counseling session with him and then draw blood for HIV screening by an ELISA test with reflex Western blot study for confirmation. (Reflex testing is only run by the laboratory based on defined results of the first test; in this case, a reactive ELISA would trigger a reflex Western blot assay.)

Results. The next day, the ELISA is reported as reactive; one week later, the confirmatory Western blot assay is

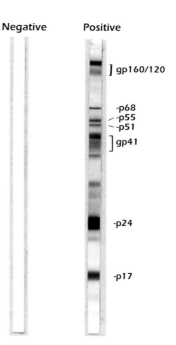

Figure 9.2. HIV-1 Western blot. Negative HIV Western blots have no reactive bands. Positive HIV Western blots have antibodies that recognize two or more of the indicated bands. As indicated, the positive Western blot may react with a series of HIV proteins. Indeterminate Western blots represent any Western blot that is not either negative or positive. The most common indeterminate pattern is an aberrant reactivity with p24. The numerous reasons for indeterminate Western blot results are listed with the mnemonic "indetermine."

Positive Western blot

Any two of the following bands: gp160/120, gp41, p24

Causes of Indeterminate Western blot

Infections (shistosomiasis, HIV-2)
Neoplasms
Dialysis
Ethnicity—Africans
Thyroiditis
Elevated bilirubin
Rheumatologic diseases
Multiple pregnancies
Immunization (tetanus)
Nephrotic proteinuria (massive)
Error in laboratory

reported positive. You call William and ask him to come to your office to discuss the test results.

Follow-Up Evaluation

William is understandably upset when you tell him the test results. Over the past week, though, he has done extensive reading on HIV (getting a jump on his medical school education) and is quite prepared to start a program of therapy and monitoring. You draw blood samples for CBC, chemistries, and T-cell subset analysis. In addition, although he seems quite knowledgeable, you set up a counseling and informational session for a discussion of the disease.

Results. No abnormalities are found in the CBC or chemistries. However, the T-cell subset analysis discloses a decreased CD4$^+$ T-cell count of 350 cells/μL (reference range 1000–4000 cells/μL) and a reduced CD4:CD8 ratio of 0.6 (reference range >1). HIV RNA titer is 50,000 copies/ml.

How do you interpret the test results in conjunction with William's history and physical exam?

*The combination of the physical exam and history, which did not reveal any unusual, AIDS-defining (see below) conditions as is seen in the crisis phase or any viral symptoms as is seen in acute infection, suggests that William is in the chronic phase. He may have passed through an acute phase and not distinguished it from any other viral or "flu-like" illness or he may have been totally asymptomatic when he became infected. The reduced CD4$^+$ T-cell count (which results in the inverted CD4:CD8 ratio) and viral titers in the peripheral blood (notice that they are lower than Jack's) are typical of the chronic "latent" phase. Although it is within the criteria of the chronic latent phase, the low CD4$^+$ T-cell count suggests the need to start triple-agent **highly active antiretroviral therapy (HAART)** to delay advancement to the **crisis phase**.*

You relate these results to William, explaining that he is in the chronic phase, and begin him on HAART and a schedule of monitoring.

TESTS FOR THE DIAGNOSIS AND MONITORING OF HIV INFECTION

Three different tests for HIV: ELISA, Western blot, and NAT, were used to diagnose and evaluate Jack and William. These assays are actually names of techniques that can be and are applied to the investigation of any number of disorders, particularly infectious diseases. The assays are used here to detect components of the HIV virus (nucleic acid:

NAT; protein: ELISA) or serologic responses to the virus (ELISA and Western blot; see also Unit V).

Typical screening for HIV infection involves sequential serologic testing using the extremely sensitive ELISA for detection of antibody to the whole virus followed by a highly specific Western blot assay for detection of antibody to specific individual proteins of the virus (Figs. 9.2 and 9.3). The two-step process, ELISA and Western blot, is essential. Sensitivity (number of patients who HAVE the disease and who test POSITIVE) at the initial stage is critical, since any patients missed on the screening test represent individuals with undiagnosed HIV infections. The sensitivity of HIV ELISA testing is >99.5% once the patient has seroconverted (developed antibodies). While detecting nearly all HIV infections, the consequence of using an extremely sensitive assay is a significant false-positive rate, that is, patients who test positive but who do not have HIV infection. The false-positive rate of HIV ELISA in low-risk populations such as blood donors is as high as 10%. This is why ELISA results alone are not sufficient to make a diagnosis of HIV infection and why results for HIV ELISA tests are reported as "reactive" or "nonreactive" and **not** "positive" or "negative." Western blot assays are used to confirm HIV diagnoses in patients with reactive ELISA results.

In the Western blot for detection of antibodies, viral proteins are separated on a nitrocellulose membrane, and the presence and amount of antibody in the patient's serum to each individual protein component are measured. Western blots have the highest specificity of any HIV test (proportion of patients with NEGATIVE tests who DO NOT have HIV infection). This ensures that patients without the disease are not incorrectly identified as HIV infected. However, Western blots are only useful in a population with a high probability of infection, such as those who are ELISA positive. Western blots are interpreted as negative (no reactive bands), positive (a series of bands reflecting an immune response to more than one component of the virus), or indeterminate (Fig. 9.2). Antibody to the viral protein p24 is often the first one detected, but this alone is not sufficient to call the test positive. Indeterminate Western blots may arise from the presence of single-band reactivity and do not indicate infection; instead, they suggest the presence of nonspecific cross reactivity in patient sera. Numerous causes of indeterminate Western blots have been described and are shown in the form of a mnemonic in Figure 9.2.

Very early in infection (as in the acute HIV seroconversion syndrome), the humoral immune response (antibodies) may not be sufficiently developed to register the presence of HIV infection (Fig. 9.1). ELISA assays approved by the Food and Drug Administration (FDA) are available to detect the structural component of the HIV virion, p24, which is present in high levels early in infection. In addition, the presence or level of HIV RNA or complementary DNA (cDNA) may be measured through amplification technology and NAT. Although this is not FDA approved for

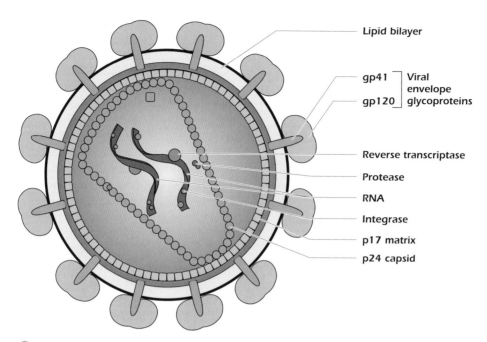

Lipid bilayer

gp41 ⎤ Viral
⎥ envelope
gp120 ⎦ glycoproteins

Reverse transcriptase

Protease

RNA

Integrase

p17 matrix

p24 capsid

Figure 9.3. Structure of HIV-1 showing two identical RNA strands (the viral genome) and associated enzymes including reverse transcriptase, integrase, and protease packaged in a cone-shaped core composed of p24 capsid protein with surrounding p17 protein matrix, all surrounded by a phospholipid membrane envelope derived from the host cell. Virally encoded membrane proteins (gp41 and gp120) are bound to the envelope.

first diagnosis of HIV infection, judicious application may be useful in identifying early cases such as Jack's. NAT testing is routinely used to ensure the safety of the blood supply in this country, and a quantitative NAT test is employed to follow viral titers (copies per milliliter in plasma) in known HIV+ patients. In general, HIV RNA levels are relatively high in acute HIV infection (>100,000 RNA copies/ml plasma). In the evaluation of patients with suspected acute HIV infection, a low HIV RNA level (5000–10,000 copies HIV RNA/ml plasma) in the absence of supporting serologic evidence should prompt concern about a possible false-positive viral RNA test result.

Laboratory testing of HIV infection is a serious undertaking and requires confidentiality, pre- and post-test counseling, and patient consent, often in written form. Confidentiality, counseling, and consent are three characteristics that are derived directly from paramount concern for patient dignity and represent nonnegotiable physician responsibilities. For this reason, various medical and governmental agencies, including the World Health Organization, have rejected mandatory testing under any circumstances. Certain instances, including mandatory testing of patients upon inadvertent exposure of health care workers, remain under discussion but have been supported by the American Medical Association. Mandatory testing for HIV has been approved in federal prisons and some state prisons; in some states, it is required for all newborns.

What test results would you expect in the event of accidental exposure?

An individual who is inadvertently "stuck" with a contaminated needle would be expected to be negative or nonreactive in all three tests (as might a patient in the eclipse phase). Certainly they would not yet have formed antibodies, a process which requires 5–10 weeks, and would likely have too low a level of viral particles to be confidently considered positive. The level may even be below detectability. Triple-agent therapy as prophylaxis is administered immediately in an attempt to prevent establishment of infection in the event that there was exposure, and the individual is then closely monitored to determine whether infection has occurred.

In addition to quantitative viral loads, HIV+ patients are monitored by following their peripheral blood CD4+ T-cell counts, since this reflects their degree of immune competence. The peripheral T cells are comprised of two alternative subsets, one expressing CD4 and one expressing CD8; commonly, although not accurately, these are referred to as helper (CD4+) and cytotoxic or "suppressor" (CD8+) T cells. The peripheral T cells are quantitated using a flow cytometer and fluorescent monoclonal antibodies to detect the CD surface markers, along with CD3 to identify the total T-cell population. The absolute number of CD4+ T cells and the percent of CD4+ T cells (also known as the CD4:CD8 ratio) are monitored in HIV+ patients.

LIFE CYCLE OF HIV

In order to understand the clinical features of HIV infection, it is important to first review the structure and life cycle of the virus.

HIV is an enveloped retrovirus, an RNA virus with a cDNA intermediate stage, which is part of the lentivirus family. Two strains, HIV-1 and HIV-2, have been described; HIV-1 is the more virulent strain. The viral particle contains two identical single strands of genomic RNA that, along with three enzymes (integrase, protease, and reverse transcriptase), are packaged in the p24 core antigen with the nucleoproteins p7 and p9 and surrounded by the p17 matrix protein (Fig. 9.3). The viral envelope consists of the host cell membrane, which contains inserted viral glycoproteins. The most important of these is gp120 noncovalently bound to gp41; the latter is a transmembrane protein. It is the gp120 that has high affinity for CD4 and that governs the target specificity of HIV. All cells expressing CD4 are potential targets for the virus; these include macrophages/monocytes and dendritic cells, as well as $CD4^+$ T cells.

Glycoprotein 120 binds to CD4, undergoes a conformational change, and then must bind a second coreceptor molecule, one of several chemokine receptors, to gain entry into the target cell. Molecular variations in the gp120 molecule determine which chemokine coreceptor is used and thus dictate the tropism of the virus, that is, the $CD4^+$ target cell that can be infected by that viral particle. Macrophage tropic HIV uses the chemokine receptor CCR5, expressed by macrophages, dendritic cells, and activated T cells, and requires only a low level of CD4 on the host cell. Lymphotropic HIV uses the chemokine receptor CXCR4 that is found on T cells and requires a high density of CD4 on the cell surface. HIV variants using CCR5 exclusively are termed R5, while those using CXCR4 are termed X4; variants able to bind both chemokine coreceptors are referred to as R5X4. Mutations in the gp120 gene, leading to alterations in its amino acid sequence, change the tropism of the virus produced within the infected individual over time.

Recently, $\alpha_4\beta_7$, an integrin receptor, was identified as a target molecule for gp120. The binding of $\alpha_4\beta_7$ by HIV also results in the activation of leukocyte function-associated antigen 1 (LFA-1), an integrin on the T cells involved in immunologic and virologic synapses between cells. This may facilitate HIV transfer from one cell to the next. In addition, the targeting of T cells with activated $\alpha_4\beta_7$, which is the gut mucosal homing receptor, may explain the predilection of HIV to home to gut-associated lymphoid tissue.

Following the binding of gp120 to CD4 and its coreceptor, gp41 penetrates the host cell membrane; this causes fusion of the viral envelope with the membrane and results in viral entry and uncoating of the viral core. Using its own enzyme, reverse transcriptase, the viral RNA is replicated to a cDNA copy in the host cell. The cDNA may enter the nucleus, where it is integrated into the host genome as a provirus with the help of another viral enzyme, integrase.

The HIV genome has a long terminal repeat (LTR) region at each end (Fig. 9.4), which is required for viral integration and for the binding of regulatory proteins. Although viral replication can continue at a low level for years, when a T cell is activated by antigen, a cascade of reactions is initiated that leads to activation of the transcription factor NF-κB. In infected T cells, NF-κB binds to the promoter region in the LTRs, activating host transcription of the provirus. The provirus is transcribed as a long mRNA transcript that can be spliced at alternative sites for the synthesis of different proteins. Tat and Rev

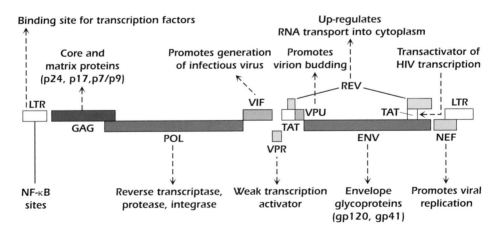

Figure 9.4. The Genes and proteins of HIV-1. The HIV-1 RNA genome is flanked by LTRs required for viral integration and regulation of the viral genome. Several viral genes overlap resulting in different reading frames, thus allowing the virus to code for many proteins in a small genome. The functions of the gene products are listed.

are the first two proteins made. Tat enters the nucleus where it acts as a transcription factor, binding to the LTR region of the proviral DNA and increasing the rate of viral transcription. Rev also acts in the nucleus but binds to the Rev-responsive element in the viral mRNA transcript, causing the viral mRNA to be transported more rapidly into the cytoplasm. As a result of this rapid movement into the cytoplasm, less splicing of the mRNA occurs in the nucleus and different proteins can be synthesized. The structural components of the viral core and envelope are produced in precursor form during this second wave of viral protein synthesis. In the third wave, unspliced RNA is transported to the cytoplasm and serves as the RNA for packaging into the new viral particles and for the translation of *gag* and *pol*. Gag and pol are first produced as a polyprotein product that is then cut into the individual proteins by the HIV protease, the third enzyme that the virus brought with it into the cell. *Gag* codes for p24, p17, p7, and p9. *Pol* codes for the viral protease, reverse transcriptase, and integrase.

Release of virus from CD4$^+$ T cells frequently results in lysis of the cell. Macrophages and dendritic cells are generally not killed by HIV but serve as a reservoir, transporting virus to other parts of the body [lymphoid tissue and central nervous system (CNS)], with macrophage producing a small number of particles without cytopathic consequences.

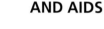

EPIDEMIOLOGY AND CLINICAL FEATURES OF HIV INFECTION AND AIDS

Epidemiology

In 1981 several cases of an unusual pneumonia caused by *Pneumocystis jiroveci* [pneumocystis pneumonia (PCP)] were reported in homosexual males in the San Francisco area of California. This was followed in that same year by the recognition of an aggressive form of Kaposi sarcoma in a similar population in New York City. These cases of unusual diseases were rapidly identified as manifestations of a severe immunodeficiency state and thus heralded the recognition of the AIDS epidemic. From 1981 until today, over 20 million people have died worldwide of AIDS and over 30 million are currently infected with HIV.

AIDS is the end result of infection with HIV, which is transmitted by contact with blood and body fluids from an infected individual. Blood, semen, vaginal secretions, breast milk, and (to a small extent) saliva of an infected individual contain free virus or cells harboring virus. Transmission can occur through sexual contact, sharing of needles, transfusion of blood or blood products, placental transfer, passage through the birth canal, and breast feeding. Two major forms of HIV exist: HIV-1 and the related but distinct virus, HIV-2. The more virulent strain, HIV-1 is pandemic throughout the world, whereas HIV-2 has a geographic distribution limited to West Africa, some European countries, and India.

Although sexually active homosexual males in large U.S. cities were the first demographic group identified with AIDS, HIV infection and AIDS have no sexual preference. In fact, worldwide, heterosexual transmission is more common than homosexual transmission. In addition, while homosexual males and intravenous drug abusers still constitute the major infected groups in the United States, the greatest increase in the rate of HIV infection is now among heterosexual women and minorities (African-Americans and Hispanics). The risk of acquiring the virus through transfusion of blood and blood products has been virtually eliminated in the United States through screening of donors, testing of collected blood units, and heat inactivation of clotting factor concentrates. A dangerous "window period" still exists when infection of blood units or organs cannot be detected, but this has been narrowed by NAT testing for viral RNA. Transplacental transmission, which accounts for >80% of the pediatric cases, has been greatly diminished by antiviral treatment of the mother and the avoidance of vaginal childbirth and breast feeding. However, these positive statements exist almost as a footnote to an epidemic that continues to spread throughout the world without signs of abating, particularly in Africa and Southeast Asia.

Clinical Features of HIV Infection

The clinical course of HIV infection can be divided into three phases: the acute infection phase, the chronic latent phase, and the crisis or AIDS phase. Jack's scenario illustrates the first *acute infection phase*, while William's illustrates the *chronic latent phase*. It is the third phase that is defined as AIDS. We will describe, but chose not to illustrate by a clinical scenario, this *crisis*, or *AIDS*, *phase*, hoping that the course of the disease will continue to be altered, at least in developed countries where therapy is accessible.

Acute HIV Infection. Infection with HIV may have a spectrum of presenting symptoms. Acute HIV-1 infection syndrome, an illness similar to infectious mononucleosis or influenza, is thought to occur in 40–70% of patients after primary HIV-1 infection. The prognostic significance of clinically significant symptoms with primary infection is unknown, but it has been postulated that more intense symptoms at presentation may correlate with more rapid disease progression.

Presenting symptoms may consist of fever, headache, sore throat, a rash that may include erythematous exanthema (rash associated with viral infection) and enanthem (mucous membrane eruption), arthralgia (joint

◉ TABLE 9.1. Signs and Symptoms Associated with Acute Retroviral Syndrome

Signs and Symptoms	Frequency (%)
Fever	96
Lymphadenopathy	74
Pharyngitis	70
Rash	70
Myalgia or arthralgia	54
Diarrhea	32
Headache	32
Nausea and vomiting	27
Hepatosplenomegaly	14
Weight loss	13
Thrush	12
Neurologic symptoms	12

Source: From the U.S. Department of Health and Human Services (Aug. 2001): *Guidelines for the Use of Antiretrovirals in Adults and Adolescents.* Washington, DC: DHHS.

aches), myalgias (muscle aches), diarrhea, and generalized lymphadenopathy (Table 9.1). Laboratory tests may be normal but common abnormalities include leukopenia (decreased WBC), anemia, thrombocytopenia (low platelet count), atypical lymphocytosis (large, reactive, and increased numbers of lymphocytes), elevated liver enzymes, and hypergammaglobulinemia. The peripheral blood CD4$^+$ T-cell count and the CD4:CD8 ratio are usually decreased. Acute illness typically manifests two to four weeks after infection and resolves spontaneously within two to three weeks. During primary infection, the CD4$^+$ T-cell count drops and is occasionally low enough to allow opportunistic infections. Though the CD4$^+$ T-cell count rebounds with the resolution of acute infection, it usually does not return to baseline.

Because the symptoms of acute HIV infection are nonspecific and common to many other viral illnesses, the diagnosis of primary HIV infection is challenging. HIV diagnosis proceeds from history and physical examination to laboratory studies. In one retrospective review, more than 50% of patients with acute retroviral syndrome required at least three visits to health care providers before the diagnosis was made. Only 15% of patients were diagnosed at their first visit to a health care professional. To make the diagnosis, health care providers must maintain a high index of suspicion, obtain an accurate exposure history, and be prepared to discuss HIV and test the patient for the virus.

The typical, florid presentation for HIV infection will not occur in all patients and will completely resolve even in those who are symptomatic. Their infection can then proceed in an asymptomatic fashion, and patients may not

realize for years that infection has occurred (see the section on the chronic latent phase below). Early diagnosis leads to appropriate treatment, monitoring, and counseling; may prevent lethal complications in the patient; and hopefully will interrupt subsequent cycles of HIV transmission to others. Delayed diagnosis results in progressive immune destruction and in the potential of unknowingly transmitting infection through high-risk behavior. Patients will have seroconverted, producing antibodies specific for HIV by the end of the acute phase.

Chronic Latent Phase. Clinically, the chronic latent phase can be relatively quiet, characterized more often by its *lack* of symptoms. In reality, as we will see below in the immunopathophysiology section, HIV infection is never truly latent; there continues to be a great deal of activity with regard to the virus's effects on the immune system. As mentioned above, without knowledge of being infected, the individual risks transmitting the virus and not receiving treatment that might delay destruction of their immune system and entry into the final crisis stage. The "latent" phase, which may last as long as 15 years, is associated with a low level of viral replication and a gradual decline in CD4$^+$ T-cell numbers, heralding in the crisis phase.

Current antiviral therapies have been successful in extending the chronic latent phase, making it almost truly latent in some patients, at least as determined by peripheral blood viral titers, thus changing the prognosis of HIV from an imminent death sentence to a chronic illness. Even so, complications of the viral infection do occur in a significant number of patients during this phase. There is a high incidence of renal dysfunction and failure in HIV-infected patients due to the viral infection itself resulting in focal segmental glomerular sclerosis (partial fibrosis of renal glomeruli) and is sometimes complicated by the nephrotoxic side effects of some medications. In addition, there are characteristic maturational changes in bone marrow precursor cells, correlating with mildly to moderately decreased peripheral blood platelet levels, anemia, and neutropenia (decreased neutrophils), as well as nonspecific reactive changes in the lymph nodes resulting in lymphadenopathy. In the chronic latent phase, patients' CD4$^+$ T-cell levels and viral RNA titers must be monitored closely and they must be treated aggressively in the event of infection with other organisms.

Crisis Phase, or "AIDS." The appearance of unusual infections and malignancies that led to the original description of AIDS continues to be the hallmark of the full-blown disease. The illnesses that the Centers for Disease Control (CDC) have identified as AIDS associated fall into three categories: unusual malignancies, opportunistic infections, and general debilitating syndromes. These reflect the primary effects of HIV on the immune

TABLE 9.2. AIDS-Associated Diseases Defined by CDC

Infections: frequently disseminated

    Fungal: candidiasis, cryptococcosis, histoplasmosis, coccidioidomycosis, cryptosporidiosis

    Parasitic: toxoplasmosis, pneumocystis, cryptosporidiosis, isosporiosis

    Bacterial: mycobacteriosis, including atypical; salmonella

    Viral: cytomegalovirus, herpes simplex virus, progressive mutifocal leukoencephalopathy

Malignancies

    Sarcoma: Kaposi sarcoma

    Lymphoma: Burkitt lymphoma, diffuse large B-cell lymphoma, effusion-based lymphoma, primary CNS lymphoma

    Carcinoma: invasive cancer of uterine cervix

General conditions

    HIV encephalopathy and dementia

    Wasting syndrome

    $CD4^+$ T-cell count $<200/\mu L$ (is AIDS defining)

Note: Selected illnesses are discussed in the text.

system and CNS (Table 9.2). Their relative frequencies and time course have changed in the last decade with the now common practice of prophylactic treatment for infections, first PCP and more recently tuberculosis (TB). Diagnosis of any of these identified illnesses (or a defined threshold $CD4^+$ T-cell level of <200 cells/μL or $<14\%$ of T cells) changes the patient's status from merely being HIV^+ to having AIDS.

Malignancies. During the early years of the AIDS epidemic in the United States, it was noted that the specific AIDS-associated illnesses emerging in an individual partially correlated with the mode of transmission of HIV to that patient—that is, sexual transmission versus intravenous drug use (IVD). Differences in the infections and malignancies seen among AIDS patients with different HIV exposure and between AIDS patients and other immunosuppressed individuals (i.e., transplant patients) suggested that HIV^+ individuals may be coinfected with other organisms depending on their route of HIV exposure. That this observation applied to the malignancies (which are unusual and very aggressive), as well as the infectious complications, was particularly intriguing at the time and led to the discovery of a previously unrecognized oncogenic virus in Kaposi sarcoma (KS) in HIV^+ patients. KS is an abnormal proliferation of small blood vessels. In its usual form (in the absence of immunodeficiency), KS manifests as a slow growth on the skin of the lower extremities of elderly men. In HIV-infected patients, it is aggressive and not limited to the lower extremities. This aggressive behavior of KS is virtually unique to AIDS patients and is rarely seen in other immunodeficient individuals. In addition, it usually occurs

in HIV^+ male homosexuals (rather than IVD patients) and tends to manifest relatively early in the course of HIV infection. KS might now be regarded as an "infectious" disease, since human herpes virus 8 (HHV-8), a DNA oncogenic virus, has been identified in KS from AIDS patients (as well as the elderly gentlemen). This virus is also associated with an unusual form of aggressive lymphoma seen in AIDS patients called primary effusion lymphoma. The latter is also more common in male homosexual AIDS patients; some have the lymphoma and KS concurrently.

In fact, many of the malignancies seen in AIDS patients are associated with oncogenic DNA viruses; their manifestation as aggressive malignant growths is presumably due to the patient's reduced host defense against the causative viral agent. For example, cervical cancer in women, a malignancy associated with specific types of human papillomavirus (HPV), occurs with markedly increased frequency and aggressiveness in HIV^+ women. As a result, the CDC includes invasive cervical cancer as an AIDS-associated malignancy (see Table 9.2).

The incidence of aggressive B-cell lymphomas, many of them associated with EBV, is increased in AIDS patients (both male homosexual and IVD patients) as it is in immunosuppressed transplant patients. This is not surprising given that EBV is a ubiquitous virus that establishes infection in B cells that, in normal individuals, are controlled by T-cell mediated host defense mechanisms. Therefore, exposure to EBV and an inability to control the EBV infected cells (usually B cells) would be seen in all T-cell immunodeficient populations. Burkitt and diffuse large B-cell lymphomas are the common types of lymphomas in AIDS patients and are often, but not always, EBV associated and often involve sites outside the lymph nodes (extranodal). Primary CNS lymphoma, very unusual in the general population, is also seen in HIV^+ patients. Lastly, although not currently listed as AIDS-defining, two other malignancies—squamous cell carcinoma of the head and neck region (also possibly associated with HPV) and atypical Hodgkin lymphoma (possibly EBV associated)—have more aggressive courses in AIDS patients.

Infectious Diseases. As in any patient with defective T-cell-mediated immunity (see Cases 2 and 3), AIDS patients are subject to **opportunistic infections**, infections caused by organisms (usually viral and fungal) that are not pathogenic in healthy individuals. As mentioned above, PCP was an early and major cause of lethal infection in AIDS until the institution of prophylactic antibiotic therapy and it remains a feared complication. Other frequent opportunistic infections in HIV include widespread fungal infections, particularly candidiasis and uncontrolled and unusual mycobacterial infections such as infection with Mycobacteria avium intracellulare—M. avium is not normally a human pathogen and can cause overwhelming infection in AIDS patients due to their deficient capacity to develop granuloma, a classical T-helper-cell function. Opportunistic infections of the gastrointestinal (GI) tract with *Cryptosporidia, M. avium*, and cytomegalovirus (CMV) are common, causing diarrhea in AIDS patients and adding to their debilitated state while infection of the CNS with cryptococcus, toxoplasmosis, or CMV results in neurologic complications. Infection of the retina with CMV is a significant problem as it can cause blindness and is seen in approximately 25% of late-stage AIDS patients.

General Debilitating Illnesses. Patients with AIDS often exhibit general debilitating illnesses reflecting either systemic or organ-specific dysfunction. A prime example of this is the cachexia or wasting syndrome associated with AIDS that transcends the weight loss and fatigue that can be attributed to their concurrent illnesses that are known to be associated with cachexia in non-HIV$^+$ patients. One theory of the origin of this syndrome is that the GI tract serves as a major reservoir of HIV and chronic infection of cells in the mucosa leads to loss of epithelial cell barrier function and thus increased access of gut flora. This in turn results in systemic activation of macrophages and an increase in their production of cytokines, such as tumor necrosis factor (TNF), that mediate cachexia. Alternatively, it is possible that the same end result ensues from direct stimulatory effects of HIV on macrophages. Many patients with AIDS exhibit a syndrome known as "AIDS enteropathy" that is characterized by atrophy of the small intestines and varying degrees of malabsorption and diarrhea.

The CNS is another organ implicated in the general debilitation that accompanies HIV. Infection of neural tissue with the virus presumably occurs via transport by infected macrophages that penetrate the blood–brain barrier. The virus infects microglia cells (bone marrow–derived cells in the same lineage as the macrophage), oligodendrocytes, and astrocytes. Ultimately, such infection may lead to AIDS-related dementia and progressive encephalopathy. In total, up to 50% of AIDS patients show CNS symptoms and >70% have CNS changes at autopsy.

In addition to the AIDS-defining illnesses described above, patients in the crisis stage may have a host of other problems arising from their immunodeficient state; they are subject to serious infections with ordinary (nonopportunistic) pathogens. Thus, although AIDS patients appear to have abundant B-cell activity and antibody production, they are unable to mount effective antibody responses to newly encountered pathogens, perhaps due to the T-cell defect. This problem extends to T-cell-independent B-cell responses to encapsulated organisms, which still require T-cell-derived cytokine secretion. In addition, AIDS patients may have increased susceptibility to bacterial

infections, such as *Pseudomonas aeruginosa* pneumonia, as a result of their neutropenia.

A collateral problem is the continuous cell necrosis (death) caused by multiple infections: bacterial, viral, fungal, as well as HIV itself. These organisms and the cell debris provide a rich source of antigens causing chronic antigenic stimulation of B cells, which can result in polyclonal hypergammaglobulinemia (elevated serum immunoglobulins), circulating immune complexes, and markedly increased plasma cell production. Thus, patients can have problems due to immune complex deposition and even a hyperviscosity syndrome due to the increased levels of circulating immunoglobulins (see Cases 22 and 26).

Fortunately, this described clinical course of HIV infection has changed for the better, at least for individuals in developed countries with access to medication. The first dramatic improvement was the result of early, aggressive, and now prophylactic treatment of *Pneumocystis jiroveci*. Whereas at the beginning of the epidemic many patients died early from PCP, with effective therapy of this infection, more patients began surviving the early stages of HIV. However, this longer survival with HIV led to an increase in the incidence of malignancies and these took prominence among AIDS patients. The second improvement came with the introduction of increasingly effective antiviral therapies that prolonged the chronic phase of HIV infection, delaying progression to full-blown AIDS and delaying the occurrence of AIDS-associated malignancies (see below). The spectrum of chronic conditions that long-surviving AIDS patients suffer from now is first beginning to be recognized.

IMMUNOPATHOPHYSIOLOGY OF HIV INFECTION

What explains the three clinical stages of HIV infection? To answer that question we have to correlate the life cycle of HIV with its effects on the body's immune system.

If an individual is first exposed to HIV via the urogenital or gastrointestinal tract, infection can be established in the macrophages and dendritic cells of the mucosal associated lymphoid tissue with a macrophage tropic variant (R5 or R5X4) of the virus. CCR5 is thought to be the major coreceptor for establishing primary infection, since individuals with mutations in CCR5 appear to be at least partially protected. These infected antigen-presenting cells (APCs) then provide a *reservoir* of virus both locally and distally, since they are not killed by the infection and are capable of migrating throughout the body. Dendritic cells carry the virus mostly on their surface, whereas the macrophages internalize the virus and then allow a constant low level of viral production without cell lysis. Exposure to an unrelated antigen promotes increased HIV viral replication in the macrophages and a switch to the lymphotropic form

(X4) that can enter T cells. The activation of both infected macrophages and T cells by cytokines or antigen results in increased viral replication (as stimulated by the increased NF-κB in the host cells) and the productive phase of the virus life cycle.

During the asymptomatic (early) phase of infection, extensive dissemination of virus occurs. In lymphoid tissues, virus becomes trapped in the follicular dendritic cell network and establishes an initial site of high viral concentration and significant replication (Fig. 9.5). At this early time higher levels of virus exist in lymph nodes than in the blood. Once HIV has become established in lymphoid tissues, significant viral replication takes place (still in the absence of a detectable adaptive immune response), resulting in the high-level HIV viremia, as was seen in Jack's case. Peak viremia is thought to occur 7–14 days after the onset of symptoms (acute phase), with viral levels reaching as high as 100 million copies per milliliter. After several days, HIV infection induces first a cellular immune response to HIV proteins followed shortly thereafter by an antibody response. Evidence of this response becomes manifest in the physical signs of early infection, including lymphadenopathy, splenomegaly, and rash.

A viral "setpoint" (sustained level of virus in the blood) is established at around 12–18 months following infection. Exact determinants of the viral setpoint are not known, but contributing factors may include the immune response of the host, the number of available target CD4+ T cells, the host's degree of immune activation, the extent of trapping and sequestration of HIV and infected CD4+ T cells in the germinal centers of lymphoid tissue, as well as the replicative capacity of the viral strain. The setpoint predicts the rate of disease progression, suggesting

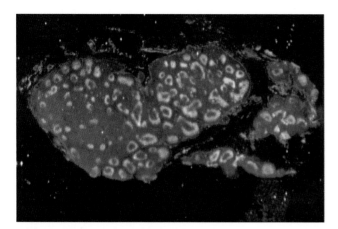

Figure 9.5. Identification of HIV-infected cells in lymph node. HIV-infected cells were identified by *in situ* hybridization using nucleic acid probes complementary to the HIV genome. Infected cells (light areas) were present surrounding germinal centers and in interfollicular areas. (Photo courtesy of Michael A. Polis, NIAID, NIH.)

that this initial viral–host interaction is critical in HIV immunopathogenesis. It is likely that HIV immunity controls the extent of viremia and the numbers of infected cells to some degree; however, despite persistent evidence of an immune response (both cellular and humoral), the immune response to HIV is ultimately ineffective.

Why does the immune response merely contain rather than eradicate the virus? The first likely answer to this question is that the virus is inherently capable of an extremely high rate of mutation and thus produces altered proteins that evade the immune response. In addition, as the patient becomes progressively more immunodeficient with time through the death of the T cells, the ability to mount an effective immune response decreases. Meanwhile, the reservoir of infected cells, macrophages and dendritic cells, remains and is capable of hiding the virus from view and generating more virus as the immune response wanes.

An examination of the lymph nodes during the course of the disease illustrates the sequence of immune depletion. The viral infection at first causes the lymphadenopathy seen clinically and due to a follicular or germinal center hyperplasia in response to the virus. However, as HIV results in progressive destruction of the T cells, there is follicular center lysis and eventual depletion of the lymph nodes. The end result is a disrupted lymph node architecture characterized by few and poorly formed germinal centers along with fibrosis at later stages of the disease.

The T cells undergo a slow rate of lysis as evidenced by involutional changes in the lymph nodes and by the gradual decline in peripheral CD4+ T-cell counts. Both naive and memory CD4 T cells are affected, although naive cells are particularly affected. Estimates of the proportion of infected cells range from 1:50 to 1:10,000 cells, and it is unlikely that this lymphodepletion is due to HIV infection alone. A number of probable causes of CD4+ T-cell depletion have been proposed:

- Production of virus in the T cells is itself a cause of cell lysis.
- The infected cell seems to be intrinsically more susceptible to apoptosis.
- Cytotoxic T lymphocytes (CTLs) specific for virally infected cells may kill at least some of the infected cells.
- Uninfected CD4+ T cells may also be killed in an antibody-dependent cell-mediated cytotoxicity (ADCC)–like mechanism as a result of binding of soluble gp120 and anti-gp120 antibody to their surface CD4 molecules.
- T cells may undergo activation-induced cell death as a result of activation even without encountering their specific cognate antigen. Such activation-induced cell death may therefore be responsible for the death of

large numbers of uninfected cells, eventually exhausting the immune system.

- Cells physically close to infected cells (bystander cells) have also been shown to undergo cell death, suggesting that local effects may be important influences on lymphodepletion.
- Activation of HIV-infected T cells (and macrophages) by infectious agents other than HIV induces the provirus to initiate the productive and lytic cycle with stimulation by the host transcription factor, NF-κB.

Regardless of the mechanism of cell depletion, as the number of CD4$^+$ T cells reaches progressively lower values, the patient becomes symptomatic and enters the final phase of HIV infection, AIDS.

In summary, several factors may act to bring the patient to the crisis phase. The gradual drop in CD4$^+$ T cells eventually results in an immunodeficient state that leaves the individual susceptible to opportunistic infections. Activation of virally infected T cells by antigen results in stimulation of viral transcription and progeny formation. This leads to T-cell death and exacerbation of the immunodeficient state. Rapid viral replication also increases the viral mutation rate, allowing escape from any immune controls that may still remain.

 ## TREATMENT OF AIDS

Highly Active Antiretroviral Therapy

The development of antiretroviral therapy would not have been possible without knowledge of the HIV life cycle and the identification of viral-specific proteins that could be the targets of therapy. These include proteins necessary for viral entry into the host cell (gp120 and gp41) as well as those necessary for viral integration and replication once inside the cell (reverse transcriptase, integrase, and protease). To date, agents used in an attempt to treat HIV infection have included inhibitors of virally encoded enzymes essential for HIV replication (reverse transcriptase or protease) and inhibitors of virus–cell fusion. Azidothymidine (AZT), a nucleoside inhibitor of reverse transcriptase, was the first drug developed and shown to have efficacy in preventing HIV replication. AZT was used as a sole therapy for several years. Later, protease inhibitors and nonnucleoside reverse transcriptase inhibitors were developed. There are no drugs currently in use against integrase.

It soon became apparent that single-agent treatment was ineffective presumably because of the capacity of the virus to mutate into a drug-resistant form. The current approach is therefore to use triple-agent antiviral therapy referred to as highly active antiretroviral therapy. HAART combines three drugs from at least two of the inhibitor classes directed against HIV's reverse transcriptase and

protease in the expectation that the triple-agent therapy will delay the appearance of mutant strains resistant to all three agents. It should be noted, however, that this therapy results in suppression but not elimination of HIV since it does not affect integrated provirus. Thus, while the therapy prevents successful infection of new cells by blocking the activity of reverse transcriptase and prevents the formation of productive viral particles by blocking protease, previously infected cells are left undisturbed until they are lysed. Thus, initiation of HAART therapy results in a rapid and dramatic fall in viral titers, but a small baseline titer almost always remains.

In practice, the goal of HAART therapy is to achieve maximal suppression of plasma HIV viral RNA levels. In effect, this may mean reducing levels to below that measurable with common detection techniques (50 copies/ml plasma); however, HIV replication can still be demonstrated in all infected patients using more sensitive techniques. Therefore, the popular description of HIV suppression to "undetectable" levels is a misleading characterization of the true situation. It is encouraging, though, that application of effective antiretroviral therapy and suppression of viral replication result in a sustained increase in CD4$^+$ T-cell numbers and decreases in rates of opportunistic infections and mortality. Most patients using HAART therapy experience viral suppression for years and thus have significantly prolonged and active lives. As one might expect, discontinuation of the drugs for a prolonged period results in a resurgence of virus.

The question of when to initiate antiretroviral therapy in a given patient with HIV infection has no clear answer. Such therapy is generally lifelong and has significant adverse side effects. Current guidelines recommend HAART therapy and prophylactic PCP treatment for patients with CD4 cell numbers ≤200 cells/μL or for patients with a diagnosis of AIDS. In many centers, therapy is initiated in asymptomatic patients with CD4 cell counts between 200 and 350 cells/μL or viral RNA levels >55,000 copies/ml.

Treatment in the acute stage of HIV infection remains controversial. The potential benefit of preserving immunity (and prolonging life) before viral destruction proceeds is, at present, an unproven hypothesis. It is possible that early therapy may diminish dissemination of HIV within the individual and decrease transmission of the virus to others as well. However, treatment in acute HIV infection may turn into lifelong therapy, which could lead to cumulative toxicity and the potential for the emergence of HIV drug resistance. Some recommend initiating therapy during the acute stage, discontinuing after one year or so, and then basing the decision to restart therapy on HIV RNA levels and CD4$^+$ T-cell numbers measured while off therapy. Acute HIV infection represents a severe psychological stress and any decision to initiate therapy must be balanced with an honest discussion of the risks and benefits of such a strategy.

The Reality and Hopes for the Future

In spite of the current success of HAART, the ready ability of the virus to undergo mutation and escape suppression requires an expanded repository of available drugs. Additional pharmacological approaches involve targeting CD4 and coreceptors on host cells to block viral entry, development of integrase inhibitors, and nonspecific stimulation of the immune system to partake in resistance. However, the ultimate goal is to develop an HIV vaccine that can both prevent infection and control an already established infection. The history of medicine is replete with examples of successful vaccination development against viral infection and, theoretically at least, a vaccine for HIV should likewise be possible.

Possible, but difficult! First, we are hampered by a paucity of animal models in which to develop and test potential vaccines (or even study the disease) because of their lack of susceptibility to the virus. The monkey provides the best model since it develops a disease similar to AIDS after infection with the related virus, simian immunodeficiency virus (SIV). Second, potential targets for immunization, the viral proteins that govern infectability, are highly mutable due to the inaccurate nature of the reverse transcriptase activity. It is estimated that the mutation rate is so high that numerous variants of HIV are generated within an individual patient every single day, making HIV proteins a "moving" target. Third, the ability of the virus to "hide out" in reservoir cells allows easy escape from the immune response and is in fact part of the reason why the body cannot eliminate the virus on its own. Fourth, because it is unclear which type of immune response (antibody, cytotoxic, etc.) will be effective in preventing HIV infection or fighting one that has already been established, it is difficult to design vaccination protocols. Lastly, clinical testing of any potential vaccine is fraught with more ethical problems than have ever before been encountered.

In the absence of an HIV vaccine (and even in the event of vaccine development), the best approach is prevention and control of the spread of HIV. This can be accomplished by avoiding unprotected contact with blood and body fluids from infected individuals. Education and public awareness of both what to avoid and what is safe (such as casual contact) are required to control the disease and to prevent unreasonable prejudice.

Starting in 1985, all blood donations in the United States have been tested for antibodies to HIV. Because the development of an antibody response after exposure to HIV can take up to five weeks, this testing still left a long window period during which a recently infected individual might not be detected. Blood donors were—and still are—screened by an interview and questionnaire process in which they are asked direct questions (orally and in writing) about high-risk behaviors. Although testing for viral RNA, which uses an amplification step, is very sensitive and has significantly decreased the window period, it has not been eliminated; thus the need to interview donors remains. Even after collection of their blood, potential donors are given an opportunity to indicate privately and in writing not to use their blood.

HIV$^+$ pregnant women are placed on anti-viral therapy to decrease viral load and thereby diminish the risk of transplacental transfer of virus. Cesarean sections are performed to eliminate infection during passage through the birth canal. In some states, all newborns are tested so that they can be treated immediately if found to be positive. Finally, exposure through breast milk is avoided. For individuals who are accidentally exposed to infected blood, therapy is administered as soon as possible after exposure to prevent establishment of infection.

Thanks to the efforts of many, people in underdeveloped countries are just beginning to have access to medication, but this is still minor compared to the overwhelming problem in these nations. Although amazing strides have been made, the goal of stopping this worldwide pandemic of HIV has not yet been reached.

REFERENCES

Arthos J, Cicala C, Martinelli E, Macleod K, Van Ryk D, Wei D, Xiao Z, Veenstra TD, Conrad TP, Lempicki RA, McLaughlin S, Pascuccio M, Gopaul R, McNally J, Cruz CC, Censoplano N, Chung E, Reitano KN, Kottilil S, Goode DJ, Fauci AS (2008): HIV-1 envelope protein binds to and signals through integrin a4b7, the gut mucosal homing receptor for peripheral T cells. *Nature Immunol* 9:301–309.

Borrow P, Lewicki H, Hahn BH, Shaw GM, Oldstone MB (1994): Virus-specific CD8+ cytotoxic T-lymphocyte activity associated with control of viremia in primary human immunodeficiency virus type 1 infection. *J Virol* 68:6103–6110.

Branson BM (2007): State of the art for diagnosis of HIV infection. *Clin Infect Dis* 45(Suppl 4):S221–S225.

Busch MP, Satten GA (1997): Time course of viremia and antibody seroconversion following human immunodeficiency virus exposure. *Am J Med* 102(Suppl 5B):117–124.

Centers for Disease Control and Prevention (2007): Rapid HIV testing in outreach and other community settings—United States, 2004–2006. *MMWR Morb Mortal Wkly Rep* 56:1233–1237.

Chan DC, Fass D, Berger JM, Kim PS (1997): Core structure of gp41 from the HIV envelope glycoprotein. *Cell* 89:263–273.

Cicala C, Arthos J, Censoplano N, Cruz C, Chung E, Martinelli E, Lempicki RA, Natarajan V, VanRyk D, Daucher M, Fauci AS (2006): HIV-1 gp120 induces NFAT nuclear translocation in resting CD4+ T-cells. *Virology* 345:105–114.

Cooper DA, Gold J, Maclean P, Donovan B, Finlayson R, Barnes TG, Michelmore HM, Brooke P, Penny R (1985): Acute AIDS retrovirus infection. Definition of a clinical illness associated with seroconversion. *Lancet* 1:537–540.

Dalgleish AG, Beverley PC, Clapham PR, Crawford DH, Greaves MF, Weiss RA (1984): The CD4 (T4) antigen is an essential component of the receptor for the AIDS retrovirus. *Nature* 312:763–767.

Deng H, Liu R, Ellmeier W, Choe S, Unutmaz D, Burkhart M, Di Marzio P, Marmon S, Sutton RE, Hill CM, Davis CB, Peiper SC, Schall TJ, Littman DR, Landau NR (1996): Identification of a major co-receptor for primary isolates of HIV-1. *Nature* 381:661–666.

Dhasmana DJ, Dheda K, Ravn P, Wilkinson RJ, Meintjes G (2008): Immune reconstitution inflammatory syndrome in HIV-infected patients receiving antiretroviral therapy: Pathogenesis, clinical manifestations and management. *Drugs* 68:191–208.

Doranz BJ, Rucker J, Yi Y, Smyth RJ, Samson M, Peiper SC, Parmentier M, Collman RG, Doms RW (1996): A dual-tropic primary HIV-1 isolate that uses fusin and the β-chemokine receptors CKR-5, CKR-3, and CKR-2b as fusion cofactors. *Cell* 85:1149–1158.

Dragic T, Litwin V, Allaway GP, Martin SR, Huang Y, Nagashima KA, Cayanan C, Maddon PJ, Koup RA, Moore JP, Paxton WA (1996): HIV-1 entry into CD4+ cells is mediated by the chemokine receptor CC-CKR-5. *Nature* 381:667–673.

Embretson J, Zupancic M, Ribas JL, Burke A, Racz P, Tenner-Racz K, Haase AT (1993): Massive covert infection of helper T lymphocytes and macrophages by HIV during the incubation period of AIDS. *Nature* 362:359–362.

Fidler S, Fox J, Porter K, Weber J (2008): Primary HIV infection: To treat or not to treat? *Curr Opin Infect Dis* 21:4–10.

Gürtler L, Mühlbacher A, Michl U, Hofmann H, Paggi GG, Bossi V, Thorstensson R, G-Villaescusa R, Eiras A, Hernandez JM, Melchior W, Donie F, Weber B (1998): Reduction of the diagnostic window with a new combined p24 antigen and human immunodeficiency virus antibody screening assay. *J Virol Meth* 75:27–38.

Hammer SM, Katzenstein DA, Hughes MD, Gundacker H, Schooley RT, Haubrich RH, Henry WK, Lederman MM, Phair JP, Niu M, Hirsch MS, Merigan TC. (1996): A trial comparing nucleoside monotherapy with combination therapy in HIV-infected adults with CD4 cell counts from 200 to 500/ μl. *N Engl J Med* 335:1081–1090.

Kaufmann DE, Bailey PM, Sidney J, Wagner B, Norris PJ, Johnston MN, Cosimi LA, Addo MM, Lichterfeld M, Altfeld M, Frahm N, Brander C, Sette A, Walker BD, Rosenberg ES (2004): Comprehensive analysis of human immunodeficiency virus type 1-specific CD4 responses reveals marked immunodominance of gag and nef and the presence of broadly recognized peptides. *J Virol* 78:4463–4477.

Kearney M, Palmer S, Maldarelli F, Shao W, Polis MA, Mican J, Rock-Kress D, Margolick JB, Coffin JM, Mellors JW (2008):

Frequent polymorphism at drug resistance sites in HIV-1 protease and reverse transcriptase. *AIDS* 22:497–501.

Liu R, Paxton WA, Choe S, Ceradini D, Martin SR, Horuk R, MacDonald ME, Stuhlmann H, Koup RA, Landau NR (1996): Homozygous defect in HIV-1 coreceptor accounts for resistance of some multiply-exposed individuals to HIV-1 infection. *Cell* 86:367–377.

Maldarelli F, Palmer S, King MS, Wiegand A, Polis MA, Mican J, Kovacs JA, Davey RT, Rock-Kress D, Dewar R, Liu S, Metcalf JA, Rehm C, Brun SC, Hanna GJ, Kempf DJ, Coffin JM, Mellors JW (2007): ART suppresses plasma HIV-1 RNA to a stable set point predicted by pretherapy viremia. *PLoS Pathog* 3:e46.

Owen SM, Yang C, Spira T, Ou CY, Pau CP, Parekh BS, Candal D, Kuehl D, Kennedy MS, Rudolph D, Luo W, Delatorre N, Masciotra S, Kalish ML, Cowart F, Barnett T, Lal R, McDougal JS (2008): Alternative algorithms for human immunodeficiency virus infection diagnosis using tests that are licensed in the United States. *J Clin Microbiol* 46:1588–1595.

Palmer S, Wiegand AP, Maldarelli F, Bazmi H, Mican JM, Polis M, Dewar RL, Planta A, Liu S, Metcalf JA, Mellors JW, Coffin JM (2003): New real-time reverse transcriptase-initiated PCR assay with single-copy sensitivity for human immunodeficiency virus type 1 RNA in plasma. *J Clin Micro* 41:4531–4536.

Panel on Antiretroviral Guidelines for Adults and Adolescents. Guidelines for the use of antiretroviral agents in HIV-1-infected adults and adolescents. *Department of Health and Human Services*. January 29, 2008: 1–128. Available: http://www.aidsinfo.nih.gov/ContentFiles/AdultandAdolescentGL.pdf.

Pantaleo G, Graziosi C, Demarest JF, Butini L, Montroni M, Fox CH, Orenstein JM, Kotler DP, Fauci AS (1993): HIV infection is active and progressive in lymphoid tissue during the clinically latent stage of disease. *Nature* 362:355–358.

Popovic M, Tenner-Racz K, Pelser C, Stellbrink HJ, van Lunzen J, Lewis G, Kalyanaraman VS, Gallo RC, Racz P (2005): Persistence of HIV-1 structural proteins and glycoproteins in lymph nodes of patients under highly active antiretroviral therapy. *Proc Natl Acad Sci USA* 102:14807–14812.

Rosenberg ES, Altfeld M, Poon SH, Phillips MN, Wilkes BM, Eldridge RL, Robbins GK, D'Aquila RT, Goulder PJ, Walker BD (2000): Immune control of HIV-1 after early treatment of acute infection. *Nature* 407:523–526.

Soria A, Lazzarin A (2007): Antiretroviral treatment strategies and immune reconstitution in treatment-naive HIV-infected patients with advanced disease. *J Acquir Immune Defic Syndr* 46(Suppl 1):S19–S30.

Volberding PA, Lagakos SW, Koch MA, Pettinelli C, Myers MW, Booth DK, Balfour HH Jr, Reichman RC, Bartlett JA, Hirsch MS, et al. (2000): Zidovudine in asymptomatic HIV infection. A controlled trial in persons with fewer than 500 CD4-positive cells per cubic millimeter. *N Engl J Med* 322:941–949.

Unit II

IMMEDIATE HYPERSENSITIVITY AND MAST CELL DISORDERS

INTRODUCTION: WHEN ANTIGENS BECOME ALLERGENS

WARREN STROBER and SUSAN R. S. GOTTESMAN

Diseases of immediate hypersensitivity encompass the various conditions in which the major pathologic event is an allergic reaction. An ***allergic reaction*** is essentially an immune response in which the stimulating antigen is a type of antigen known as an allergen. An allergen is defined by its ability to elicit an IgE antibody response. Allergens bound to IgE antibodies form complexes that have a special propensity to bind to Fc receptors on mast cells via the IgE–Fc domain. This binding or cross-linking of IgE on the surface of mast cells results in their activation and the release of mast cell mediators. These mediators have multiple effects that are characteristic of allergic reactions. This type of immune response is called an ***immediate hypersensitivity response*** because the interaction of allergen with IgE and the subsequent activation of mast cells occur quickly (immediately), as do the pathologic disease manifestations. Because immediate hypersensitivity depends on the production of IgE antibodies by B cells, it also depends on cytokine-producing T cells, which support B-cell responses. These cytokines belong to the T_H2 family of cytokines and include IL-4, IL-5, and IL-13. Thus, diseases of hypersensitivity are typically T_H2 T-cell mediated. Recently it has been shown that antigen-presenting cells (dendritic cells) that produce thymic stromal lymphopoietin (TSLP) are necessary for the induction of T_H2 T cells. Thus, allergic reactions are ultimately dependent on certain types of inducing cytokines.

A major question relating to allergic reactions is why certain antigens are allergens specifically capable of eliciting immediate hypersensitivity responses whereas other antigens do not have this property and are not allergens. Recently it has been shown that allergens are proteases, enzymes with properties that lead to the recruitment of basophils to draining lymph nodes and the activation of these cells at this site. The activated basophils release IL-4, a key cytokine that favors the differentiation of T_H2 cells and the production of IgE. These data thus suggest that antigens are allergens when they have the capacity to activate basophils and that the latter cells have an unexpected role in the genesis of the allergic response.

In this unit, three immediate hypersensitivity diseases are considered—mastocytosis, anaphylaxis, and asthma. The vasculitides, which are actually a complex set of diseases with varying underlying and often unknown etiologies are also included.

Mastocytosis is a disease in which the mast cell is hyperactive in the absence of IgE triggering; thus, this disease is a type of hypersensitivity disease uncoupled from the immune response. Indeed, we extend our discussion of mastocytosis to include its malignant counterpart which is characterized by uncontrolled proliferation of mast cells. We use this chapter to familiarize you with mast cell biology.

Immunology: Clinical Case Studies and Disease Pathophysiology, By Warren Strober and Susan R. S. Gottesman
Copyright © 2009 John Wiley & Sons, Inc.

Anaphylaxis is the prototypic allergic disease; it is due solely to an IgE–allergen interaction and has potentially catastrophic consequences resulting from massive mediator release. In Unit I on immunodeficiency diseases, we discussed C1 esterase inhibitor deficiency. This is a disease of the complement system, not an allergic disease, because it does not involve IgE antibodies. Nevertheless, it is a related disease because it also results in the release of mediators and symptoms that may mimic anaphylaxis.

Asthma, one of the most common and important of the immediate hypersensitivity diseases, is in reality only partly an allergic disease. In this case, the allergic reaction is a frequent trigger for asthmatic symptoms, but the disease is more complex in that it also involves other pathophysiologic mechanisms dependent on the T_H2 T-cell response but not on IgE.

Certain forms of vasculitis are the result of immune complex deposition, some of which may be the consequence of exogenous antigen exposure and which lead to an inflammatory response. Other types could have easily been discussed in the autoimmune section of this book (Unit III), although the possible autoantigens involved (if such is the case) have not been identified.

10

MASTOCYTOSIS

CEM AKIN*

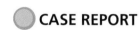

CASE REPORT

"I have a rash that won't go away!"

History and Physical Examination

Tom, a 35-year-old male, comes to your office with the chief complaint of a rash, which he noticed about two years ago. He first thought that the rash was freckles; however, it gradually spread, covering most of his stomach, back, legs, and arms. Although they are flat, he noticed that they become slightly raised and itchy when he takes a hot shower, exercises, or rubs his skin. He also describes recurrent episodes of flushing accompanied by rapid heart rate, lightheadedness, nausea, and itchy eyes. These episodes, which have occurred over the past year, last anywhere from about 30 min to several hours. He can not identify any apparent triggers.

On physical examination you find a diffuse maculopapular, hyperpigmented rash covering most of his trunk and extremities but seeming to spare his face, hands, and other sun-exposed areas. [*Maculopapular lesions* are small (1–2 cm maximum diameter), discolored, circumscribed, and slightly elevated.] When you scratch the skin with a tongue depressor, the lesions become more erythematous (red), raised, and palpable (*Darier's sign:* hiving of skin

upon firm rubbing or stroking). Abdominal examination reveals mild epigastric tenderness to deep palpation with no peritoneal irritation signs. The tip of the spleen is palpable, indicating slight enlargement. The rest of the physical examination is normal.

Differential Diagnosis

What is the differential diagnosis based on the history and physical findings?

*The chief complaints of persistent skin rash and episodic flushing with increased heart rate and lightheadedness suggest an excess release of histamine or other specific neuroendocrine mediators and lead to a differential diagnosis of an allergic or anaphylactic reaction, a hormone-secreting tumor, or a proliferation of the cells normally responsible for histamine secretion: mast cells and basophils. The specific appearance of the rash and associated Darier's sign, which is the result of local release of mast cell mediators, are characteristic of **urticaria pigmentosa**, a disorder due to accumulations of abnormal mast cells in the skin.*

Narrowing It Down: Although mastocytosis is your primary diagnosis, the other possibilities must be investigated.

Allergic/Anaphylactic Reactions. The patient reports that he underwent an allergy evaluation when he

*With contributions from Warren Strober and Susan R. S. Gottesman

Immunology: Clinical Case Studies and Disease Pathophysiology, By Warren Strober and Susan R. S. Gottesman
Copyright © 2009 John Wiley & Sons, Inc.

first complained of the rash. A combination of serum testing for IgE to common allergens and skin testing failed to identify any food or aeroallergen hypersensitivity (see Case 11).

Hormone-Secreting Tumor. Similarly, Tom's internist had done an endocrine workup to elucidate the cause of flushing and rapid heart rate. Results did not suggest a hormone-secreting tumor such as a carcinoid or pheochromocytoma (tumors that may produce serotonin and catecholamines, respectively).

Mast Cell Excess. Urticaria pigmentosa and episodes of unexplained flushing and lightheadedness are suggestive of mastocytosis as the underlying diagnosis. Mastocytosis results in an excess of mast cells in many tissues, such as the skin, bone marrow, liver, spleen, gastrointestinal tract, and lymph nodes. Infiltration of and mediator release in different organs explain the diverse symptomatology, for example, rash, flushing, tachycardia (rapid heart beat), gastrointestinal cramping, diarrhea, bone and soft tissue pain, and signs of bone marrow disease (Table 10.1). In addition, it explains the variety of possible radiologic findings, including osteoporosis (decreased bone mineral density), lytic or sclerotic bone lesions, abnormal bone scans indicative of increased bone turnover, hepatomegaly, splenomegaly, and lymphadenopathy. However, mast cells are part of the body's innate and adaptive immune systems and may be elevated in various tissues and may degranulate in response to a variety of stimuli (see below). Therefore, true mastocytosis must be distinguished from a reactive process.

Definitive Diagnosis and Workup

Mastocytosis is defined as the uncontrolled proliferation and accumulation of a hematopoietic derived cell. In those cases involving more than one organ, it is considered a clonal disorder (derived from a single founder cell) and is characterized by the World Health Organization (WHO) as a hematopoietic tumor. Several clinical subtypes are defined (Table 10.2).

For the Diagnosis. To confirm your diagnosis of mastocytosis, you order a skin biopsy and a serum test of tryptase levels. Further analysis is needed to subtype Tom's disease. Results are discussed below.

Skin Biopsy. A punch biopsy of a skin lesion from Tom shows an infiltration of mast cells in the papillary dermis and in a perivascular pattern (adjacent to blood vessels) deeper in the dermis (Fig. 10.1).
Interpretation: Mast cells are normally found in small numbers in the skin and are increased in inflammation. The cells are most often located adjacent to blood vessels. The finding of involvement of the papillary dermis or sheets of mast cells without other inflammatory cells supports a diagnosis of **cutaneous mastocytosis**, rather than a reactive process resulting from allergen exposure.

Tryptase Levels. Tom has a significantly elevated serum tryptase level of 115 ng/ml (reference range generally less than 12 ng/ml).
What is the significance of an elevated serum tryptase level?

Tryptase, a protease enzyme, is one of many mediators synthesized and stored by mast cells, its primary source. It is often elevated in the circulation of patients with mastocytosis and is therefore valuable as a surrogate and diagnostic marker. Human basophils also contain tryptase, but their levels are 300- to 700-fold less than those in lung or skin mast cells. Therefore, tryptase levels in serum are considered a marker for systemic mast cell activation.

Mast cell tryptase (molecular weight 134,000 Da) is a serine esterase with four subunits, each with an enzymatically active site. When dissociated from heparin, tryptase rapidly degrades into its monomers and loses enzymatic activity. Enzymatically mature forms of tryptase (β-tryptase) are believed to be stored in mast cell granules, whereas proenzyme forms (α-tryptase) are routed directly to the cell membrane for extracellular release. Both forms are present in the serum and are detected by the fluorescent immunoassay. α-Protryptase levels serve as a measure of total mast cell number while β-tryptase levels are a measure of the extent of mast cell activation.

Mast cells that have been activated during an IgE-mediated hypersensitivity reaction release proteases, including tryptase, along with prestored histamine and

TABLE 10.1. Signs and Symptoms of Mastocytosis

Skin	Episodic flushing, itching, hyperpigmented maculopapular lesions [urticaria pigmentosa (UP)]
Cardiovascular	Episodic tachycardia, hypotension, lightheadedness
Gastrointestinal	Abdominal cramping, diarrhea, heartburn, nausea, vomiting, peptic ulcer, hepatomegaly, ascites
Musculoskeletal	Osteoporosis, osteosclerosis, diffuse soft-tissue pain
Hematologic	Splenomegaly, lymphadenopathy, signs and symptoms of associated hematologic disorder, if present
Constitutional	Fatigue, headache

CASE REPORT   **131**

TABLE 10.2. WHO Classification of Mastocytosis

Cutaneous mastocytosis

Indolent systemic mastocytosis

Mastocytosis associated with clonal hematologic non–mast cell lineage disorder

Aggressive systemic mastocytosis

Mast cell leukemia

Mast cell sarcoma

Extracutaneous mastocytosis

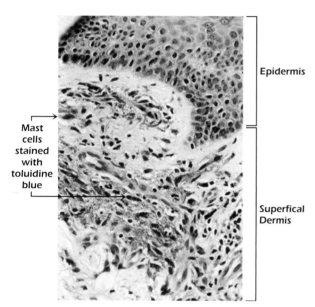

Mast cells stained with toluidine blue

Epidermis

Superfical Dermis

Figure 10.1. Toluidine blue staining of skin biopsy in urticaria pigmentosa. Epidermis at upper portion of photomicrograph. Mast cell infiltrate in upper or superficial dermis.

newly generated vasoactive mediators into surrounding soft tissue. Serum tryptase levels are elevated after mast cell degranulation in severe allergic reactions or anaphylaxis. Therefore, these enzyme levels may aid in two aspects of the workup: first as a surrogate marker of total mast cell burden when measured at the patient's baseline and, second, to clarify the involvement of mast cells in the etiology of the patient's recurrent flushing and hypotensive episodes if determined within 4 h after an episode. The normal median total tryptase level is approximately 5 ng/ml; a baseline tryptase level of greater than 20 ng/ml is suggestive of mastocytosis. The levels will increase even further after an anaphylactic episode. This increase will be detected within 15–30 min of an allergen challenge and will decline with a half-life of 2 h, therefore necessitating collection of sample within 30 min to 4 h after exposure to a stimulus.

Elevated tryptase levels are also found in other hematologic disorders, such as certain hypereosinophilic syndromes, myelodysplastic syndromes, or myeloid

leukemias. As you can surmise, it cannot be used alone to establish the diagnosis.

Additional Studies. Although the skin biopsy and tryptase results suggest a diagnosis of UP/mastocytosis and the symptoms suggest systemic involvement, Tom requires further evaluation to determine the subtype of his disease. A complete blood count and white blood cell differential, enzyme levels indicative of liver function, and coagulation (clotting) studies are ordered. In addition, because of the epigastric tenderness and splenomegaly, abdominal imaging, bone densitometry, and upper and lower gastrointestinal evaluation are needed. The tests relating to hematologic function are particularly important because mastocytosis frequently involves the bone marrow in adult patients. In contrast, children experience onset of skin lesions within the first two years of life and generally have a disease limited to the skin.

Tom's blood counts and liver function values prove normal; nevertheless, you arrange a consult with a hematologist to obtain a bone marrow study.

A bone marrow biopsy and aspiration are performed. The pathology report states the following:

• Biopsy is 55% cellular.

• Tryptase staining of the biopsy shows mast cell aggregates in excess of 15 cells in perivascular and paratrabecular (adjacent to the bone spicules) locations. More than 25% of the mast cells have an elongated shape.

• No dysplastic changes (abnormal maturation features) are noted in other hematopoietic cells in the aspirate smear.

Which features support a diagnosis of mastocytosis in the bone marrow as opposed to a reactive process or other hematologic disorder?

Normal mast cells have a round shape with a central nucleus and a fully granulated cytoplasm. In mastocytosis, the mast cells in the bone marrow are usually clustered, are elongated with cytoplasmic projections and fewer granules, and may be difficult to recognize as mast cells in both biopsies and aspirate smears (Fig. 10.2). Therefore, the core biopsy sections are stained either with toludine blue, a metachromatic stain, or immunohistochemically for tryptase in order to highlight the mast cells (Fig. 10.2). The lack of dysplastic changes in the other lineages and the normal cellularity of the bone marrow help exclude other hematologic disorders.

Putting It All Together. Specific criteria have been established to help physicians confirm or rule out the diagnosis of systemic mastocytosis. These consist of one major and four minor criteria. The patient meets the diagnostic

Bone spicule

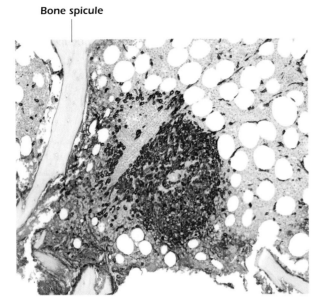

Figure 10.2. Tryptase immunohistochemical staining (brown-colored stain) of a bone marrow core biopsy section in systemic mastocytosis. Mast cells are present as dense paratrabecular and perivascular aggregates.

criteria if he has the major criterion and one minor criterion or three minor criteria in the absence of the major criterion:

Major criterion:

Presence of multifocal mast cell aggregates consisting of 15 or more mast cells in bone marrow or other extracutaneous organs.

Minor criteria:

1. Elongated "spindle" shapes or atypical morphology in more than 25% of mast cells
2. Expression of CD2 and/or CD25 by mast cells
3. Consistently elevated serum tryptase level greater than 20 ng/ml
4. Detection of a point mutation at codon 816 of *c-kit* gene (see below)

Do the findings in Tom obtained thus far satisfy the criteria for a diagnosis of systemic mastocytosis?

The pathology and laboratory findings for Tom support the major criterion as well as two minor criteria (abnormal mast cell morphology and elevated serum tryptase level), and therefore fulfill the diagnostic criteria for systemic mastocytosis. Flow cytometry to define the surface markers of the mast cells and a mutational analysis of the c-kit gene were not performed. Although not necessary to establish the diagnosis in this particular case, they should be done if possible.

TABLE 10.3. WHO Criteria for subtyping Mastocytosis

B Findings

1. Bone marrow biopsy: >30% mast cell infiltration and/or serum tryptase >200 ng/ml
2. Dysplasia or proliferation of non–mast cell lineage but insufficient for diagnosis of non–mast cell hematopoietic tumor and approximately normal blood counts
3. Hepatomegaly, splenomegaly, and/or lymphadenopathy without impaired function

C Findings

1. Peripheral blood cytopenias (low blood cell counts) without non–mast cell malignancy
2. Hepatomegaly with impaired function
3. Skeletal involvement
4. Splenomegaly with impaired function
5. GI involvement with malabsorption and weight loss

Seven subtypes of mastocytosis exist according to the WHO classification (Table 10.2). These range from localized skin disease (solitary mastocytoma of the skin) to an aggressive mast cell leukemia. Tom has indolent systemic mastocytosis. The prognosis of indolent systemic mastocytosis is good, with no significant impact on life expectancy, although a small percentage (estimated to be <5%) may progress into a more aggressive category (Table 10.3).

Treatment Plan

You meet with Tom to explain his disease and to develop a treatment plan. Currently, treatment of indolent systemic mastocytosis remains aimed at controlling symptoms. This is due to the fact that most of these patients have good prognoses and are not candidates for aggressive treatment approaches with potentially life-threatening adverse effects. In addition, there is at present no treatment specifically directed at the abnormal mast cells carrying the *c-kit* mutation (see below).

You recommend two types of antihistamines and instruct him on the use of an Epi-Pen in case of a systemic mast cell degranulation episode (see Case 11). You ask him to return in a few weeks to see if this approach is improving his quality of life.

Antihistamines, both H1 receptor blockers to control itching and H2 receptor blockers for gastrointestinal symptoms, are commonly used to treat systemic mastocytosis. Proton pump inhibitors may be added if gastrointestinal symptoms related to gastric acid hypersecretion are not sufficiently controlled by H2 blockers alone. Epinephrine injection (Epi-Pen) is critical during acute episodes of impending vascular instability and anaphylaxis. Steroids or glucocorticoids are used in patients with frequent episodes of anaphylaxis or when the disease is more aggressive than in Tom's case, presenting with signs of organ dysfunction such as diarrhea with malabsorption or liver disease with ascites. Bisphosphonates, in combination with calcium and vitamin D, are used in an attempt to delay bone density loss in patients with osteoporosis or significant osteopenia (see Case 26).

Cytoreductive therapies such as interferon-α or 2-chlorodeoxyadenosine are aimed at reducing mast cell number and proliferation, and are considered in patients in aggressive categories of disease with poor prognosis. Bone marrow transplantation may be considered in patients with an associated hematologic disorder if indicated for the treatment of that hematologic disease. In these patients, the associated hematologic disease should be treated regardless of the mast cell disease. Future investigational therapies will include signal transduction inhibitors capable of inhibiting Kit carrying the D816V mutation.

NORMAL MAST CELL BIOLOGY

Mast cells are derived from precursors in the bone marrow and migrate to and continue to mature in the peripheral tissues. They are similar to basophils, a type of circulating granulocyte which release many of the same mediators in allergic and anaphylactic reactions. The electron-dense basophilic granules filling the mast cell's cytoplasm contain biogenic amines (histamine and serotonin), proteoglycans (heparin and chondroitin sulfate), neutral proteases (tryptase, chymase, cathepsin G-like protease, and carboxypeptidase), acid and alkaline phosphatases, and eosinophil chemotactic factor of anaphylaxis (ECF-A), some of the most potent inflammatory molecules (Fig. 10.3).

Two subsets of mast cells are identified based on their protease contents. Mucosal mast cells are present in the lung alveoli and intestinal mucosa. Their maturation is dependent on T cells, presumably interleukin-3 (IL-3) produced by these cells and stem cell factor (see below). They contain tryptase but lack the other neutral proteases. Connective tissue mast cells are present in the skin and intestinal submucosa. They are not dependent on T cells for development and contain chymase, carboxypeptidase, and cathepsin G as well as tryptase. These are not distinct lineages but alternative phenotypes which are interchangeable in response to environmental stimuli. Both tend to preferentially localize around blood vessels and near sites of contact with the outside environment.

Both mast cell types express FcεRI on their surface and bind monomeric IgE from the serum and interstitial fluid (Fig. 10.4). In addition they express Mac-1 (CD11b/CD18), an integrin which is a receptor for complement fragment iC3b, microbes, and intercellular adhesion molecule 1 (ICAM-1), the integrin ligand on endothelial cells. Human skin mast cells also have receptors for the anaphylatoxin C5a on their surface. Although mast cells may be activated in a variety of ways, the predominant path is through FcεRI. When the bound IgE is cross-linked by its specific antigen (allergen), the mast cell responds as follows: It releases its preformed soluble mediators; it synthesizes and secretes lipid mediators (leukotrienes, prostaglandins, and thromboxanes); and it synthesizes and secretes cytokines such as IL-4, IL-5, IL-6, IL-8, IL-9, tumor necrosis factor α (TNF-α), and granulocyte–macrophage colony-stimulating factor (GM-CSF) (see Case 12) (Fig. 10.5).

Exocytosis results from the signaling cascade initiated by cross-linking of FcεRI, which causes phosphorylation of a series of tyrosine kinases, leading to phosphorylation of phosphatidylinositol-specific phospholipase C (PLC$_\gamma$). This

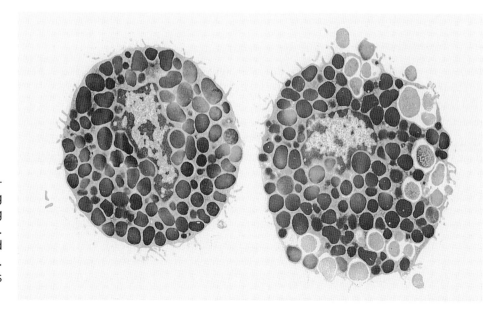

Figure 10.3. Electron micrograph of mast cells showing electron-dense granules filling cytoplasm and overlying nuclei. Cell on right has been triggered and is releasing its granules. (Courtesy of T. Theoharides, Tufts Medical School.)

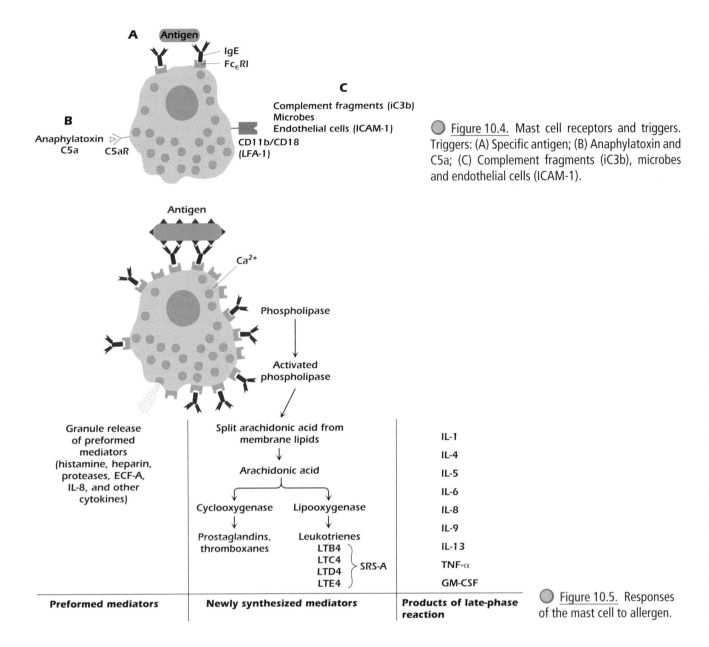

Figure 10.4. Mast cell receptors and triggers. Triggers: (A) Specific antigen; (B) Anaphylatoxin and C5a; (C) Complement fragments (iC3b), microbes and endothelial cells (ICAM-1).

Figure 10.5. Responses of the mast cell to allergen.

enzyme then catalyzes the breakdown of phosphatidylinositol bisphosphate (PIP$_2$) in the membrane to diacylglycerol (DAG) and inositol triphosphate (IP$_3$). DAG then activates protein kinase C (PKC), and IP$_3$ raises intracellular calcium. PKC and Ca^{2+} together phosphorylate the myosin light chain. This change in the actin–myosin cytoskeleton moves granules to the cell membrane where fusion is regulated by activated Ras-related Rab protein. The mediators are released from the proteoglycans in the granule. The biogenic amines (histamine and serotonin) cause vascular permeability and smooth muscle response and the proteolytic enzymes cause tissue damage. The release of the preformed mediators causes this rapid or immediate response, hence the term *immediate hypersensitivity*.

The tyrosine kinase signaling molecules that are phosphorylated as a result of FcεRI cross-linking also activate mitogen-activated protein kinases (MAPKs). These enzymes activate the two remaining pathways: one leading to the synthesis of lipid mediators and the other to cytokine production. MAP kinases and Ca^{2+} combine to activate phospholipase A$_2$ (PLA$_2$), which in turn catalyzes the breakdown of membrane phospholipids to arachidonic acid. This leads ultimately to leukotrienes, prostaglandin, and thromboxane synthesis and secretion. Activation of MAPKs also leads to the translocation and activation of various transcription factors (NF-AT, NF-κB, AP-1) which move from the cytoplasm to the nucleus and there initiate transcription of cytokine genes.

The clinical consequence of these intracellular events is that the immediately released biogenic amines and newly synthesized lipid mediators cause vascular leak, bronchial constriction, and intestinal hypermotility (see Case 12) with the location of the activated mast cell determining the reaction. The immediately released enzymes can cause tissue damage. The cell's propensity for perivascular distribution in all the organs ensures the release of these mediators into the bloodstream. TNF-α and the lipid mediators also cause inflammation. Interestingly, the activated mast cell produces IL-4 and IL-5. IL-4 is a major stimulus for the production of T_H2 cells leading to an IgE response, and IL-5 is a chemoattractant for eosinophils. Mast cells will thus respond by both contributing to a pathway which leads to more IgE production and calling in eosinophils, another major player in allergic reactions (see Case 12). In addition to antigen specific for the bound IgE resulting in mast cell activation, non-antigen-specific signals, such as common stimulators of the innate immune system (i.e., microbes or complement fragments), may activate the cell. Since mast cell cytokine production contributes to the T_H2 response pathway, you can see that mast cells can provide one of the links between the innate and adaptive immune systems. What is also notable is that degranulation of the mast cell does not result in cell death. Not only does the cell go on to synthesize the lipid mediators and cytokines, but it can also replenish and repackage the mediators found in the granules. Mast cells are relatively long-lived cells, surviving for several months.

In summary, mast cells may be activated either specifically through binding of its IgE receptors, or nonspecifically via its complement and microbe receptors. The activated mast cell then further interacts with both the innate and adaptive arms of the immune system.

Mast cells also express CD117 (c-Kit; stem cell factor receptor) and normally lack T- and B-cell associated markers, specifically CD2 and CD25 (IL-2Rα chain). The expression of c-Kit on normal mast cells is of more than academic interest. c-Kit is a membrane-bound cellular protooncogene protein that functions as a tyrosine kinase when activated by its ligand, stem cell factor (SCF). SCF is produced in either a membrane-bound or a soluble form by bone marrow stromal cells. SCF acts on pluripotential hematopoietic stem cells in the bone marrow and is required for hematopoiesis as well as for mast cell growth, development, and activation. Activation of c-Kit by SCF occurs through the phosphorylation of tyrosine residues in the c-Kit protein itself, which in turn act as docking sites for downstream signal transduction molecules. The result is mast cell proliferation and activation.

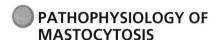

PATHOPHYSIOLOGY OF MASTOCYTOSIS

Neoplastic Mast Cells

The intracellular portion of c-Kit has a domain that acts as a tyrosine kinase and is involved in autophosphorylation of c-Kit after binding of its ligand, SCF. Because of its significance for mast cell functions, c-Kit has been the target of studies seeking to identify a genetic cause for mastocytosis. These studies have indeed demonstrated somatic point mutations in *c-kit* in the lesional tissue samples obtained from patients with systemic mastocytosis. The mutation most commonly observed in mastocytosis involves the codon 816 of the gene and results in substitution of a valine for aspartic acid (D816V). Codon 816 lies within the tyrosine kinase domain of the protein and results in constitutive activation of c-Kit, regardless of its binding of SCF.

An interesting observation is that the D816V *c-kit* mutation is found not only in mast cells but also in other non–mast cell lineages in the peripheral blood and bone marrow cells of some patients with extensive mast cell disease. This indicates the involvement of an early hematopoietic progenitor cell giving rise to multiple lineages in disease pathogenesis.

From the practical aspect, detection of D816V *c-kit* mutation carries significant implications for therapy. Recent years have witnessed the emergence of targeted therapy and pharmacogenomics in the treatment of neoplastic disorders. These approaches utilize the knowledge gained from functional genomics to select drugs that specifically inhibit the protein altered by a mutation in a given disorder. In mastocytosis, the therapeutic target has been the inhibition of the constitutively activated tyrosine kinase function of c-Kit. Imatinib is a tyrosine kinase inhibitor that is effective against the *bcr–abl* oncogene product in chronic myeloid leukemia. Imatinib has also been shown to inhibit mutated c-Kit, although the D816V mutation in mastocytosis is not targeted by this drug. Therefore, patients with mastocytosis bearing the D816V *c-kit* mutation are not considered candidates for imatinib therapy. However, rare cases lacking the D816V *c-kit* mutation and associated with a favorable response to imatinib have been described. Newer tyrosine kinase inhibitors capable of binding to c-Kit carrying the D816V mutation are currently in preclinical and clinical development.

Categories of Mastocytosis

Mastocytosis is a heterogeneous disease. There are seven categories of disease with different clinical presentations and prognosis according to the latest classification document adopted by the WHO (Table 10.2).

- *Cutaneous mastocytosis* without systemic (bone marrow) involvement is commonly diagnosed in children. Cutaneous mastocytosis, in the absence of systemic involvement, has a good prognosis, and the skin lesions usually regress or improve by the time the child reaches adolescence.

- *Indolent systemic mastocytosis* is the most common category diagnosed in adults. Patients with indolent systemic mastocytosis generally have urticaria pigmentosa skin lesions and meet the WHO criteria for systemic involvement, as discussed above. Although pathologic mast cell collections are present in bone marrow in this category, hematopoietic bone marrow function is not compromised and there is no evidence of end-organ damage due to mast cell infiltration. The prognosis of indolent systemic mastocytosis is good, although a small percentage may progress into a more aggressive category.

- *Systemic smoldering mastocytosis* is a subcategory of systemic indolent mastocytosis, which presents with extensive mast cell involvement of the bone marrow (greater than 30%) and high tryptase levels but no other evidence of tissue dysfunction (see Table 10.3, B findings). The possibility that patients with systemic smoldering mastocytosis are more likely to advance into a more aggressive category of mastocytosis is currently under investigation.

- *Mastocytosis with an associated clonal hematologic non–mast cell lineage disorder* affects approximately 10–15% of the patients with systemic disease. In addition to meeting WHO criteria for systemic mastocytosis, these patients also have evidence of a second bone marrow disorder, usually a myelodysplastic syndrome or a myeloproliferative disorder. Acute leukemias and lymphomas have also been reported to be associated with mast cell disease. Prognosis of this category depends on the prognosis of the associated hematologic disorder.

- *Aggressive systemic mastocytosis* is diagnosed when there is evidence of end-organ dysfunction due to mast cell infiltration. Examples of such dysfunction include malabsorption in the presence of intractable diarrhea, hepatic involvement with ascites (collection of fluid in the peritoneal cavity), cytopenias (low peripheral blood cell counts) due to bone marrow dysfunction or hypersplenism, and pathologic bone fractures with osteolytic or osteosclerotic lesions (see Table 10.3, C findings). These patients are generally considered for cytoreductive therapies.

- *Mast cell leukemia* is a rare condition manifested by the presence of more than 20% immature mast cells in bone marrow aspirate or more than 10% in peripheral blood. Mast cells are tissue-resident cells and are not normally found in peripheral circulation. Prognosis of mast cell leukemia is poor, as there are no consistently effective therapeutic options.

- Mast cell collections can be rarely observed as a solid tumor in noncutaneous tissue sites. These could have malignant or benign cytologic features and are termed *mast cell sarcoma* and *extracutaneous mastocytoma*, respectively.

REFERENCES

Akin C, Kirshenbaum AS, Semere T, Worobec AS, Scott LM, Metcalfe DD (2000): Analysis of the surface expression of c-kit and occurrence of the c-kit Asp816Val activating mutation in T cells, B cells, and myelomonocytic cells in patients with mastocytosis. *Exp Hematol* 28:140–147.

Akin C, Metcalfe D (2002): Surrogate markers of disease in mastocytosis. *Int Arch Allergy Immunol* 127:133–136.

Castells M, Austen KF (2002): Mastocytosis: Mediator-related signs and symptoms. *Int Arc Allergy Immunol* 127:147–152.

Escribano L, Akin C, Castells M, Orfao A, Metcalfe DD (2002): Mastocytosis: Current concepts in diagnosis and treatment. *Ann Hematol* 81:677–690.

Feger F, Ribadeau Dumas A, Leriche L, Valent P, Arock M (2002): Kit and c-kit mutations in mastocytosis: A short overview with special reference to novel molecular and diagnostic concepts. *Int Arc Allergy Immunol* 127:110–114.

Hartmann K, Henz BM (2002): Cutaneous mastocytosis—Clinical heterogeneity. *Int Arch Allergy Immunol* 127:143–146.

Horny H, Valent P (2001): Diagnosis of mastocytosis: General histopathological aspects, morphological criteria, and immunohistochemical findings. *Leuk Res* 25:543–551.

Li C (2001): Diagnosis of mastocytosis: Value of cytochemistry and immunohistochemistry. *Leuk Res* 25:537–541.

Schwartz L, Sakai K, Bradford TR, Ren S, Zweiman B, Worobec AS, Metcalfe DD (1995): The alpha form of human tryptase is the predominant type present in blood at baseline in normal subjects and is elevated in those with systemic mastocytosis. *J Clin Invest* 96:2702–2710.

Tefferi A, Pardani A (2004): Clinical, genetic, and therapeutic insights into systemic mast cell disease. *Curr Opin Hematol* 11:58–64.

Valent P, Akin C, Sperr WR, Escribano L, Arock M, Horny HP, Bennett JM, Metcalfe DD (2003): Aggressive systemic mastocytosis and related mast cell disorders: Current treatment options and proposed response criteria. *Leuk Res* 27:635–641.

Valent P, Akin C, Sperr W, Mayerhofer M, Födinger M (2005): Mastocytosis: Pathology, genetics, and current options for therapy. *Leuk Lymph* 46:35–48.

Valent P, Horny HP, Escribano L, Longley BJ, Li CY, Schwartz LB, Marone G, Nunez R, Akin C, Sotlar K, Sperr WR, Wolff K, Brunning RD, Parwaresch RM, Austen KF, Lennert K, Metcalfe DD, Vardiman JW, Bennett JM (2001): Diagnostic criteria and classification of mastocytosis: A consensus proposal. Conference Report of "Year 2000 Working Conference on Mastocytosis. *Leuk Res* 25:603–625.

11

ANAPHYLAXIS

ROBERT G. HAMILTON*

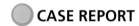

CASE REPORT

"Yikes. I just got stung and I feel faint, warm and itchy all over"

Emergency Room Visit

Adam, a 29-year-old dentist, has had chronic problems with allergies over many years. He has been premedicating routinely with Loratadine (an antihistamine) to manage his perennial rhinitis (runny nose!). One Saturday, Adam went golfing with his friends and on hole 3 he got stung by an insect. Previous stings while playing golf on the same course had produced a local area of irritation, swelling, and itching that was confined to the sting site. It would hurt for minutes and then vanish after only minor itching. With each subsequent sting, however, Adam noticed an increase in the area of swelling and duration of itching. This occurred only with some stings, others causing essentially no swelling and itching.

On this day, however, the sting on the right side of Adam's face produced a feeling of warmth and itching all over his body within minutes. His face felt flushed, and within 15 min he had difficulty breathing, as though there was a baseball lodged in his throat. At this point, Adam's

*With contributions from Warren Strober and Susan R. S. Gottesman

friends quickly rushed him to the local hospital. By the time he reached the emergency room, his right eye was completely shut as a result of the swelling, and he continued to have difficulty breathing. In addition, he was disoriented and was experiencing cardiac arrhythmias.

What is the differential diagnosis of these symptoms?

The constellation of chief complaints of itching, swelling, respiratory distress, and cardiac symptoms suggests a release of histamines. Although similar to the presentation seen in mastocytosis (see Case 10) and therefore having the same differential diagnosis, in this case the episode is acute and temporally related to the insect sting. The urgency of Adam's condition necessitates immediate action based on the assumption that one is dealing with an anaphylactic reaction to a specific instigating agent—insect toxin.

What is the definition of anaphylaxis?

Anaphylaxis, *as originally identified by Portier and Richet in 1902, is a heightened, serious, potentially fatal immunologic response following exposure to a foreign protein that has been previously seen by the patient's immune system. The term* ***anaphylaxis (ana*** *= against or without;* ***phylaxis*** *= protection) was used to describe the condition that is the antithesis of prophylaxis and is a type I hypersensitivity reaction.*

Immunology: Clinical Case Studies and Disease Pathophysiology, By Warren Strober and Susan R. S. Gottesman
Copyright © 2009 John Wiley & Sons, Inc.

This anaphylactic event is due to the rapid and massive release of mediators from mast cells and basophils. Both IgE-mediated immunologic mechanisms (anaphylaxis or allergen induced) and non-IgE-mediated mechanisms (anaphylactoid, e.g., exercise induced) exist and are indistinguishable by symptoms. This case involves an individual who was exposed to stinging insects and with each subsequent sting, developed an incrementally increasing response to specific proteins in the venom. The increasing sensitivity can be correlated with an increase in allergen-specific IgE antibody with each new event.

What symptoms might a patient present with during an anaphylactic reaction?

Allergen-induced anaphylaxis is diagnosed by first identifying a spectrum of nonspecific signs and organ-based changes in response to the exposure of a predisposed individual to an allergen to which they have been sensitized (and are therefore IgE antibody positive). The reaction occurs rapidly, within 15–30 min and almost always within 2 h of allergen exposure. Individuals report a sense of internal and cutaneous warmth associated with flushing and pruritus (itching). Some report a metallic taste in their mouth and a sense of impending doom. Nearly all individuals have cutaneous changes such as flushing of the upper chest, face, and ears and itching often accompanied by urticaria (wheals or hives) and angioedema (swelling due to vascular changes). Laryngeal edema can lead to upper airway obstruction and lower airway obstruction that may present as wheezing, cough, hoarseness, difficulty speaking or swallowing, or asthma. Cardiovascular changes related to anaphylaxis include hypotension, changes in cardiac rhythm and rate and cardiovascular collapse. If the allergen is ingested, gastrointestinal symptoms such as diarrhea, vomiting, nausea, and cramps may occur. Rhinitis, nasal and oral itching, and conjunctival swelling have also been reported as symptoms associated with anaphylaxis.

Upon Adam's arrival at the emergency room, you quickly assess him, checking his airway, level of consciousness, and vital signs. Notably, Adam has tachycardia (heart rate of 120), low blood pressure (BP 70/50), and rapid respirations of 28/min. Epinephrine and oxygen are immediately administered to Adam, who is put in a supine position with his legs elevated. Peripheral intravenous fluids are started as well as cardiac monitoring. Adam is stabilized and transferred to intensive care for observation and further management. Other interventions that you consider upon his arrival in the emergency room include histamine (H1, H2) antagonists, vasopressors, corticosteroids, and glucagon. Given the rapid recognition of anaphylaxis, he receives only H1 and H2 antagonists and systemic corticosteroids in addition to the epinephrine and fluids. You enter a diagnosis of anaphylaxis induced by an insect sting in the chart.

Why were fluids and epinephrine immediately necessary?

The reaction results in the rapid and massive release of vasoactive amines, specifically histamine. One of histamine's actions is to bind to H1 receptors on endothelial cells causing separation of the cells and increased permeability. As the fluid leaves the vascular space for the tissue, the blood pressure plummets while swelling occurs. Fluid is given to maintain the blood pressure. Epinephrine works rapidly to cause constriction of vascular tissue and, as the blood is restricted from entering some vascular beds, the overall pressure increases. Epinephrine also increases the force and rate of cardiac contraction; these changes combine to restore normal blood pressure.

Definitive Diagnosis of Anaphylactic Reaction

Once Adam is stabilized, a blood sample is sent to the clinical immunology laboratory for a mast cell tryptase analysis. Although a complete workup of Adam's allergic triggers will be done later the definitive diagnosis of an anaphylactic reaction can and should be confirmed at the present time.

Why is tryptase being measured?

Anaphylaxis is the result of the release of mediators of mast cells and basophils, usually through an IgE-dependent mechanism. Although it is histamine which wreaks the most immediate havoc, tryptase levels are the most useful marker of mast cell degranulation (see Case 10).

Adam's total tryptase ($\alpha + \beta$ forms), as measured by a fluorescent immunoassay on a blood sample collected 2 h after the onset of his reaction, was 15 ng/ml. This elevated level of total serum tryptase (>10 ng/ml) is consistent with levels that are seen 30 min to 4 h after the onset of systemic anaphylaxis with hypotension. More importantly, Adam's β-tryptase level was elevated at 4.2 ng/ml, indicating recent mast cell activation (normal <1 ng/ml). These tryptase measurements support the conclusion of mast cell activation and the diagnosis of systemic anaphylaxis.

Completing the Workup: Appointment with the Allergist

Once well enough, Adam is released and referred to the allergy clinic for further workup and management. Your part as emergency room doctor is over and, although thankful, Adam is quite certain that he never wants to see you again!

At allergy clinic, Adam is presented with a long questionnaire to complete. He provides his general allergy history, which includes lifelong perennial rhinitis to a number of outdoor aeroallergens (weeds, grasses, and trees). The insect that stung him on the day he experienced anaphylaxis looked like a yellow jacket. It came out of a hole in the ground. Adam gives a history of progressively larger areas

TABLE 11.1. Medically Important Sting Insects

Family	Subfamily	Genus–Species	Common Name
Apideae	Apinae	*Apis mellifera*	Honeybee
		Bonbus pennsylvanicus	Bumble bee
Vespidae	Polistinae	*Polistes annularis*	Wasp
	Vespinae	*Vespula vulgaris*	Yellow jacket
		Dolichovespula arenaria, D. maculate	Hornet
Formicidae	Myrmicinae	*Solenopsis invicta*	Fire ant
Hemiptera	Reduviidae	*Triatoma*	Kissing bug
	Cimicidae	*Cimex*	Bedbug
Diptera	Culicidae	*Culex, Aedes, Anopheles, Culiseta*	Mosquito
	Simuliidae	*Simulium vittatum, Simulium venustum, Simulium jenningsi, Prosimulium sp.*	Blackfly
	Tabanidae	*Tabanus*	Horsefly
		Chrysops	Deerfly
	Muscidae	*Glossina*	Tsetse fly
Siphonaptera	Pulicidae	*Ctenocephalides*	Flea

of skin swelling with more recent stings. He is confused by the fact that this was not always consistent, since some stings produced no apparent itching or swelling.

How can Adam's reported history be explained?

A number of stinging insects produce IgE responses and can induce allergic reactions (Table 11.1). Hymenoptera (yellow jacket, yellow hornet, white faced hornet, Polistes wasp, and honeybee, bumble bee, and the fire ant in southern parts of the United States) are the immediate suspects in Adam's case. His history suggests that he was sensitized to proteins in yellow jacket venom. The apparent absence of any itching or swelling with certain stings suggests that insects other than yellow jackets may have stung him (e.g. bees) at those times. The vespids (yellow jacket, hornets, and wasps) share venom proteins that are structurally similar and thus cross-reactive; however, honeybee venom proteins are essentially antigenically distinct. Thus, if Adam is stung by an occasional honeybee, he will not have a systemic or even a large local reaction since (in theory) he has no premade IgE antibody to honeybee venom proteins. The progressive increase in reactions is consistent with repetitive vespid stings that elicit increasing levels of IgE antibody in the skin and blood and increase his sensitivity to vespid venoms.

The allergist concludes that Adam's clinical history supports the diagnosis of stinging insect hypersensitivity and requests skin testing to confirm the presence and specificity of the IgE antibody.

Adam asks if the skin testing is necessary or only of academic interest. Although he is usually a willing patient, since he is quite shaken by his experience, he is nervous about having the "protagonist" injected. The allergist explains the results will form the basis for immunotherapy and assures him of the safety measures taken.

The definitive diagnosis of human allergic disease (including insect sting allergy) rests on an unambiguous clinical history of an allergic reaction that is temporally correlated within minutes of exposure. Several confirmatory tests may be performed to detect specific IgE antibody in the skin (skin test) or blood (serology). There are two basic forms of skin testing used to identify the specific allergen: puncture and intradermal.

Puncture skin testing involves placing a drop of allergen on the forearm and introducing it into the epidermis with a needle puncture. An immediate reaction is read by measuring the diameter of the **wheal** (swelling) and ***erythema*** (redness) at 15–20 min as it reaches maximum size. Histamine injection is used as a positive control and as a measure of maximum wheal formation.

Intradermal skin testing is reportedly 1000–10,000 times more sensitive than a puncture skin test. As such, it is analytically more sensitive (fewer false negatives) but less specific (more false positives). To maximize sensitivity, the intradermal skin test is routinely used for evaluation of venom allergic patients. For hymenoptera venom skin testing, four 10-fold concentrations from 0.001 to 1 μg/ml are sequentially injected intradermally every 15 min to ensure maximum safety. Skin testing results (wheal and erythema mean diameter) are graded.

Why do skin testing when you can just measure levels of specific IgE antibody in the serum?

*Every test has its virtues and drawbacks and, in many situations, multiple modalities are used. Specific IgE levels, which will be discussed below, are certainly less uncomfortable both physically and mentally for the patient. Skin testing, however, provides a **biologically relevant** response. It is a functional assay which demonstrates the end point of complex interactions in the patient. It is also*

TABLE 11.2. Clinical Diagnostic Sensitivity of Assays for IgE-Mediated Systemic Reactions

Systemic Reactions	Serum IgE Antibody (RAST)[a]	Prick/Puncture Skin Test	Intradermal (ID) Skin Test
Venom allergy	Complementary to ID skin test	Not sufficient	Preferred
Drug allergy	"	"	"
Latex allergy	Inadequate	Preferred	Not needed[b]
Food allergy	Acceptable	Acceptable	False positives

[a]RAST = radioallergosorbent test.
[b]Availability of a high-concentration extract renders the prick puncture sufficiently sensitive.

rapid (15–45 min) and semiquantitative. Intradermal skin testing is believed to be the most sensitive IgE antibody confirmatory test available. Thus it is the diagnostic confirmatory test of choice for evaluating patients suspected of having hymenoptera venom allergy. The downside of a functional assay conducted in the patient is that recent events may affect the results. Antihistamines and some other medications may interfere with the activation of skin mast cells. In addition, systemic anaphylaxis, the result of generalized mast cell activation and mediator release, may lead to false-negative results if the patient is skin tested soon after the event. Moreover, days and weeks after an anaphylactic reaction associated with a sting, skin test results can appear negative due to a refractory period of anergy. If a negative skin test occurs in an individual who has experienced a systemic reaction after a sting, it should be repeated after four to six weeks. The diagnostic sensitivity of skin testing has been contrasted to serology for allergens that are known to induce anaphylaxis (see Table 11.2).

When Adam is asked to provide his medication history, including β blockers, antihistamines, or tricyclic antidepressants within the past week or antihistamine within the past month, he indicates that he took Loratidine a number of days prior but cannot remember the precise date. Most antihistamines need to be held for at least 72 h prior to any skin testing to minimize the risk of false-negative skin test results.

How do you control for medication use and recent history?

A histamine (positive control) and saline (negative control) are applied at the same time as the test allergen extracts. If medications known to interfere with skin testing have been withheld for a specified period and the histamine skin test wheal is <3 mm in diameter, then this indicates possible continued interference (Table 11.3). The saline negative control aids in identifying individuals who have false-positive skin reactions that result from dermographism in response to the physical stimulus of injection. (Dermatographism is wheal and erythema upon irritation of skin due to non-allergen-induced mast cell release; see Case 10.)

Adam shows no detectable response with the 1.8 mg/ml histamine positive control when compared to the saline control (Table 11.3). This lack of responsiveness indicates that either Adam's recent anaphylactic reaction or the medication he had taken may be interfering with the skin test.

The allergist asks Adam to return in several weeks to have the skin test repeated. However, it is important to obtain confirmatory IgE antibody data as soon as possible to verify Adam's sensitivity to venoms. Therefore, an IgE antivenom serology panel is ordered and Adam's serum is tested for total IgE, IgE for multiple allergens, and IgE specific for a variety of individual insect venoms by radioabsorbent assay (Table 11.4).

Antihistamines or other allergy medications do not generally interfere with serologic testing for IgE antibody, which can be performed within a short time interval after a systemic anaphylactic reaction. IgE antibody can even be measured in postmortem blood specimens that are grossly hemolyzed to investigate a cause of death.

What information is obtained from these assays (Table 11.4)?

Adam's total serum IgE level combined with the multiallergen screen gives an indication of his general allergic nature. The multiallergen screen is a single qualitative test measuring IgE antibody specific for 15 aeroallergens, including weeds, grasses and tree pollens, mites, molds, and pet epidermal allergens but not foods. This panel covers those specificities that induce 80–90% of aeroallergen-related allergic disease in adults. It therefore may be considered the single best laboratory test for documentation of the atopic (allergic) state of an individual. Adam's total serum IgE of 4368 ng/ml (Table 11.4) is four standard deviations from the mean and in the 99th percentile for an age-adjusted nonatopic population. His IgE anti-multiallergen screen is positive, supporting his general atopic nature.

It is necessary to know which specific antigens Adam is sensitive to in order to develop a treatment plan. The two clinical assays available both use a RAST design. In the RAST-type assays, the antigen, allergosorbent, is immobilized in a solid phase and binds the venom-specific antibody in the serum. The secondary antibody in this sandwich technique is labeled antihuman IgE which quantitatively detects bound IgE antibody.

In general, Adam's serology confirms his atopic status and supports his sensitivity to a number of vespid venoms.

⬤ TABLE 11.3. Adam's First Intradermal Skin-Testing Results

Preparation	Concentration	Wheal (mm)	Erythema (mm)	Positive or Negative
Saline (negative control)	NA	0	2	Negative
Histamine (positive control)	1.8 mg/ml	0	3	Negative[a]

[a]Apparent false-negative result induced by premedication or by a recent systemic anaphylaxis event.

⬤ TABLE 11.4. Adam's Serology Results[a]

A. Overall IgE Serology

Test Description	Pharmacia CAP System	Age-Dependent Nonatopic Mean	Percentile
Total serum IgE	4368 ng/ml	48.5 ng/ml	4.0
Adult multiallergen screen	Positive	Negative	NA
B. Levels of Specific IgE Antibody	Pharmacia CAP	RAST	Positive or
Specificity	System (kIUa/L)	(ng/ml)	Negative
IgE anti–yellow jacket venom (YJ)	2.06	13	Positive
IgE anti–honeybee venom (HB)	<0.35	<1	Negative
IgE anti–bumble bee (BB)	not done[b]	<1	Negative
IgE anti–white face hornet venom (WFH)	0.51	3	Positive
IgE anti–yellow hornet venom (YH)	0.67	4	Positive
IgE anti–*Polistes* wasp venom (PW)	0.49	3	Positive

[a]Three weeks after his systemic reaction.
[b]not done because BB crossreacts with HB.

Adam's IgE antibodies are specific for the vespid venoms (yellow jacket, white face hornet, yellow hornet, and *Polistes* wasp) whereas they are nonreactive to bumble bee venom. Since anti-IgE is used to detect the reaction, only the IgE isotype is being measured in this assay. The highest level of IgE is against yellow jacket venom, suggesting that yellow jacket is the culprit insect that induced Adam's symptoms of anaphylaxis. The other IgE antibody specificities may simply be the result of cross-reactivity. Moreover, the fact that yellow jackets live in holes in the ground, is consistent with Adam's impression of where the insect came from on the golf course.

It is important to note that the level of venom-specific IgE antibodies that is measured serologically or in the skin does not reliably allow one to predict the severity of a future reaction. Some individuals with the most severe systemic reactions have minimal venom-specific IgE antibodies in their skin and/or blood. The half-life of IgE is only a few days and is found mostly bound to its cellular receptor.

Once three months had passed, Adam returns for a skin test evaluation. To ensure maximum safety so as not to incite an anaphylactic reaction, an intradermal skin test titration is performed, starting with the most dilute venom concentrations (0.001 μg/ml) and moving to the next higher concentration after 15-min intervals. Adam is evaluated for immediate hypersensitivity to each of the common hymenoptera: yellow jacket, honeybee, bumble bee, white faced hornet, yellow hornet, and *Polistes* wasp. Results of this skin testing are presented in Table 11.5.

The intradermal skin testing (Table 11.5) supports the earlier serology results. They indicate that Adam is IgE antibody positive to the vespid venoms and negative to the bee venoms. The 4+ reaction to yellow jacket venom and 2+ skin reactions to the hornets also indicate that the yellow jacket is most probably the offending insect that induced the systemic anaphylaxis. It is likely that the weak sensitivity (1+ reaction) to *Polistes* wasp venom is a result of antigenic cross-reactivity with proteins in yellow jacket venom. These data, together with the positive clinical history and positive IgE anti–yellow jacket venom serology, complete the diagnostic testing. They provide evidence for the definitive diagnosis of systemic anaphylaxis secondary to vespid venom sensitivity.

Treatment Plan

The allergist explains that there are three general approaches to the treatment of human allergic disease: avoidance, pharmacotherapy, and immunotherapy. At present, there is no clinical indication for the use of the newest treatment modality, antihuman IgE, for treating

TABLE 11.5. Adam's Intradermal Skin Testing Results

Preparation	Concentration (mg/ml)	Wheal (mm)	Erythema (mm)	Positive or Negative
Saline (negative control)	NA	0	2	Negative
Histamine (positive control)	1.8	9	20	Positive
Yellow jacket venom	0.001	19[a]	52	4+ Positive
	0.01	ND[b]	ND	ND
	0.1	ND	ND	ND
	1.0	ND	ND	ND
Honeybee venom	0.001	0	2	Negative
	0.01	0	3	Negative
	0.1	0	1	Negative
	1.0	0	2	Negative
Yellow hornet venom	0.001	0	2	Negative
	0.01	0	3	Negative
	0.1	5	7	± Equivocal
	1.0	9	21	2+ Positive
White-faced hornet venom	0.001	0	2	Negative
	0.01	0	3	Negative
	0.1	6	9	± Equivocal
	1.0	8	29	2+ Positive
Polistes wasp venom	0.001	0	2	Negative
	0.01	0	3	Negative
	0.1	0	2	Negative
	1.0	8	11	1+ Positive

[a] with pseudopods.
[b] ND = not done because the less concentrated venom produced a positive response.

allergies to hymenoptera venom. Avoidance is not always possible, especially when one is dealing with stinging insects. Pharmacotherapy, self-treatment with an injectable dose of epinephrine, commonly called an Epi-Pen, is another approach, but alone is not ideal. Obviously, anaphylaxis is a shock to the body and not something you want your patient to experience if avoidable. However, the patient should be prepared with an Epi-Pen in an emergency. Overall, however, immunotherapy is advised in individuals who have experienced systemic anaphylaxis.

What does immunotherapy in this situation try to accomplish?

Immunotherapy is designed to stimulate an antigen-specific IgG response in the patient. The objective is to exchange one immunoglobulin isotype (IgG) for another (IgE) in the response. For overall objectives of immunotherapy see Case 12.

Adults such as Adam with a history of a systemic allergic reaction to a sting and children with severe generalized urticaria and cutaneous angioedema are candidates for immunotherapy to those venoms to which they have been shown to have specific IgE antibody. Venom immunotherapy involves injecting increasing quantities of each purified venom to which the patient is sensitive until a maintenance dose of 100 μg of each is successfully tolerated. Once at maintenance, patients are commonly treated monthly, and after 6–12 months the dosage interval may be lengthened to 6–8 weeks. Venom immunotherapy from 3 to 5 years produces protection, although anaphylaxis to hymenoptera venoms during immunotherapy can sometimes occur even after maintenance dose is reached and is not uncommon during the buildup period. Other agents that are known to induce IgE-mediated systemic anaphylaxis include antibiotics (e.g., β lactams), natural rubber latex, and food allergens (eggs, milk, wheat and soy in children, and shellfish, tree nuts, and peanuts in older children and adults).

After reaching the maintenance dose, Adam remains faithfully on maintenance immunotherapy injections every four weeks for one year. At his one-year visit, the allergist sends a serum specimen for quantification of venom-specific IgG antibody levels. Adam's preimmunotherapy and one-year immunotherapy data are presented in Table 11.6.

The allergist comments that Adam's IgG antivenom levels are well above the 3 μg/ml target level, indicating an appropriate humoral immune response. Rather than change

TABLE 11.6. Adam's Preimmunotherapy and One-Year Postmaintenance Immunotherapy IgG Antivenom Serology

Description	Preimmunotherapy IgG Antivenom (μg/ml)	Post 1 Year of Immunotherapy IgG Antivenom (μg/ml)
IgG anti–yellow jacket venom	1.9	10.1
IgG anti–honeybee venom	<1	<1
IgG anti–bumble bee venom	<1	<1
IgG anti–white face hornet venom (WFH)	1.2	6.2
IgG anti–yellow hornet venom	1.4	7.8
IgG anti–*Polistes* wasp venom	1.3	8.8

Note: Measurement of IgG antivenom is performed with a solid-phase radioimmunoassay using anti-IgG for detection.

the frequency or dose of the treatments, the allergist chooses to continue the same regimen because of the severity of the initial reaction. He indicates that at some point they may decide to increase the interval between maintenance injections from monthly to every six weeks.

Several months later Adam recounts to the allergist that he received a field sting by a yellow jacket while playing his favorite game of golf. He had his Epi-Pen ready this time; however, he did not use it since the sting induced none of the symptoms he had experienced previously. After 15 min, he had one small area (<5 mm) of swelling, redness, and itching at the site of the sting. It went away after 25 min. The allergist indicated that the venom immunotherapy should afford him this type of protection; however, he encouraged continued vigilance and reminded Adam to continue carrying his Epi-Pen and to always be prepared to use it.

PATHOPHYSIOLOGY

Normal Biology

IgE Biology and Function. IgE is composed of two light chains and two heavy chains connected by disulfide bonds. Like all immunoglobulins, the molecule can be divided by treatment with proteolytic enzymes into two regions with different biologic properties (Fig. 11.1). The Fab (fragment antigen binding) portion is composed of one light chain and the amino terminal portion of the heavy chain, whereas the Fc portion (crystalline fragment) is composed of the carboxy-terminal regions of the two heavy chains. As the name suggests, the Fab portion, which contains the variable regions of both the heavy and light chains, binds the specific antigen. The Fc portion, which contains the constant regions of the heavy chains, is responsible for

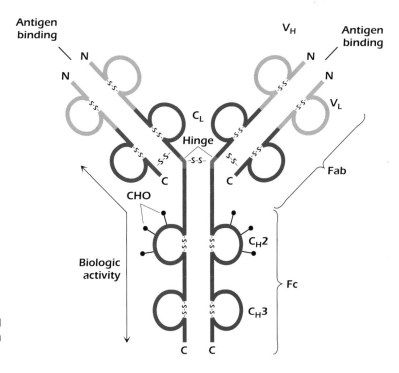

Figure 11.1. Immunoglobulin molecule showing immunoglobulin fold domains formed by intrachain disulfide bonds.

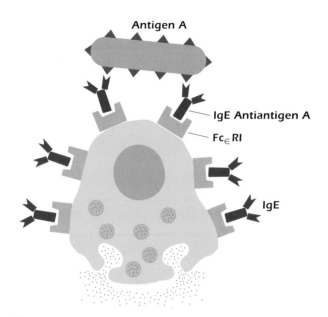

Figure 11.2. Mast cell degranulation mediated by antigen cross-linking of IgE bound to IgE Fc receptors (FcεRI).

the biologic properties of the particular heavy-chain isotype, in this case epsilon (ε).

IgE has two binding sites for antigen, as does IgG. IgE's half-life in serum is only two days and its concentration is quite low. Most of the body's IgE is bound to its Fcε receptors present on mast cells and basophils, where it is retained for extended periods (months). The binding of specific antigen to the Fab portions of the IgE molecules causes cross-linking of adjacent IgE molecules on the cell surface with resulting degranulation of the cell (Fig. 11.2). This response is "immediate" upon antigen binding, hence the term type I immediate hypersensitivity reaction.

IgE is the body's primary defense against parasites. Parasites are susceptible to the products of mast cells, basophils, and eosinophils. Eosinophils are called in by mediators released from mast cells, specifically eosinophil chemotactic factor A. Eosinophils participate in the late-phase reaction, a reaction developing over several days, and release major basic protein, which is particularly potent in leading to the death of the worm (see also Case 12). The eosinophils can bind to the worm via their Fc receptors for IgG and their low-affinity Fc receptors for IgE (FcεRII or CD23), a form of passive binding (Fig. 11.3). Both immunoglobulin isotypes coat the invading organisms. Thus IgE serves at two points in this defense mechanism. One, mast cell bound IgE specifically binds small antigens released from worms, resulting in cross-linking of the IgE, degranulation, and all its downstream consequences (see Case 10). And two, IgE directly coats the organisms, along with IgG, resulting in passive binding of eosinophils.

Contrast with IgG. IgG has the longest half-life of all the immunoglobulin isotypes and has the highest concentration in the serum. It is distributed throughout the intra- and extravascular spaces. IgG binds its specific antigen and the complex binds to Fcγ receptors on phagocytic cells (monocytes, macrophages, and neutrophils).

Control of IgE and IgG Synthesis: The Role for T Helper Cells. T helper 1 (T_H1) cells, with their production of interleukin-2 (IL-2), interferon γ (IFN-γ), and tumor necrosis factor β (TNF-β), are active in helping cells involved in cell-mediated immunity. They also interact with B cells via IFN-γ to stimulate isotype switching (the rearrangement of immunoglobulin heavy-chain gene to allow the production of a different isotype; see Case 4) to IgG2 (Fig. 11.4). T_H2 cells, on the other hand, produce IL-4, IL-5, IL-10, and IL-13 and, via IL-4 and IL-13, are very potent in stimulating isotype switching to IgE and IgG4. The cytokines cross-inhibit so that IFN-γ inhibits T_H2 cells and thus IL-4 production, whereas IL-4 and IL-10 inhibit T_H1 cells (see Case 12).

Manipulations of Normal: Exchanging the "Bad" for the "Good"

It is generally believed that the benefit of stimulating antigen-specific IgG antibodies by immunotherapy rests in their ability to bind and eliminate the allergen before it has a chance to engage its specific IgE bound to mast cells and basophils. IgG's long half-life and high concentration in the serum combine to help achieve this goal.

To be effective in producing IgG responses, immunotherapy may actually work via the stimulation of alternative T helper subsets; that is, it may stimulate T_H1 cells as opposed to T_H2 cells. The resulting IFN-γ production, in contrast to IL-4 and IL-13, will lead to IgG rather than IgE production. In addition, one must not forget the possibility of a role for tolerance, whether cellular or humoral, in decreasing the IgE and mast cell response.

Can we prove our hypothesis concerning the underlying mechanism?

Allergen injections during immunotherapy are known to enhance the production of specific IgG "blocking" antibodies. As a general rule, quantitative measurements of allergen-specific IgG (or IgG subclass) antibodies in studies of allergic rhinitis have not correlated well with improvement in clinical symptoms of individual patients on immunotherapy. Moreover, the presence or levels of IgG antibodies specific for food antigens have not shown any correlation with the diagnostic results of positive double-blind placebo-controlled food challenges. However, clinically successful immunotherapy is almost always accompanied by high serum levels of allergen-specific IgG. One application of allergen-specific IgG antibody measurements is in their use as an aid to document

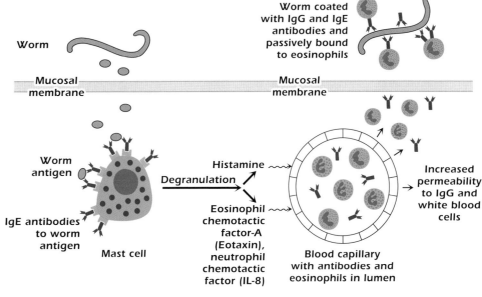

Figure 11.3. Destruction of a worm by eosinophils that have migrated to the area and been activated after IgE- and antigen-mediated mast cell degranulation.

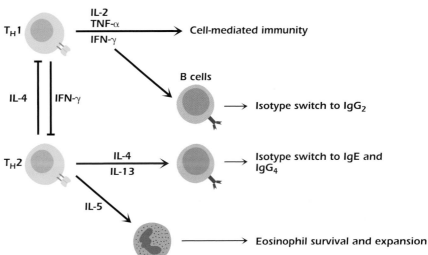

Figure 11.4. Balance between T_H1 and T_H2 responses leading to different immunoglobulin isotypes.

immunotherapy in patients with hymenoptera venom sensitivity. In a prospective study of venom allergic patients, systemic allergic symptoms occurred in 16% of those with <3 μg/ml of venom-specific IgG antibody and in only 1.6% of those with venom IgG levels >3 μg/mL. The highest rate of allergic reactions (26%) occurred among patients who had both a venom-specific IgG antibody level of <3 μg/ml and less than four years of venom immunotherapy. Quantitative venom-specific IgG antibody levels therefore may be of value for individualizing the dose and frequency of injections while maximizing the protective effects in individuals who have undergone up to four years of venom immunotherapy.

Pathogenesis

In anaphylaxis, mast cells and basophils become activated and degranulate through cross-linking of IgE bound to surface epsilon Fc receptors by allergen (IgE dependent, anaphylactic pathway). A variety of non-IgE-dependent stimuli can also induce direct activation and degranulation (anaphylactoid pathway). The chapter on mastocytosis (Case 10) discussed the degranulation of neoplastic mast cells in response to nonspecific stimuli. Whatever the mechanism, when these cells are activated, preformed histamine, tryptase, and heparin are released from ruptured granules. Other mediators such as prostaglandins, leukotrienes, and cytokines are also synthesized in response to cell activation; however, this takes more time to develop. The severity of the reaction in the patient depends on the number and location of activated mast cells. The explosive release of the preformed mediators from cells throughout the body produces systemic pathophysiological events of vascular dilatation, bronchoconstriction, laryngeal edema, and smooth muscle contraction that lead to the symptoms of an anaphylactic reaction. Although systemic anaphylactic reaction can easily be recognized as life threatening, even a localized reaction can be fatal depending on the location, laryngeal edema being the most worrisome. Exposure to food allergens may occur either via the gastrointestinal tract and/or by aerosol of food molecules. Similarly, latex, a potent allergen in some individuals, reaches its target by inhalation. Thus, the response in the body's defense against parasites when usurped to respond to an environmental antigen and expanded by repeated exposures to that antigen becomes a life-threatening situation.

REFERENCES

Golden DB (1989): Epidemiology of allergy to insect venom and stings. *Allergy Proc* 10:103–107.

Hamilton RG, Adkinson Jr NF (2003): Clinical laboratory assessment of IgE dependent hypersensitivity. *J Allergy Clin Immunol* 111:S687–701.

Norman PS (1982): In Middleton E, Ellis EF, Reed CF (eds): *Allergy: Principles and Practice*, 2nd ed. St. Louis: CV Mosby.

Portier P, Richet C (1902): De l'action anaphylactique de certain venins. *CR Soc Biol (Paris)* 54:170–.

Schartz LB, Yunginger JW, Miller J, Bokhari R, Dull D (1989): Time course of appearance and disappearance of human mast cell tryptase in the circulation after anaphylaxis. *J Clin Invest* 83:1551–1555.

Valentine MD (1992): Anaphylaxis and stinging insect hypersensitivity. *JAMA* 268:2830–2833.

Wolf BL, Hamilton RG (1998): Near fatal anaphylaxis after Hymenoptera venom immunotherapy. *J Allergy Clin Immunol* 102:527–528.

12

ASTHMA

KARI C. NADEAU and DALE T. UMETSU*

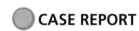

CASE REPORT

"My son's asthma is not well controlled."

Seeing the Specialist

Timothy, an eight-year-old boy who is actively wheezing, arrives at your office with his parents. The father explains that his son's current breathing difficulty started after a cold three weeks ago and has not responded to treatment with his albuterol inhaler (β-adrenergic agonist). Timothy has had two wheezing episodes over the past week, including a severe one at night. In addition to albuterol, he is on a corticosteroid inhaler and an antihistamine for intermittent, clear nasal discharge. Until one month ago, he was also using a corticosteroid nasal spray for his allergic rhinitis (hay fever), caused by grass and tree pollens. Timothy does not have fever, shakes, or chills at this time but complains of a chronic cough, especially in the morning, at night, and when running.

The parents are looking for help in managing Timothy's asthma over the long and short term and hope that he can have a normal active childhood.

Long-term management of asthma patients requires taking an extensive history—medical, social, and family—to

*With contributions from Warren Strober and Susan R. S. Gottesman

understand both the pattern and severity of the disease and the triggers that result in exacerbations.

Medical History

Timothy was the product of a full-term vaginal delivery, with a birth weight of 7 lb 3 oz and excellent APGAR scores. Developmental milestones were achieved on time. As an infant he had frequent skin rashes (eczema/atopic dermatitis), but this has not been a problem since age 2 and the parents had managed them with over-the-counter skin products. At age 3 the first episode of wheezing occurred, apparently precipitated by an upper respiratory viral infection. By age 4, these episodes were more frequent, occurring four to five times a year, particularly during the spring. They were generally responsive to albuterol inhaler at home, although one episode required an emergency hospital visit with a short course of oral steroids added to the albuterol. Often the wheezing attacks were associated with **purulent** nasal discharge (containing pus, a mixture of viable and dead white blood cells, usually with bacteria), headache, cough, and sometimes, fever. At those times, a diagnosis of sinusitis (bacterial infection of the sinus cavities) was made and he was treated with oral antibiotics. In addition, since age 5 he has had intermittent sneezing episodes associated with a clear nasal discharge when outdoors. Timothy misses about seven days of school a year; nevertheless he is doing well.

Social and Family History

The patient lives with his mother, father, and younger sister in a 10-year-old house. His sister is 9 months old and has been diagnosed with "colic" and eczema. The father had a history of asthma as a child. The family acquired a cat 5 years ago, but he is kept outdoors because of the possibility that exposure might worsen Timothy's symptoms. The house has wood and tile floors throughout, with the exception of the bedrooms, which are carpeted, and an area rug in the living room.

Timothy enjoys playing sports and is able to participate in Little League baseball. However, he becomes frustrated trying to keep up with his friends when playing soccer, particularly in the late fall when the weather gets colder.

Physical Exam

On physical examination you find that Timothy is in mild respiratory distress marked by easily audible wheezing, a respiratory rate of 24/min (normal 12–15/min) and a heart rate of 100/min (normal 70–80/min). He is not using accessory muscles to exchange air and apparently has good blood oxygenation since his color is normal and his nail beds are not cyanotic or clubbed (indicative of chronic oxygen deprivation). This is confirmed by a pulse-oximeter reading showing 98% oxygen saturation on room air. As previously noted, Timothy is afebrile, but he has swollen and congested **turbinates** (part of nasal septa) and purulent discharge from both nasal passages. In addition, his throat is mildly erythematous (red) and he has mild lymph node enlargement in the anterior cervical chain of the neck. Pulmonary auscultation reveals both inspiratory and expiratory wheezing in both lungs but no rhonchi or rales (low-pitched continuous sounds and crackling sounds, respectively). The rest of the examination is normal, although you note that Timothy is in the 25th percentile for his age in both height and weight.

The Obvious Diagnosis: Asthma

What is the definition of asthma?

> **Asthma** can be defined as an abnormal inflammatory response to specific and/or nonspecific stimuli in the bronchial lining, resulting in obstruction of the small and large airways. This obstruction has two components: (1) the inflammatory infiltrate itself, associated with the overproduction of mucus, and (2) airway hyperreactivity or bronchospasm (contraction of the muscle around the bronchiole tree) in response to mediators released from the inflammatory cells or the activation of neural signals. These causes of bronchospasm lead to intermittent obstruction.

How does this correlate with the physical findings and basic course of Timothy's disease?

> The obstruction leads to the physical findings of wheezing, breathlessness, chest tightness, and coughing. The

> inflammation can, at least in earlier stages of disease, undergo rapid and complete resolution and the mediators causing bronchospasm can quickly dissipate. Therefore, the symptoms of asthma are usually episodic and reversible. However, because the bronchospasms correlate with increasing instability of lung function, repair by fibrosis, and thus with more severe, frequent and persistent symptoms, there is permanent obstruction to airflow and reduced oxygenation of blood over time.

This pattern is precisely what we see in Timothy, whose clinical course is marked by episodic bouts of airway obstruction that are controlled by albuterol, a substance that blocks the action of β-adrenergic mediators, effectors of bronchospasm in asthma.

What is the basis of Timothy's asthma?

> Within the population of patients with asthma, there are several subgroups, each with a somewhat different pathologic basis. The major subgroup consists of those patients in whom the asthma has an immunologic basis.
>
> In this form of asthma the airway inflammation is the result of a T helper 2 cell (T_H2)–biased response to aeroantigens and is thus characterized by infiltration of the peribronchiolar and bronchiolar space by T cells producing T_H2 cytokines [such as interleukin-4 (IL-4) and IL-13] as well as other cells infiltrating in response to these soluble mediators—cells such as neutrophils, mast cells, basophils, and eosinophils. Perhaps most importantly, this T-cell response leads to B cells producing IgE; indeed, the tendency to develop an IgE-mediated allergic response to indoor and outdoor allergens is recognized as a major risk factor in the development of the disease.
>
> Timothy's asthma can be presumed to fall into this subgroup on clinical grounds alone since he has a history of atopic dermatitis, an allergic condition associated with a high risk for later development of aeroallergen sensitization and allergic rhinitis. In addition, his allergic rhinitis and asthma have a seasonal pattern, suggesting induction by seasonal allergens.

Subtypes of Immunologically Mediated Asthma

There are two subtypes of **immunologically mediated asthma**, extrinsic and intrinsic, based on the inciting agents.

Persistent wheezing in patients with **"extrinsic" asthma** (asthma brought on by external agents) is associated with allergy to specific inhalant antigens, particularly indoor allergens such as dust mite, cockroach, and cat antigens and outdoor allergens such as tree and grass pollens. Eighty to 90% of children and 70–80% of adults with asthma have environmental allergies. Because inhaled allergen doses are generally very low, sensitization requires several years of exposure and is generally not detected until after two years of life, increases in prevalence during later childhood and adolescence, and peaks in the second decade of life. This corresponds to the pattern of onset and severity of asthma.

In *"intrinsic" asthma*, the inciting agent is believed to be an endogenous component of the lung, such as a substance associated with chronic lung infection. However, the association of asthma with allergic responses in all age groups suggests that even intrinsic asthma is, at least in part, fundamentally due to an IgE-mediated reaction.

Identification of the specific allergen is sometimes easy to establish by history, for example, diagnosing cat allergy in a child who develops wheezing soon after visiting the house of a cat owner. It is, however, more difficult when the immediate reaction is blunted or suppressed by chronic exposure to allergen or when the major symptoms result from late-phase reactions (see below), hours after allergen exposure. A more reliable way of identifying an allergen is by skin testing for specific sensitivities. As an alternative to the skin test reaction, a RAST (RadioAllergoSorbent Test) can be performed. This test measures allergen-specific IgE in the blood (see Case 11).

Other Potential Triggers and Subtypes of Asthma.

Other major precipitants important in the induction of asthma in the overall patient population usually aggravate preexisting asthma due to allergic sensitization and need to be considered in Timothy's case. However, in some patients they define a category of asthma that occurs in the apparent absence of allergic sensitization.

Asthma Precipitated by Nonsteroidal Anti-Inflammatory Drugs (NSAIDs).

A small percentage of patients with asthma have an acute exacerbation when exposed to NSAIDs, particularly aspirin. This is probably related to drug-induced changes in arachidonic acid metabolism, which are characterized by suppression of the cyclooxygenase pathway and thus the enhancement of the lipooxygenase pathway and the overproduction of leukotrienes. Asthma due to NSAID sensitivity can occur as a distinct syndrome, typically in patients who also have nasal polyps, vasomotor rhinitis, and eosinophilia (increased eosinophils in blood) but who lack evidence of allergic sensitization.

Exercise-Induced Asthma.

Bronchospasms can be triggered by heat loss or changes in osmolality in the respiratory tract because of the increased pulmonary ventilation that occurs during exercise. Such exercise-induced asthma can occur as an isolated phenomenon or as a trigger for preexisting allergic asthma. The latter is the case with Timothy's asthma and probably contributes to his difficulty in playing soccer.

Asthma Precipitated by Gastroesophageal Reflux Disease (GERD).

Relatively recently, gastroesophageal reflux has been associated with the precipitation or exacerbation of asthma. The mechanism of this association is not yet understood.

Other environmental precipitants of asthma that need to be borne in mind are *food additives*, *occupational substances*, and *pollutants*.

Workup and Management of Current Episode

You explain to Timothy's parents that in order to avoid or modulate his responses to the triggers that initiate his asthma, these triggers must first be identified. In addition to avoiding exacerbations, any acute episodes that do occur need to be managed more effectively by medication than has previously been done.

The immediate need is to control the current episode. Pulmonary function tests are conducted and cultures to identify a source of infection are sent.

The peak respiratory flow, which shows the degree of obstruction due to permanent damage and bronchospasm, is found to be about 200 L/min, or 75% of the predicted value for his height. Thus, he has a moderate amount of pulmonary obstruction. Spirometer studies, which measure FEV_1/FVC (forced expiratory volume in first one second of expiratory effort/forced vital capacity), are performed before and after administration of agents that ameliorate bronchospasm to evaluate the reversibility of the obstruction and response to therapy.

Culture of Timothy's nasal discharge reveals a sinus infection with *Streptococcus pneumoniae* that is sensitive to the antibiotic augmentin. You therefore prescribe a three week antibiotic treatment for the sinusitis. Based on the spirometer tests, you treat him with nebulized albuterol inhalation to reduce his wheezing (an inhaler of corticosteroid derivatives to reduce the bronchial inflammation). You also ask the father to make a follow-up visit in three weeks so that you may determine the effectiveness of your current management course.

At the follow-up visit, repeat culture reveals that the infection has been eradicated and examination shows that Timothy is breathing comfortably.

Summary of Factors That Led to the Current Exacerbation.

Timothy's acute attack was apparently triggered by a viral infection. **Respiratory viral infections** (e.g., those caused by rhinovirus, parainfluenza, influenza, coronavirus, or respiratory syncytial virus) cause 60–80% of exacerbations in asthmatics. *Chlamydia* and *Mycoplasma* organisms have also been implicated. Viral infections are thought to act by inducing cytokines that aggravate the underlying T_H2-mediated inflammation. They can also damage the respiratory epithelium, increasing exposure of underlying mast cells to allergens or exposure of nerve endings to stimuli that evoke bronchospasm. This is particularly true of respiratory syncytial virus (RSV) infections in infants.

Timothy's *sinus infection*, a condition known to have an adverse effect on asthma by mechanisms not fully understood, also contributed to his persistent acute attack. In patients with asthma, sinus infections can cause increased airway hyperreactivity, cough, and wheezing that is often unresponsive to bronchodilators or corticosteroids. They can go unrecognized and become chronic, resulting in symptoms primarily related to asthma with absence of fever or other signs of acute infection. Sinusitis is difficult to eradicate even with antibiotics and is often undertreated. As in Timothy's case, viral respiratory infections typically trigger the development of asthma symptoms and also set the stage for a bacterial infection of the sinuses which, if untreated, prolongs and intensifies asthma symptoms.

Treatment Plan and Future Management

Timothy's parents are eager to get his condition under better control. Pulmonary function tests are repeated to assess for permanent lung damage, and an investigation of Timothy's allergic triggers is undertaken. Many of Timothy's allergens are obvious from the history; however, as in anaphylaxis, precise delineation is needed for future immunotherapy. The results of skin testing Timothy using a large panel of allergens demonstrate reactions to dust mites, cat dander, and grass pollen.

Does this prove that these are the allergens causing Timothy's asthma?

The skin tests do not prove that his episodes of asthma are triggered by the allergens giving positive reactions, but it indicates that these allergens have the potential of inducing an immediate sensitivity response in Timothy. As you recall, skin testing measures an immediate-phase reaction due to IgE–mast cell degranulation and requires preexisting, prebound, antigen-specific IgE. The late-phase reaction, which is characteristic of asthma, develops 4–6 h later, lasts for 3–24 h, and is due to the infiltration of inflammatory cells; in the skin it is characterized by induration (thickening), brawniness, and intense pruritis (itching). In addition to those delineated by the skin testing, there may be other nonspecific triggers as immediate causes of exacerbations in Timothy. His history suggests that exercise, particularly in the cold weather, can trigger an attack.

Based on these results you recommend environmental control measures to obviate the potential sources of asthma triggering. You also discuss long-term immunotherapy for desensitization (see Case 11 and below) and make the parents aware of other factors known to lead to exacerbations that you think might apply in Timothy's case. You suggest a schedule of immunotherapy treatments to desensitize Timothy to his known allergens. In addition, you instruct his parents to administer inhaler prior to athletic events and to be particularly vigilant about preventing infections.

THE PATHOPHYSIOLOGY OF ASTHMA

Immediate and Late-Phase Asthmatic Responses

As diagrammed in Figure 12.1, an asthmatic attack involves an acute or *immediate phase response* (*IPR*) as well as a chronic or *late-phase response* (*LPR*).

The *IPR* occurs within minutes of allergen exposure and is the result of allergen binding and cross-linking of antigen-specific IgE on mast cell surfaces leading to degranulation and release of factors in the respiratory tract (see Case 11). The mast cell–derived mediators critical to the IPR consist of histamine, prostaglandin D_2, the sulfidopeptide leukotrienes (LTC_4, LTD_4, and LTE_4), and possibly tryptase and chymase. Histamine release leads to increased vascular permeability and fluid extravasation into the bronchial tissues, causing obstruction and wheezing. The release of mediators at this site may directly affect smooth muscle cells, resulting in bronchospasm (see Case 10). The mast cells originate from bone marrow precursors and mature locally in pulmonary tissue in response to stem cell factor. They mediate the IPR and remain resident in bronchial tissues of asthmatic patients long after the acute response to aeroallergens has ended.

The *LPR* occurs 4–12 h after the IPR and is due to the accumulation of activated T cells, eosinophils, basophils, and other cells in the bronchial lining. In essence, the LPR represents the maturation of a recurrent response to an asthma-inducing allergen and results from exuberant T_H2-mediated inflammation. This inflammation includes the induction of T cells to produce the cytokines IL-4, IL-5, IL-9, and IL-13, which in turn stimulate the production of chemokines such as RANTES (CCL5), eotaxin (CCL11), and TARC (CCL17). These soluble mediators and the cells they attract and activate characterize the T_H2 response. As shown in Figures 12.1 and 12.2, these factors cause excess mucous secretion (IL-13) and recruitment of inflammatory cells such as eosinophils [IL-5, eotaxin, RANTES, and intercellular adhesion molecule (ICAM)] and mast cells (IL-4 and IL-13) that are critical to the development of a more chronic asthmatic state. Early on, chronic asthma is characterized by denudation of airway epithelium, mucous plugging and edema of bronchi and bronchioles, infiltration by inflammatory cells, and smooth muscle hypertrophy/hyperplasia, all of which are still reversible. Excess mucous production is an important factor in the pathophysiology of asthma, as it can lead to mechanical narrowing of the airway lumen and, in severe and/or chronic asthma, to the formation of tenacious plugs that obliterate the airway. Later, chronic asthma is associated with airway remodeling and collagen deposition in the sub–basement membrane region (lamina reticularis) of the bronchioles. This fibrosis leads to irreversible changes and permanent loss of pulmonary function.

Immediate phase response (IPR)

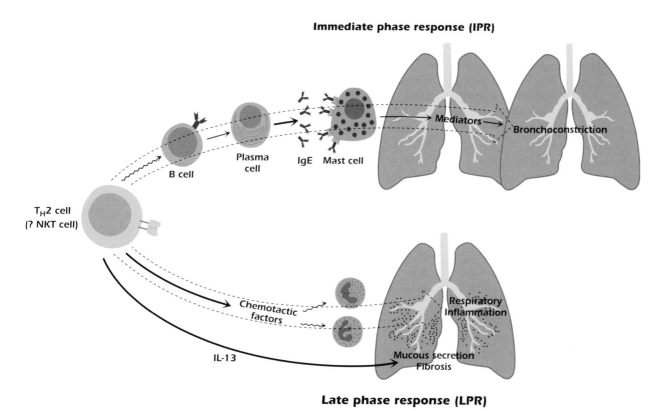

Figure 12.1. Asthmatic attack: Acute or immediate and chronic or late-phase response.

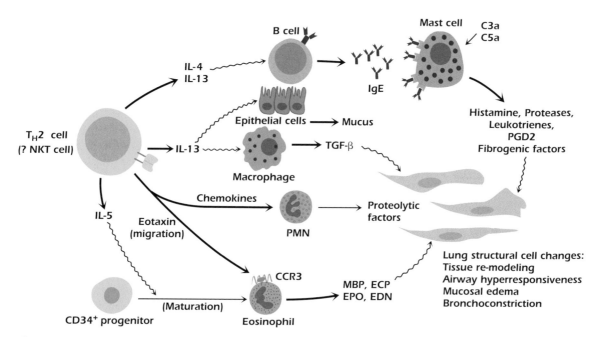

Figure 12.2. Schematic representation of the effector phase in asthma. Cytokines derived from $CD4^+$ T_H2 cells orchestrate the asthmatic response through effects on other cells such as B cells, mast cells, and eosinphils and by direct interactions with lung structural cells; epithelial cells, mesenchymal cells, fibroblasts, and smooth muscle cells.

Airway Hyperreactivity

Airway hyperreactivity is another important factor in asthma pathogenesis and contributes to both the IPR and the LPR. *Airway hyperreactivity (AHR)* is defined as the tendency of the bronchi to undergo bronchospasm and thus cause asthmatic symptoms in response to a large array of stimuli, including those that do not evoke an IgE-mediated immune response. AHR may be an independent factor in asthma pathogenesis; that is, it may have a genetic basis separate from that underlying the immune response. However, the dominant view is that AHR is secondary to the T_H2 inflammation and thus a consequence of the release of substances in the bronchial mucosa that render the bronchi sensitive to environmental stimuli. Examples of these mediators include major basic protein from eosinophils and histamine from mast cells. The main significance of AHR is that asthmatic symptoms can occur in the absence of allergen when the airways are exposed to certain nonspecific environmental stimuli. These include such disparate factors as viral infections, cold air, and irritant smoke. AHR correlates well with the frequency of asthmatic symptoms and thus this, rather than triggering of the T_H2 response, is most frequently the proximate cause of asthmatic exacerbations. In addition, AHR may underlie the association of asthma with exposure to NSAID agents, exercise, and gastrointestinal reflux as mentioned above.

Pulmonary Structure and Pathogenesis of Asthma

Not all individuals with allergic sensitization develop asthma, suggesting that mechanisms intrinsic to the lung also contribute to the pathogenesis. One such mechanism involves epithelial and mesenchymal cell interactions and epithelial cell responses to injury. Normally, the pulmonary epithelium and underlying mesenchymal cells communicate via cytokines and growth factors [transforming growth factor (TGF) β and epithelial growth factor (EGF)] to coordinate growth and respond to damage. In asthma, the mesenchymal cells differentiate into myofibroblasts and the latter deposit interstitial collagen, leading to thickening of the subepithelial basement membrane. Other intrinsic lung mechanisms involve the capacity of the epithelium to undergo repair, the tendency of smooth muscle cells to undergo hypertrophy, and the ability of bronchial tissue to support neovascularization. These responses together lead to structural remodeling that is only partially reversible and thus account for the deterioration in lung function associated with persistent disease (Fig. 12.2).

The Immunologic Basis of Asthma

Previous chapters dealt in succession with various features and consequences of the T_H2 immune response. First, mast cell biology and the effects of its mediator release were discussed in Mastocytosis (Case 10), a malignant proliferation of mast cells essentially independent of external control. Second, an abnormal IgE response and the subsequent antigen-specific triggering of mast cell degranulation was discussed in Anaphylaxis (Case 11). That case also touched on the T_H1/T_H2 paradigm and the role of skewed T_H2 T cell differentiation in generating the IgE response and the recruitment of eosinophils. Here, in the discussion of asthma, the complexities of the T_H2 immune response and its control will be discussed in greater detail.

The Normal Immune Response in Respiratory Mucosa and Its Derangement in Asthma

Origin of IgE Responses Responsible for the Development of Asthma. Immune responses in the respiratory mucosa appear more oriented to a T_H2-biased response than in other organs, setting the stage for T_H2-mediated immunopathology in that organ. The basis for this T_H2 bias is poorly understood. One possibility that is gaining increasing support is that the respiratory response is conducive to the development of subsets of NKT cells, cells that bear surface markers of both natural killer (NK) and T cells (see Fig. 12.3). These cells normally respond to glycolipid antigens as part of an early "innate" immune response and can produce either T_H1 or T_H2 cytokines. Respiratory tract conditions are such that the NKT cells produce T_H2 cytokines (perhaps in response to aeroallergens that cross-react with self-antigens) and thus drive a T_H2 response that leads to IgE production (unless controlled by regulatory T cells).

Components of the T_H2 Inflammatory Response. As shown in Figure 12.4, the T_H2 cell response is a multifaceted reaction that brings many cells and inflammatory elements derived from those cells into dynamic interplay. In the sections below we outline the major components of this reaction, beginning with the four most relevant T_H2 cytokines (IL-4, IL-13, IL-5, and IL-9) and continuing with the major inflammatory elements that participate in but are not exclusive to the T_H2 response.

IL-4. IL-4 is critical for the induction of IgE synthesis and for the up-regulation of IgE receptor expression on B cells (low-affinity receptor, CD23), mast cells, and basophils (high-affinity receptor, FcεRI). IL-4 increases leukotriene production from IgE-primed mast cells (see Fig. 12.2) and induces expression of adhesion molecules such as vascular cell adhesion molecule 1 (VCAM-1) on endothelium. VCAM-1 attracts eosinophils, basophils, and lymphocytes expressing the VCAM-1 ligand, VLA-4. In addition, IL-4 induces expression of eotaxin by lung cells, a chemokine essential to the migration of eosinophils into the asthmatic airway. Finally, IL-4 increases mucous production and may have direct effects on smooth muscle

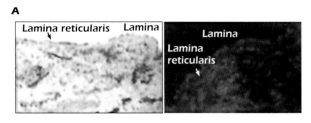

Figure 12.3. CD4$^+$-invariant NKT cells in airways of patients with asthma. (A) Left side: Endobronchial biopsy specimen obtained from a patient with asthma has typical features of chronic asthma, including thickening of the basement membrane (lamina reticularis) (arrow), epithelial disruption, and cell infiltrates in the submucosa and lamina propria. Right side: A section from the same specimen shows staining of cells immediately beneath the lamina reticularis with fluorescein isothiocyanate conjugated (FITC) antibody (monoclonal antibody 6B11) against the invariant NKT cell receptor (arrow). (B) Laser confocal images of bronchial biopsy specimens from a patient with asthma. The CD4$^+$ cells in asthmatic patients are invariant NKT cells. A lung biopsy specimen was stained with phycoerythrin-conjugated CD4 (red) and FITC-conjugated 6B11 monoclonal antibody (blue). The overlay results (pink) indicate that nearly all of the CD4$^+$-infiltrating lymphocytes from the patient with asthma coexpressed the invariant T-cell receptor.

cells, but its role in causing AHR and mucous production is complex and overlaps with that of IL-13. These activities of IL-4 notwithstanding, short-term treatment of patients with an IL-4-neutralizing monoclonal antibody or soluble receptor has been disappointing. This suggests that other cytokines (e.g., IL-13) also play important effector roles in asthma.

IL-13. IL-13 has 30% homology with IL-4, and the receptors for both share the chain (IL-4Rα) involved in signal transduction. Accordingly, IL-4 and IL-13 have several common functions, including promotion of isotype switching to IgE, and utilize some of the same signal transduction pathways. Nevertheless, IL-4 and IL-13 are functionally distinct in several important ways. IL-4 is able to induce T$_H$2 cell differentiation, but IL-13 is not. IL-13 has more profound effects on epithelial cell and muscle cell function than IL-4. High IL-13 levels are observed in bronchial biopsies, bronchoalveolar lavage fluid, and serum of atopic patients with asthma. Selective overexpression of IL-13 in the lungs of mice results in pulmonary inflammation,

epithelial and goblet cell hyperplasia, increased mucous production, increased collagen deposition, and increased eotaxin levels. In addition, overexpression of IL-13 in mice is associated with the occurrence of AHR, and IL-13 knockout mice are characterized by an inability to develop AHR. IL-13's direct actions on lung epithelial (goblet) cells (causing mucous secretion) and on airway smooth muscle cells (causing increased contractility) suggest that IL-13 is the most critical cytokine in the development of asthma.

IL-5. IL-5, together with IL-3 and granulocyte–macrophage colony-stimulating factor (GM-CSF), promotes the differentiation and maturation of eosinophil progenitor cells in the bone marrow and induces their release into the circulation, thereby amplifying and prolonging allergic inflammation. Although IL-3 and GM-CSF promote the differentiation of multiple cell lineages, IL-5 promotes only the terminal differentiation of eosinophils. IL-5 is important for the survival of eosinophils once in the tissues and for priming eosinophils for response to several stimuli. Although eosinophils in the airways (and in the circulation) are closely associated with the symptoms of asthma, recent studies show that AHR in both mice and humans was not reduced after depletion of eosinophils (through neutralization of IL-5 with anti-IL-5), suggesting that neither eosinophils nor IL-5 are absolutely necessary for the development of asthma.

IL-9. IL-9 participates in mast cell maturation and potentiates IgE production elicited by IL-4. IL-9 and IL-9 receptor expression is increased in bronchial tissue of atopic asthmatic subjects, and constitutive overexpression of IL-9 in experimental asthma is associated with AHR, inflammation, mucous production, and increased numbers of tissue mast cells. Although IL-9-deficient mice have significantly decreased goblet cell hyperplasia and mast cell proliferation in a pulmonary granuloma model, they have only minimal reductions in a model of allergen sensitization. The activities of IL-9 are mediated through IL-4 and IL-5, as shown by the ability of neutralization of these cytokines to inhibit the effects of overexpressed IL-9 in a model of experimental asthma.

IL-17 CYTOKINE FAMILY. The IL-17 family of cytokines is comprised of a group of structurally related proteins with similar or overlapping properties. Specifically, IL-17E induces T$_H$2-type cytokine production, eosinophilia, and increased IgE and IgG$_1$ production. The precise cell types that produce IL-17E are not known. IL-17 is expressed in high amounts in sputum and bronchioalveolar lavage fluid of asthmatics. Introduction of human IL-17 into rat tracheas induces airway epithelial cells to produce the chemokine macrophage inflammatory protein 2 (MIP-2)/CXCL2, which acts to attract neutrophils to the airways.

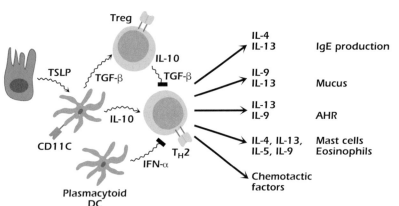

Figure 12.4. T$_H$2 cell as conductor of multi-faceted reaction.

IL-25. IL-25 is a member of the IL-17 family of cytokines that is produced by T$_H$17 cells. It has functions similar to IL-4 and IL-13, promoting increased IgE synthesis, T$_H$2 cytokine production, and blood eosinophils and causing epithelial cell hyperplasia and mucous production. Like IL-9, IL-25 mediates its effects through the induction of T$_H$2 cytokine production (IL-4, IL5, and IL-13).

THYMIC STROMAL LYMPHOPOIETIN (TSLP). Human lung and skin epithelial cells produce TSLP. This cytokine is unique in that it triggers dendritic cells to produce the T$_H$2-attracting chemokines, TARC (CCL17) and MDC (CCL22) and to induce T$_H$2 cytokine production (IL-4, IL-5, IL-13), while down-regulating IL-10 and interferon-γ (IFN-γ). These functions of TSLP may help localize allergic inflammatory responses to the respiratory mucosa and skin of atopic individuals. TSLP is also produced in the thymus, where it participates in the development of regulatory T cells.

BRONCHIAL EPITHELIAL-CELL-DERIVED MEDIATORS. Bronchial cells produce several mediators, including cytokines (IL-5 and GM-CSF), chemokines (RANTES/CCL5, eotaxin/CCL11, and MCP-1/CCL2), growth factors [platelet-derived growth factor (PDGF), fibroblast growth factor (FGF), and endothelins], and other inflammatory mediators such as nitric oxide.

In addition to the above T$_H$2-associated inflammatory elements, there are others which are not strictly T$_H$2 related but are components of many types of immune responses:

NK CELLS AND NKT CELLS. NK cells, lymphocytes that do not express B-cell markers, surface CD3, the T-cell receptor (TCR), CD4, or high-density CD8, are part of the innate immune system, important in controlling certain microbial infections and killing virus-infected cells and tumors. They rapidly produce large quantities of IFN-γ in response to IL-12, IL-18, or CpG oligonucleotides, and may produce other cytokines, including tumor necrosis factor (TNF) α, TGF-β_1, IL-5, and IL-10. Depletion of NK cells

in a murine model resulted in a reduction in pulmonary eosinophilia, suggesting that NK cells normally exacerbate airway inflammation and increase T$_H$2 cytokine production. However, IFN-γ may also protect against the development of asthma.

NKT cells are a subset of lymphocytes that express characteristics of both NK cells and $\alpha\beta$ T cells ($\alpha\beta$ refers to the particular type of chains used for the TCR). NKT cells are also part of the innate immune system, in that they rapidly (within hours of stimulation) produce IFN-γ as well as IL-4 in response to self–glycolipid antigens, microbial components, and even glycolipids in plant pollens (that might cross-react with glycolipids). Although animals deficient in NKT cells develop normal T$_H$2 responses, these animals are incapable of developing airway hyperreactivity or experimental forms of colitis, suggesting that NKT cells play a critical role in regulating immune responses at mucosal surfaces, such as in the lungs and intestinal system. This is supported by recent data showing that NKT cells form a major component of the inflammatory infiltrate in the asthmatic lung (see Fig. 12.3). Subsets of NKT cells exist, some producing IFN-γ but not IL-4 (CD8α^+ NKT cells), whereas others produce IFN-γ as well as IL-4 and IL-13 (CD4$^+$ NKT cells). The CD4$^+$ NKT cell subset may be preferentially recruited and/or enriched in the lungs, thereby enhancing T$_H$2 differentiation and asthma, whereas the CD8α^+ NKT cell subset may inhibit T$_H$2 differentiation.

CHEMOKINES. Increased levels of the chemokines CCL2, CCL3, CCL5 (RANTES), CCL7, CCL11 (eotaxin), and CXCL8 (IL-8) have been demonstrated in bronchoalveolar lavage and biopsy samples of asthmatic patients compared with control subjects. In murine models of asthma, CCL2, CCL5, and CCL11 contribute to airway hyperresponsiveness and cellular emigration. Since the chemokine family can recruit eosinophils, T cells, and monocytes to regions of inflammation, small-molecule drugs that block certain chemokines and their receptors are now being tested in human trials to determine their effectiveness in blocking allergy symptoms (Fig. 12.5).

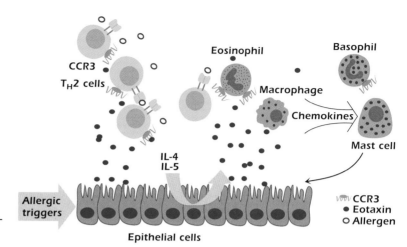

 Figure 12.5. Chemokine recruitment of eosinophils, T cells, and mast cells.

COMPLEMENT. Complement appears to be important in the development of asthma, although its precise role is controversial. Activated C5a and C3a fragments, anaphylatoxins, participate in the anaphylaxis reaction. They induce smooth muscle contraction, increase blood vessel permeability, and cause histamine release from mast cells and basophils. In addition, C5a fragment is a chemoattractant for neutrophils and monocytes. C3a receptor–deficient mice have reduced AHR, although they can develop airway inflammation, increased IgE levels, and T_H2-type cytokine production. Similar results were observed in a naturally occurring guinea pig strain with a defective C3a receptor which manifest reduced AHR but no reductions in eosinophil infiltration. To the contrary, C5 may protect against asthma because C5 deficiency in mice is associated with susceptibility toward AHR.

Factors Governing an Individual's Response to Respiratory Challenge.

If the major immunologic abnormality underlying asthma is a T_H2-biased T-cell response, one needs to ask: Why do asthma patients have such a response in their airways whereas normal individuals do not?

Several factors have been proposed to account for the development of asthma in only certain individuals. These include a lack of or disruption in tolerance mechanisms, an early decrease in exposure to infections (the hygiene hypothesis), genetic susceptibility to the induction of increased T_H2 responses, and an association with an inherited resistance to hepatitis A.

Lack of Tolerance.

Lack of tolerance to aeroallergens may explain the development of asthma.

What is the evidence for the presence of tolerance in normal individuals?

*Studies of murine models of asthma strongly suggest that the answer to this question lies in the fact that tolerogenic (also called regulatory) mechanisms dominate immune responses on all mucosal surfaces, including those in the respiratory tract. In these murine models, test antigens administered via the respiratory route normally induce **T regulatory** (T_{reg}) **cells** that suppress nascent T_H2 T-cell responses and the IgE responses that would subsequently ensue from these T_H2 responses. Two kinds of regulatory T cells have been described. One is a T cell (designated a Tr-1 cell) that produces large amounts of IL-10 and appears to arise in response to exogenous antigens that enter the respiratory mucosal system. The second is a T cell (designated a "natural" suppressor cell) that originates in the thymus and appears to have specificity for endogenous self-antigens; this cell is present in many tissues and is distinguished by its expression of an intracellular transcription factor known as foxp3. In contrast to the IL-10 producing suppressor cell, this suppressor cell relies on TGF-β as its suppressor cytokine (see Unit III for further discussion). The basis of development of either type of regulatory T cell in mucosal tissues is still poorly understood. However, it is commonly believed that both arise in relation to dendritic cells that produce cytokines favoring suppressor cell development, such as IL-10 or TGF-β. Finally recent evidence indicates that a certain type of dendritic cell, the plasmacytic dendritic cell, is a major cellular component of the respiratory mucosa and that, upon reacting to aeroallergens, they have a direct tolerogenic effect on T cells.*

On the basis of these experimental findings, we may tentatively say that in patients with asthma the tolerance mechanism is disrupted, either because of an abnormality in the development of regulatory T cells or an abnormality that leads to an unusually robust IgE response resistant to down-regulation by a normal regulatory T-cell response. The development of T_{reg} cells may be the normal response on exposure to mucosal antigen, and aberrant or lack of generation of T_{reg} cells in atopic individuals may instead result in T_H2 cell development.

The Hygiene Hypothesis.

While the prevalence of asthma and allergies has greatly increased over the past two decades, the incidence of many infections (tuberculosis, measles, mumps, hepatitis A) in industrialized countries has decreased, suggesting that some infections may have the potential to prevent the development of allergic disease and asthma. This is the basis for the ***"hygiene hypothesis"*** which proposes that good public health measures, use of vaccinations and antibiotics and thus decreased incidence of infections, led to the increasing prevalence of asthma and allergies. Infection would normally protect against the development of atopy. A number of epidemiologic and biological studies indirectly support the hygiene hypothesis. The risk of developing asthma is decreased in children with older siblings or those who entered daycare at an early age (before six months); both situations presumed to increase exposure to infections. Asthma incidence is also decreased in children exposed to farm animals or to cats and dogs in the first year of life. The specific infectious pathogens or immunologic mechanisms responsible are not well defined. Some data suggest that endotoxin exposure (e.g., from cow manure) or other bacterial products (e.g., CpG DNA) reduces allergic asthma. Alternatively, infections associated with T_H1-polarizing immune responses (e.g., tuberculosis or viral infections) might be important for protection against asthma and allergy. However, T_H1 cytokines are proinflammatory and exacerbate rather than inhibit inflammation in the airways. Furthermore, the prevalence of T_H1-associated autoimmune diseases (e.g., diabetes mellitus, multiple sclerosis, rheumatoid arthritis) has also increased dramatically over the past two decades. Therefore, the environmental changes have adversely affected both T_H1- and T_H2-mediated diseases.

A better explanation may be that the ability to mount regulatory T-cell responses in the respiratory mucosa (as well as other organs) depends on environmental exposure to specific antigens, particularly those associated with certain pathogenic agents. This is based on evidence that regulatory T cells generally recognize self-antigens and environmental antigens that cross-react with self-antigens. Thus, in the absence of exposure to certain environmental antigens, that is in the situation of improved hygiene, one loses the capacity to rapidly develop high levels of regulatory T cells.

The Genetics of Atopy/Asthma. Atopic diseases, which include asthma, allergic rhinitis, atopic dermatitis, and some food allergies, are grouped because they are T_H2-driven inflammations and are generally inherited together, implying common genetic elements. The tendency toward atopy is complex, involving both environmental and genetic factors. Genetic polymorphisms in asthma susceptibility genes may result in the predisposition toward asthma by amplifying inflammatory mechanisms, increasing the likelihood of responses to environmental factors or sensitization to environmental allergens, or enhancing airway remodeling. (Recall that in Timothy's case there is a family history of asthma and atopy.) Human genome–wide scans have linked asthma/atopy to more than a dozen chromosomal regions, including chromosome

5q23–35 [total IgE and eosinophil levels; IL-4, -5, and -13; CD14 (endotoxin receptor)], chromosome 6p21–23 [major histocompatibility complex (MHC), TNF complex], chromosome 11q13 (FcεRI), chromosome 12q (asthma) and chromosome 13q (atopy and asthma), among others (see Table 12.1 for details).

Recently, the ***ADAM33*** gene on chromosome 20 was found to be strongly associated with airway hyperreactivity but not elevated serum IgE. *ADAM33* codes for a metalloprotease, a protein that may regulate the response of the respiratory epithelium to damage and stress. In addition, ***Tim-1***, a gene located at chromosome 5q33.2 that regulates cytokine production, is associated with the development of atopy, presumably by regulating the T_H2 inflammatory response. Other genes that have been linked to asthma include *DPP10*, which encodes a dipeptidyl peptidase (DPP) homolog, and *PHF11*, which probably regulates transcription.

Gene Product and Microbe: The TIM-1 Protein and Its Relation to Hepatitis A Virus. One of the asthma-associated genes mentioned above, *Tim-1*, is of particular interest because its protein product is a receptor for hepatitis A virus (HAV) and elevated HAV antibody titers are associated with a reduced risk for the development of allergic rhinitis or asthma. The gene product of *Tim-1*, TIM-1 protein, is preferentially expressed on T_H2 cells (and liver cells) and may play a role in the regulation of T_H2 cell development. It is possible, for instance, that HAV interaction with TIM-1 leads to clonal deletion of allergen-specific T_H2 cells and thus prevents the development of atopy and asthma. This would fit with the observation that certain genetic variants of *Tim-1* are associated with protection against the development of atopy, particularly in individuals who have been exposed to HAV.

TREATMENT OF ASTHMA

Therapeutic strategies for asthma fall into two categories: acute interventions (measures to stop acute symptoms) and maintenance therapies (measures to prevent symptoms).

Treatment of Acute Symptoms of Asthma

Patients with acute, severe symptoms are treated immediately to prevent progression toward respiratory failure. In the emergency room, they are given supplemental oxygen and several doses of a β_2 agonist by inhalation (albuterol) if they are capable of effective inhalation, or by injection (epinephrine) if they are severely dyspneic, to counter the bronchospasm due to release of mediators. They should also receive high-dose corticosteroids (orally or intravenously) to limit airway inflammation. Eosinophils and T cells are particularly sensitive to corticosteroids

TABLE 12.1. Linkages with Asthma and Allergy

Chromosome	Candidate Genes or Products
1p	IL-12 receptor
2q	IL-1, cytotoxic T-lymphocycle-associated antigen 4. CD28
3p24	B-cell lymphoma 6 (STAT-6 binding inhibition), Chemokine cell receptor 4
5q23–35	IL-3, IL-4, IL-5, IL-9, IL-13, GM-CSF
	LTC4S
	Macrophage colony-stimulating factor receptor
	β_2-Adrenergic receptor
	Glucocorticosteroid receptor
	Tim-1, *Tim-3*
6p21–23	MHC
	TNF-α
	Transporters involved in antigen processing and presentation (*TAP1* and *TAP2*)
	Large multicatalytic proteolytic particles
7q11–14	TCR γ chain, IL-6
11q13	High-affinity IgE receptor (FcϵRI) β chain
	Clara cell protein 16
	FGF-3
12q14–24	IFN-γ
	Stem cell factor
	Nitric oxide synthetase (constitutive)
	β Subunit of nuclear factor Y [transcription factor for human MHC genes]
	Insulinlike growth factor 1
	Leukotriene A_4 hydrolase
	STAT-6 (IL-4 STAT)
13q21–24	Cysteinyl leukotriene 2 receptor
14q11–13	TCR α and δ chains
	Nuclear factor κB (NF-κB) inhibitor
16p11–12	IL-4 receptor
17p12–17	CC chemokine cluster
19q13	CD22, TGF-β_1
20p13	ADAM-33

Source: Shearer and Li, (2003).

(see Fig. 12.6). In addition, cytokine production by and activation of the pulmonary epithelium and vascular endothelium are greatly inhibited by corticosteroids. Corticosteroids function by inhibiting the effects of proinflammatory transcription factors, such as NF-κB and AP-1, possibly via inhibition of histone acetylation and stimulation of histone deacetylation (Fig. 12.6).

Early patient follow-up is important since pulmonary inflammation may not respond fully to corticosteroid therapy, particularly if an underlying viral respiratory infection or sinusitis is not improved. Respiratory failure is indicated by a rising pCO_2 in the blood, particularly with an O_2 saturation of <90% in room air or with severe dyspnea or retraction.

Treatment of Chronic Asthma

The major goal in the treatment of chronic asthma is to prevent severe acute exacerbations. In addition, such treatment is directed at normalizing pulmonary function, preventing asthma from interfering with activities including competitive athletics or sleep, and achieving this with minimal side effects from medications. These goals are generally obtained by reducing the T_H2-driven inflammatory response in the airways and by anticipating or avoiding the triggers of asthma exacerbations.

Because the severity of disease varies greatly, treatment regimens must be tailored to the individual's clinical pattern. These patterns include ***intermittent asthma***, characterized by episodic illness interspersed with extended symptom-free periods, and ***persistent/chronic asthma***, with frequent episodes of symptoms. Symptoms of intermittent asthma will occur episodically, for example, following acute respiratory viral infections, sinusitis, and bronchitis or with exposure to allergens or respiratory irritants (solvent fumes, cold air). This asthma pattern can be treated solely with symptomatic use of bronchodilators ("rescue medications"), such as inhaled albuterol.

On the other hand, patients with chronic persistent asthma need maintenance medication to prevent symptoms in addition to rescue medications. Chronic persistent asthma (classified as mild, moderate, or severe disease) is generally treated with anti-inflammatory therapy, such as inhaled corticosteroids, as maintenance therapy. Oral corticosteroids are also effective but are associated with much more severe side effects (immunosuppression, endocrinologic complications, bone loss), which limit its use to severe exacerbations. Maintenance anti-inflammatory therapy minimizes symptoms and the need for rescue medications and reduces the frequency of exacerbations. The severity of persistent asthma can change over time, necessitating periodic reevaluation.

Although inhaled corticosteroids are very effective and are not generally associated with severe side effects, long-term studies suggest that they can reduce growth velocity in children and after prolonged use can cause cataracts and glaucoma in rare patients. Therefore, the lowest possible dose is used, and additional, possibly safer therapies are considered. These other therapies (Fig. 12.6) include the following: ***Long-acting bronchodilators*** synergize with inhaled corticosteroids and reduce the dose required. ***Leukotriene antagonists*** inhibit the effects of cysteinyl leukotrienes, mediators produced by mast cells, eosinophils, and basophils that cause bronchospasm and enhance leukocyte chemotaxis. Montelukast (Singulair), an LTC_4 receptor antagonist, is effective in mild to moderate asthma and in exercise- and aspirin-induced asthma. **Cromones** (cromolyn sodium and nedocromil), which are thought to prevent mast cell degranulation, function as mild anti-inflammatory agents and block both immediate- and late-phase reactions. ***Phosphodiesterase inhibitors*** (theophylline) increase intracellular cyclic adenosine monophosphate (cAMP) levels, resulting in bronchodilation and some anti-inflammatory effects, and are sometimes used as adjunctive agents. However, first-generation phosphodiesterase inhibitors have many side effects (nausea, vomiting, gastritis, arrhythmias) and may enhance T_H2 cytokine production (as shown in Fig. 12.6). Newer phosphodiesterase-4-specific inhibitors with fewer side effects are being investigated. ***Calcineurin inhibitors*** (cyclosporine, FK506/tacrolimus) have been used experimentally for the treatment of severe asthma. These agents inhibit NFAT (Nuclear Factor of activated T cells)-mediated transcription (required for IL-2 and IL-4

synthesis in T cells and mast cells). The side effects of cyclosporine (nephrotoxicity, neurotoxicity, and hirsutism) have limited its use, although topical forms of these agents are now used for treatment of mild to moderate atopic dermatitis. Other therapies that may be helpful include **antibiotics** for bacterial sinusitis, **neuraminidase inhibitors** for acute therapy of influenza, **influenza vaccines** to prevent infections, and ***therapies for GERD***.

Allergen Immunotherapy

Allergen immunotherapy is commonly referred to as "allergy shots." As conventionally performed, allergen immunotherapy consists of the subcutaneous administration of increasing doses of allergen (see Case 11). Whereas pharmacologic agents (corticosteroids, bronchodilators, etc.) treat symptoms only, allergen immunotherapy seeks to modify the underlying adaptive immune response leading to asthma. The mechanisms by which it does so are not fully understood. Initially, it was thought that immunotherapy induced blocking IgG antibodies that bound allergen, thereby preventing mast cell degranulation. More recently, it has been thought that allergen immunotherapy induces allergen-specific T_H1 cells, which prevent the development of allergen-specific T_H2 cells. However, IFN-γ production by T_H1 cells cannot block T_H2 cell function at mucosal surfaces and may in fact exacerbate inflammatory responses. Recent focus is on the possibility that immunotherapy induces anti-inflammatory regulatory T cells. Regulatory T cells induced by immunotherapy may be similar to those that are normally found in nonatopic individuals. In particular, Tr-1 or T_{reg} cells that produce IL-10 or TGF-β are induced by allergen immunotherapy, appear to suppress T_H2 inflammatory function, and induce allergen-specific tolerance that prevents airway hyperreactivity.

Allergen immunotherapy, although effective in allergic rhinitis and preventing progression to asthma, is rather inefficient, requiring more than 100 shots given over three to five years. This has limited its use in the treatment of asthma. Increased understanding has led to the development of methods that will hopefully be more efficient. For example, adjuvants are being attached or added to the injected allergens to induce protective immunity more rapidly. These include CpG oligonucleotides, which activate Toll-like receptor 9 (TLR9) and induce allergen-specific IFN-γ and IL-10 production. In addition, oral administration of allergen immunotherapy is being studied to take advantage of the observation that the gastrointestinal tract is an effective route for tolerance induction. These forms of therapy are likely to lead to more efficient treatment and possibly to effective cures for allergy and asthma.

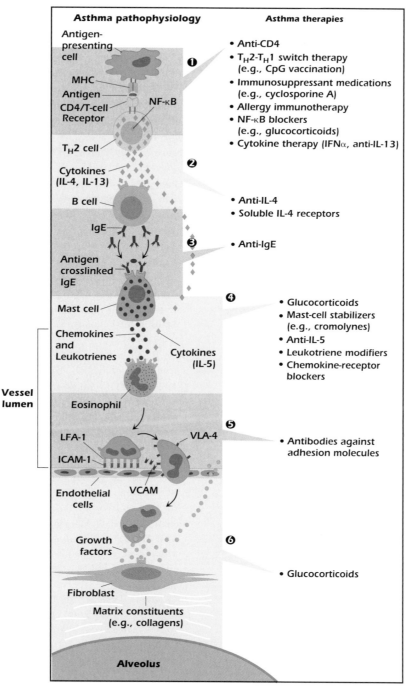

Figure 12.6. Existing and proposed asthma pharmacotherapies are designed to target biomolecular events at numerous points in the disease's pathogenesis, thus interfering with lymphocyte, mast cell, and eosinophil activities. The asthmatic process beginning with allergen presentation to T cells (1) causes release of T_H2 cytokines such as IL-4, IL-5, and IL-13 (2) Some of these trigger B cells to elaborate IgE, which, in the presence of antigen, cross-links receptors on mast cells (3) Mast cells release inflammatory mediators, including some that lead to eosinophil chemotaxis (4) Eosinophils interact with adhesion molecules on endothelial cells (5) resulting in eosinophil migration into airway perivascular tissue (6) There, eosinophils and constituent airway cells secrete growth factors that activate fibroblasts. Consequent buildup of collagens and other matrix macromolecules leads to airway remodeling.

Novel Asthma Therapies

Anti-IgE monoclonal antibody (omalizumab, Xolari) has recently become available for patients 12 years and older with moderate to severe asthma. Since Timothy is 8 years old, you mention to his father that this might be available to him in the future should his asthma symptoms worsen. This is a humanized mouse monoclonal antibody (mAb) (see Case 25), which contains the complementarity-determining regions (CDRs) of the mouse in the framework of a human antibody and is about 90% human. This antibody binds to the Cε3 region on IgE, reducing the level of circulating free IgE and inhibiting the binding of IgE to its high-affinity receptor (FcεRI) on mast cells and basophils. It does not cross-link IgE on the surface of mast cells and therefore does not cause mast cell degranulation. The reduction in free IgE levels results in a decrease in the expression of FcεRI receptors on basophils and mast cells. Thus, it gradually reduces the frequency of asthma exacerbations and concomitantly reduces the need for corticosteroids. Unfortunately, therapy with anti-IgE is expensive and currently is reserved for patients with moderate to severe asthma. In addition, when treatment with omalizumab is discontinued, serum IgE levels return to pretreatment levels, and symptoms of asthma and allergy reappear.

Other Immunomodulators

Just as humanized mAbs may be directed against IgE, mAbs can be used against T_H2 cytokines, including IL-4, IL-5, and IL-13. However, use of anti-IL-4 mAb as well as soluble IL-4 receptor (sIL-4R), have been disappointing. Treatment with anti-IL-5 antibodies in humans reduces eosinophilia but has no apparent effect on limiting AHR. Treatment with the cytokine IL-12 also reduces eosinophilia but does not reduce AHR. Treatments to reduce the influx of inflammatory cells into the lungs with mAbs against leukocyte function-associated antigen 1 (LFA-1), ICAM-1, very late antigen VLA-4, or Vascular cell adhesion molecule VCAM-1 are being investigated.

REFERENCES

Akbari O, Meyer E, Stock P, Kronenberg M, Sidobre S, Nakayama T, Taniguchi M, Grusby MJ, DeKruyff RH, Umetsu DT (2003): Essential role of NKT cells producing IL-4 and IL-13 in the development of allergen induced airway hyperreactivity. *Nature Med* 9:582–588.

Barnes PJ (1996): Mechanisms of action of glucocorticoids in asthma. *Am J Respir Crit Care Med* 154:521–527.

Barnes PJ, Adcock IM (2003): How do corticosteroids work in asthma? *Ann Intern Med* 139:359–370.

Clark TJH, Cagnani CB, Bousquet J, et al. (2002): Global initiative for asthma. Global strategy for asthma management and prevention. *NIH Publication* No. 02-3659:1–176.

Cockcroft DW (2001): How best to measure airway responsiveness. *Am J Respir Crit Care Med* 163:1514–1515.

Cookson WO (2002): Asthma genetics. *Chest* 121(3 Suppl): 7S–13S.

Fenech A, Hall IP (2002): Pharmacogenetics of asthma. *Br J Clin Pharmacol* 53:3–15.

Harding SM (1999): Gastroesophageal reflux and asthma: Insight into the association. *J Allergy Clin Immunol* 104:251–259.

Kuchroo VK, Umetsu DT, DeKruyff RH, Freeman GJ (2003): The TIM gene family: Emerging roles in immunity and disease. *Nature Rev Immunol* 3:454–462.

Lamanske RS, Bussy WW (2003): Asthma. *J Allergy Clin Immunol* III suppl 2:S502–S519.

Macaubas C, Umetsu DT (2003): Immunology of the asthmatic response. In *Pediatric Allergy: Principles and Practice*. St. Louis D.Y.M. Leung, R. Geha, H.A. Sampson, S.J. Szefler (eds): Mosby.

Malo JL, Chan-Yeung M (2001): Occupational asthma. *J Allergy Clin Immunol* 108:317–328.

O'Hollaren MT, Yunginger JW, Offard KP, Somers MJ, O'Connell EJ, Ballard DJ, Sachs MI (1991): Exposure to an aeroallergen as a possible precipitating factor in respiratory arrest in young patients with asthma. *N Engl J Med* 324:359–363.

Perrin JM, Homer CJ, Berwick DM, Woolf AD, Freeman JL, Wennberg JE (1989): Variations in rates of hospitalization of children in three urban communities. *N Engl-J Med* 320:1183–1187.

Stein RT, Sherrill D, Morgan WJ, Holberg CJ, Halonen M, Taussig LM, Wright AL, Martinez FD (1999): Respiratory syncytial virus in early life and risk of wheeze and allergy by age 13 years. *Lancet* 354:541–545.

Stock P, Akbari O, Berry G, Freeman G, Dekruyff R, Umetsu D (2004): Induction of T helper type 1-like regulatory cells that express Foxp3 and protect against airway hyperreactivity. *Nature Immunol* 5:1149–1156.

Szczeklik A, Stevenson DD (1999): Aspirin-induced asthma: Advances in pathogenesis and management. *J Allergy Clin Immunol* 104:5–13.

Umetsu SE, Lee W-L, McIntire JJ, Downey L, Sanjanwala B, Akbari O, Berry GJ, Nagumo H, Freeman GJ, Umetsu DT, DeKruyff RH (2005): TIM-1 induces T cell activation and inhibits the development of peripheral tolerance. *Nature Immunol* 6:447–454.

Wright RJ, Rodriguez M, Cohen S (1998): Review of psychosocial stress and asthma: An integrated biopsychosocial approach. *Thorax* 53:1066–1074.

13

THE VASCULITIDES

CAROL A. LANGFORD and MICHAEL C. SNELLER*

The following is a series of case presentations which have in common an inflammation of the blood vessel walls, so they all fall under the designation *vasculitis*. However, both the etiology and the types of vessels affected vary. The presentation of vasculitis depends on the location of the vessels under attack: rash when the subcutaneous vessels are involved, renal disease or glomerular nephritis when the small vessels in the glomeruli are affected, or pulmonary disease and neurologic symptoms when vessels in those organs are involved. These different presentations therefore give rise to disparate differential diagnoses for the individual patient. The underlying causes or etiologies of these vascular inflammatory attacks also fall into several groups: They may be primary or secondary vascular diseases; they may be the result of infectious agents, either due to direct attack or indirectly; or they may be autoimmune in nature. Vasculitis can therefore be classified according to the several different schemes: size of vessels involved (small, medium, or large), primary versus secondary, or etiology (see Tables 13.1–13.3). We have chosen to present four cases representing vasculitides of different etiologies, some of which are unknown or still being debated.

TABLE 13.1. Vasculitis Syndromes Categorized by Involved Vessel Size

Large Vessels
Giant cell (temporal) arteritis: aorta and major branches, especially carotid artery branches; granulomatous
Takayasu arteritis: aorta and major branches
Medium-Sized Vessels
Polyarteritis nodosa: medium or small arteries only
Kawasaki disease: large, medium, and small arteries, coronaries often affected
Small Vessels
Wegener's granulomatosis: small to medium vessels in respiratory tract and kidneys
Churg–Strauss syndrome: small to medium vessels in respiratory tract
Microscopic polyarteritis: small vessels mostly in kidney, sometimes pulmonary
Henoch–Schönlein purpura: small vessels in skin, gut, kidney
Connective tissue disease: small vessels in connective tissue
Essential cryoglobulinemia: small vessels in skin and kidney
Cutaneous leukocytoclastic angiitis: small vessels isolated to the skin

Source: Chapel Hill Consensus Conference on the Nomenclature of Systemic Vasculitis. Chapel Hill, N. Careline, 2001.

*With contributions from Warren Strober and Susan R. S. Gottesman.

Immunology: Clinical Case Studies and Disease Pathophysiology, By Warren Strober and Susan R. S. Gottesman
Copyright © 2009 John Wiley & Sons, Inc.

TABLE 13.2. Vasculitis Syndromes: Primary vs Secondary

Primary Vasculitis Syndromes
Wegener's granulomatosis
Microscopic polyangiitis
Polyarteritis nodosa
Churg–Strauss syndrome
Giant cell (temporal) arteritis
Takayasu's arteritis
Isolated central nervous system vasculitis
Henoch–Schönlein purpura
Essential mixed cryoglobulinemia
Cutaneous vasculitis
Kawasaki disease
Inflammatory bowel disease
Secondary Vasculitis Syndromes
Vasculitis associated with infection: *Neisseria*, Rocky Mountain
　spotted fever, etc.
Vasculitis associated with malignancy
Vasculitis associated with connective tissue disease: systemic
　lupus erythematosus, rheumatoid arthritis
Drug-induced vasculitis
Vasculitis associated with organ allograft rejection

 TABLE 13.3. Vasculitides Categorized by Pathophysiology

Direct Infection
Bacterial: *Neisseria*, syphillis
Rickettsial: Rocky Moutain spotted fever
Viral: herpes zoster varicella
Fungal: *Mucormycosis*, *Aspergillus*
Immune Complex Mediated
Serum sickness
Essential mixed cryoglobulinemia: hepatitis infection induced
　immune complex
Henoch–Schönlein purpura
Vasculitis associated with connective tissue disease
Drug—induced vasculitis
ANCA Associated
Wegener's granulomatosis
Microscopic polyangiitis
Churg–Strauss syndrome
Miscellaneous
Direct antibody: Goodpasture's syndrome
Superantigen: Kawasaki disease
Cell-mediated immunity: organ allograft rejection
Paraneoplastic: malignancy associated
Unknown: polyarteritis nodosa, giant cell (temporal) arteritis,
　Takayasu's arteritis, isolated central nervous system arteritis,
　cutaneous arteritis

VASCULITIS DUE TO IMMUNE COMPLEX DEPOSITION: ESSENTIAL MIXED CRYOGLOBULINEMIA

 CASE REPORT 1

"I have spots on my legs."

Initial Evaluation

Ms. Georges, a 45-year-old female, is referred to you for a rheumatologic evaluation because of joint pains and rash. She was well until 2–3 months ago when she noted the insidious onset of fatigue and joint pains involving her hands, knees, ankles, and feet. Over the past four weeks, she had also developed a skin rash on both legs. Her only current medication is acetaminophen, which she takes intermittently for the arthralgias. Her past history is remarkable for cardiac surgery at age 10 years to repair an atrial septal defect.

On physical examination you note some tenderness to palpation over the wrists, knees, ankles, and small joints of both hands and feet. However, no swelling of the joints is detected. Examination of the skin reveals palpable *purpura* (small, reddish, nonblanching nodules) over both lower extremities (Fig. 13.1).

Initial laboratory studies are remarkable for: normal complete blood count (CBC) with normal platelets of 234,000/μL; an elevated erythrocyte sedimentation rate (ESR) of 42 mm/h (reference range 0–25); normal serum creatinine; normal blood urea nitrogen (BUN); elevated aspartate aminotransferase (AST) of 97 units/L (reference range 9–34); elevated alanine aminotransferase (ALT) of 112 units/L (reference range 6–41); normal bilirubin and alkaline phosphatase; and a urinalysis revealing 2+ protein and 5–10 RBC/HPF (red blood cells/high power field) with rare red cell casts.

What do these lab results tell you?

*The normal platelet count is significant since thrombocytopenia is a common cause of **petechiae** (minute hemorrhages) and purpura. You expect the platelet count to be normal since Ms. Georges has purpura without petechiae.*

ESR measures the rate at which the RBCs settle in a tube. It is a nonspecific test that is increased in inflammatory and infectious diseases and in some neoplasms. It may also be increased in hypercholesterolemia or anemia.

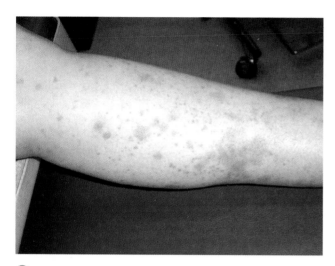

Figure 13.1. Case 1: Purpura (skin lesions) of lower extremities characteristic of vasculitis.

The urine analysis showing 2+ protein, RBCs, and red cell casts is consistent with glomerular disease. The normal creatinine suggests that the damage is not severe.

AST and ALT, although frequently used as indicators of liver disease and hepatocellular damage, may be increased as a result of damage to other cell types. The bilirubin, which is more specific to obstruction of the hepatobiliary tracts, is normal, as is the alkaline phosphatase.

How does her physical examination, combined with her laboratory data help you arrive at a diagnosis?

In the absence of thrombocytopenia or systemic infection, the most common cause of palpable purpuric skin lesions is vasculitis (inflammation of the blood vessel walls) involving the small vessels in the dermal layer of the skin. Ms. Georges has clinical and laboratory evidence of damage to small vessels not only in the skin (purpura) but also in the kidneys (glomerular disease). Evidence of an inflammatory response (elevated ESR), synovitis causing her joint pain, and probable hepatocellular damage in the absence of obstruction (elevated AST and ALT) also support the conclusion that she has vasculitis.

You refer Ms. Georges to a dermatologist who performs a biopsy of one of the skin lesions on her lower extremity and you order additional laboratory studies.

Test Results and Definitive Diagnosis

The pathology report of the skin biopsy reads: "Small vessel vasculitis with PAS (periodic acid Schiff) staining material occluding the lumen of multiple vessels."

Results of the laboratory studies are as follows:

	Result	Reference Range
Complement assays		
C3	59 mg/dL	69–175 mg/dL
C4	<10 mg/dL	13–38 mg/dL
Serological testing		
Rheumatoid factor	600 IU/mL	0–20 IU/mL
Antinuclear antibody (ANA)	Negative	Negative
Antineutrophil cytoplasmic antibody (ANCA)	Negative	Negative
Hepatitis B surface antigen	Negative	Negative
Anti–Hepatitis A virus	Negative	Negative
Anti–Hepatitis C virus (HCV)	Positive	Negative
Cryoglobulins[a]	6%	<3%

[a]Immunoglobulins or antigen-antibody complexes that precipitate at temperatures below 37°C.

Interpretation: The skin biopsy report confirms that Ms. Georges has an inflammation of the small vessels with necrosis and fibrin thrombi, thus accounting for the rash and, by extension, her glomerular disease. The decrease in complement levels is likely due to consumption of complement components. Thus, the positive HCV serology, elevated serum cryoglobulins, and hypocomplementemia (low levels of complement components) combined with the AST and ALT suggest ***essential mixed cryoglobulinemia*** associated with chronic HCV infection as the underlying cause of the vasculitis. Rheumatoid factor is not specific for rheumatoid arthritis but is elevated in many inflammatory conditions, both autoimmune and infectious. The ANA negativity helps rule out systemic lupus erythematosus (see Case 22), while ANCA negativity rules out ANCA-associated vasculitis (Table 13.3). There is no evidence of exposure to hepatitis A or chronic hepatitis B infection; rather, the positive HCV serology suggests chronic infection with HCV.

Treatment Plan

You inform Ms. Georges that her test results indicate that she has chronic hepatitis due to infection with HCV. She most likely acquired HCV from a transfusion received during the cardiac surgery she had as a child, which occurred prior to the development of screening tests for HCV contamination of blood. You explain that her skin lesions and other current symptoms are related to an aberrant immunologic response to the chronic HCV infection as evidenced by the cryoglobulin levels and presenting symptoms and refer her to a gastroenterologist for treatment of her HCV.

Differential Diagnosis of Vasculitis Affecting Skin

The differential diagnosis of a skin rash was briefly touched upon above. Knowing that it is due to a vasculitis leads to consideration of the underlying causes of vasculitis. These may be divided into two broad categories: vasculitis as the result of direct attack of vessel walls by an organism or vasculitis by an immune-mediated scenario. The immune-mediated variety also may have an underlying infectious agent causing immune complex formation or cross-reactivity or may be one aspect of a systemic autoimmune disease. Infectious agents which directly infect vessels run the spectrum of microorganisms and include bacterial (Neisseria), rickettsial (Rocky Mountain spotted fever), fungal (aspergillus, mucor mycosis), and viral (herpes zoster varicella) organisms. Systemic vasculitis syndromes (especially microscopic polyangiitis, Henoch–Schönlein purpura, and idiopathic cutaneous vasculitis) as well as other systemic autoimmune diseases such as systemic lupus erythematosus enter into the differential diagnosis with HCV-associated essential mixed cryoglobulinemia. The latter can usually be distinguished from other forms of small-vessel vasculitis by the presence of circulating cryoglobulins combined with evidence of active HCV infection.

● PATHOPHYSIOLOGY OF IMMUNE COMPLEX VASCULITIS

Vasculitis: A General Definition

Vasculitis is a clinicopathologic process characterized by inflammation of and damage to blood vessels. The vessel lumen is usually compromised, and this may cause ischemia of the tissues supplied by the involved vessel. Vasculitis may occur as a primary process or as a component of another underlying disease (Table 13.2). In years past, most forms were considered to fall within the category of *immune complex diseases*, which includes serum sickness and certain connective tissue diseases of which systemic lupus erythematosus is the prototype (Table 13.3).

Immune Complex Vasculitis: General Considerations

The consequences of pathogenic *intravascular immune complex* formation were first appreciated in patients with

infectious diseases (such as diphtheria and scarlet fever) who had been treated with horse-derived antisera. Horse antiserum treatment frequently resulted in "serum sickness" characterized by fever, arthralgias, lymphadenopathy, urticarial rash, and occasionally nephritis. Animal models of acute serum sickness were then developed in which vasculitis was a prominent feature. In these models, a single intravenous injection of foreign protein resulted in circulating immune complexes which were deposited in vessel walls and induced inflammatory vascular lesions that resembled human *polyarteritis nodosa*. Evidence for immune complex involvement in the pathogenesis of human vasculitis was inferred from these early observations of serum sickness and animal models.

The study of animal models has delineated the mechanisms by which immune complex deposition can result in vasculitis. The ability of immune complexes to activate complement is believed to be of primary importance in initiation of vascular damage. Immune complexes containing activated complement components are deposited in vessel walls at sites of increased vascular permeability, which is thought to result from the release of vasoactive amines by platelets and mast cells triggered by IgE. Once the immune complexes are deposited, vessel damage can occur by a number of interacting mechanisms. The activation of complement by immune deposits can lead to endothelial damage through formation of the C5b9 membrane attack complex (see Case 8 for complement pathways). Complement activation also produces complement fragments (e.g., C5a) that are chemotactic for (recruit) neutrophils and monocytes and stimulate the clotting and kinin pathways. This stimulation leads to further inflammation and vessel thrombosis. Immune complexes deposited in vessel walls can also interact directly with inflammatory cells through Fcγ receptors present on neutrophils and monocytes (see Coico and Sunshine, Chapter 15). This interaction leads to cellular activation and release of cytokines, oxygen radicals, and proteolytic enzymes, which further escalates the inflammatory vascular damage.

While immune complex formation clearly plays a primary role in serum sickness pathogenesis, evidence that it has a similar role in the human vasculitic syndromes is indirect. In fact, in many systemic vasculitis syndromes there is little evidence that immune complexes are involved. Specifically, elevated levels of circulating immune complexes, systemic complement depletion, and deposition of complement and immunoglobulin in vasculitic lesions are usually not found in Wegener's granulomatosis, microscopic polyangiitis, Takayasu's arteritis, or giant cell arteritis, and the underlying pathophysiology of each of these disorders remains unknown. In other primary vasculitic syndromes (see Table 13.2), routine findings of elevated circulating immune complex levels, hypocomplementemia, and deposits of complement and immunoglobulin in the lesions imply that immune complexes play a primary role in their pathogenesis. In most of these, the specific antigen that elicits pathogenic immune complex formation is unknown. The exception is essential mixed cryoglobulinemia in the setting of chronic infection with HCV.

Essential Mixed Cryoglobulinemia: A Specific Type of Immune Complex Vasculitis

Essential mixed cryoglobulinemia is a syndrome in which vasculitis is associated with circulating cryoprecipitable immune complexes. These complexes usually contain monoclonal IgM with anti-IgG (rheumatoid factor) activity and polyclonal IgG. They precipitate at temperatures below 37°C. Evidence suggests that HCV infection plays an important role in their formation and may be the triggering antigen. First, there is a high prevalence (>90%) of HCV infection in patients with this syndrome. Second, HCV RNA and antibodies to HCV are present in the serum cryoprecipitates. Third, HCV-associated antigens are demonstrated in the vasculitic skin lesions. Finally, antiviral therapy with interferon-α is effective in the treatment of essential mixed cryoglobulinemia (see below). Thus, current evidence suggests that essential mixed cryoglobulinemia occurs when an aberrant immune response to HCV infection leads to the formation of immune complexes consisting of HCV antigens, polyclonal HCV-specific IgG, and monoclonal IgM anti-IgG rheumatoid factor. Deposition of the complexes in vessel walls triggers an inflammatory cascade that results in the clinical syndrome of essential mixed cryoglobulinemia. This does not exclude the possibility that in individual patients other antigens may serve as the inciting agent.

 ## CLINICAL FEATURES OF ESSENTIAL MIXED CRYOGLOBULINEMIA

The most common clinical manifestations of essential mixed cryoglobulinemia are cutaneous vasculitis, arthritis, peripheral neuropathy, and glomerulonephritis. Although renal disease develops in 10–30% of patients, life-threatening, rapidly progressive glomerulonephritis is infrequent, as is vasculitis of the central nervous system, gastrointestinal tract, or heart.

The presence of circulating cryoprecipitates is the fundamental laboratory finding. Rheumatoid factor and hypocomplementemia are almost always found. An elevated ESR and anemia occur frequently. Evidence for hepatitis C infection and chronic hepatitis (elevated hepatic transaminases) is present in the vast majority of patients.

 ## TREATMENT OF ESSENTIAL MIXED CRYOGLOBULINEMIA

In patients in whom essential mixed cryoglobulinemia is associated with HCV infection, treatment with interferon-α and ribavirin can prove beneficial. Clinical improvement is dependent on the virologic response. Patients who clear HCV from the blood have objective improvement in their vasculitis, along with significant reductions in levels of circulating cryoglobulins, IgM, and rheumatoid factor. Sustained suppression of viral replication presumably removes the stimulus for immune complex formation, resulting in resolution of the vasculitis. However, a substantial proportion of patients will not have a sustained virologic response, and the vasculitis typically relapses with the return of viremia.

For patients who do not respond to antiviral therapy, there are few good therapeutic options. The role of HCV infection in the pathogenesis has particular relevance when considering the use of immunosuppressive therapy. Plasmapheresis (filtering the patient's blood) has been used with the thought that rapid removal of cryoprecipitates may result in clinical improvement. While there are anecdotal reports of short-term responses, such treatment is not practical for long-term management of a chronic condition. Immunosuppressive agents have formed the foundation of treatment for most forms of systemic vasculitis, particularly in the case of life-threatening disease. Clinical improvements have been reported; however, there are no data from controlled trials. Immunosuppressive drugs may transiently decrease the inflammatory manifestations but in suppressing the immune response they can cause an increase in HCV viremia. Ongoing viral replication drives further immune complex formation and subsequent vasculitis. Thus, the use of standard immunosuppressive therapy in essential mixed cryoglobulinemia usually does not result in sustained improvement or long-term remission in most patients.

ACUTE-ONSET VASCULITIS IN CHILDHOOD: SUPERANTIGEN HYPOTHESIS—KAWASAKI DISEASE

 ## CASE REPORT 2

"My child has a high fever and seems very sick."

Physical Examination and Diagnosis

A mother brings her two-year-old son, Ryan, to your office for evaluation of high fevers. She first noted that the child was febrile five days ago. His fevers have been as high as 38.5–39°C and are associated with extreme irritability. In your office, Ryan's temperature is 39.5°C, his pulse is elevated at 130/min, and his respiratory rate and blood pressure are normal. His physical examination is remarkable for bilateral conjunctival injection (redness of eyes), cervical lymphadenopathy, a polymorphous rash on the trunk, and erythema (redness) of the palms and soles. You also note significant erythema of the oral mucosa and tongue with fissuring of the lips. You admit the child to the hospital for further evaluation.

Initial laboratory studies are remarkable for the following:

	Result	Reference Range
White blood cells (WBC)	23,000/μL	5500–15,000/μL
Hematocrit	34%	33–42%
Platelets	450,000/μL	130,000–400,000/μL
ESR	75 mm/h	0–25 mm/h
C-reactive protein (CRP)	2.8 mg/dL	<0.8 mg/dL
Antistreptolysin O (ASO) IgM	Negative	Negative

Urinalysis reveals trace protein and 5–10 WBC/HPF. Cultures of blood, urine, and throat are all reported negative 24 h, 48 h, and one week later.

Based on the above clinical features and laboratory findings, what is the most likely diagnosis?

The differential diagnosis of fever and rash in a young child is broad and includes a number of infectious childhood exanthems (rash due to viral infection) and certain autoimmune diseases (see below). The findings of a slightly elevated WBC and platelet counts along with elevated ESR and CRP (an acute-phase reactant), all point to an inflammatory reaction. The mucocutaneous findings in this patient combined with the negative (bacterial, mycobacterial, and fungal) cultures and negative ASO titer strongly suggest the diagnosis of **Kawasaki disease (KD)**, *an arteritis of large, medium, and small vessels which is a diagnosis of exclusion. It is associated with mucocutaneous inflammation and lymphadenopathy and usually occurs in children.*

Treatment Plan

Due to the likelihood of a diagnosis of KD and its association with coronary artery vasculitis, you begin treatment with high-dose intravenous immunoglobulin (IVIG) and aspirin. Over the next 48 h Ryan's fever resolves and

he is discharged from the hospital on daily baby aspirin. You see him in the office a week later and he is doing well. He has remained afebrile, the mucosal lesions have resolved, and the skin on his hands and feet has begun to desquamate. Two weeks later, repeat laboratory studies show that his ESR and CRP have decreased but are not yet normal. You schedule the patient for a transthoracic two-dimensional echocardiogram to rule out cardiac complications of KD (see below).

DIFFERENTIAL DIAGNOSIS OF MUCOCUTANEOUS LESIONS AND FEVER IN CHILDREN

A number of childhood exanthems such as measles, echovirus, or adenovirus may produce some of the clinical features of KD. However, these diseases are not generally associated with the severe systemic inflammation that is characteristic of KD. In addition, induration and subsequent desquamation of the skin on the hands and feet are not usually a feature of these infectious childhood exanthems. Toxin-mediated syndromes associated with β-hemolytic streptococcal infections should be considered, but these are usually associated with evidence of streptococcal infection and do not produce the ocular manifestations typical of KD. Finally, drug reactions and other rare forms of systemic vasculitis, such as polyarteritis nodosa, need to be considered in the differential diagnosis of KD. Since no organism has been isolated as the causative agent for KD, in the final analysis this is a diagnosis of exclusion based on clinical presentation and negative laboratory findings for other causes.

PATHOPHYSIOLOGY OF KAWASAKI DISEASE

KD is an acute, self-limited systemic necrotizing vasculitis of unknown etiology that primarily affects the medium-sized vessels, occurs in young children, and is associated with myocarditis and coronary artery vasculitis. The acute self-limited nature of the disease, seasonal variation in incidence, geographic clustering of outbreaks, and unique susceptibility of young children all suggest an infectious etiology. Although multiple infectious agents have been implicated, none have been conclusively demonstrated to cause KD.

Some features of KD are similar to those found in syndromes caused by toxin-producing bacteria, such as toxic shock syndrome and scarlet fever. The clinical manifestations of these syndromes are mediated by microbial toxins that behave as **superantigens**; proteins that bind to specific Vß chains of the T-cell receptor (TCR) irrespective of the receptor's antigen specificity, inducing activation and proliferation of large numbers of T cells. Superantigens can activate all T cells expressing a particular Vβ gene product and thus are capable of activating large numbers of T cells (see Case 19 on psoriasis for further discussion).

The acute phase of KD is associated with abnormalities indicative of intense immunologic activation, including increased serum levels of interleukin-1 (IL-1), tumor necrosis factor (TNF), IL-6, interferon (IFN) γ, and soluble CD25; increased numbers of activated CD4⁺ T cells in the peripheral blood; polyclonal B-cell activation; and circulating antibodies that are cytotoxic to cultured endothelial cells. These immunologic abnormalities, along with the epidemiologic features described above led to the hypothesis that a superantigen produced by an infectious agent causes KD. Initial reports of selective expansion of Vβ2⁺ T cells and, to a lesser extent, Vβ8⁺ T cells in patients with KD seemed to support the superantigen hypothesis. However, other studies failed to find evidence of selective Vβ expansion or toxin production. Thus, it remains unclear whether KD is mediated by a microbial toxin with superantigen properties.

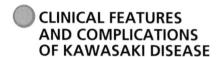

CLINICAL FEATURES AND COMPLICATIONS OF KAWASAKI DISEASE

Kawasaki disease is a disease of childhood with at least 80% of cases occurring in children under five years of age. The peak incidence is in children two years of age and younger with boys being affected 1.5 times as often as girls. The principal diagnostic criteria for KD are listed in Table 13.4. Since, as stated above, this is a diagnosis of exclusion based on certain clinical manifestations in the absence of evidence for infectious, autoimmune, and neoplastic diseases, five of six principal diagnostic criteria must be present to establish the diagnosis. Fever is an absolute criterion for diagnosis of KD. Some clinicians feel that "atypical" cases of KD may be diagnosed when less than five criteria are present and associated

TABLE 13.4. Kawasaki Disease: Principal Diagnostic Criteria

Fever persisting for five or more days

Conjunctival injection

Changes in peripheral extremities; erythema of palms and soles, indurative edema (initial stage); desquamation of skin of hands and feet (convalescent stage)

Polymorphous exanthema

Cervical adenopathy

Oropharyngeal changes: erythema, swelling and fissuring of lips, diffuse erythema of oropharyngeal mucosa, strawberry tongue

with coronary artery aneurysms. In addition to the features listed in Table 13.4, patients with KD may exhibit other clinical manifestations including arthritis, sterile pyuria (WBCs in urine without organisms), hydrops of the gallbladder, uveitis, aseptic meningitis, and diarrhea.

The most serious clinical feature of KD is cardiac disease. During the acute phase of the disease, up to 30% of patients may develop pericarditis (inflammation of the pericardial sac) or myocarditis (inflammation of cardiac muscle). The latter may give rise to congestive heart failure, arrhythmias, and mitral regurgitation. Vasculitis involving the coronary arteries is responsible for most of the morbidity and mortality. Coronary artery involvement developed in 20–25% of patients prior to the widespread use of intravenous immunoglobulin IVIG but now occurs in less than 10% of patients. It is usually manifested by aneurysmal dilatations of the proximal artery, which develop one to four weeks after the onset of fever. These lesions are most easily detected by two-dimensional transthoracic echocardiography. Small- and medium-sized aneurysms usually regress, but giant aneurysms (>8 mm) rarely do so and are frequently associated with thrombotic occlusion and resulting myocardial infarction, the most common cause of death in KD.

TREATMENT OF KAWASAKI DISEASE

Randomized controlled trials have shown that high-dose IVIG given within the first 10 days of illness reduces myocardial inflammation and the incidence of coronary artery aneurysm formation and leads to rapid defervescence and normalization of acute-phase reactants. Administration of aspirin is generally continued until the platelet count and other markers of acute inflammation have normalized.

VASCULITIDES OF UNKNOWN ETIOLOGY: GIANT CELL ARTERITIS

CASE REPORT 3

"I have headaches all the time and my jaw hurts with chewing."

Presentation and Initial Workup

Ms. Simmons, a 72-year-old woman, comes to your clinic because of headaches that have been increasing in frequency. She has also noticed pain in her jaw that begins after she starts chewing (claudication). For the past month she has felt unwell with fatigue and pain in her shoulders and hips.

Her physical examination is notable for nodularity and tenderness over both temporal arteries. Her teeth, temporomandibular joints, and neurologic assessment appear normal, as does the remainder of her examination.

Laboratory studies reveal the following:

	Result	Reference Range
WBC	12,900/μL	4800–10,800/μL
Hemoglobin	10.0 g/dL	12–16 g/dL
Platelets	399,000/μL	130,000–400,000/μL
ESR	89 mm/h	0–25 mm/h

Serum chemistries, liver function tests, urinalysis, and chest radiograph are all within expected reference range.

What is the differential diagnosis of headache with jaw claudication?

*Since headaches have a wide variety of causes, the accompanying clinical and laboratory features need to guide the differential diagnosis. This patient is over 50 years of age and has weight loss, fatigue, arthralgias, mild leukocytosis (elevated WBC count), anemia, and an elevated ESR, all of which could occur in the setting of malignancy, infection, or a connective tissue or inflammatory disease. However, the concomitant occurrence of jaw claudication and abnormal temporal arteries more selectively directs the differential toward a vasculitic disease, **giant cell arteritis (GCA)**.*

Based upon your patient's symptoms and signs, you consider GCA a strong diagnostic possibility. You begin treatment with prednisone (a steroid) and refer her to a surgeon for a temporal artery biopsy.

Definitive Diagnosis

One week later, you receive a copy of the pathology report, which states: "The temporal artery demonstrates a focal panmural mononuclear cell infiltration with histiocytes and giant cells forming nonnecrotizing granuloma. There is proliferation of the intima and fragmentation of the internal elastic lamina. These changes are compatible with giant cell arteritis" (Fig. 13.2).

What does the pathology report mean?

The pathology report describes a lesion in which a cell-mediated-type immune reaction is attacking the vessel wall, causing thickening of the intima (inner layer) and therefore narrowing of the lumen. The lesion also causes a disruption of the structural components of the wall, including the internal elastic lamina. These create the potential for thrombosis and aneurysm (a ballooning out and weakening of the wall), respectively.

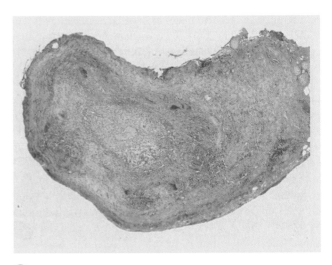

Figure 13.2. Case 3 Temporal artery biopsy demonstrating active arteritis with panmural inflammation and giant cells. The lumen is greatly narrowed.

Treatment Plan

Ms. Simmons returns to your clinic 10 days later. She reports that within 2 days of beginning prednisone she no longer had shoulder or hip discomfort and after one week her headaches and jaw claudication had also resolved. You continue her prednisone treatment and see her in 1–2 weeks for repeat evaluation, further laboratory tests, and consideration of prednisone tapering (see Case 14 for a discussion of the side effects of steroid use).

DIFFERENTIAL DIAGNOSIS OF HEADACHE AND JAW PAIN

In a patient over the age of 50 who presents with headaches, the differential diagnosis is broad and includes a wide range of vascular diseases, such as atherosclerosis, infection, and infiltrative processes such as amyloidosis as well as other forms of primary and secondary vasculitis (Table 13.2). In addition, a space-occupying lesion needs to be considered. The concomitant symptoms of joint pain and, particularly, jaw claudication suggest GCA. GCA is a granulomatous vasculitis that preferentially affects the extracranial branches of the carotid artery.

PATHOPHYSIOLOGY OF GIANT CELL ARTERITIS

Vascular inflammation in GCA is hypothesized to be a T-cell-dependent process that occurs as a consequence of inappropriate activation of the cell-mediated adaptive immune system. Granuloma formation is considered the hallmark of a T_H1 response (see Case 18 for detailed discussion of T_H1 response). Sequence analysis of the TCRs of tissue-infiltrating T cells in GCA indicates restricted clonal expansion, suggesting the presence of an unknown antigen residing in the arterial wall that is being recognized by these T cells. T cells enter the artery through the vasa vasorum (capillary blood supply to walls of large arteries) and migrate to the adventitia, where they encounter stimulatory signals, undergo clonal expansion, and release IL-2 and IFN-γ. These cytokines attract macrophages, which are recruited to the vessel wall and produce the granulomatous inflammation seen in this disease. Macrophages also produce IL-1 and IL-6 and contribute to arterial injury by producing metalloproteinases and nitric oxide in the media and intima, respectively. These changes ultimately lead to the degradation of the internal elastic lamina and to occlusive luminal hyperplasia.

 ## CLINICAL FEATURES OF GIANT CELL ARTERITIS

Symptoms of GCA include headache, jaw or tongue claudication, scalp tenderness, fatigue, weight loss, and fever. Polymyalgia rheumatica, which is characterized by aching and morning stiffness in the proximal muscles of the shoulder and hip girdles, occurs in 40–50% of patients. Findings on physical examination include nodularity, tenderness, or absent pulsations of the temporal arteries or other involved vessels. Involvement of the main branches of the aorta occurs in 15% of cases and can present with limb claudication. Aneurysms of the thoracic aorta can develop as a late complication and result in dissection and mortality.

The most significant complication of GCA is vision loss due to ischemic optic neuropathy from arteritis involving the ophthalmic blood vessels. Ocular involvement may present as diplopia, ptosis, and/or transient or permanent blindness.

 ## TREATMENT OF GIANT CELL ARTERITIS

Glucocorticoids are the foundation of treatment in GCA, improving symptoms and reducing the risk of vision loss. When GCA is strongly suspected and there is no evidence of active infection, prednisone should be administered immediately to protect vision while workup continues. Most patients require treatment for at least two years, and relapses occur in a large percentage. Glucocorticoids have significant toxicity and cause treatment-related morbidity.

ANCA-ASSOCIATED VASCULITIDES: WEGENER'S GRANULOMATOSIS

 ## CASE REPORT 4

"I am coughing up blood!"

Physical Examination and Initial Workup

Larry, a 30-year-old male patient of yours, presents to your office with a two-day history of hemoptysis (blood in sputum) with expectoration of approximately one tablespoon of blood on four or five occasions. He has had a six-month history of nasal congestion and facial pain that he attributed to dust in his home. For the past week he has also noted dyspnea (shortness of breath) on exertion, migratory joint pain, and profound fatigue. There was no antecedent illness and he denies fever or sore throat. Prior to this, he was in good health without recent travel or exposures. He is on no medication and denies recreational drug use.

On physical examination, Larry appears pale and unwell. His nasal mucosa has an ulcerated appearance and he has a small nasal septal perforation. His right knee and left wrist are swollen and appear fluid filled, suggesting inflammation of the joint (synovitis). The remainder of his examination is normal.

Laboratory evaluation reveals the following:

	Result	Reference Range
WBC	17,000/μL	4800–10,800/μL
Hemoglobin	8.8 g/dL	14–18 g/dL
Platelets	670,000/μL	130,000–400,000/μL
ESR	95 mm/h	0–25 mm/h
Creatinine	1.9 mg/dL	0.7–1.3 mg/dL

The WBC count, which is slightly elevated, shows a normal differential cell percentage (subpopulation distribution). Urinalysis shows 3+ protein, 20–40 dysmorphic (abnormal shaped) RBCs, and red blood cell casts. A chest computerized tomography (CT) scan reveals bilateral ground-glass pulmonary infiltrates (Fig. 13.3).

What do these laboratory findings indicate?

The patient is significantly anemic with a leukocytosis and a thrombocytosis (increased WBCs and platelets). The ESR is markedly elevated, indicating inflammation, neoplasm, or infection. There is renal insufficiency with evidence of significant glomerular damage, as documented by the presence of RBC casts (see Case 20 for discussion of renal failure). Chest X-ray and hemoptysis indicate pulmonary

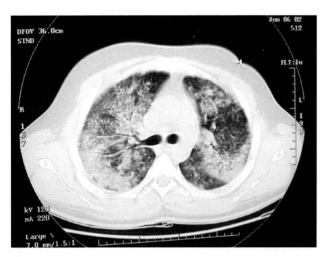

🔵 Figure 13.3. Case 4 Chest CT showing ground-glass infiltrates characteristic of pauci-immune glomerulonephritis.

disease, while the findings of nasal septal damage suggest that the upper respiratory tract is involved as well.

What is the differential diagnosis of hemoptysis with renal insufficiency?

Hemoptysis from the lower respiratory tract can originate from disease involving the airways, the vasculature, or the pulmonary parenchyma. This patient has radiographic evidence of pulmonary infiltrates, suggesting a parenchymal source. Causes include infection, coagulopathies, cocaine abuse, or an inflammatory immunologic disorder. The differential diagnosis in this patient is narrowed by the presence of glomerulonephritis, characterized by renal insufficiency and an active urine sediment. This combined picture of ground-glass infiltrates, which is consistent with alveolar hemorrhage, and glomerulonephritis suggests a pulmonary–renal syndrome from an immunologically mediated disease. In this setting, the differential diagnosis would include a primary small-vessel vasculitis, anti–glomerular basement membrane (anti-GBM) antibody disease (Goodpasture's syndrome), or systemic lupus erythematosus.

You admit Larry to the hospital for further evaluation of what you recognize to be a potentially life-threatening process. The following day, his creatinine has risen to 2.2 mg/dL. A bronchoalveolar lavage confirms alveolar hemorrhage and yields negative results for microorganisms. You send additional serological studies, begin treatment with high-dose methylprednisolone, and arrange for a renal biopsy.

Definitive Diagnosis

The renal biopsy report reads: "focal segmental necrotizing glomerulonephritis with abundant crescents. Electron

microscopy reveals no evidence for immune complex deposits; immunofluorescent staining is negative for immunoglobulin and complement. These findings are consistent with a pauci-immune glomerulonephritis."

The absence of immunoglobulin and complement deposits in the kidney helps rule out Goodpasture's syndrome; this is confirmed by the absence of anti-GBM antibody in the serum. ANA characteristic of systemic lupus erythematosus is also negative; however, antineutrophil cytoplasmic antibody (proteinase 3-ANCA) is positive. ANCA can be measured by indirect immunofluorescence or target antigen-specific testing. ANCA directed against proteinase 3 results in a cytoplasmic immunofluorescence pattern (cANCA) on ethanol-fixed neutrophils, while myeloperoxidase ANCA generates a perinuclear immunofluorescence pattern (pANCA).

The presence of upper airway disease, migratory arthritis, alveolar hemorrhage, pauci-immune glomerulonephritis, and proteinase 3-ANCA supports a diagnosis of *Wegener's granulomatosis*.

Treatment Plan

Larry is given a three-day course of methylprednisolone and then begins treatment with prednisone. Daily cyclophosphamide is added. He is also placed on antibiotics as prophylaxis against *Pneumocystis jiroveci* (formerly *Pneumocystis carinii*) pneumonia; the concern is that the immunosuppressive therapy could open the door to opportunistic infection. The hemoptysis resolves with the immunosuppressive treatment and there is improvement of the pulmonary infiltrates. His creatinine peaks at 2.5 mg/dL and then declines steadily. Following discharge, you arrange for weekly laboratory tests and follow-ups in your office. After one month, if his pulmonary and renal disease continues to improve, you plan to lower his prednisone dose while continuing his other medications.

🔵 DIFFERENTIAL DIAGNOSIS OF PULMONARY–RENAL SYNDROMES

The differential diagnosis of pulmonary–renal syndromes includes the primary small vessel-vasculitides, anti-GBM antibody disease (Goodpasture's syndrome), and systemic lupus erythematosus. These diseases vary with regard to their clinical features and renal histology. In contrast to both systemic lupus erythematosus and anti-GBM antibody disease, the glomerular pathology seen in primary small-vessel vasculitides is a focal segmental necrotizing glomerulonephritis that has few to no immune complex deposits, frequently referred to as a *pauci-immune glomerulonephritis*. This histology is typically seen in conjunction with circulating ANCA that targets proteinase 3 or myeloperoxidase. Because of this association, diseases that have this serologic and histologic picture are often collectively referred to as ANCA-associated vasculitides.

Pauci-immune ANCA-associated glomerulonephritis with alveolar hemorrhage can occur in three primary vasculitic diseases: Wegener's granulomatosis, microscopic polyangiitis, and Churg–Strauss syndrome. Although these are all characterized by the presence of vasculitis involving the small to medium-sized vessels, they possess individual clinical and laboratory features that identify them as unique disease entities (Table 13.5).

Churg–Strass syndrome is characterized by eosinophilia and symptoms of asthma, in contrast to the other two entities. Microscopic polyangiitis is associated with lower airway, not upper airway, disease and is more often associated with myeloperoxidase-associated ANCA than the other syndromes.

Wegener's granulomatosis is characterized by necrotizing, granulomatous inflammation involving the upper and lower respiratory tract, vasculitis of the small to medium-sized vessels, and glomerulonephritis. When renal disease accompanies other typical features, Wegener's granulomatosis is usually readily differentiated from other diagnoses. However, in the setting of isolated upper and/or lower airways disease, Wegener's granulomatosis needs to be distinguished from tumors of the upper airway or lung, infections, as well as noninfectious granulomatous processes.

 PATHOPHYSIOLOGY OF WEGNER'S GRANULOMATOSIS

The pathogenesis of Wegener's granulomatosis remains poorly understood. The presence of granulomatous inflammation of the upper airways and lungs suggests an aberrant cell-mediated immune response to an antigen that enters through or is located in the airways. Peripheral blood CD4+ T cells from patients with active Wegener's granulomatosis demonstrate increased secretion of IFN-γ and TNF compared to normal controls. These findings, combined with the granuloma formation, suggest that an unbalanced T_H1 pattern of cytokine production may play a role in pathogenesis of this disease.

A high percentage of patients with Wegener's granulomatosis develop ANCA. These autoantibodies are directed against proteins in the cytoplasmic granules of neutrophils and monocytes. There are two major categories of ANCA based on their target antigens. More than 90% of patients with typical active Wegener's granulomatosis have antibodies directed against proteinase 3, a 29-kDa serine proteinase present in the azurophilic granules of neutrophils. ANCA that targets the enzyme myeloperoxidase occurs in 5–20% of patients. A number of *in vitro* observations suggest possible mechanisms whereby ANCA could contribute to the pathogenesis of vasculitis. Proteinase 3 and myeloperoxidase reside in the azurophilic granules and lysosomes of resting neutrophils

TABLE 13.5. Comparison of Three Forms of ANCA-Associated Vasculitis

Characteristic: % Occurrence in Each Form	Wegener's Granulomatosis	Microscopic Polyangiitis	Churg–Strauss Syndrome
Upper airway disease	95	No	50–60
Asthma	No	No	90–100
Pulmonary nodules/infiltrates	70–85	15–70	40–70
Alveolar hemorrhage	5–15	10–50	<5
Glomerulonephritis	70–80	75–90	10–40
Gastrointestinal	<5	30	30–50
Peripheral nervous system	40–50	60–70	70–80
Central nervous system	5–10	10–15	5–30
Cardiac	10–25	10–15	10–40
Ocular	50–60	<5	<5
Arthralgias/arthritis	60–70	40–60	40–50
Skin	40–50	50–65	50–55
Proteinase 3 ANCA	75–90	10–50	3–35
Myeloperoxidase ANCA	5–20	50–80	2–50
Eosinophilia	Rare	Rare	80–100
Granulomatous inflammation	Present	Absent	Present

Note: Frequencies reflect data compiled from different series.

and monocytes, where they are normally inaccessible to serum antibodies. However, when TNF or IL-1 primes neutrophils or monocytes, proteinase 3 and myeloperoxidase translocate to the cell membrane where they can interact with these extracellular autoantibodies. The neutrophils then degranulate and produce reactive oxygen species that can cause tissue damage. ANCA-activated neutrophils can also adhere to and kill endothelial cells *in vitro*. Further evidence for a direct pathogenic role of ANCA has been provided by mouse models in which glomerulonephritis and vasculitis resulted in recipients receiving serum containing high-titer anti-myeloperoxidase antibody (passive transfer) or lymphocytes obtained from myeloperoxidase "knockout" mice that had been immunized with myeloperoxidase. Arguing against a primary pathogenic role for ANCA is the occurrence of patients with Wegener's granulomatosis who lack ANCA, the absence of a direct temporal association between a rise in ANCA and relapse, the clinical observation of patients who remain in remission despite high levels of circulating ANCA, and the uncertainty about how ANCA, an antibody, could produce granulomatous inflammation.

CLINICAL FEATURES OF WEGENER'S GRANULOMATOSIS

Wegener's granulomatosis is a multisystem disease that has a predilection to involve the upper and lower respiratory tracts and kidneys (Table 13.5). Over 90% of patients first seek medical attention for upper and/or lower airway symptoms. Nasal and sinus mucosal inflammation may result in perforation of the nasal septum and/or collapse of the nasal bridge. Pulmonary disease occurs in 85% of patients with radiographic abnormalities, including single or multiple nodules or infiltrates, cavities, and ground-glass infiltrates suggestive of alveolar hemorrhage. Renal involvement is present in 20% of patients at the time of diagnosis but occurs in 80% during the course of the disease. Glomerulonephritis, which is detected by the presence of an active urine sediment with microscopic hematuria and RBC casts, has the potential to be rapidly progressive while being asymptomatic.

TREATMENT OF WEGNER'S GRANULOMATOSUS

Active Wegener's granulomatosis that is life threatening is treated with cyclophosphamide in combination with prednisone. With such treatment, >90% of patients demonstrate marked improvement, 75% achieve complete remission, and an 80% survival rate has been observed. In the setting of alveolar hemorrhage with respiratory failure, rapidly progressive glomerulonephritis, or other fulminant

manifestations, high-dose intravenous methylprednisolone is given in combination with cyclophosphamide. While cyclophosphamide is very effective, it is associated with toxicity including bone marrow suppression, opportunistic infections, and hematologic malignancies.

SUMMARY

In conclusion, we have presented four cases of vasculitis, the vasculitides being a group of diseases which have in common an inflammatory attack of vessel wall. **Essential mixed cryoglobulinemia** is a small-vessel vasculitis which is ***immune complex mediated*** and for which the usual antigen is known (chronic HCV infection). It usually manifests as cutaneous, joint, neurologic, and/or renal disease. **Kawasaki disease**, an inflammation of the medium-sized vessels (as well as large and small vessels) may be the result of a ***superantigen*** from an as yet unidentified infectious agent. This form of vasculitis, although presenting as an acute mucocutaneous syndrome, frequently has coronary artery involvement with potentially serious consequences. **Giant cell arteritis** affects large vessels, particularly the branches of the carotid artery, and is a ***granulomatous inflammation***. It is of ***unknown etiology***, possibily due to direct attack by T cells. **Wegener's granulomatosis**, a vasculitis of the small vessels of the lung and kidneys, is another granulomatous inflammation, in this instance associated with ***anti-neutrophil cytoplasmic antibodies***. All of these vasculitides have the potential of serious consequences to the affected organ(s).

REFERENCES

Barron KS (2002): Kawasaki disease: Etiology pathogenesis and treatment. *Cleve Clin J Med* 69(Suppl 2): SII–69.

Hoffman GS, Kerr GS, Leavitt RY, Hallahan CW, Lebovics RS, Travis WD, et al. (1992): Wegener's granulomatosis: An analysis of 158 patients. *Ann Intern Med* 116: 488.

Jennette JC, Falk RJ (1997): Medical progress: Small vessel vasculitis. *N Engl J Med* 337:512–523.

Langford CA, Sneller MC (2001): Update on the diagnosis and treatment of Wegener's granulomatosis. *Adv Intern Med* 46: 177.

Sneller MC, Fauci AS (1997): Pathogenesis of vasculitis syndromes. *Med Clin North Am* 81: 221.

Vassilopoulos D, Calabrese LH (2002): Hepatitis C virus infection and vasculitis: Implications of antiviral and immunosuppressive therapies. *Arthritis Rheum* 46: 585.

Weyand CM, Goronzy JJ (2003): Giant-cell arteritis and polymyalgia rheumatica. *Ann Intern Med* 139: 505.

Unit III

AUTOIMMUNE DISORDERS

INTRODUCTION: OVERVIEW OF AUTOIMMUNE DISORDERS AND MECHANISMS OF TOLERANCE

WARREN STROBER and SUSAN R. S. GOTTESMAN

The many factors controlling the development of lymphocytes from precursors to mature cells now ready to protect the body from harmful pathogens were reviewed in Unit I in the discussion of immunodeficiency disorders. However, an important aspect of the generation of mature T and B cells not covered so far includes the processes ensuring tolerance or anergy to self-antigens. Breakdown of these mechanisms results in an immune attack on the body's own cells and proteins and the development of autoimmune disease.

This unit is devoted to autoimmunity and the various autoimmune disorders that result from this immune abnormality. These disorders comprise a surprisingly common group of diseases in that they have a combined prevalence of about 3% of the total population. In addition, they are usually life-long afflictions with frequently serious consequences for the affected patient. In the chapters that follow, individual diseases will be discussed in which one or more of the protective mechanisms against self-attack have been breached. The discussions of these diseases will focus on the prevailing hypothesis of the unique mechanism(s) operating in and the destructive processes characteristic of each disease. Before we proceed to these specific abnormalities, however, we review the common principles of tolerance and the general mechanisms by which such tolerance may be broken. A more detailed analysis may be found in Chapter 12 of Coico and Sunshine, *Immunology: A Short Course*, sixth edition.

CENTRAL AND PERIPHERAL TOLERANCE

An understanding of autoimmunity begins with knowledge of how the immune system learns to distinguish between foreign (exogenous) antigens to which it must respond and self (endogenous) antigens to which it must be unresponsive (tolerant) to avoid autoreactivity and autoimmune disease. We therefore begin our overview of autoimmunity with a discussion of the mechanisms of self-tolerance that develop first during differentiation, mostly in the central lymphoid organs, the thymus and the bone marrow, and then discuss the mechanisms operating on mature cells in the periphery, the lymphoid and nonlymphoid tissue outside the thymus and bone marrow. Later we will discuss how these mechanisms can be subverted in the various autoimmune diseases.

Central Tolerance

Central tolerance refers to tolerance (immune nonreactivity) that develops during the early maturation of lymphoid

Immunology: Clinical Case Studies and Disease Pathophysiology, By Warren Strober and Susan R. S. Gottesman

cells—T cells in the thymus and B cells in the bone marrow. However, since B cells also undergo further maturation in peripheral organs, central tolerance also refers to B-cell anergy which develops in peripheral lymphoid tissues.

T-Cell Tolerance. The generation of unresponsiveness in the T-cell compartment begins early in T-cell development in the thymus. As discussed more fully in Chapter 3 on DiGeorge syndrome (congenital thymic aplasia), thymocytes are subject to both positive and negative selection: *positive selection* to expand cells that recognize antigens only when presented by self–major histocompatibility complex (MHC) molecules and **negative selection** to delete cells that recognize, with high affinity, self-antigens presented by self-MHC molecules. This second selection process removes most autoreactive T cells from the nascent T-cell population but leaves a residual T-cell population that reacts with low affinity with self-antigens presented by self-MHC and high affinity with cross-reactive nonself-antigens (foreign antigens) presented by self-MHC.

It seems logical to conclude that the induction of T-cell tolerance via negative selection in the thymus is a first line of defense against the development of T-cell autoimmunity. One piece of evidence supporting this concept is the discovery of a nuclear factor known as AIRE (autoimmune regulator), a molecule that appears to be necessary for the transcription of genes encoding certain peripheral tissue antigens in thymic stromal cells; thus AIRE appears to be involved in the expression of self-antigens in cells that are critical to the negative selection of thymocytes reactive to these self-antigens. Mutations in AIRE manifest as autoimmune inflammations of multiple endocrine organs. Thus, such mutations illustrate that, in principle, failure of thymic negative selection can lead to autoimmunity. It should be noted, however, that AIRE controls a restricted set of antigens, affecting autoimmune reactivity in some organs and not others. This leads to the possibility that molecules like AIRE which govern negative selection to additional sets of antigens may yet be discovered.

While the generation of central tolerance in the thymus may eliminate the bulk of the self-reactive T cells, it cannot and does not eliminate all such T cells (see Fig. UIII.1). Many self-antigens either are sequestered in peripheral organs and never reach the thymus to induce negative selection or contain cryptic determinants that are not normally exposed to the immune system either centrally in the thymus or in the periphery. Thus, it is not surprising that T cells with self-reactivity can be readily identified in the peripheral organs and can even be induced to cause disease upon appropriate activation. Regulatory T cells, which will be discussed below at greater length, also develop in the thymus (or the periphery) and function in the periphery to suppress autoimmune responses. As

we shall see, such cells are one of several mechanisms that guard against the development of autoimmunity despite the presence of imperfect thymic negative selection.

B-Cell Tolerance. B cells also undergo steps to remove autoreactive cells, but in this case the steps are not tied to a specific organ such as the thymus. In discussing this process it is useful to characterize a number of "checkpoints" occurring first in the bone marrow and then in peripheral tissues (see Fig. 22.3). At these checkpoints, encounter with a self-antigen and consequent B-cell receptor (BCR) signaling leads either to deletion of autoreactive B cells or to a permanent state of anergy. In the bone marrow, such BCR signaling by self-antigen induces "receptor editing," with one of two results: (1) the B cell rearranges an alternative immunoglobulin light-chain gene and changes its specificity or (2) the developing B cell is deleted.

After a B cell emerges from the marrow, it passes through "transitional" stages of development where it is subjected to additional checkpoints that can lead to anergy or deletion. It is here that BCR signaling causes permanent changes in the topology of the BCR signaling apparatus that render the cell unable to signal. Interestingly, at this stage T-cell cosignaling (via CD40L) or B-cell growth factors such as BAFF (B-cell activation factor) can prevent B-cell anergy and lead to the emergence of autoreactive B cells. Another series of checkpoints involves the mature cells of the B-cell subsets known as B1 cells and marginal zone B cells. These B cells not infrequently display specificity for autoantigens. Nevertheless, they do not normally produce pathologic autoantibodies; instead, they make low-affinity antibodies because they have not undergone somatic mutation and class switching. The checkpoints in this case involve mechanisms that prevent the maturation of B cells in germinal centers, which would lead to high-affinity antibodies, perhaps accompanied by alterations in specificity that generate pathologic autoreactive antibodies. A final checkpoint occurs in the germinal centers, the main site where B cells (B2 cells or conventional B cells) encounter foreign antigens. The mechanisms involved in the deletion of autoreactive cells at this stage of B-cell development are poorly understood. However, the fact that such deletion can occur in germinal centers can be inferred from the observation that autoantibodies with characteristics indicating that they are products of germinal center B cells, such as antibodies showing evidence of somatic mutation and class switch differentiation, are found. Recent studies indicate one possible germinal center checkpoint mechanism: B cells are negatively signaled via their Fc receptors (FcγRIIB) when these receptors bind antigen–antibody complexes (see Case 22).

Mechanisms of T-cell tolerance or unreactivity

Figure UIII.1. Central and peripheral T cell tolerance mechanisms guarding against autoimmunity.

Peripheral Tolerance

As already mentioned, several mechanisms are in place in the periphery to prevent autoimmune pathology arising from the action of autoreactive cells, particularly T cells that have escaped deletion. One such mechanism, called T-cell "ignorance," refers to the fact that the potentially self-reactive T cells are unaware of the existence of autoantigens to which they can react because the latter exist in "privileged" sites that either bar entry of lymphocytes or eliminate them upon penetration. The eye, testes, and brain are examples of privileged sites protected by barriers at the level of the blood vessels and by their normal lack of resident lymphoid tissue.

A second mechanism relates to the fact that the autoreactive cell usually encounters its specific antigen under conditions that tend not to result in cell activation. Recall that T cells respond to antigens when they receive two signals. Signal 1 is delivered by antigen in the context of MHC and signal 2 is delivered by costimulatory molecules [such as B7 (CD80 and CD86)] interacting with CD28 and CTLA-4 on the T cell. There is considerable evidence that cells stimulated by antigen in the absence of costimulation (in the absence of signal 2) become anergic or die. The two-signal requirement for activation (versus one signal for anergy) applies to B cells as well as T cells. Thus it may be that many or most self-antigen reactive T cells that have escaped from the thymus are anergized or eliminated in the periphery because they encounter self-antigen on cells that cannot provide costimulation.

A third mechanism that acts in the periphery to control potential autoimmunity is the action of regulatory (T_{reg}) cells. In recent years it has become known that induction of "passive" tolerance in the thymus, in which self-reactive cells are deleted from the T-cell repertoire, is accompanied by the generation of "active" tolerance in the form of T_{reg} cells that suppress potential responses to self-antigens in the periphery.

Regulatory T cells (largely $CD4^+$ cells) develop in the medullary area of the thymus via a poorly understood process that allows them to escape negative selection, despite their relative high affinity for self-antigen. IL-2 is necessary for such development, thus accounting for the fact that mice lacking IL-2, lack T_{reg} cells and are susceptible to autoimmunity. Various costimulatory molecules are also necessary for T_{reg} development, but T_{reg} cells have not been associated with a specific cytokine milieu. T_{reg} development occurs in the presence of AIRE mutations, suggesting that passive and active tolerance develop as distinct and separate processes. T_{reg} cells emerging from the thymus bear distinct cell surface markers and comprise about 5–10% of the peripheral T-cell population. CD25, the α chain of the IL-2 receptor, was the first such marker identified but suffered from the fact that it is also present on activated non-T_{reg} T cells. CTLA-4, $\alpha_4\beta_7$ integrin, and GITR [glucocorticoid-induced tumor necrosis factor (TNF) receptor (R) a member of the TNF family] were also found on T_{reg} cells, but these markers were found on only a subpopulation of T_{reg} cells and, again, on other cell populations as well. Subsequently it was found that latent transforming growth factor (TGF) β_1 (TGF-β_1 bound to latency-associated protein) is present on all T_{reg} cells (and *not* on non-T_{reg} cells), especially after activation. This protein not only marks T_{reg} cells but, as indicated below, operates as an effector mechanism of T_{reg} suppressor function.

The intracellular markers known as Foxp3 and LAG-3 (lymphocyte activation gene 3) have been identified as T_{reg} markers and, in fact, Foxp3 has emerged as the molecule that defines T_{reg} cells. This designation is supported, in part, by the fact that mutations in Foxp3 result in the IPEX syndrome (immunodysregulation, polyendocrinopathy, and enteropathy, X-linked syndrome), which is characterized by severe multisystem autoimmunity. However, the role of Foxp3 in T_{reg} function is by no means clear, and it is known that cells not expressing Foxp3 have regulatory function (see further discussion below). In addition, there is an emerging consensus that the main mechanism used by

T_{reg} cells to mediate suppressor function is surface expression and secretion of TGF-β_1, but as yet there are no data supporting the idea that Foxp3 influences the expression of this molecule.

While it is well established that Foxp3-positive T_{reg} cells develop in the thymus and that such cells have specificity for self-antigens, it has become apparent that Foxp3 positivity can also be induced from naive $CD4^+$ T cells (T_H0 cells) in the periphery by T-cell receptor (TCR) stimulation in the presence of TGF-β_1. Thus, TGF-β_1 is both an inducer of T_{reg} cells and a mediator of its regulatory function. Because T_{reg} cells can be induced in the periphery as well as in the thymus, they are elements of both peripheral and central tolerance. In addition, the fact that inducible T_{reg} cells have specificity for exogenous antigens as well as self-antigens, they are also involved in the regulation of responses to nonself, exogenous antigens such as those encountered during infections.

A related discovery concerning TGF-β_1 is that this cytokine induces T_H17 effector T cells from T_H0 cells in the presence of interleukin-6 (IL-6) and perhaps other cytokines. Thus, whether a naive $CD4^+$ T_H0 cell becomes a proinflammatory T_H17 effector cell or an anti-inflammatory T_{reg} cell depends on whether TGF-β_1 acts in association with other cytokines or alone on the naive cell. Finally, this dependence of inflammation on small changes in the cytokine environment is heightened by that fact that T_H17 and T_{reg} cells are "plastic" and can interconvert as the environment changes (see Multiple Sclerosis Case 15 and the discussion below).

A second type of regulatory T cell functional in the periphery is the Tr1 cell. This negative regulatory cell expresses neither Foxp3 nor the surface markers associated with Foxp3-bearing cells such as CD25. Tr1 cells are generated in the periphery (and not in the thymus) by exposure to exogenous antigens rather than to self-antigens; their induction at peripheral sites requires the presence of IL-10 [or IL-10 plus interferon (IFN)-α in humans]. In addition, Tr1 mediates suppression by secreting IL-10 (and to a lesser extent TGF-β_1). Thus, Tr1 cells constitute a second type of peripherally induced regulatory T cells whose function overlaps that of Foxp3 T_{reg} cells.

⬤ GENERAL FEATURES OF AUTOIMMUNE DISEASES

Autoimmune diseases are usually categorized as either *organ-specific diseases* or *systemic diseases*. While this has some validity on a descriptive level, it does not necessarily predict the immunopathologic mechanism of the disease. Organ-specific diseases of the thyroid and the nerve ending (myasthenia gravis; see Case 14) are mediated by antibodies produced by B cells, whereas organ-specific diseases of the islet cells (type I diabetes mellitus; see Case 16) and the central nervous system (multiple sclerosis; see Case 15) are mediated by cytokines produced by T cells. Systemic autoimmune diseases such as systemic lupus erythematosus (SLE; see Case 22) are mediated primarily by B cells producing antibodies that form immune complexes, in contrast to rheumatoid arthritis (see Case 21), which is more likely caused by pathogenic T cells. However, all autoimmune diseases are likely to involve autoimmune T cells at some level. This is true even when the major disease manifestation is due to pathologic autoantibodies, since the presence of the latter usually implies that abnormal T-cell function allowed their generation.

In some cases of autoimmune disease, such as myasthenia gravis (see Case 14), the target antigen consists of a single antigen, or more precisely a specific **epitope** (the smallest immunogenic fragment of the antigen recognized by an immune effector cell). In other instances, such as SLE (see Case 22), the disorder is the result of an immune response to multiple self-antigens. This usually correlates with the fact that diseases caused by a single epitope or a limited number of epitopes are organ-specific autoimmunities, whereas multiple antigen autoimmunities are global diseases affecting many organ systems.

Like immunodeficiency diseases, autoimmune diseases have a strong *genetic basis*. However, the genetic influence usually consists, not of gene mutations occurring only in individuals with the disease, but of genetic polymorphisms that occur in both normal and affected individuals and only result in disease when they are present in association with other gene polymorphisms. This introduces at least two barriers to the determination of the molecular mechanism of disease. First, if the disease requires the separate input of several genes, the contribution of each is diluted and humans (or animals) that express a polymorphism in only one of the genes will not necessarily manifest disease or even abnormal function. Second, the group of genes causing disease may vary from one individual to another individual, although some are likely to overlap.

While family studies and twin studies have indicated that genetic factors are a substantial risk factor in the development of autoimmunity, in virtually all cases genes cannot be held entirely responsible for the disease. By default this means that *environmental factors* also play a role. By far the most important of these factors are infectious organisms that are thought to "trigger" autoimmunity in susceptible individuals. A possible mechanism is the release of normally sequestered autoantigens by these organisms, which then stimulate preexisting autoreactive cells. Alternatively, since infections induce the production of cytokines which increase the ability of cells to express surface molecules (such as MHC class II antigens), the cytokines may enable cells to present autoantigens to

autoreactive cells (along with a second signal; see below). Finally, antigens associated with the infecting organism may cross-react with autoantigens, inducing responses both to the invader and to self-antigens in a process called molecular mimicry; this process is described in more detail below. Some of these possibilities are discussed in relation to specific autoimmunities in the chapters that follow.

Autoimmunity has been very fruitfully studied in *experimental animals* (usually mice) that develop diseases resembling those in humans. In general, these "autoimmune mouse models" are either inbred strains that spontaneously develop disease because of genetic defects or mice that are induced by some manipulation to develop disease. The manipulation usually consists of infection with an organism or immunization with an antigen that elicits responses from preexisting autoreactive cells. Some of the best studied models are strains with susceptibility to the development of SLE, such as New Zealand black and MRL/lpr mice; strains that spontaneously develop type 1 diabetes mellitus, such as NOD mice (nonobese diabetic) mice; and mice immunized with type II collagen or myelin protein, which develop arthritis and experimental allergic encephalomyelitis (EAE), respectively. Models such as these have been used quite successfully to study genetic and environmental factors underlying autoimmunity, the nature of the effector cells involved (such as the specific T-helper-cell subset or T cells vs. B cells), and whether or not the autoimmunity results from decreased regulatory T-cell function. Finally, and perhaps most importantly, these models can be used to test new therapies for control of autoimmunity. Bear in mind, however, that murine models of autoimmunity rarely if ever display all aspects of the human illness; at best, they capture one or two features of human disease which can be regarded as a composite of parts of several animal models.

It has been apparent for many years both in humans and in experimental animal models that the *MHC has a major influence on the occurrence of autoimmune disease;* the MHC is at least partly responsible for the genetic basis of these diseases. As mentioned above, the development and activation of T cells normally involve presentation of antigen in the context of MHC molecules. In the thymus, the stimulation of $CD4^+CD8^+$ (double-positive) T cells by antigen associated with MHC class I and MHC class II results in $CD8^+$ T cells and $CD4^+$ T cells, respectively. These cells subsequently recognize antigen in the periphery only when the antigen is presented in relation to those MHC molecules (see Case 3 for detailed description of thymic events). Since antigens are preferentially presented by certain MHC alleles both in the thymus and in the periphery, it is easy to envision the preferential presentation of self-antigens by specific MHC alleles; thus, the occurrence of autoimmunity depends on the presence of these MHC alleles. For example, in rheumatoid arthritis (RA; see Case 21) a particular MHC amino acid sequence in the DR β chain (called the shared epitope) is associated with RA and determines its severity. This MHC sequence may allow the binding of arthritogenic peptides and thus the development of disease-inducing arthritogenic T cells either in the thymus (where it defeats negative selection) or in the periphery (where it induces autoreactive T-cell clones). Alternatively, the MHC sequence may negatively affect the development of regulatory T cells that would prevent autoimmunity. Thus the normal way T cells recognize and respond to antigen may explain some genetic susceptibility to autoimmune disease.

IMMUNOLOGIC MECHANISMS LEADING TO TISSUE DAMAGE IN AUTOIMMUNE DISEASES

Most autoimmune diseases are in some way dependent on the activity of CD4$^+$ T cells that recognize and respond to autoantigens. This is easy to see in organ-specific autoimmunities such as multiple sclerosis (see Case 15) and Crohn's disease (see Case 18), where the effector cell is clearly a CD4$^+$ T cell producing cytokines that mediate the inflammation. However, it is also true of diseases such as myasthenia gravis (see Case 14) and SLE (see Case 22), in which the final effector cell is a B cell that produces a pathologic antibody. This arises from the fact that the B cell requires T-cell help to produce antibody or that T cells are required for the activation of a normally anergic B cell. In addition, it is true of diseases in which the final effector is a CD8$^+$ cytotoxic T cell such as type 1 diabetes mellitus (see Case 16), where again the CD8$^+$ T cell requires CD4$^+$ T-cell help. An interesting variation on this theme occurs in RA (see Case 21), where the CD4$^+$ T cell plays an essential role as an initiator and sustainer of disease but the full-blown inflammation requires cytokine production by nonimmune cells, synoviocytes, and possibly B cells.

The CD4$^+$ T cells, T$_H$1, T$_H$2, T$_H$17, and T$_{reg}$ cells, discussed above are all generated from T$_H$0 cells; each produces a characteristic cytokine profile (see Case 15). On the other hand, T$_H$2 T-cell responses are not generally implicated in autoimmune disease development. An exception to this rule is systemic sclerosis (see Case 23), a fibrotic disease clearly mediated by IL-4 and IL-13 responses that drive the development of fibrosis. In SLE (see Case 22), levels of T$_H$2 cytokines are elevated, but T$_H$1 cytokines are also increased. In addition, in SLE there is evidence that IFN-α is overproduced and that this cytokine is important in driving antigen-presenting cells to become effectors of damage. Finally, in ulcerative colitis (see Case 18), the key effector cell appears to be a natural killer T cell (NKT cell) that produces IL-13 but not IL-4.

IL-13 has detrimental effects on the gut epithelium and stimulates the NKT cells to become cytotoxic cells that kill epithelial cells.

Initially it was thought that the above CD4$^+$ T-cell responses that induced autoimmunity were T$_H$1 responses that led to the production of IFN-γ. T$_H$1 cells are derived from T$_H$0 cells under the influence of IL-12p70. More recently, studies of murine models of autoimmunity, as well as limited studies in humans, have suggested that perhaps a more important cytokine response involves T$_H$17 cells giving rise to the cytokines IL-17 and IL-22; such responses are driven (or sustained) by IL-23. However, although it is fair to say that this latter cytokine system undoubtably plays a role in autoimmunity, it is too early to dismiss the role of the T$_H$1 response. The most likely possibility is that both cytokine systems can and do participate in the pathologic autoimmune process, perhaps in different phases of the inflammatory response.

Both the T$_H$1 and T$_H$17 cytokine responses prompt a secondary round of cytokine (and chemokine) production that is the more proximal cause of tissue injury. This includes but is not limited to IL-6, tumor necrosis factor (TNF) α, and IL-1β as well as a host of chemokines. These in turn bring in monocytes (macrophages) and granulocytes that release other inflammatory mediators. Pinpointing the T-cell subsets responsible for the production of cytokines that initiate autoimmune responses, as well as those cytokines more directly responsible for damage, identifies potential targets for therapy.

In many autoimmune diseases, antibody-mediated pathologic effects are due to antibody–antigen complexes that cause pathology via fixation of complement, followed by the release of inflammation-inducing complement components. For example, the deposition of such complexes is responsible for the kidney damage occurring in patients with SLE (see Case 22). However, antibodies can also cause direct tissue injury and/or functional abnormalities by binding to key receptors and inhibiting receptor signaling (as in myasthenia gravis; see Case 14) or by the activation of nonspecific inflammatory cells via binding to their Fcγ receptors (as in SLE; see Case 22).

MECHANISMS UNDERLYING LOSS OF TOLERANCE IN AUTOIMMUNE DISEASES

Many mechanisms have been proposed to explain the emergence of pathologic autoreactive cells and, indeed, it is unlikely that one mechanism explains all forms of autoimmunity. In many or most instances these mechanisms involve to some extent the dysfunction of central and peripheral tolerance induction discussed above.

Thymic Events

Autoimmune T cells could arise from a failure of negative selection in the thymus; as already discussed, mutations in the AIRE gene may represent a prototype of this type of abnormality. Because individual genes encoding self-antigens under the control of the AIRE transcription factor are variably sensitive to the level of AIRE, patients with mutations resulting in reduced levels of AIRE will exhibit variability in the expression of these antigens in the thymus. Indeed, polymorphisms in the promoter regions of the genes for self-antigens determine their sensitivity to AIRE levels. The resulting pattern of self-antigen expression may not be sufficient to direct effective negative selection. This could explain the fact that AIRE mutations lead to multiple autoimmune syndromes on the one hand and account for the potential selectivity of defects in central tolerance and the genetic basis of individual autoimmune diseases of the endocrine system such as diabetes mellitus (see Case 16) on the other. We have also discussed how certain types of MHC class II antigens may predispose to failure of negative selection in the thymus and even in the periphery by determining the strength of response and specific epitopes of self antigens presented.

Further support for the role of a defect in central tolerance and negative selection in some forms of autoimmunity is observed in cases of myasthenia gravis accompanied by thymoma or thymic follicular hyperplasia (see Case 14). The proliferative process occurring in this situation may disrupt intrathymic development and lead to the escape of T cells from the thymus prior to their normal deletion by negative selection.

Central B-Cell Tolerance

A process that subverts the elimination or tolerization of B cells occurring at various checkpoints of B-cell development can lead to B-cell autoimmunity. A number of processes fall into this category. These range from the overproduction of type 1 IFN, which directly or indirectly prevents the induction of B-cell anergy, to the formation of self-antigens such as DNA and RNA, that have intrinsic stimulatory properties via Toll-Like Receptors, (a part of our innate immune system; see Case 22 for immunopathogenesis of SLE). Interestingly, defects in processes such as apoptotic mechanisms, which normally dispose of such intracellular molecules upon cell death, may actually contribute to the accumulation and exposure of such molecules.

Breaching Peripheral Tolerance

Finally, peripheral mechanisms contribute to the prevention of autoimmune responses by T cells or B cells that escape central (developmental) tolerization processes; these may be disrupted and lead to autoimmunity. Defects in antigen sequestration or disruptions of natural barriers can lead to entry of potentially autoreactive cells into immunologically privileged sites. An excellent example of this is **sympathetic ophthalmoplegia**, where injury to one eye results in release of normally sequestered eye antigens and/or sensitization of potentially eye-antigen reactive cells, which then cause inflammation of the other (uninjured) eye.

Anergy of the T cell occurs when only one signal is delivered to the cell; delivery of a second signal via a co-stimulatory molecule may break tolerance. Autoreactive T cells exposed to potential self-antigens on cells that normally lack co-stimulatory molecules (such as epithelial cells) may therefore fail to either be stimulated or will be tolerized by the self-antigen. The epithelial (or other) cells may then gain the capacity to both present self antigen and deliver a second signal, thus inducing autoreactivity and/or becoming targets of immune attack. This newly gained capacity to stimulate T cells may be induced by local production of cytokines or by abnormal cell-cell stimulation events.

A variation on this theme involves inhibitory second signals that are normally delivered by antigen-presenting cells to the T cells in some situations. Antigen-presenting cells that stimulate T cells, not via CD28 (a positive second signal) but through CTLA-4, deliver a negative second signal. Thus, it can be speculated that a defect in the delivery of negative signals via co-stimulatory molecules could also lead to autoimmunity. In support of this notion, mice that lack the ability to express CTLA-4 develop severe, systemic autoimmunity.

A related mechanism operative in some autoimmune diseases is a phenomenon known as ***molecular mimicry*** wherein an antigen associated with a microbe that is either colonizing the body or causing an infection resembles a self-antigen. Such antigens elicit a response that in part involves normally dormant cells that have escaped thymic deletion and can react with self-antigens. In effect, the cells responsive to self-antigen "cross-react" with the microbial antigen and are stimulated because the microbial antigen is presented by an antigen-presenting cell with the "equipment" to induce a robust immune response, MHC class II and costimulatory molecules. This scenario has long been considered the basis for the development of rheumatic heart disease (rheumatic fever) following inadequate treatment of group A ß-hemolytic streptococcal pharyngitis (common strep throat). This mechanism has also been proposed to underlay the development of psoriasis (see Chapter 19), the occurrence of arthritis in patients expressing the human leukocyte antigen (HLA) B27 MHC antigen who develop arthritis following certain gastrointestinal infections (see Chapter 21), and the development of Guillain–Barré syndrome, a demyelinating peripheral nervous system disease in some patients following infection with *Campylobacter jejuni*. In addition, molecular mimicry has been evoked as a possible initiator of type 1 diabetes mellitus (see Chapter 16). Along similar lines, infections may induce autoimmune responses, not because they express antigens that mimic self-antigens, but rather because the infectious agent (or drugs) modifies self-antigens and renders them immunogenic to reactive cells that eventually respond to unmodified self-antigens as well.

The phenomenon of *"epitope spreading"* may perpetuate or aggravate the cross-reactive autoimmune response resulting from molecular mimicry. The original autoimmune response to an individual epitope on a single antigen becomes enlarged to include responses to many epitopes in this antigen or to epitopes in other antigens. This may occur because the tissue damage attending the initial autoimmune response can cause the release of new cell antigens into an inflammatory milieu that permits presentation of these antigens to potentially autoreactive cells. Again, the salient feature of this milieu is the induction of antigen-presenting cells that have the capacity to successfully present autoantigens and to stimulate cells. Epitope spreading complicates any attempt to treat autoimmune disease by modulation of the response to a single antigen.

A final and quite important potential mechanism leading to autoimmunity is a failure of the regulatory T cell system. This possibility is dramatically supported by the observation that humans with IPEX syndrome due to a mutation in the important T_{reg} cell transcription factor Foxp3 develop a severe, multisystem autoimmune disorder. In addition, in experimental animal models, defects in regulatory T cell development have been assumed to be the origin of the autoimmunity. These include a mouse model of inflammatory bowel disease, colitis which can be successfully treated by the provision of regulatory T cells (see Case 18), mice lacking IL-10 (a recognized anti-inflammatory cytokine), mice lacking IL-2 (a cytokine necessary for the development of T cells in the thymus), and NOD mice (see Case 16) that have an unexplained defect in regulatory T cell development. Despite the evidence cited above derived from models of autoimmunity, in actuality there is as yet insufficient evidence for this mechanism in humans. In particular, although there are reports that defects in regulatory T cell function do occur in various autoimmune diseases, it has yet to be shown that these defects are actually the cause of human disease.

AUTOIMMUNE DISEASE CASE HISTORIES DISCUSSED IN THIS UNIT

We begin this section of the text with a group of diseases for which the self-antigens are well identified and are usually protected from attack as a result of clonal deletion in the thymus. We have chosen myasthenia gravis (Case 14), multiple sclerosis (Case 15), and type I diabetes mellitus (Case 16) to represent this group; other representative disorders include Graves disease and Hashimoto's thyroiditis. Myasthenia gravis is considered the prototypic autoantibody disease, whereas multiple sclerosis is likely the consequence of autoreactive T_H1 and T_H17 cells and a cell-mediated (delayed-type hypersensitivity) immune attack. Type I diabetes mellitus may well have several possible autoimmune effector mechanisms in individual patients, but it is generally considered a T-cell autoimmune disease and is an important and common human disease deserving of detailed consideration.

In the next group of diseases, an environmental agent more clearly contributes to the breakdown in self-tolerance; in each disorder the specific agent has been identified or is at least highly suspected. This group includes celiac disease (Case 17), inflammatory bowel disease (Case 18), and psoriasis (Case 19). Among other disorders in this same category are some of the vasculitides (see Unit II).

We end the unit with systemic autoimmune diseases in which numerous autoantibodies against multiple self-antigens attack targets. Much of their pathology is the result of immune complex formation, antigen–antibody deposition throughout the body. These include IgA nephropathy and kidney transplant (Case 20), rheumatoid arthritis (Case 21), SLE (Case 22), and systemic sclerosis (Case 23).

For each disease, we describe current knowledge about the target of immune attack, the antigen or antigens responsible, how the breach of immune tolerance occurs, and which normally adaptive immune response is believed to go awry. Not surprisingly, some themes will repeat from chapter to chapter or disease to disease, such as the events that can result in autoimmune disease; only by attempting to dissect these reactions can we hope to control or even prevent these diseases in a manner less damaging than current strategies.

14

MYASTHENIA GRAVIS

CAMILLA BUCKLEY and ANGELA VINCENT*

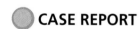

CASE REPORT

"I am seeing double"

History and Initial Evaluation

Meg, a 25-year-old student teacher, is referred to you, a neurologist, by her general physician. As indicated by her chief complaint, she has been experiencing intermittent episodes of double vision (diplopia) that seem to be worse at the end of the day. These symptoms had their onset at the start of the school year about six weeks ago. Two weeks ago they started to worsen; in addition to seeing two images side by side (horizontal displacement), she now occasionally sees two images one above the other (vertical displacement). Over the last several weeks Meg's husband has noticed that her left eyelid droops occasionally. Meg says that she has been otherwise well but is naturally distressed by these somewhat alarming symptoms.

On examination you find that Meg has ptosis (drooping) of the left eyelid that is worse upon sustained upgaze (fatigable ptosis). She also has horizontal diplopia with bilateral restriction of abduction (movement of gaze

outward) and adduction (movement of gaze inward) and restricted ability to gaze upward with the left eye. You also note that Meg has mild bilateral weakness of the eyelids upon eye closure. The rest of Meg's neurologic examination is normal, as is her general examination.

What is the differential diagnosis of diplopia and ptosis? (See Table 14.1.)

*Diplopia can be caused by disorders affecting the intraocular muscles, and **ptosis** can be caused by disorders affecting the levator palpebrae muscle. The combination of ptosis and diplopia (as in Meg's case) may be the result of impairment of the nerve supply to the muscles, weakness of the muscles, or impaired neuromuscular transmission.*

*Neuronal causes include lesions of the third cranial nerve and Horner's syndrome (oculosympathetic paralysis). Muscular causes include mitochondrial cytopathies such as chronic progressive external opthalmoplegia, myotonic dystrophy, and rare ocular muscular dystrophies. Neuromuscular causes include **myasthenia gravis (MG)** restricted to the eye muscles (ocular MG) or MG affecting bulbar, respiratory, and limb muscles (generalized MG); the **Lambert–Eaton myasthenic syndrome (LEMS)**; and rare genetic disorders of neuromuscular transmission. In addition, local disorders of the orbit may also cause diplopia and apparent ptosis; these include tumors of the*

*With contributions from Warren Strober and Susan R. S. Gottesman

Immunology: Clinical Case Studies and Disease Pathophysiology, By Warren Strober and Susan R. S. Gottesman
Copyright © 2009 John Wiley & Sons, Inc.

◉ TABLE 14.1. Differential Diagnosis of Myasthenia Gravis

Presenting Symptoms	Possible Diagnosis
Generalized myasthenia (ocular/bulbar/limb weakness to varying extents)	Lambert–Eaton myasthenic syndrome
	Hereditary myasthenic syndromes
	Acute or chronic inflammatory demyelinating polyradiculoneuropathies
	Myopathies (inflammatory, metabolic, dystrophies)
	Neurotoxins:
	Botulism
	Venoms (e.g., snakes, scorpions, spiders)
Bulbar myasthenia	Brain stem stroke
	Motor neuron disease (pseudobulbar palsy)
Ocular myasthenia	Mitochondrial cytopathy (chronic progressive external ophthalmoplegia)
	Oculopharyngeal muscular dystrophy
	Thyroid ophthalmopathy
	Other causes of ptosis, such as contact lens syndrome
	Brain stem lesions

orbit, skull fractures, or the ocular manifestations of Graves disease (autoimmune thyroiditis).

From this list of possible disorders, your leading diagnosis is MG, but you need to rule out LEMS, Graves disease, and muscular dystrophies. Meg is not so incapacitated by her symptoms that she demands immediate treatment. She is rather taken aback by the list of diagnostic possibilities, as she has no family history of autoimmune disease and she has no constitutional symptoms. For these reasons she consents to undergo extensive diagnostic testing to establish a definite diagnosis before starting treatment.

In the initial workup you order a series of blood tests, including a complete blood count (CBC), serum chemistries, creatine kinase (a muscle enzyme), and thyroid function tests [T3 and T4 levels and thyroid-stimulating hormone (TSH) levels]. At the same time, you obtain serum for detection of circulating antibodies to acetylcholine receptor (AChR) and TSH receptor (TSHR) and arrange for Meg to have outpatient electrophysiologic studies of muscle and nerve conduction.

What are the definitions of Graves disease, LEMS, and MG, and how will the tests listed above help you distinguish among them?

While all three disorders are autoimmune diseases, the antigen targeted by the autoimmune process differs in each case. Graves disease is an autoimmune disease of the thyroid gland in which autoantibodies, usually specific for the TSHR, cause stimulation of this endocrine organ and the symptoms of hyperthyroidism. These autoantibodies, as well as autoreactive T cells, frequently react with fibroblasts surrounding the ocular muscles (as well as thyroid cells) and thus cause swelling and inflammatory edema of orbital tissue. This leads, in turn, to proptosis or protrusion of the

orbit. Since proptosis can give rise to symptoms similar to those seen in LEMS and MG, Graves disease must be considered in the differential diagnosis of these diseases.

LEMS and MG are both autoimmune diseases in which the immune targets are elements of the neuromotor conduction system. The neuromuscular junction (NMJ), the synapse between the motor nerve terminal and the muscle membrane, is specialized to facilitate rapid, reversible transmission of electrical signals from the nerve to the muscle (Fig. 14.1). Action potentials arriving at the end of the nerve terminal cause ACh-containing vesicles to fuse with the cell membrane of the presynaptic button and release ACh into the synaptic cleft. ACh diffuses across the cleft and binds to AChRs on the muscle cell membrane, leading to depolarization and initiation of a muscle action potential. This mobilizes intracellular calcium stores and initiates muscle contraction. Acetylcholinesterase in the synaptic space degrades ACh, thus ensuring fine control of neuromuscular transmission. In normal individuals, repeated stimulation leads to depletion of ACh-containing vesicles, which is quickly followed by increased calcium secretion and increased efficiency of vesicle release. Thus, sufficient overall availability of ACh is maintained for continued muscle function.

LEMS is characterized by IgG antibodies that interact with proteins in the calcium channels of the presynaptic motor nerve terminal; in so doing, they interfere with the release of ACh. MG is marked by IgG antibodies that bind to the AChRs on the muscle cell and block the binding of ACh to the AChR. Signaling is impaired in both cases. However, in LEMS repeated stimulation will increase ACh release and therefore increase transmission of signal through the unblocked (normal) AChRs. In contrast, in MG initial stimulation may lead to the release of a sufficient number of ACh-containing vesicles to overcome the AChR block, but repeated stimulation leading to a normal decrement in

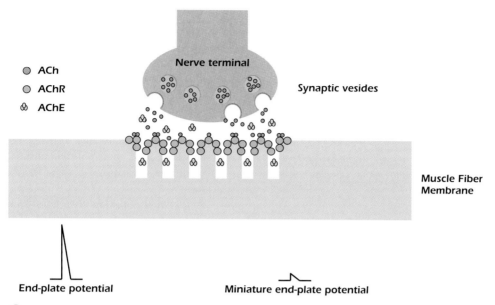

○ Figure 14.1. The Neuromuscular junction. Transmission depends on calcium-induced release of acetylcholine (ACh) from the motor nerve and its interactions with the AChRs on the surface of the muscle fiber. ACh is hydrolyzed by the enzyme acetylcholinesterase, which is present in the neuromuscular junction.

vesicle release is not sufficiently compensated by increased efficiency of vesicle release to overcome the receptor blockade, so there is further decrease in signal transmission.

The three disorders described above may be distinguished by assays for the specific autoantibodies associated with each disease. In addition, Graves disease can be distinguished from LEMS and MG by the presence of abnormal thyroid function tests, and LEMS and MG can be distinguished from each other by differing clinical presentations. Most patients with LEMS present with limb weakness, and the majority of patients with MG present with ocular difficulty. Lastly, LEMS and MG give rise to different results in muscle and nerve conduction studies (see below).

Meg's CBC, serum chemistries, creatine kinase level, and thyroid function tests are available the next day and prove to be normal. AChR antibody levels are available one week later and are detected at a concentration of 10 nM (reference range <0.5 nM); her TSHR antibodies are not elevated.

How are AChR antibodies measured and what is the significance of a positive result?

*AChR antibodies are detected using a sensitive and robust radioimmunoassay that relies on the high affinity and specificity of a snake venom toxin, α-bungarotoxin. This toxin binds to a site on α subunit of AChR that is different from the site (epitope) on the same subunit that is usually recognized by the autoantibody in patients with MG. (Recall that an **epitope** is the smallest region within an antigenic molecule that is specifically recognized by an antibody or the antigen receptor of a lymphocyte.) To detect the*

autoantibody, AChRs extracted from human muscle are incubated with ^{125}I-α-bungarotoxin, forming ^{125}I-α-bungarotoxin–AChR complexes. The test serum is then added and any IgG–^{125}I-α-bungarotoxin–AChR complexes formed are precipitated by addition of an antiserum to human IgG. The amount of ^{125}I-α-bungarotoxin in the precipitate is proportional to the amount of AChR antibody and can be counted on a gamma radioactivity counter. AChR antibodies are demonstrated in approximately 50% of patients with ocular MG, in approximately 85% of patients with generalized MG, and only rarely in patients with no clinical evidence of MG. Thus the presence of AChR antibodies is a sensitive (85%) and highly specific (>99%) test for generalized MG.

Meg's electrophysiology studies are reported as showing abnormal decrement on repetitive stimulation and increased jitter.

How do you interpret the abnormal nerve and muscle electrophysiology results?

In normal individuals, repetitive nerve stimulation at a frequency of 3 Hz can result in a reduction in the amplitude of the evoked muscle action potential (decrement). However, when this reduction exceeds 15% within the first five repetitive stimuli, a defect in neuromuscular transmission is likely to be present. This is the case in MG patients where, as discussed above, the reduced number or availability of AChRs is the cause of reduced muscle responses, which become worse upon repetitive stimulation. In generalized MG the sensitivity of this test approaches 90%. False-negative results can occur in ocular MG because the test is usually performed in a peripheral muscle, which may be unaffected in this variant of the illness.

   Single-fiber electromyography is a more sensitive, although less specific, diagnostic tool. It involves recording the action potentials in pairs of muscle fibers supplied by branches of a single nerve fiber. As a consequence of the delayed or blocked transmission at the NMJ caused by reduced numbers of AChRs, the times between responses of the two muscle fibers differ or the second of the two may not occur; these differences are known as jitter or blocking, respectively. The more severe the MG symptoms are, the longer the potential delay, and therefore the greater the degree of jitter or blocking.

The results of anti-AChR antibody study and electrophysiologic tests strongly suggest that Meg does indeed have MG and further suggest that she has generalized MG currently presenting with ocular involvement only. You convey these conclusions to Meg and ask her to return to you in a week for further evaluation and formulation of a therapeutic plan. At this point you also tell her that MG is frequently associated with thymus gland enlargement and to manage her effectively you will need to perform studies to determine if she has such enlargement.

Evolution of Symptoms and Further Evaluation

Meg finds it difficult to return to you at the agreed time because of her student teaching obligations. When she does return, one month after the diagnostic workup, the diplopia and ptosis have progressed and are present throughout the day to a variable extent. In addition, Meg now notices that her speech begins to slur by the end of a long telephone conversation or while teaching. She has no difficulty swallowing and has not noticed any choking or shortness of breath. She does have to rest while washing her hair and finds it difficult to climb stairs. All her symptoms fluctuate and tend to worsen at the end of the day or after activity and to improve after rest.

On reexamination you find that Meg has bilateral fatigable ptosis, more pronounced on the left than the right, with limitation of eye movements in all directions of gaze. She has clearly demonstrable weakness of the facial muscles and is unable to smile properly (Fig. 14.2). She has dysarthria (slurring and slowing of speech), which worsens during the course of the consultation, and she has mild fatigable weakness of shoulder abduction and hip flexion.

You explain to Meg that her localized ocular MG has now progressed to a generalized disease. You arrange a computerized tomography (CT) scan of the chest; meanwhile to provide symptomatic relief, you commence treatment with pyridostigmine, an agent that inhibits the enzyme acetylcholinesterase and thus increases the level of acetylcholine at the NMJ. Meg notices a marked improvement in her symptoms within 30 min of taking the first dose, with virtually complete resolution of her diplopia and ptosis.

Unfortunately, after a week on pyridostigmine, Meg's symptoms recur at a level that limits her day-to-day activities, although she continues to notice some benefit. The CT scan showed an enlarged thymus gland, although there was no radiologic evidence of a thymic tumor (thymoma). After discussion of treatment options, Meg decides to undergo thymectomy (surgical removal of the thymus) to try to attain complete remission and avoid long-term immunosupressive treatment.

What is the role of thymectomy in young patients with MG?

An association between thymic abnormalities and MG has been recognized since early in the last century (see below), and thymectomy has been part of the standard treatment of

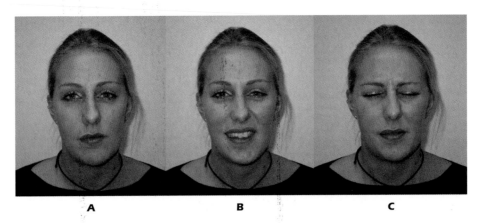

                    A   B   C

◯ Figure 14.2. Typical early-onset patient with MG. (**A**) At rest, the expression is somewhat flat and there is noticeable ptosis. (**B**) When asked to smile, there is minimal upturning of the corners of the mouth and no creasing around the eyes. (**C**) When asked, she is unable to screw up her eyes despite efforts to do so (note lowered eyebrows).

MG since 1939, although there has never been a randomized controlled trial to test its benefit. In patients under the age of 40 years without a thymoma and with AChR antibodies, thymectomy probably results in medication-free remission in approximately 25%, improvement in MG symptoms in 50%, and no benefit in the remaining 25% of patients. In patients with thymoma, thymectomy does not usually relieve the MG but is still an indicated treatment since the tumor may be locally invasive.

Over the next several days, Meg undergoes assessment in preparation for thymectomy. However, her condition during this short period deteriorates and she now complains of increased dysarthria, occasional difficulty with swallowing, and shortness of breath on exertion. On examination you find that her facial weakness is more marked and she has delayed swallowing. You have pulmonary function tests performed and learn that her vital lung capacity (total amount of air that can be forcefully exhaled after maximum inspiration) is reduced to 1.5 L (30% of the level predicted for her age and sex), suggesting active involvement of respiratory muscles. You therefore postpone the thymectomy and arrange for her to be admitted for a course of plasmapheresis, a plasma exchange procedure.

What is plasmapheresis?

Plasmapheresis is an exchange transfusion during which a defined volume of the patient's plasma is removed and replaced by plasma from healthy donors. Typically, 50 ml of plasma per kilogram of body weight is replaced each day for five consecutive days. The rationale of this procedure in the treatment of MG (as well as other autoimmune diseases) is that plasmapheresis is a method of removing pathogenic antibodies in the patient's plasma and replacing the latter with antibody-free plasma from healthy donors. Maximum

benefit is observed within a few days after the last exchange when AChR antibody levels have been maximally reduced, but the disease symptoms return six to eight weeks later as levels are replenished by the synthesis of new antibodies.

As expected, the plasmapheresis results in a dramatic clinical improvement; within 10 days Meg's vital capacity increases to 4 L (80% of normal). She is now able to undergo thymectomy, and the procedure is promptly performed without complications. Her thymus gland is found to be enlarged. Histologic examination confirms the diagnosis of thymic follicular hyperplasia (Fig. 14.3; also see below). No microscopic evidence of thymoma is found.

Clinical Progression

Upon follow-up one year after the operation, Meg reports that her symptoms have improved since the plasmapheresis and the surgery, but her dysarthria still disrupts her work as a teacher, and she still suffers from shortness of breath. You suggest initiating steroid therapy to control the symptoms of MG, since steroids suppress the immune response and could therefore reduce production of the anti-AChR antibodies. You also indicate that in view of the severity of her persistent symptoms that she should begin such therapy, in spite of the fact that it has potentially serious side effects (see below). Meg discusses this treatment option with her husband, and they agree to begin steroid therapy. You have Meg admitted to the hospital, as the initiation of corticosteroid treatment can induce a life-threatening exacerbation of bulbar and respiratory weakness in patients with MG. In the hospital she is begun on prednisone treatment, initially at a dose of 10 mg on alternate days; over the next

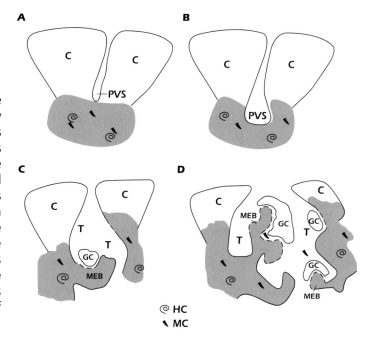

Figure 14.3. The thymus in myasthenia gravis. (A) The normal thymus has clearly distinct cortical and medullary regions. Within the medulla, there are Hassall's corpuscles (HCs) and a few myoid cells (MCs). (B) In normal adults and some patients with seronegative MG, there may be some expanded perivascular spaces (PVSs). (C) In typical AChR antibody-positive early-onset MG, germinal centers (GCs) form within these perivascular spaces. These contain T-cell areas (T), and the laminin border between the true medullary epithelial areas (pink areas) and PVS may be fenestrated (dotted lines). Myoid cells and germinal centers may occur near these fenestrations. (D) The epithelium of the medulla becomes distorted into medullary epithelial bands (MEBs) and changes illustrated in (C) expand. (Courtesy of I. Roxannis and N. Willcox.)

two weeks the dose is gradually increased to 100 mg on alternate days.

What are the common effects of treatment with corticosteroids?

Corticosteroids inhibit the immune response by affecting the distribution, number, and function of T and B cells as well as other bone marrow–derived cells. The change in the distribution of lymphocytes leads to a decreased number of cells in the periphery. This, plus steroid-induced lymphocyte death, results in a reduced ability of these cells to accumulate and cause inflammation at tissue sites. These effects are then magnified by the ability of steroids to inhibit several key leukocyte functions, particularly the cells-ability to produce proinflammatory factors. Since steroids cause demargination of neutrophils from vessel walls, steroid administration causes a rapid rise in the circulating white blood cell count and a decrease in the neutrophils that are poised to infiltrate tissues.

The price of these sought-after immunosuppressive activities of corticosteroid therapy is a broad range of adverse side effects. Short-term therapy can cause hypertension and diabetes characterized by increases in blood glucose levels. In addition, it can cause increased appetite and associated weight gain (particularly around the face and upper back); altered mood and psychiatric disturbances including mania or depression; difficulty sleeping; atrophy of the skin; easy bruising; and dyspepsia associated with gastrointestinal bleeding in predisposed individuals. Finally, the immunosuppressive effect that treats the autoimmunity may also predispose the patient to infection, including infection with "low-grade" opportunistic organisms. Corticosteroid therapy also has long-term effects, including inhibition of endogenous adrenal steroid leading ultimately to iatrogenic Addison's disease, premature cataracts, osteoporosis, and steroid-induced myopathy.

To prevent many of these side effects of corticosteroid therapy, Meg is also put on a "steroid-sparing" agent called azathioprine. Azathioprine is a purine analogue that inhibits purine metabolism and DNA and RNA synthesis, thus inhibiting the rapid proliferation of immune cells during an inflammatory process.

Three months after commencing prednisone/azathioprine treatment, Meg is symptom free and has no limitations on her activities. She gradually reduces and stops the pyridostigmine and then slowly reduces her corticosteroid dose until she notices a recurrence of mild symptoms. She then remains on the lowest dose of prednisone that maintains remission in conjunction with azathioprine.

Two years later Meg comes to you for advice about the possibility of becoming pregnant. You respond positively but emphasize that it will be critically important that her MG remain well controlled during the pregnancy. This is necessary both for her own health and that of the developing fetus, particularly in the later stages of pregnancy when there may be transplacental transfer of pathogenic IgG antibodies. Meg is concerned about azathioprine use during pregnancy, as she has read that it interferes with DNA synthesis. You reassure her that there is good evidence in the medical literature that azathioprine use is safe in pregnancy, and there is no evidence to suggest an increased risk of fetal abnormalities. In addition, you tell her that you have had several patients with MG who have given birth to healthy babies while taking prednisone and azathioprine. In fact, a much larger group of patients, those treated with azathioprine for other indications (such as prevention of renal transplant rejection), have been similarly successful. Meg then decides to become pregnant, continues on prednisone and azathioprine during her pregnancy, and starts taking folic acid supplements on the recommendation of her obstetrician. Later in the year she gives birth to a healthy baby boy.

The Diagnosis of MG

The diagnosis of MG is usually made clinically with a typical history of fatigable weakness especially affecting proximal limb, neck, bulbar, and respiratory muscles. The most sensitive and specific diagnostic test is the detection of circulating antibodies to the AChR. While 15% of patients with generalized MG do not have circulating AChR antibodies and are termed "seronegative," it is now known that this latter designation is not precisely accurate; antibodies against another neuromuscular junction protein, the muscle-specific tyrosine kinase (MuSK), are present in up to 50% of this "seronegative" group. Thus, if AChR antibodies are not detected in a case of suspected generalized MG, a radioimmunoassay to detect MuSK antibodies should be performed.

Other tests are available for the diagnosis of MG, such as the electrophysiologic tests performed as part of Meg's workup. These tests do not have the high specificity of the antibody assays; results may be abnormal in other disorders of neuromuscular transmission and occasionally in motor nerve or muscle diseases. However, electrophysiologic tests are the best diagnostic approach for patients who do not have AChR or MuSK antibodies. These tests are sometimes supplemented with a "tensilon" test to confirm the diagnosis. This involves an objective measurement of weakness followed by the injection of a short-acting acetylcholinesterase inhibitor (edrophonium/tensilon; see below) and another measurement to discern significant improvement. The patient is often pretreated with atropine, which counteracts the muscarinic side effects of edrophonium. It should be noted that there is a risk of precipitating cardiorespiratory arrest with the tensilon test, as edrophonium disrupts systemic neuromuscular function ("depolarization block"). Thus, the tensilon test is rarely used unless other diagnostic modalities are inconclusive; when it is used, it is performed under controlled circumstances with the ready availability of resuscitation equipment.

CLINICAL ASPECTS OF MYASTHENIA GRAVIS

Epidemiology

The approximate prevalence of MG is 15–20 per 100,000 in the United Kingdom and the United States. MG affects all races and can develop at any age, although there are two peaks in the age of onset, one between 20 and 30 years and the other over age 70. In the early-onset age group, women are more frequently affected, while patients in the late-onset group are more frequently men.

Symptoms and Signs

Because MG is a disorder of neuromuscular transmission, any skeletal muscle may be affected, and patients can develop a diverse range of symptoms. These include ptosis and diplopia; impaired swallowing, speaking, and chewing; breathing difficulties; and weakness of the trunk and limbs. Extraocular muscles are weak at presentation in 60% of cases and become weak in 90% of patients at some stage. The feature that differentiates MG from other causes of weakness is fatigability: Patients with MG typically complain that their symptoms are worse after exertion or at the end of the day. Symptoms also worsen after infections, in postpartum and premenstrual periods, and in hot weather. Myasthenic crisis is a life-threatening acute exacerbation of muscle weakness that may progress rapidly to respiratory arrest, may be precipitated by any of the factors mentioned above, or may occur on initiation of treatment with corticosteroids, after thymectomy, or spontaneously.

Classification

Patients with generalized MG are often divided into four subgroups depending on age at onset, thymic pathology, and presence of circulating AChR antibodies (Table 14.2). The optimal treatment strategies are slightly different for each subgroup, reflecting differences in the site and nature of the underlying autoimmunizing process.

 IMMUNOPATHOLOGIC MECHANISMS UNDERLYING MYASTHENIA GRAVIS

General Considerations

MG is a prototype of a group of autoimmune diseases in which the pathology is a direct result of production of pathogenic autoantibodies with specificity for defined epitopes on self-antigens. As discussed in the introduction to this Unit, the precise cause of such autoimmune responses is not understood in most autoimmune diseases (including MG). It is likely to involve either a failure of the thymic mechanisms (resulting in the inability to exclude cells with the potential to respond to self-antigens) or a defect in the central or peripheral mechanisms (that normally would result in the elaboration of regulatory cells that suppress responses to self-antigens). In recent years there has been increasing recognition of the influence of the innate immune system, which has its own set of control factors; a defect in these control factors could lead to excess responses to self-antigens. Thus, the general if somewhat imprecise answer to the question of why autoimmune diseases occur is that genetic and environmental factors lead to inadequate tolerogenic and/or regulatory functions of the immune system that would normally limit or even forbid responses to self-antigens.

A major goal of autoimmune disease investigators has been the establishment of detailed knowledge of the structure of the self-antigen, in particular the epitope of the self-antigen, toward which the autoimmune response is directed. With this knowledge, immunologically based treatments could be devised to restore tolerance to a particular autoantigen, even if the underlying cause of the lack of tolerance is unknown. One tell-tale feature suggesting that an autoimmune response to a particular epitope has occurred is the excess use of particular variable-region segments in the antigen-combining sites of the antigen receptors on the responding T cells. This is seen in MG, where T cells specific for AChR epitopes exhibit limited Vβ-region usage. This type of finding has raised the possibility that MG (and other autoimmune states with similar findings) occurs in response to a single (dominant)

 TABLE 14.2. Subgroups of MG

Subgroup	Age at Onset (years)	Sex Incidence	Thymus[a]	Predominant HLA[b] Association	AChR Antibody Levels	Response of MG to Thymectomy
Early-onset MG	<40	1M:3F	Hyperplasia	B8 DR3	High	75% improve
Late-onset MG	>40	2M:1F	Atrophy	B7 DR2	Low	No significant improvement
Thymoma and MG	Any age	M = F	Thymoma	No consistent association	Intermediate	No significant improvement
Seronegative MG	Any age	M = F	Atrophy	No consistent association	Absent	No significant improvement

[a]Typical histologic findings at thymectomy, if performed.
[b]HLA: human leukocyte antigen.

epitope that can be treated by the induction of inhibitory antibodies specific for the antigen-binding region of the T-cell receptor (TCR) or with inhibitory antigens that likewise bind to this TCR. However, individual patients may be responding to different dominant epitopes. Even in the same individual the autoimmune response may exhibit the phenomenon of "epitope spreading," in which an initial autoimmune response to a particular epitope is later joined by responses to new epitopes on the original antigen or to new epitopes on antigens exposed as a result of the initial immunologic onslaught. These factors force consideration of the control of a panoply of pathologic responses and tend to compromise immunologic approaches focused on a single epitope.

The Autoantibodies

AChR Autoantibodies.   The importance of AChR antibodies in the pathogenesis of MG was initially supported by an animal model of the disease created by immunizing rabbits with purified AChR from electric eels. Upon such immunization, the rabbits developed antibodies that inhibited AChR activity; more importantly, they developed flaccid muscle paralysis associated in electrophysiologic testing with decrement in neuromuscular transmission. In addition, both the flaccid paralysis and decrement were improved by the administration of acetylcholinesterase inhibitors. From this animal model it became evident that the presence of anti-AChR was sufficient to induce a myasthenic syndrome and that the syndrome was probably due to the presence of such antibodies. Later studies showed that the transfer of patient plasma to mice caused myasthenic symptoms in the animals and that plasmapheresis of patients with MG, which caused a reduction of antibody levels, led to

symptomatic improvement in the disease, providing strong confirmation of this conclusion.

Binding of autoantibodies to AChRs on the muscle membrane reduces the efficiency of neuromuscular transmission in three possible ways (Fig. 14.4): (1) the antibody causes accelerated degradation of AChRs by antibody-mediated cross-linking of the receptors, which induces endocytosis of the receptors and reduction in their cell surface expression; (2) the antibody competes with ACh for binding to the AChRs and thereby directly blocks receptor function; and (3) the antibody causes loss of AChR via complement-mediated damage to the NMJ. The third of these mechanisms is probably the major mechanism in most MG patients.

AChR antibodies are usually of the IgG class and may consist of any of the four IgG subclasses, although IgG$_1$ and IgG$_3$ predominate. They have extremely high avidity, with K_D values between 5 and 100 pM, and are heterogeneous, binding to many different sites on the AChR molecule. The heterogeneity may be a consequence of somatic mutation and epitope spreading, so that while the initial immunogenic epitope is located in a major conformation-dependent site that includes amino acids 67–76 on the α subunit, antibodies appear later that are non-cross-reactive with the original epitope. This process is facilitated by immune damage to muscle, which may provoke subsequent immune responses against newly exposed AChR epitopes, including the γ subunit of the fetal form of the receptor. The heterogeneous nature of AChR antibodies may explain why there is such poor correlation between antibody titers and disease severity across the population of MG patients but a relatively good correlation over time within individual patients. Finally, bear in mind that other poorly understood immune factors may influence the effect of the antibodies in individual patients. This could explain why AChR

Mechanisms of damage to neuromuscular junction in myasthenia gravis

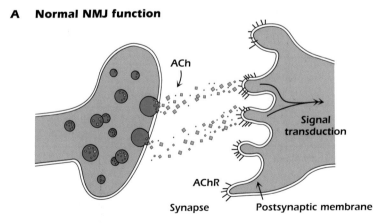

Figure 14.4. Antibodies to ACh receptors can interfere with neuromuscular transmission in several ways: (A) normal (continued on next page).

B Mechanisms of antibody mediated damage

1 Antibody-induced receptor internalization and degradation

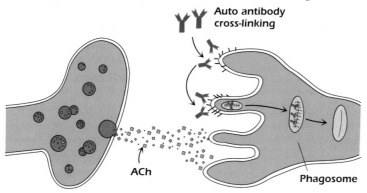

2 Antibody blockade of signal transduction

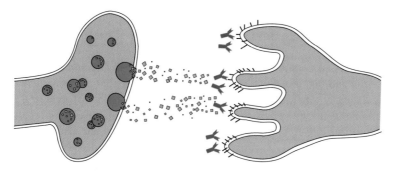

3 Complement mediated damage to NMJ

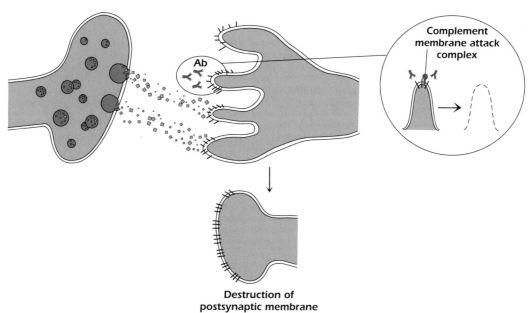

Figure 14.4. (*Continued*) (B) mechanisms of antibody damage: (1) cross-linking of AChR followed by its internalization and destruction in phagosomes leading to decreased AChR expression; (2) binding to AChR resulting in blocking of ACh access to AChR; (3) antibody recruitment of complement followed by formation of membrane attack complex and membrane loss.

antibodies are detected in the serum of almost all babies born to mothers with seropositive MG, even though only about 10–15% of the babies have demonstrable muscle weakness.

MuSK Antibodies. MuSK is a receptor tyrosine kinase with four immunoglobulin-like domains, a cysteine-rich extracellular domain, and an intracellular kinase domain. It is expressed exclusively in muscle and is localized to the NMJ in mature skeletal muscle. Up to 50% of "seronegative" patients have antibodies to MuSK, which are mostly of the IgG_2 and IgG_4 isotypes. *In vitro*, these antibodies inhibit agrin-induced clustering of AChR; their *in vivo* role remains undefined. It is estimated that 85% of Caucasian populations with generalized MG have antibodies to AChR and 6% have antibodies to MuSK, leaving 9% with identical clinical and electrophysiologic characteristics in whom no relevant autoantibodies have yet been identified.

T-Cell Responses in Myasthenia Gravis

Given the role of the thymus in the generation of central T-cell tolerance and regulatory T (T_{reg}) cells and the association of MG with thymic pathology, is it simply a defect in these functions that results in disease? The histology of the thymus itself may provide an answer to this question. (Also see DiGeorge syndrome, Case 3.)

Thymus in Myasthenia Gravis. Myasthenis gravis is associated with two distinct thymic abnormalities, thymic hyperplasia and thymic tumor (thymoma).

Thymic Hyperplasia. Thymic hyperplasia is seen in early-onset MG and is characterized by infiltration of the medulla by B-cell-rich germinal centers surrounded by T-cell areas, which are similar to those found in lymph nodes (Fig. 14.3). Myoid cells, which are immature muscle–like cells that express the complete fetal form of the AChR molecule on their cell surface, can be detected adjacent to the germinal centers in thymic hyperplasia. In some cases, the laminin-containing connective tissue layer, which usually separates the T-cell areas from the medullary epithelium, may be broken down.

The hyperplastic thymus is enriched with AChR-reactive T cells that appear to have been induced in the above-described thymic germinal centers by the numerous AChR-presenting dendritic cells that are also present in the lesion. These may have acquired the AChR for presentation from fetal AChR normally associated with thymic myoid cells. Evidence for thymic antibody induction comes from studies in which thymic cells derived from patients with MG and thymic hyperplasia are cultured *in vitro* to study their production of autoantibodies. Thymic B cells spontaneously produce AChR antibody in

about 65% of such cases, and the magnitude of *in vitro* antibody production correlates with the serum titer of AChR antibodies and with thymic histology; in addition, the fine specificity of the antibodies produced *in vitro* closely matches that found in the patient's serum. These findings support the view that the thymus is the site of autoantibody production. Additional support comes from the observation that AChR antibody levels decline after thymectomy, particularly if performed early in the disease process.

In recent studies, cells phenotypically characteristic of T_{reg} cells ($CD4^+$ $CD25^+$ cells) are located in the regions surrounding the thymic germinal centers, but such cells localize mainly in the medullary areas of the normal thymus. However, given the evidence of autoantibody generation in the thymus noted above, the functional ability to down-regulate responses seems inadequate at best. Thus the possibility that there is a defect in the differentiation and/or function of T_{reg} cells remains open.

Thymoma and Myasthenia Gravis. The role of thymomas in MG is somewhat different from that of thymic hyperplasia. ***Thymomas*** are benign tumors originating from the epithelial component of the thymus that contain variable numbers of maturing T lymphocytes (Fig. 14.5). MG is found in 30% of patients with this type of tumor. Thymomas are also associated with other paraneoplastic autoimmune diseases; in fact, they are the tumors most frequently associated with these conditions. [***Paraneoplastic diseases*** are clinical syndromes that are caused by (often unexpected) products of tumor cells.] Thymoma-associated diseases include ***red cell aplasia*** (lack of production of red blood cells) and a form of ***hypogammaglobulinemia*** (low immunoglobulin levels) distinct from common variable hypogammaglobulinemia; whether these associations have an autoimmune basis is not yet known.

Although the pathologic basis of the association between thymomas and autoimmune diseases is unknown, thymic mechanisms for depleting autoreactive cells and promoting T-cell tolerance may well be defective in thymomas, which are unique among human neoplasms in their ability to generate mature T cells. Thus, in the abnormal environment of the tumor, aberrant negative selection may permit autoreactive T cells to persist. Alternatively, aberrant positive selection may produce novel autoreactive T cells. Although thymomas are associated with specific autoimmune diseases, the presence of this tumor is not heralded by generalized autoimmunity to many self-antigens; this has led some researchers to suggest that the association is most likely the result of aberrant positive selection or even active immunization.

In culture, the thymoma-derived epithelial cell can present AChR peptides to T-cell lines expressing the

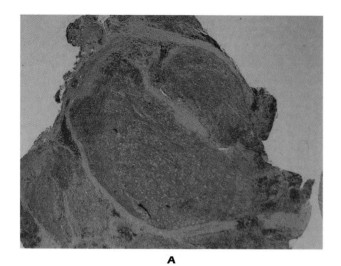

A

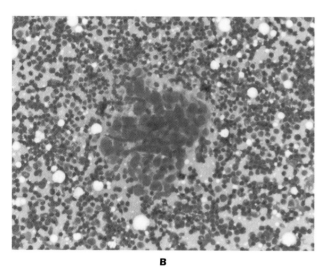

B

Figure 14.5. Photomicrographs of thymoma: **(A)** low-power view; **(B)** high-power view showing association of epithelial cells clustered in center and surrounding normal thymocytes.

appropriate TCR and costimulatory molecules for antigen presentation are expressed in thymomas, suggesting the presence of an environment conducive for the production of autoreactive T cells. Reduced levels of major histocompatibility complex (MHC) class II expression relative to normal cortical epithelium are frequently seen, which may allow "false-positive selection" to occur; the signal to the T cell will not be too strong, and therefore not result in negative selection or clonal deletion. Indeed, while thymomas are selectively enriched for AChR-reactive T cells, they have a reduced capacity to generate other mature CD4$^+$ cells. Moreover, there is evidence that T-cell maturation is abnormal within the thymoma, with reduced proportions of some T-cell subsets.

Messenger RNA (mRNA) transcripts for most AChR subunits have been detected within thymomas, but there is minimal overlap between AChR epitopes encoded by these transcripts and those recognized either by AChR antibodies or by AChR-specific T-cell lines isolated from MG patients. Despite extensive effort, expression of the whole AChR molecule has not been detected in thymomas, and B cells are rarely found within the tumors. Thus the entire autoimmunizing process probably does not occur within the thymoma itself. More likely, AChR-specific T cells migrate into the periphery, where they stimulate B cells to produce antibody in the presence of the whole AChR in its native conformation. This explanation is consistent with the observation that MG does not usually improve after removal of the thymoma, and indeed some patients develop symptoms for the first time several years after thymectomy.

Peripheral T Cells in Myasthenia Gravis. The IgG antibodies isolated from MG patients have such a high affinity and specificity for AChR (a complex protein) that T-cell help is likely to play a role in autoantibody production. Given that T$_{reg}$ cells in these patients appear to be unable to suppress the anti-AChR response, the helper T cells may provide uncontrolled "help" for the B cells, leading to the production of high-affinity autoantibodies. Several clinical observations support the pivotal role of helper T cells in the generation of anti-AChR antibodies. One is that cyclosporin A, an agent that suppresses the clonal expansion of activated helper T cells, is an effective treatment for MG. Another is that treatment of patients with anti-CD4 monoclonal antibodies both abolishes the *in vitro* T-cell response to AChR and brings about clinical and electrophysiologic improvement of the disease.

Autoreactive T cells may also develop in the periphery as a result of molecular mimicry by infectious organisms or by alterations of antigens (such as by proteases during apoptosis). Evidence for molecular mimicry has been found in multiple sclerosis (see Case 15), and alterations of antigens are documented in celiac disease (see Case 17).

Despite the findings mentioned above implicating T cells as having a key role in the pathogenesis of MG, a precise understanding of T-cell involvement in the pathogenesis of MG has remained elusive. It is still possible that, in some patients, the defect lies mainly but not wholly with the B cells producing the anti-self-antibodies; thus, in the MG patient group as a whole the underlying mechanism may differ in individual patients, and several roads may lead to anti-AChR antibodies and disease.

TREATMENT OF MYASTHENIA GRAVIS

Medical Treatment

Acetylcholinesterase Inhibitors. By delaying the metabolism of ACh, acetylcholinesterase inhibitors increase the effective ACh concentration at the NMJ and partially overcome the loss of AChR. The short-acting inhibitor, edrophonium, is mainly used diagnostically in the tensilon test (see above), while pyridostigmine, which has a longer duration of action and fewer muscarinic side effects, is used for symptom relief, particularly in mildly affected patients. Indeed, in these patients, it remains the first line of treatment.

Immune Therapies. Most patients do not become symptom free on acetylcholinesterase inhibitors and require additional treatments directed against the autoimmune process. These include corticosteroids and/or "steroid-sparing" immunosuppressive agents such as azathioprine and cyclosporin. Plasmapheresis or intravenous immunoglobulin (IVIG) are short-term measures that are used acutely in severely affected patients, often in conjunction with respiratory support and nasogastric feeding.

Corticosteroids. These are the mainstay of treatment and are extremely effective in inducing remission, although they do have numerous side effects (see above), especially when used in high doses over a prolonged period. The introduction of corticosteroid treatment for MG has transformed a previously life-threatening and life-destroying illness into one that is compatible with near normal life in the majority of patients.

Alternative Immunosuppressive Therapy. To reduce the dose of corticosteroids, "steroid-sparing" agents, such as azathioprine, cyclosporin A, or methotrexate, are often used. Approximately 10% of patients are acutely intolerant of azathioprine, developing fever, rash, gastrointestinal symptoms, and abnormal liver function tests upon initiation of therapy. In addition, these therapies are associated with a dose-dependent risk of bone-marrow suppression, so the CBC should be monitored regularly. Bone marrow suppression is partly determined by the patient's thiopurine methyltransferase (TPMT) level. Low TPMT levels are found in up to 1 in 300 individuals; these individuals may have an increased risk of pancytopenia. Methotrexate use may also cause fibrosis of the liver and lungs after prolonged use, and hypertension, renal damage, hirsutism (male hair distribution), and gingival hypertrophy can develop with the use of cyclosporin A.

Plasmapheresis and IVIG. Plasmapheresis (described above) is an effective short-term treatment that is used in a myasthenic crisis, to minimize symptoms prior to thymectomy, and to prevent the deterioration that is often seen during the initiation of corticosteroid therapy. However, plasmapheresis is not available at all centers and is not appropriate for all patients. An alternative that is probably just as effective is the infusion of IVIG over five days.

Surgical Treatment: Thymectomy

Current estimates suggest that 40% of patients with MG have a hyperplastic thymus and 10% have an associated thymoma; however, both of these figures may be revised with increased recognition of MG in older patients with thymic atrophy. As discussed above, removing the thymus may have beneficial effects on the MG in early-onset patients (<40 years) with thymic hyperplasia and AChR antibodies. In patients with MG and a thymoma, thymectomy has no clearly beneficial effect on the MG but is performed to treat the thymoma, which can compress or invade important local thoracic structures, although it rarely metastasizes outside the thorax. In thymectomies of patients who do not have AChR antibodies ("seronegative MG"), no specific thymic pathology has been found and generally there is no convincing evidence of improvement in their MG. In older patients without an enlarged thymus, thymectomy is not beneficial; when it is performed, the thymus is usually found to be atrophic, although occasionally a microscopic thymoma may be discovered.

The Future of Myasthenia Gravis Therapy

The goal of specific modulation of the immune system to control or prevent disease may be more realistic for those autoimmune diseases in which the pathogenic antibody is directed against a specific and defined antigen. Thus, attempts are being made in experimental models to vaccinate animals in a manner that induces tolerance rather than immunity (such as low-dose oral administration of AChR fragments), to induce a response against the dominant determinant on the TCR (idiotype) of the autoreactive T helper cells, or to stimulate the generation of specific negative regulatory cells.

REFERENCES

Berrih-Aknin S, Fuchs S, Souroujon MC (2005): Vaccines against myasthenia gravis. *Expert Opin Biol Ther* 5:983–995.

Gronseth GS, Barohn RJ (2000): Practice parameter: Thymectomy for autoimmune myasthenia gravis (an evidence-based review): Report of the Quality Standards Subcommittee of the American Academy of Neurology. *Neurology* 55:7–15.

Lan RY, Ansari AA, Lian ZX, Gershwin ME (2005): Regulatory T cells: Development, function and role in autoimmunity. *Autoimmun Rev* 4:351–363.

Vincent A (2002): Unravelling the pathogenesis of myasthenia gravis. *Nat Rev Immunol* 2:797–804.

Vincent A, Bowen J, Newsom-Davis J, McConville J (2003): Seronegative generalized myasthenia gravis: Clinical features, antibodies and their targets. *Lancet Neurol* 2:99–106.

Vincent A, Palace J, Hilton-Jones D (2001): Myasthenia gravis. *Lancet* 357:2122–2128.

15

MULTIPLE SCLEROSIS

DERIC M. PARK and ROLAND MARTIN*

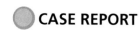

CASE REPORT

"My vision is blurry."

Initial Presentation and Evaluation

Stephanie, a 22-year-old office clerk, has arranged an urgent appointment with you, her internist, for evaluation of blurred vision in one eye. Two days ago she noticed a change in the vision of her left eye that she describes as "looking through a shower curtain," which you interpret as a decrease in contrast and brightness. In addition, she remarks that she has pain over that eye and has been trying to limit her eye movements in an attempt to decrease it.

On examination you find that the visual acuity of the left eye is so limited that she sees only hand motion; however her light perception is intact. A swinging flashlight test reveals an afferent pupillary defect (Marcus Gunn pupil) involving the left eye (paradoxical papillary dilatation in response to increased light). In contrast, vision and pupillary responses in the right eye are unaffected. Funduscopy (visual assessment of retina and retinal vessels) of both eyes is normal. The remainder of your neurologic exam shows patchy but consistent **hypoesthesia** (decreased feeling) to pin and light touch over the right limbs. On questioning she informs you of a self-limiting episode of right-sided

numbness and tingling a few months ago. The remainder of the physical examination is normal.

Review of systems is significant only for an abnormal level of fatigue, particularly at the end of the day. She denies depression, cognitive dysfunction, diplopia (double vision), focal weakness, clumsiness, falls, bladder disturbance, and history of diabetes or hypertension. The family history is unrevealing.

You refer Stephanie to an ophthalmologist to help you understand her problem. In the interim you obtain blood samples for tests to rule out the more common disorders that present with neurologic symptoms. These tests include a complete blood count, vitamin B_{12} level, and Lyme disease antibody titer. You decide to wait on additional testing until hearing from the ophthalmologist.

Stephanie sees the ophthalmologist the next day and he makes a diagnosis of retrobulbar optic neuritis with recommendations for corticosteroid treatment and a cranial magnetic resonance imaging (MRI) study with gadolinium. In view of the possibility that she may suffer permanent visual loss, Stephanie is immediately started on systemic corticosteroids, and her MRI is scheduled. Over the next week her vision improves.

What is optic neuritis?

Optic neuritis *is inflammation of the optic nerve that may be caused by infections, tumors, chemical exposure, or allergic*

*With contribution from Warren Strober and Susan R. S. Gottesman

Immunology: Clinical Case Studies and Disease Pathophysiology, By Warren Strober and Susan R. S. Gottesman
Copyright © 2009 John Wiley & Sons, Inc.

*reactions; it is also a common initial manifestation of **multiple sclerosis (MS)**. Demyelinating optic neuritis associated with MS occurs in three forms: acute, chronic, and asymptomatic. Acute optic neuritis is the best recognized form and is characterized by sudden loss/impairment of vision in one or occasionally both eyes. In most cases retro-orbital pain exacerbated by eye movement accompanies the visual symptoms. The range of visual dysfunction varies from absence of light perception to minimal loss of color contrast. Patients like Stephanie with monocular involvement will exhibit an afferent pupillary defect, and funduscopy can be unrevealing if the site of optic nerve involvement is retrobulbar (area behind the globe of the eye).*

The blood tests you ordered show no abnormalities. However, the MRI indicates the presence of multiple deep white matter lesions scattered throughout the brain, some demonstrating contrast (gadolinium) enhancement indicative of an active area of inflammation. The suspected radiologic diagnosis, depending on the clinical profile, is a demyelinating disorder, possibly MS.

What is MS?

Multiple sclerosis is a disease of the central nervous system (CNS) characterized by multiple discrete foci of inflammation and destruction of the myelin sheath (Fig. 15.1). These foci result in single or multiple neurologic deficits occurring in defined, periodic episodes that sometimes lead to permanent abnormalities. Since lesions may occur anywhere in the CNS, symptoms are widespread and varied. MS is generally believed to be the result of an autoimmune inflammatory attack on cells in the CNS.

Further Workup for Diagnosis

You relate the MRI finding to Stephanie and refer her to a neurologist for further workup and treatment. Several days later, Stephanie is seen by the neurologist, who explains that she will need to have a test of evoked potentials (EPs) and a lumbar puncture (LP) to reach a diagnosis. The neurologist explains that in the EP test peripheral nerves will be stimulated and a record will be made of how quickly and how completely the signals reach the brain. She reassures Stephanie that it is a noninvasive procedure with minimal if any discomfort and explains that it is more sensitive that a neurologic examination or even an MRI in detecting abnormalities. The lumbar puncture involves the insertion of a long needle through the vertebral space into the paraspinal space to obtain a small sample of cerebrospinal fluid (CSF) for examination. While this test is accompanied by some short-term discomfort, it is also a safe procedure.

The visual EP shows prolongation of the visual pathway conduction on the left side of the brain. On the other hand, somatosensory EP and brain stem auditory EP are normal on both sides.

Analysis of Stephanie's CSF reveals normal total leukocyte count and protein content but an elevation of the IgG index (ratio of IgG concentration in the CSF to the IgG concentration in the blood). In addition, gel electrophoresis of the CSF proteins reveals the presence of oligoclonal bands (OCBs) (IgG arrayed on the gel in a few bands rather than a diffuse smear; see Unit V for detailed description of this assay).

What is the meaning and significance of the IgG index and OCB?

Because the CSF level mirrors the activity of cells in the neural tissue, elevation of the IgG index indicates increased intrathecal synthesis of immunoglobulins (antibodies) by plasma cells in the CNS. OCBs indicate that there are several, rather than one (monoclonal) or many (polyclonal), B-cell clones producing the immunoglobulins, consistent with the presence of a B-cell response directed at a very

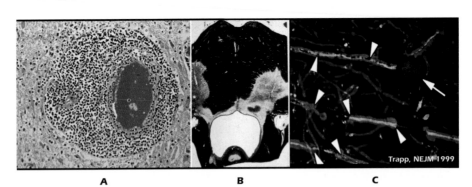

● Figure 15.1. Major pathologic findings in multiple sclerosis. (**A**) Inflammation: dense lymphomononuclear infiltrate in perivascular location in MS brain; these are the lesions that are visualized by contrast-enhanced MRI. (**B**) Demyelination and gliosis: demyelinating lesions in light blue in the brain stem of an MS patient. (**C**) Axonal injury and loss: confocal microscopic image demonstrating axonal transections (arrow) and areas of demyelination (arrowheads). [Reprinted with permission from Trapp B, et al. (1998): *N Engl J Med* 338:278–285].

limited set of antigens. OCBs may also be seen in infections and other inflammatory conditions, so they are therefore not specific for MS; however, because they are seen in approximately 90% of MS patients, in the proper clinical setting, their presence strengthens the diagnosis of MS. In spite of this, the exact specificity and significance of the elevated CSF immunoglobulins in MS remain unknown.

The neurologist now has completed her workup and is thus in a position to consider whether or not Stephanie has MS. She recognizes that while there is no definitive clinical profile of this disease, its presence is favored by Stephanie's visual symptoms, which are quite typical of MS, and by the fact that the symptoms have occurred as, at least, two temporally distinct events (numbness and visual changes). The involvement of different areas of the body (left eye and right limbs) is consistent with a disease causing multifocal involvement of the CNS, which also suggests the diagnosis of MS. These clinical facts mesh well with results of the ancillary tests; the MRI, the EP, and the LP are all consistent with a diagnosis of MS. At this point the neurologist considers the relevant differential diagnosis of MS.

Differential Diagnosis

Although MS often presents with a set of typical symptoms (as in Stephanie's case), its multifocal nature can also lead to a wide variety of symptoms that cannot be easily ascribed to MS. As indicated in Table 15.1, the diseases that may have to be considered in the differential diagnosis of MS are wide ranging and fall into a number of broad and disparate categories, including infectious, inflammatory/autoimmune, metabolic, neoplastic, spinal, and traumatic states. These categories by no means delimit the diseases that must be considered in each case. The diagnosis of MS may at times be difficult to make in those patients with an atypical background, unusual symptoms and signs, or a single symptom event.

TABLE 15.1. Differential Diagnosis of Multiple Sclerosis

Category of Disease	Disease Entities
Infectious	HTLV-1 infection
	Lyme disease
	Progressive multifocal leukoencephalopathy
	Syphilis
Inflammatory	Behcet's disease
	Sarcoidosis
	Sjogren's syndrome
	Systemic lupus erythematosus
	Vasculitis
	Whipple's disease
Metabolic/Genetic	Adrenoleukodystrophy
	Cerebral autosomal dominant arteriopathy with subcortical infarcts and leukoencephalopathy
	Familial spastic paraparesis
	Friedrich's ataxia
	Lysosomal disorders
	Metachromatic leukodystrophy
	Mitochondrial encephalopathy
	Olivopontocerebellar atrophy
	Spinocerebellar ataxia
	Vitamin B_{12} deficiency
Neoplastic	Optic nerve glioma or sheath meningioma
	Primary CNS lymphoma
Spinal	Degenerative: spondylotic myelopathy
	Subacute necrotic myelitis: Foix–Alajouanine syndrome
	Syringomyelia
	Vascular malformations
Traumatic	Nonspecific signal on long TR sequence resulting from head trauma

After putting together all of the available evidence and considering some of the possible alternative diseases, the neurologist comes to the conclusion that Stephanie does have MS. Depending on the particular clinical presentation, patients may be considered to have **definite MS** or **probable MS** or to be **at risk for MS**; the neurologist assigns Stephanie to the definite MS category or, more completely, to a diagnosis of definite relapsing–remitting MS (RRMS).

Stephanie's Treatment Plan

After two weeks, Stephanie returns to you in a much improved state. The corticosteroids have accelerated the near recovery of her vision and she is feeling generally well. However, in consideration of the fact that the MRI indicated widespread, albeit clinically inapparent disease, you believe she should be on long-term, disease-modifying therapy. After consulting with the neurologist, you start Stephanie on glatiramer acetate. This drug is a mixture of peptides that mimic the antigen myelin and has been proven to inhibit MS inflammation early in the course of the disease.

CLINICAL FEATURES OF MULTIPLE SCLEROSIS

MS affects young adults, with women outnumbering men 2:1. In the United States, 350,000 or more patients are afflicted by this debilitating condition, and worldwide estimates top one million. This makes MS the most common neurologic disorder of young adults. Specific clinical manifestations vary from patient to patient, depending on the site affected, but typical symptoms consist of sensory disturbances, monocular visual impairment (optic neuritis), diplopia, weakness, spasticity, ataxia, and sphincter dysfunction. Lhermitte's sign, a transient electric shock–like sensation radiating down the spine or limbs upon neck flexion, may indicate a cervical cord lesion. Many of these symptoms are exacerbated upon exposure to increases in ambient temperature. Finally, in some cases patients are subject to depression and other neuropsychiatric symptoms.

MS can be further categorized by its variable clinical course (Fig. 15.2). The majority of patients (~ 85%) begin with a relapsing–remitting course (Fig. 15.2B), characterized by periods of clinical inactivity punctuated by relapses (acute attacks) and remittances, which may or may not be complete. Incomplete reversal of clinical deficits translates into accumulation of residual neurologic deficit. Over time, most enter a secondary progressive form of the disease (Fig. 15.2C) in which gradual worsening is observed without overt relapses. The progressive course refers to an insidious onset of the disease and continuous progression without transient improvement of symptoms. Primary progressive MS (Fig. 15.2E) is seen in a minority of patients (~ 10%). A fraction of these patients may exhibit frank relapses superimposed on gradual deterioration.

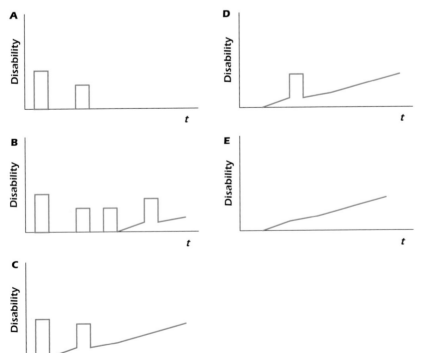

Figure 15.2. Clinical courses of multiple sclerosis: (**A**) benign MS; (**B**) relapsing–remitting MS; (**C**) secondary progressive MS; (**D**) progressive–relapsing MS; (**E**) primary progressive MS.

NORMAL TYPE IV IMMUNE RESPONSES: DTH AND T$_H$1/T$_H$17 SUBSET DIFFERENTIATION

MS is an autoimmune disease mediated by an excessive T$_H$1/T$_H$17 T-cell immune response (see the section on pathophysiology of MS below). The essence of the lesion in MS is a delayed-type hypersensitivity (DTH) reaction, a prototype immune response first described as a type IV hypersensitivity skin response to certain types of antigens and now known to be mediated by T$_H$1/T$_H$17 cytokines. We will therefore begin our discussion of the pathogenesis of MS with a brief overview of the DTH reaction and CD4$^+$ T-cell subset differentiation from CD4$^+$ T$_H$0 cells into T$_H$1 and T$_H$17 cells.

At the initiation of normal host defense immune responses stimulated by pathogenic viruses or bacteria, antigen-presenting cells (APCs; primarily dendritic cells) are stimulated by viral or bacterial components via pattern recognition receptors of the innate immune system (i.e., *Toll-like receptors*) to produce master cytokines such as

IL-12p70 and IL-23. Such cytokine production occurs during dendritic cell presentation of processed viral or bacterial antigen [in the context of major histocompatibility complex (MHC) molecules] to T cells bearing T-cell receptors (TCRs) specific for the antigen. This induces the responding CD4$^+$ T cell to differentiate into effector cells that produce either T$_H$1 or T$_H$17 cytokines (Fig. 15.3). Alternatively, the immune response is induced by antigen (usually in association with an *adjuvant*, a substance that enhances an immune response); in this case the adjuvant is the initial stimulant of dendritic cell cytokine production. In both cases, the dendritic cell is further stimulated to produce cytokines by the activated T cells themselves, which express CD40L and "back-stimulate" the dendritic cell via CD40 (see Case 4 on Hyper-IgM syndrome for detailed description).

The classical DTH skin reaction shows us how this dendritic cell–T cell interaction leads to inflammation. As originally described, this reaction was initiated by a "sensitization" step that we now know involves the dendritic cell (such as the Langerhans cell of the skin)/T-cell interaction described above, which leads to the initial generation

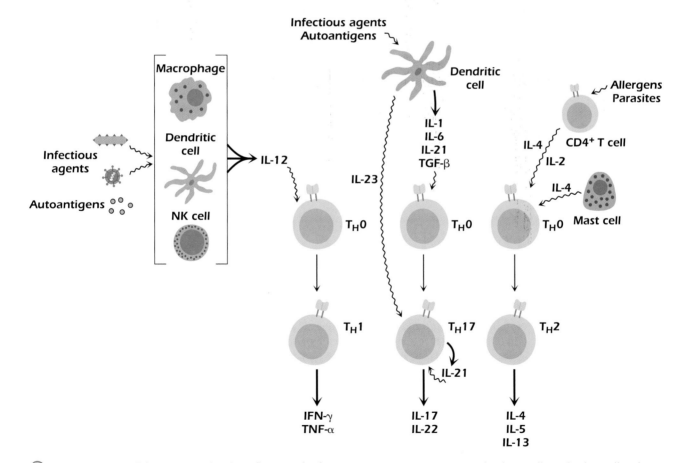

Figure 15.3. T cell lineages. Under the influence of infectious agents or autoantigens, dendritic cells and other cells release cytokines that induce naive T cells (T$_H$0 cells) to become T$_H$1, T$_H$17, and T$_H$2 cells. The latter produce particular cytokines that subserve unique immune functions.

of antigen-specific T_H1 and T_H17 T cells from T_H0 cells. This was followed by a second "elicitation" step, which we now understand is actually an extension of the sensitization step in that it involves continued or secondary exposure to the antigen and induction of an expanded number of activated T_H1 and T_H17 T cells. In a third "effector" step, these effector T cells mediate the activation and recruitment of antigen-specific and nonspecific inflammatory cells to the reaction site (Fig. 15.4), including macrophages, natural killer (NK) cells, $CD8^+$ T cells (cytotoxic T cells), neutrophils, and B cells. In the skin DTH reaction the macrophage is a major effector cell and indeed similar cells play an important role in the MS inflammatory lesion.

The macrophages are derived from circulating monocytes and become macrophages under the influence of interferon (IFN) γ and other inflammatory cytokines. They then can cause damage by secreting reactive oxygen intermediates, proteases, chemotaxic factors, tumor necrosis factor (TNF), and IL-1β.

How is the DTH reaction used clinically in the evaluation of a patient?

In addition to its value as a model of T-cell inflammation, the DTH skin response has a practical use as a measure of an individual's capacity to mount a T-cell response to environmental immunogens. It is usually elicited by skin

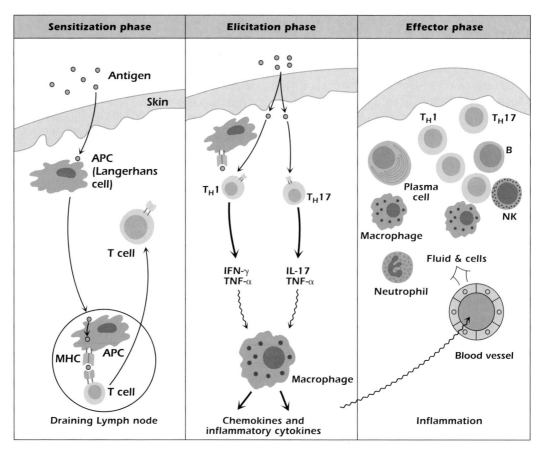

Figure 15.4. DTH reaction: a "classical" immunologic response in the skin which contains many of the features of the inflammation occurring in autoimmune states such as MS. It is called a delayed-type reaction because the inflammation requires a period of time to develop. In the initial **"sensitization" phase**, antigen enters the skin and is taken up (and processed) by local APCs (Langerhans cells in the case of a skin reaction). The APCs then migrate to the draining lymph nodes where they present antigen to T cells and induce T-cell proliferation and differentiation into T_H1 and T_H17 cells by mechanisms diagrammed in Fig. 15.3. The differentiated T cells then migrate back to the skin where they reencounter antigen in the **"elicitation" phase** of the response. At this point they are induced to produce an array of cytokines that initiate the DTH inflammation. These cytokines act on macrophages and the latter in turn produce effector cytokines and chemokines that bring other inflammatory cells into the nascent inflammatory lesion. This is the **effector or inflammatory phase** of the DTH response. In MS, T cells are induced in a sensitization phase in nonneurologic tissue and then reencounter antigen in the CNS during an elicitation phase followed by a T_H1/T_H17 inflammation.

injection of a "recall" antigen, that is, an antigen to which the individual has been previously exposed and therefore has a population of resting (memory) T$_H$1/T$_H$17 cells that were induced in the initial sensitization step. When the individual is again exposed to that antigen, an elicitation step ensues that results in local inflammation. Diphtheria or tetanus toxoid is often used to elicit a DTH reaction since nearly everyone has been exposed to these antigens during their normal childhood immunization program. Another use of the test is to determine whether there has been a history of exposure to tuberculosis by assaying for response to PPD. The DTH skin reaction derives its name from the fact that the reaction is delayed; it takes at least 48 h to unfold.

In recent years much has been learned regarding the differentiation of T cells in response to "master" cytokines derived from APCs. We now realize that naive T cells can undergo several lines of differentiation, depending for the most part on the cytokine environment in which they receive antigenic stimulation (Fig. 15.5). Such differentiation may also be influenced by other factors, such as the type of costimulation or the presence of auxiliary stimulatory factors. T$_H$1 T-cell differentiation occurs under the influence of IL-12p70, a heterodimeric molecule comprised of a p40 chain linked to a p35 chain. This cytokine induces T$_H$0 cells to express the transcription factors Stat4 and T-bet, which direct the cells to produce IFN-γ, the hallmark cytokine of T$_H$1 T cells. In contrast, T$_H$17 differentiation occurs under the influence of IL-23, another heterodimeric molecule that is comprised of the same p40 as in IL-12, in this case linked to a p19 chain. The differentiation of

T$_H$17 cells is somewhat more complex than that of T$_H$1 cells and appears to differ in mice and humans. In mice, which have been studied more thoroughly, T$_H$17 cells are initially induced by exposure to transforming growth factor (TGF) β$_1$ and IL-6, cytokines that together induce RORγt, a transcription factor necessary for the transcription of IL-17, the hallmark cytokine of T$_H$17 T cells. (T$_H$17 cells also produce IFN-γ and IL-22.) In addition, IL-6 elicits the production of IL-21, which induces IL-23R expression and allows the subsequent stimulation of the newly formed T$_H$17 cells by IL-23. Thus, in the mouse, IL-23 is only secondarily involved in T$_H$17 T-cell differentiation, but it is necessary for the expansion/survival of these cells. In humans, IL-21 acting in conjunction with TGF-β$_1$ seem to be the most important T$_H$17-inducing cytokines for naive T cells whereas IL-1β alone or in conjunction with IL-6 seem to be the most important for induction of memory T cells; again, IL-23 appears to be necessary in the maintenance of T$_H$17 cells after their induction by other cytokines. As in mice, IFN-γ is produced along with IL-17 by human T$_H$17 cells.

A third type of T-cell differentiation from the naive CD4$^+$ T cell results in regulatory T (T$_{reg}$) cells. As discussed in Case 3, T$_{reg}$ cells can differentiate in the thymus under the influence of IL-2. Naive CD4$^+$ T cells that have emerged from the thymus can also differentiate to T$_{reg}$ cells in the peripheral lymphoid tissues under the influence of TGF-β$_1$. Such "induced" T$_{reg}$ cells express Foxp3, the transcription factor uniquely associated with regulatory T cells, as well as other T$_{reg}$ markers, and function as fully capable

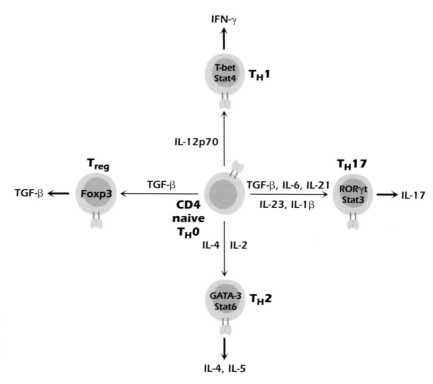

Figure 15.5. Differentiation of T$_H$ subsets and T$_{reg}$ cells. Note that T$_H$17 and T$_{reg}$ cells both require TGF-β for development, and the development of these may be reciprocal.

regulatory T cells. Because TGF-β_1 and IL-6 induce T$_H$17 cells, it is somewhat surprising that TGF-β_1 alone induces T$_{reg}$, cells that oppose rather than cause inflammation. The key difference is the activity of IL-6, a cytokine that acts through Stat3 to inhibit T$_{reg}$ induction and favor T$_H$17 production. The fact that T$_H$17 and T$_{reg}$ differentiation are both dependent on a single cytokine, TGF-β_1 (at least in mice), suggests that the molecular factors controlling their differentiation are overlapping and interrelated. This idea is supported by recent data showing that a hallmark transcription factor associated with T$_{reg}$, Foxp3, has an inhibitory effect on the function of RORγt, the transcription factor mentioned above as being necessary for T$_H$17 differentiation.

T$_H$2 T-cell differentiation is the fourth pathway of T-cell differentiation; this pathway is taken in immune responses to antigens such as allergens and those associated with parasites (Fig 15.3). These antigens elicit production of IL-4, the cytokine that is the main driving force of T$_H$2 differentiation as well as the signature cytokine of T$_H$2 T cells. In addition, there may be Notch signaling of the cells from Notch ligands expressed on the APCs. (As outlined in Case 3, Notch signaling also functions in the differentiation of pre-T cells in the thymus.) The source of the IL-4 for T$_H$2 differentiation is unclear. It may be produced by cells of the innate immune system such as NKT cells or basophils. On the other hand, it may be produced by the T cell itself, especially when stimulated by antigens at low concentrations or low affinity. The T$_H$2 cells express the transcription factors Stat6 and GATA-3; in addition to IL-4, they produce IL-5, IL-13, and in some cases IL-10.

In summary, peripheral T-cell differentiation is multifaceted and depends on the cytokines present during initial TCR stimulation of naive T cells. IL-12p70 and TGF-β_1, the latter acting in concert with IL-6 or IL-1β and IL-23, are the important cytokines governing T$_H$1 and T$_H$17 T-cell differentiation, respectively. On the other hand, TGF-β_1 alone governs T$_{reg}$ cell differentiation and IL-4 governs T$_H$2 differentiation.

Both T$_H$1 and T$_H$17 T cells involved in the DTH reaction are highly proinflammatory. The production of IL-17 results in stimulation of endothelial cells and fibroblast secretion of IL-1β, TNF-α, and, perhaps most importantly, chemokines that attract neutrophils. Most immune responses resulting in inflammation are accompanied by the differentiation of both T$_H$1 and T$_H$17 cells so that a mixture of effector cytokines is present in the inflammatory lesion. There is some evidence that T$_H$1 differentiation precedes T$_H$17 differentiation, occurring during the more acute phase of inflammation. In various mouse models of human autoimmune inflammation, including a model of MS, the T$_H$17 response is more responsible for chronic inflammation than is the T$_H$1 response. However, this has not been proven in human inflammations or human MS.

PATHOPHYSIOLOGY OF MULTIPLE SCLEROSIS

Initiation of Immunologic Dysfunction

As described above, MS is a DTH-like inflammation of the CNS mediated by autoreactive T cells responding to the self-antigen, myelin protein, or one of its components (Fig. 15.6). The inflammation results in destruction of the myelin sheath and resultant disruption of neurologic function. The most fundamental question regarding the etiology of this autoimmunity is the following: What is the origin of the breakdown in tolerance that leads to the appearance of myelin-reactive cells? The usual, albeit vague, answer to this question is that the myelin-specific autoreactive cells arise in the thymus because of a defect in negative selection specific to myelin. As discussed in Case 3 and the introduction to this unit, medullary thymic epithelial cells normally display peripheral tissue self-antigens under the influence of the transcription factor AIRE and in so doing cause the deletion (negative selection) of emerging T-cell clones that recognize the self-antigens with high affinity. Thus, an antigen-specific defect in this process could lead to the emergence of cells with the capacity to react to the self-antigen specified by the defect. The fact that mutations in the *AIRE* gene lead to an autoimmune polyglandular syndrome lends credence to this idea. However, the presence of an *AIRE* gene defect does not explain the antigen-specific nature of MS or indeed most other autoimmune syndromes, and it is likely that other genetic defects affecting thymic negative selection is the basis of autoimmune states such as MS.

Another point to consider is that in spite of the presence of negative selection for self-protein in the thymus, normal individuals can possess myelin basic protein (MBP)–specific helper T cells in the peripheral lymphoid tissue. This suggests that thymic negative selection is "leaky" and that cells with such self-reactivity are normally kept in check by myelin-specific T$_{reg}$ cells generated in the thymus by exposure to myelin or in the periphery by myelin presentation in the presence of TGF-β_1. In this scenario, the appearance of functional myelin-reactive cells causing MS would be due to antigen-specific T$_{reg}$ cell dysfunction.

One phenomenon that may facilitate the appearance of autoreactive cells in MS is referred to as "molecular mimicry."

What is molecular mimicry?

Molecular mimicry refers to a process in which cells with reactivity to self-antigens are induced by foreign, pathogen-associated antigens because of similarities between the epitopes of those foreign antigens and self-antigens. The principle of molecular mimicry has been evoked to explain some autoimmune diseases that appear to occur as a complication of infection. Perhaps the most

Proposed inflammatory cascade in MS

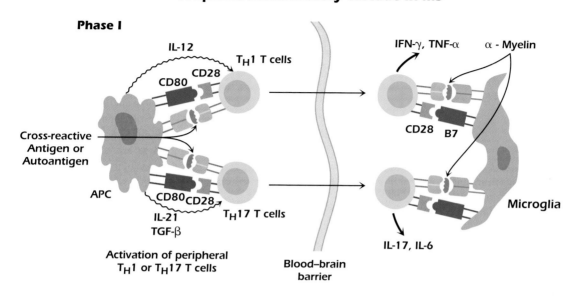

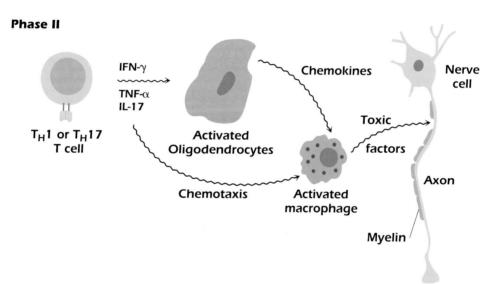

○ Figure 15.6. In phase I of MS, T_H 1 and T_H 17 T cells are activated by cells presenting antigen cross-reactive with self-antigen. These activated T cells migrate across the blood–brain barrier and into the CNS. Here they encounter self-antigen (α -myelin) and are induced to produce inflammatory cytokines. In phase II the activated T-cell production of cytokines (and chemokines) leads to activation of local oligodendritic cells which then release chemokines that call in macrophages; alternatively the T cells release cytokines and chemokines that call in macrophages. Macrophages then release cytokines and mediators that cause demyelinization of neurons. If this process persists, permanent damage to the CNS ensues.

familiar of these is the development of rheumatic fever following a pharyngeal infection with some serotypes of β-hemolytic streptococci; antibodies specific for the bacteria cross-react with cardiac muscle proteins and are the presumed initiating cause of the cardiac inflammation.

The suggestion that molecular mimicry may play a role in the pathogenesis of MS resulted from an observation in an experimental model in which the disease could be induced by a protein from hepatitis B virus, presumably because the protein bore a structural similarity to MBP. However, it has yet to be proven as a mechanism of induction in human MS. Regardless of whether molecular mimicry is a factor in MS, a more fundamental abnormality of tolerance must also be present or everyone would be subject to this disease following specific infections.

Immunopathogenesis of MS: Lessons learned from the Study of Experimental Allergic Encephalomyelitis (EAE)

In the last several decades, the study of the pathogenesis of MS has been greatly facilitated by the use of murine experimental models. The best known and most widely investigated of these is EAE.

What is EAE?

EAE is an animal model of MS characterized by an acute or chronic relapsing immune-mediated disease of the CNS. It is induced in susceptible mouse strains by immunization with myelin or its components [immunodominant peptides of MBP, myelinoligodendrocyte glycoprotein (MOG), or proteolipid protein (PLP)] accompanied by appropriate adjuvants. The disease can be induced by passive transfer of encephalitogenic CD4+ T cells but not by serum, providing proof that EAE is a CD4+ T-cell-mediated disease not dependent on an autoantibody.

The EAE model has led to many of our current ideas about the pathogenesis of MS. Perhaps the most important is that MS is an autoimmune disease. This arises from the fact that in mice specific induction of a response to a self-protein (MBP) can cause a disease of the CNS that is remarkably similar to MS. Other insights into the pathogenesis of MS originating from the study of EAE concern the type of T-cell response causing the CNS lesion. In initial studies, the inflammation was thought to be mediated by $T_H 1$ cells induced by IL-12p70 and producing IFN-γ. More recently, it was shown that $T_H 17$ cells induced by IL-23 (and other cytokines as discussed above) are also present; in fact, this latter population was more critical to the inflammatory process in the CNS. This has led to the belief that $T_H 17$ cells are also more important than $T_H 1$ cells in the development of MS, but this remains unproven.

Other contributions to our knowledge of MS from the study of EAE include information on the site of initiation of this immune response as well as the traffic of inflammatory cells across the blood–brain barrier into the CNS. Related to the latter, high levels of VLA-4 (very late antigen 4), a β_1 integrin which binds to VCAM-1 (vascular cell adhesion molecule 1) on vascular endothelial cells and is involved in cell trafficking, have been found on the disease-inducing T cells in EAE. Finally, the study of EAE has contributed to our understanding of the genetic factors underlying MS as well as the CNS antigens causing this disease. Depending on the particular mouse strain used, the encephalitogenic epitope of the myelin component is variable, and the disease phenotype and severity are a reflection of the animal's genetic background.

Immunopathologic Features of MS

The initial stimulation of cells reactive to antigens in the CNS (particularly MBP) most likely occurs in the peripheral immune system in humans; in the EAE model, the mice are immunized via foot pad injection. The activated T cells thus induced, unlike naturally occurring T cells with MBP specificity, express adhesion molecules that endow them with the capacity to traffic to endothelial sites in the CNS and pass into the CNS tissue. It is also possible that T cells with MBP specificity are activated upon recognition of antigen(s) presented by endothelial cells and then pass through the blood–brain barrier into the CNS.

Upon entering the CNS, activated T cells with MBP specificity encounter large amounts of potentially stimulatory antigen and begin to secrete an array of inflammatory cytokines, including IL-2, TNF-α, IFN-γ, and IL-17. This, in turn, results in the induction of MHC human leukocyte antigen (HLA) class II] and costimulatory molecules on local APCs, which further magnifies the stimulation of T cells. Although both astrocytes and microglial cells possess the potential to act as APCs in the CNS, evidence currently favors the view that the microglia are more important. Microglial cells are actually CNS-specific macrophages descended from the bone marrow–derived monocyte/macrophage lineage. Finally, it is important to note that the release of T-cell cytokines leads to activation of microglial cells, which now act as effector cells in the inflammatory sites and contribute to inflammation and tissue damage by the release of effector products including nitric oxide, proteolytic enzymes, and oxygen radicals.

Once the pathogenic immune reaction has been initiated by T cells specific for a particular CNS antigen (i.e., MBP), the inflammatory process may be amplified by epitope spreading. This is a phenomenon in which new epitopes begin to take part in the pathologic process as a result of initial tissue damage and the subsequent release of additional self-antigens with the potential to stimulate T cells that have migrated into the initial lesion.

The current understanding of MS pathogenesis supports a central role of CD4+ T cells in the inflammatory response, with most studies demonstrating preferential restriction of myelin-specific CD4+ T cells by MS-associated HLA-DR (class II) molecules. It should be noted, however, that CD8+ T cells are also found in lesional sites at critical locations, suggesting that these cells have at least a supportive function in the inflammation. Thus, both CD4+ and CD8+ T cells reactive against a variety of myelin antigens such as MBP, MOG, and PLP have been identified in MS lesions.

While T cells and macrophages clearly remain the major effector components in MS, there is interest in the possibility that antibodies also play a role. This is in part due to the recognition that anti-MOG antibodies have demyelinating potential. In addition, it has recently been suggested that the presence of antimyelin antibodies may have prognostic value. Thus, whether or not the antibody response in MS is intrinsically pathogenic, determining its context should help elucidate the overall disease pathogenesis and refine the disease phenotype.

CNS Pathology

Examination of acute lesions in MS reveals foci of demyelination (see Fig. 15.1B) and axonal damage (see Fig. 15.1C), the pathologic hallmarks of this disease. Demyelination due to damage to the insulating sheath surrounding nerve fibers results in impaired nerve conduction and exposure of the underlying axon to direct nerve injury. This loss of myelin can block conduction of nerve impulses and thus cause a neurologic deficit; alternatively, it can result in positive symptoms through the generation of aberrant spontaneous action potentials. Axonal insult resulting from demyelination is considered to be the major cause of irreversible neurologic disease in MS.

Environmental Factors in MS

As discussed above, MS may be triggered by an antigen associated with an environmental pathogen that resembles a self-antigen in the CNS (molecular mimicry). Indeed, this possibility is supported by the fact that MS is characterized by a distinct geographic pattern of disease prevalence, a close temporal relation of clinical relapse to viral infections, and a similarity to certain peri-infectious demyelinating diseases.

Disease Prevalence. Population studies suggest greater risk for inhabitants of areas at higher latitudes on both hemispheres, for example, people in Northern European countries or North America in the Northern Hemisphere. Environmental "priming factors" are further supported by details of migration analyses, which suggest a critical time of exposure. Those migrating prior to age 15 acquire the disease risk observed in the adopted land. In contrast, the disease risk of geographic origin is retained in those migrating after the age of 15. Disease "epidemics" have been reported, including one on the isolated Faroe Islands upon visit by nonresidents, implying introduction of a pathogen.

Clinical Relapse and Viral Infection. The well-documented temporal association between viral infection and relapse is not limited to a single viral agent. The long list of implicated viruses hints at a more generalized mechanism of immune response rather than a single critical pathway activated by a unique etiologic agent. Possibilities include triggering of immune response against self-antigens (not necessarily by molecular mimicry) and/or imparting vulnerability to myelin-producing oligodendrocytes upon viral infection.

Similarities to Viral Infections. Infectious agents are capable of directly producing and triggering immune-mediated demyelinating diseases. Conditions such as progressive multifocal leukoencephalopathy, human T-cell leukemia/lymphoma virus (HTLV) 1–associated myelopathy/tropical spastic paraparesis, demyelination associated with Theiler's murine encephalomyelitis virus or other viruses, and other diseases are well described in the neurologic literature. The possibility remains that MS is caused by an as yet unidentified organism which initiates this disease in those with the proper genetic background.

Genetic Factors in MS

MS is considered to be a disease of complex genetic background with weak contributions by multiple alleles. Epidemiologic analyses indicating disease association with Caucasians in temperate zones, particularly Northern Europe, northern reaches of North America, and southern Oceania speak to more than mere geographic exposure, since certain homogeneous racial groups such as the Lapps and Inuits residing in temperate regions are virtually "immune" to MS. More compelling evidence for genetic susceptibility stems from family studies. The complex non-Mendelian genetic influence imparts a sibling risk of 2–5%, with a higher (25–30%) concordance for monozygotic twins. Of the numerous candidate genes identified by whole-genome searches, the association with the MHC/HLA region on chromosome 6 is the strongest. Because T cells are only able to recognize antigens in the context of self-HLA molecules, rigid HLA restriction provides a possible immunogenetic susceptibility mechanism involving preferential processing and presentation of specific autoantigen(s). The most common form of MS, RRMS (see Fig. 15.2B), is closely tied to HLA-DQ6 (*HLA-DQA1*0102* and *HLA-DQB1*0602*) and HLA-DR2 (*HLA-DRB1*1501* and *HLA-DRB5*0101*). Linkage disequilibrium does not permit assessment of independent risk conferred by these HLA class II molecules. Involvement of additional class II molecules and class I molecules has been also described.

Polymorphism of the HLA gene alone is an inadequate explanation of the association of MHC with MS. Disease susceptibility may stem from neighboring genes, such as those for complement and TNFs. The most likely explanation of the central role of HLA class II molecules is in their presentation of certain self-peptides to T cells and/or the way in which they shape the T-cell repertoire of MS patients to render it particularly responsive to myelin/brain antigens.

TREATMENT OF MULTIPLE SCLEROSIS

Immunomodulation

Great strides have been made in the therapeutic approach to MS. Until recently, corticosteroids and nonsteroidal immunosuppressives were the only available options. Most experts recommend early therapeutic intervention with either IFN-β or glatiramer acetate, both immunomodulatory agents. Although a few critics cite unknown long-term effects and current inability to predict responders, these agents are believed to be particularly effective during the early inflammatory phase and to delay irreversible axonal damage. IFN-β and glatiramer acetate are almost equally effective; the higher dosed IFN preparations have a slightly stronger effect on inflammation, but glatiramer acetate is better tolerated overall.

Glatiramer acetate consists of random peptides of four amino acids (L-alanine, L-glutamic acid, L-lysine, L-tyrosine) at a fixed molar ratio. Designed to mimic myelin, glatiramer acetate was originally thought to induce disease in animals; however, it proved to be disease inhibitory. Proposed mechanisms of action include (1) inhibition of antigen-specific T cells by competing with the antigen for the class II MHC peptide binding site and (2) suppression by induction of T_H2 cells.

The rationale for initial use of IFN–β in the treatment of MS was based on the hypothesis that viral infections are involved in either inducing or maintaining the disease. IFN-β is most effective in the treatment of RRMS. Of the antiviral, antiproliferative, and immunomodulating properties of IFN–β, the latter two are believed to have therapeutic importance in MS. Suggested therapeutic effects include down-regulation of HLA class II expression, shift to T_H2 pattern, closing of the blood–brain barrier, and inhibition of matrix metalloproteinases.

Symptomatic Treatment

In most cases, relapses are addressed by a short-term pulse of corticosteroids. The exact intervening mechanism of these anti-inflammatory/immunosuppressive agents in reducing the severity and duration of clinical exacerbations is unclear but may involve closure of the blood–brain barrier, reduction of $CD4^+$ T cells, decreased cytokine release including TNF and IFN-γ, and/or decreased MHC class II expression. They do not appear to alter the long-term course of MS, and the immunosuppressive nature of corticosteroids and other extensive side effects prohibit chronic use.

Future of Therapy

There are a variety of agents currently in the development and testing phase. Ongoing experimental work is focusing on strategies to block the adhesion molecules governing lymphocyte homing to the CNS across the blood–brain barrier, block critical cytokines such as IL-12, and vaccinate against immunodominant determinants in protocols like those described for myasthenia gravis (see Case 14). Other therapeutic strategies include reconstitution of the patient's lymphocyte repertoire by hemopoietic stem cell transplantation and very preliminary efforts at nerve regeneration.

REFERENCES

Babbe H, Roers A, Waisman A, Lassmann H, Goebels N, Hohlfeld R, Friese M, Schröder R, Deckert M, Schmidt S, Ravid R, Rajewsky K. (2000): Clonal expansion of $CD8^+$ T cells dominate the T-cell infiltrate in active multiple sclerosis lesions as shown by micromanipulation and single cell polymerase chain reaction. *J Exp Med* 192:393–404.

Brisebois M, Zehntner SP, Estrada J, Owens T, Fournier S (2006): A pathogenic role for $CD8^+$ T cells in a spontaneous model of demyelinating disease. *J Immunol* 117:2403–2411.

Cassan C, Liblau RS (2007): Immune tolerance and control of CNS autoimmunity: From animal models to MS patients. *J Neurochem* 100:883–892.

Korn T, Bettelli E, Gao W, Awasthi A, Jäger A, Strom TB, Oukka M, Kuchroo VK (2007): IL-21 initiates an alternative pathway to induce proinflammatory T_H17 cells. *Nature* 448:484–487.

McFarland HF, Martin R (2007): Multiple sclerosis: A complicated picture of autoimmunity. *Nat Immunol Rev* 8:913–919.

Oksenberg JR, Hauser SL (2005): Genetics of multiple sclerosis. *Neurol Clin* 23:61–75.

Trapp BD, Peterson J, Ransohoff RM, Rudick R, Mörk S, Bö L. (1998): Axonal transaction in lesions of multiple sclerosis. *New Engl J Med* 338:278–285.

16

DIABETES MELLITUS TYPE 1

SMITA BAID and KRISTINA I. ROTHER*

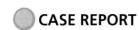

CASE REPORT

"Mommy, I wet the bed again."

Initial Presentation and Evaluation

Eric is a six-year-old boy who is brought to you, his pediatrician, by his mother for a preschool "check-up." She relates that lately Eric has been very thirsty and, much to his dismay (and hers), has had a few bed-wetting accidents. Because she had his baby brother three months ago, his mother attributes the bed wetting to psychologic stress. She relates that Eric's father disagrees because Eric has always seemed well adjusted. In any case, Eric's parents have been restricting his fluid intake in the evening without much effect on the bed wetting.

Upon further questioning, Eric's mother also recalls that when playing with his friends over the past few months he has occasionally complained about being tired and recently mentioned that he does not see well. In addition, Eric has not gained much weight; although his appetite is reported to be excellent, he has even lost some weight over the past several months. You then spend some time talking to Eric directly. He seems to be a well-adjusted six-year-old but is anxious about needing to use the bathroom so often, especially once school starts. He feels guilty about drinking so much and is trying hard to avoid it. Eric also expresses fear that he will become fat since he is always hungry and eating.

When you ask him if he can keep up with his friends, he tells you that lately he gets tired so fast that he needs to take time out to rest. When you ask about headaches and dizziness, he says that he has not experienced these symptoms.

On physical examination, Eric has some slight cervical lymphadenopathy (enlarged lymph nodes in neck) but no thyromegaly (enlarged thyroid gland). His funduscopic exam (visualization of the retina) is unremarkable. His mucous membranes appear slightly dry. Cardiopulmonary and abdominal exams are normal. He is prepubertal, as appropriate. His height is in the 75th percentile (unchanged from previous exams), but when you chart his weight, you find that it has decreased from the 50th to the 10th percentile.

From the information you have gathered, you generate a short list of possible diagnoses, including anxiety disorder, benign nocturnal enuresis, *type 1 diabetes mellitus (T1DM)*, and autoimmune endocrine disorders of the thyroid, adrenal,

*With contributions from Warren Strober and Susan R. S. Gottesman

---

or pituitary glands. Because of the symptoms of thirstiness, frequent urination, and weight loss with increased appetite, T1DM heads the list. While these symptoms can also be caused by a pituitary abnormality, there is no history of headache or neurologic problems.

To complete your initial evaluation you turn back to Eric's mother to obtain a relevant family history. What information can you obtain that might be relevant to your differential diagnosis?

> *An increased incidence of nocturnal enuresis after the birth of a sibling or at times of heightened anxiety (e.g., at the beginning of a school year) often occurs in families, so a positive history would favor this diagnosis. A family history of autoimmune disease, tumor, or an environmental insult would tip the scales in favor of a diagnosis of autoimmune disease, which usually has a genetic component.*

The mother is not aware of any family history of enuresis or autoimmune disease. However, she does recall that her husband has a cousin with early-onset diabetes. In any case, T1DM is easily ruled out (or confirmed) by simple laboratory studies. You therefore ask Eric for a urine specimen and have blood drawn to obtain a complete blood count (CBC) and determination of serum chemistries. In addition, you perform a finger stick for an immediate blood glucose reading on a glucometer.

The results are revealing and unequivocal: The serum glucose (determined by glucometer) is 375 mg/dL. Similarly, the urine sample, to which your nurse has applied a reagent strip for preliminary analysis, shows 2+ glucose, trace ketones, and slightly low specific gravity.

What do these preliminary results signify?

> *Hyperglycemia, defined as random plasma glucose >200 mg/dL on two occasions, is diagnostic for diabetes. Glucosuria, glucose in the urine, is sometimes the first sign of T1DM in asymptomatic children. Ketones are the result of breakdown of fatty acids and can be seen in the urine when there is excessive utilization of fat for energy. Eric's very high serum glucose level, which is "spilling" into the urine, is virtually diagnostic of DM. His history, age, weight, and finding of ketones in the urine support a diagnosis of T1DM rather than type 2 DM (see below).*

Eric's father has now arrived in your office; you are confident enough in your diagnosis based just on these simple laboratory tests to speak to the parents immediately. You explain that Eric most likely has type 1 diabetes mellitus, although you will obtain blood for confirmatory studies. They react with concern but also with some confusion. They have read in the newspaper about the nationwide health crisis and the rising frequency of diabetes, even among children, but thought that it was restricted to those who were overweight, which Eric clearly is not. You explain to them that this is a misconception about the form of diabetes affecting Eric.

What is T1DM?

Type 1 diabetes mellitus *is a T-cell-mediated autoimmune disorder that results in an absolute insulin deficiency secondary to the destruction of pancreatic beta (β) cells, the cellular source of insulin. It can develop at almost any age, from the first year of life to the sixth decade. Because its incidence is greatest between early school age and puberty in both males and females, it was previously called juvenile diabetes. T1DM is distinct from* ***type 2 diabetes mellitus****, which is characterized by end-organ resistance to insulin rather than decreased insulin synthesis. Another distinction is that type 2 diabetes has a later time of onset and tends to be associated with excessive weight.*

Additional Evaluation

In view of Eric's probable diagnosis, you now obtain blood samples for hemoglobin A_1C, C-peptide, and antibodies to insulin, glutamic acid decarboxylase (GAD), and islet cell antigen 512 (ICA512).

What information will these tests provide?

> *Electrolytes and a chemistry panel provide information about glucose concentration, evidence for diabetic ketoacidosis (DKA) (bicarbonate, CO_2, anion gap, and potassium), and baseline liver and kidney function. In T1DM of recent onset, it is not uncommon to find markedly elevated glucose levels (i.e., 800 mg/dL) without DKA. This is due to ingestion of beverages having high carbohydrate content such as sodas and juices in an effort to maintain hydration. A glucose tolerance test (hourly measurements of glucose levels following glucose challenge after overnight fast) is often unnecessary to confirm that the patient has diabetes in the case of T1DM.*
>
> *Although glucosuria revealed by a routine urinalysis may be the first indication of T1DM, it can occur as a result of other conditions or may be a measure of other sugars in the urine. Other causes of glucosuria include conditions such as Fanconi syndrome or other renal tubular disorders due to heavy metal intoxication, ingestion of certain drugs (e.g., outdated tetracyclines), inborn errors of metabolism (e.g., cystinosis), or nonketotic hyperglycemic syndrome, especially when associated with diarrhea and dehydration. The test usually performed to assess glucose in the urine is not actually glucose specific. Glucose is the most common sugar found in the urine, but its presence needs to be specifically confirmed; galactose, fructose, or another pentose can also yield positive results.*
>
> *Other helpful tests that will not be available for immediate review include determination of hemoglobin A_1C in the circulation. This test measures glycosylation of red blood cells and is thus an indicator of mean glucose levels over the previous three months (i.e., the lifetime of an erythrocyte). Serum C-peptide is measured to assess residual insulin production, which may be present even in patients with T1DM. Because the C-peptide is a fragment of proinsulin that is cleaved by endoproteases in the final step of insulin production in the β cells, its presence indicates*

that the β cells are producing some insulin. Although it is frequently assumed that T1DM inevitably leads to a complete loss of β cells and to a "brittle," difficult-to-control condition, many individuals with T1DM maintain some minimal endogenous insulin production for decades and therefore have a lower risk for the development of some (microvascular) complications.

Tests for the presence of antibodies against GAD (GAD65, an islet cell enzyme involved in the conversion of glutamic acid to γ-aminobutyric acid and a potential signaling molecule) and ICA512 [a protein of unknown function that is also called insulinoma-associated tyrosine phosphatase–like protein (IA-2)] may also be obtained in a T1DM work-up to help establish the presence of an autoimmune state.

As you suspected, the hemoglobin A_1C level suggests that Eric has been hyperglycemic for some time; unfortunately, the C-peptide level indicates virtual absence of insulin synthesis. Antibodies to insulin, GAD and IAC are detectable.

Treatment Plan and Early Followup

You explain to Eric's parents that his glucose levels must be controlled, both for his day-to-day well-being and to prevent or delay the long-term sequelae of diabetes (see below). Since monitoring will be difficult in a growing, active child, even with his full cooperation, you suggest that Eric's parents enroll in an educational program. Meanwhile a schedule of insulin replacement injections and glucose monitoring at home is initiated, along with a low-sugar, low-carbohydrate diet. You explain that there may be a "honeymoon period," a period of marked reduction of insulin requirements and improvement of endogenous insulin secretion at the initiation of insulin therapy. However, this period typically lasts only three to nine months, after which time ß-cell number and/or function typically decline.

At a check-up several months later, you are pleased to hear that Eric has adjusted easily to school, the bed wetting has stopped, and he is less anxious. Eric has gained an appropriate amount of weight, his finger stick glucose level in the office is 90 mg/dL, and his urine analysis is normal. You compliment Eric and his parents on their diligent monitoring of his glucose levels and insulin doses, which they have recorded in a diary. At this point you suggest that some time in the future you would like to evaluate their younger son for risk of developing the T1DM, as this disease has some genetic basis (see treatment of T1DM below).

CLINICAL FEATURES OF T1DM

By the time T1DM is clinically recognized, the autoimmune reaction has usually done its damage and the insulin-producing β cells of the pancreatic islets are destroyed or almost destroyed. Both the immediate clinical features of T1DM and the long-term effects of the disease are due to lack of insulin, the resulting metabolic imbalance, and increased glucose levels in the serum. Over the individual's lifetime this disease may affect virtually every organ in the body, mostly through damage of the microvasculature and the induction of atherosclerosis.

The day-by-day clinical features of T1DM are often a consequence of poorly controlled glucose levels. These can be either too high or too low. In Eric's case, they were too high. Frequently, patients have polyuria, polydipsia, polyphagia, weight loss (in cases of prolonged hyperglycemia), blurred vision, and fatigue. Polyuria (increased urine output) occurs because the increased filtered load of glucose exceeds the reabsorptive ability of the kidney and triggers osmotic diuresis. Polydipsia (increased fluid intake due to thirst) is a secondary symptom caused by the low extracellular fluid volume brought on by polyuria. Polyphagia (increased appetite and food intake) is a compensatory response to poor dietary fuel utilization; without insulin, glucose cannot gain access to the cell, and the body increases intake to meet energy requirements. Weight loss is secondary to excess glucose, fluid loss, and inability to use glucose; blurred vision is the result of ocular lens swelling (reversible in about two to six weeks after initiation of insulin treatment).

Diabetic ketoacidosis (DKA) is the most common and serious diabetic emergency. The symptoms described above, along with an excessive production of ketone bodies (acetone and β-hydroxybutyrate, which are weak acids) from the breakdown of fatty acids in response to unmet energy needs, lead to metabolic acidosis, hypotension, and tachycardia (increased heart rate). Patients may have a fruity breath odor secondary to the excess acetone production. Cerebral edema (swelling), complicating about 1% of pediatric cases with DKA, is the most dreaded complication; even today it is associated with a high mortality rate that has not diminished with improvement in intensive care.

Brittle or poorly controlled diabetic patients are more susceptible to infections, particularly bacterial infections, due to impaired neutrophil function; in addition, they are subject to mucormyocosis infection of the sinuses, a fungal infection due to a host defense problem that is as yet poorly understood. The ability to handle infections of any kind is compromised by microvasculature problems.

Long-term effects of T1DM include microvascular retinopathy, which results in blindness; nephropathy leading to renal failure; gangrenous necrosis of the lower extremities due to poor circulation and neuropathy, which leads to amputation; and cardiovascular disease.

IMMUNOPATHOLOGIC MECHANISMS UNDERLYING THE DEVELOPMENT OF T1DM

Type 1 diabetes mellitus is the end result of a chronic inflammatory process that causes the progressive destruction of islet β cells. There is considerable evidence that this inflammation is an autoimmune process mediated by T_H1 T cells. Within this context, several possible mechanisms of β-cell injury must be considered (Fig. 16.1):

1. CD4$^+$ T cells respond to an autoantigen associated with the β cells, resulting in the induction of

a destructive delayed-type hypersensitivity (DTH)–like response; this mechanism, which is believed to be responsible for initiating damage in other autoimmune diseases such as multiple sclerosis (MS), is reviewed in detail in Case 15.

2. The generation of CD8$^+$ cytotoxic T lymphocytes (CTLs) mediates the destruction of the β cells, most likely in conjunction with activating help from CD4$^+$ T_H1 cells

3. Local production of inflammatory cytokines, particularly tumor necrosis factor α (TNF-α), directly and indirectly causes damage to the β cells. These

Immune attack of insulin-secreting pancreatic β cells

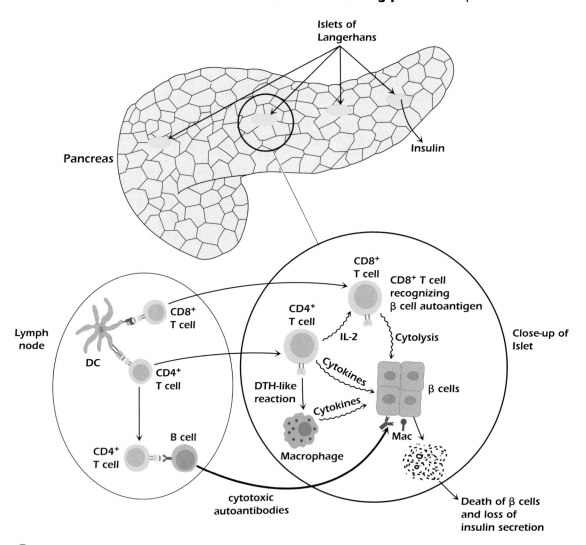

Figure 16.1. Environmental antigen(s) that cross-react with autoantigens are presented to CD4$^+$ and CD8$^+$ T cells. This sets up a cascade of reactions that result in islet cell destruction and loss of insulin secretion. CD4$^+$ T cells cause damage by direct release of inflammatory cytokines and by activation of macrophages in a DTH-like reaction. CD8$^+$ T cells cause islet cell lysis. CD4$^+$ T cells also interact with B cells to induce autoantibody formation which is an additional cause of islet cell damage.

cytokines may be the products of macrophages activated in the DTH reaction and/or products of CTLs.

4. The production of autoantibodies against β-cell-associated antigens, particularly insulin, causes complement-mediated cell damage; such pathogenic autoantibodies may also be the result of a primary T cell process as is seen in myasthenia gravis (see Case 14).

As discussed at greater length below, there is evidence that each of these four mechanisms participates, at least in part, in the pathogenesis of T1DM. In this section, we will first review some basic facts about the pancreas and insulin; then we will turn to the genetic influences on T1DM and a brief discussion of the breakdown of tolerance. The section concludes with the evidence for the mechanism(s) of cellular destruction operative in this disease.

An important clinical fact concerning T1DM has already been mentioned: By the time diabetic symptoms appear, there is already substantial (if not virtually complete) loss of β-cell function. This means that the time to institute immunologically based treatment of patients is during the "silent" preclinical phase of the disease when some β-cell function is still present. For a patient like Eric, whose studies provide evidence that all his β cells are already destroyed, it is already too late. His baby brother, on the other hand, might benefit from monitoring to detect early evidence of loss of β-cell function, particularly if he has the major histocompatibility complex (MHC) haplotype associated with the disease (see below); the appearance of such evidence should prompt consideration of intervention. There is evidence that insulin itself is a major autoantigen in T1DM. Thus, immunologically based treatment involving induction of anergy to insulin, such as that described below, could be attempted in such prediabetic cases.

Some Basic Facts about Insulin and Islet β Cells

The insulin molecule is composed of 51 amino acids arranged in two polypeptide chains (A and B) that are covalently linked by disulfide bridges. Insulin is initially synthesized as preproinsulin; it is transformed into proinsulin upon removal of the leader peptide. Proinsulin is then cleaved at two sites by endoproteases to obtain the mature insulin molecule as well as the release of C-peptide.

The insulin-producing ß cells constitute one of four cell types present in the endocrine portion of the pancreas, called islets of Langerhans. These islets also contain α cells that produce glucagon, δ cells that produce somatostatin, and pancreatic polypeptide (PP) cells that produce pancreatic polypeptide. The specificity of the damage in T1DM is underscored by the fact that other cells of the islets are not harmed. Overall, endocrine tissue makes up only 1–2% of the entire pancreas.

The Major Histocompatibility Complex (MHC)

As mentioned above, the strongest genetic factor in T1DM is its association with the MHC; however, other genetic influences exist as well. To understand the association of T1DM with the MHC, we review some basic facts about the MHC.

The MHC was discovered as an extended genetic locus containing genes that determined the outcome of skin tissue transplants. In humans, the genes are located on the short arm of chromosome 6; their products are called human leucocyte antigens (HLAs). The HLA region encodes (among other genes) class I (A, B, and C) and class II (DR, DQ, and DP) molecules. The principal differences between these two classes are as follows: (1) MHC class I molecules are expressed on all nucleated cells and interact with CD8 (cytotoxic) T lymphocytes, while class II molecules are expressed on antigen-presenting cells (APCs; such as macrophages and dendritic cells) and present antigen to CD4 (mostly helper) T lymphocytes; (2) HLA class I molecules present peptides (antigens) derived from cytosolic, usually endogenously synthesized, proteins, but class II molecules present peptides derived mainly from extracellular proteins that have undergone endocytosis (see also Case 19). Most HLA genes are highly polymorphic, meaning that the set of HLA genes (e.g., *HLA-DQ*) present in each individual is one of a large number of allelic forms present in the population as a whole. Thus, the HLA class I and class II molecules of each individual are encoded by an almost unique mixture of alleles, and most individuals have different HLA types (unless they are siblings who inherited the same haplotypes from their mother and father). Certain HLA alleles do not sort independently in a population but instead are present together on the same chromosome more frequently than would be expected by chance, a phenomenon known as linkage disequilibrium. The latter probably occurs because inheritance of certain groups of alleles together confers a certain (usually unknown) selective advantage. When a particular disease is associated with a certain HLA allele, that allele is often part of a group of HLA alleles that are in linkage disequilibrium; thus the disease is associated not only with a certain HLA allele but also with all alleles in linkage disequilibrium with that allele.

An individual's MHC (HLA) type influences positive and negative selection in the thymus (see Case 3 and the introduction to this unit.)

Finally, MHC molecules play a role in T-cell responses to antigens because CD4 and CD8 on the T-cell surface bind to invariant portions on the MHC class II and class I molecules, respectively, and thus increase the affinity of binding between the APC and the T cell.

Breakdown in Immunologic Tolerance

Central Tolerance. The development of tolerance to self-antigens is discussed in the introduction to this unit and Case 3. These discussions are relevant to T1DM because insulin is a self-peptide known to be expressed in the thymus and to direct insulin-specific negative selection and regulatory T cell (T_{reg}) generation in that central lymphoid organ. Autoimmune regulator (AIRE), a transcription factor expressed by thymic stromal cells, directs thymic expression of self antigens including insulin, in the context of MHC. An individual can have mutations in AIRE and thus in thymic selection processes for insulin and other self-peptides. Such mutations result in an autoimmune syndrome involving several endocrine organs and, in some cases, a diabetes-like condition. Although AIRE mutations do not occur in the vast majority of T1DM, they are examples of how a defect in thymic negative selection can result in the generation of insulin-specific, autoreactive T cells. A thymic abnormality involving selection could also lead to a deficiency in the generation of insulin-specific T_{reg} cells; this would allow unchecked activation of those insulin-specific autoreactive cells in the periphery that have escaped negative selection. Thus, insulin-specific autoimmunity arising from a breakdown in central tolerance can be due to the "push" of excessive autoreactive effector cell generation or the "pull" of deficient autoreactive T_{reg} cell generation.

Type 1 Diabetes Mellitus: Genes versus Environment (or Both). A defect in the development of central tolerance is only one of the many factors that could contribute to the development of T1DM. A more encompassing and realistic discussion of such development involves description of a broader group of susceptibility factors, both genetic and environmental.

The prevailing hypothesis governing the pathogenesis of T1DM is that the presence of distinct genetic and environmental factors conspires to break the state of anergy that normally exists for insulin (or perhaps other β-cell antigens). In view of the above discussion regarding the relationship of MHC to central tolerance, it should not come as a surprise that the MHC genes are the most important of the genetic factors. In fact, it has been known for several decades that these genes account for most of the inherited risk for T1DM. Many other candidate genetic factors have been proposed, but only two have been confirmed: the INS-VNTR (variable number of tandem repeat region upstream of the insulin gene) and the CTLA-4 gene. However, these genes do not contribute more than 15% of the risk for T1DM.

MHC Genes. Early positive associations between HLA and T1DM were found with the class I antigens B8 and B15. Subsequently, stronger associations were found with class II genes, and it was discovered that the initial association with class I was due to linkage disequilibrium with class II: B8 with DR3 and B15 with DR4. In Caucasians, persons carrying both DR3 and DR4 haplotypes (one inherited from each parent) have the highest risk. Approximately 3% of healthy individuals are DR3/DR4 positive, compared with 33% of Caucasians with T1DM.

There are also certain HLA alleles that are protective against T1DM. Even among islet cell antibody–positive first-degree relatives of a patient with T1DM, protection from disease is associated with a certain DQ allele (*DQA1*0102 DQB1*0602*). This may explain why approximately 85% of patients with T1DM do not have a close relative with the disorder.

Finally, it is important to note that HLA associations vary greatly in different races. For example, the presence of an amino acid other than aspartate at position 57 of the DQb chain (called "non-Asp57") confers a relative risk greater than 100 in Caucasians, but this association is not present in the Japanese population.

Additional Genes Implicated in T1DM. A significant but weaker genetic factor for T1DM has been associated with the insulin gene (*INS*), which is located on the short arm of chromosome 11. In particular, polymorphisms in the 5′VNTR region of the insulin gene are highly correlated with disease occurrence. This region determines expression levels of the insulin self-antigen in the thymus and may thus affect the shaping of the T-cell repertoire relating to insulin. This possibility is supported by the fact that insulin gene transcription levels in the thymus are inversely correlated with susceptibility to DM in both humans and transgenic models of DM.

Finally, the fact that certain genetic variants of the CTLA-4 molecule [the inhibitory receptor on T cells for the B7 costimulatory molecules (CD80 and CD86)] have been found to confer resistance to induction of DM in the NOD (nonobese diabetes) mouse model suggests that a defect in this molecule favors the development of T1DM. This idea is supported by the fact that increased expression of CTLA-4 on activated T cells is one way to turn off T-cell activity (see below); thus, this genetic factor for T1DM could contribute to autoimmunity in an antigen-nonspecific fashion.

Environmental Factors. Several environmental factors responsible for the development of T1DM have also been proposed. The strongest of these thus far is early exposure to cow's milk and viral infections with organisms such as coxsackie B and enteroviruses. The proposed mechanisms underlying these factors include direct injury to ß cells and molecular mimicry, for example, cross-reactivity between viral antigens and self-antigens (see the introduction to this unit). The fact that T1DM sometimes has an initial presentation subsequent to an acute illness (such as a viral illness of unclear etiology) has long been noted. However, in most cases of T1DM, β-cell destruction has been an ongoing process for months to years prior to diabetic decompensation. Thus, an initiating viral infection leading to a loss of tolerance must have occurred long before the onset of clinically evident disease. Childhood vaccines have also been under scrutiny as environmental triggers. However, a recent Danish study that evaluated 681 genetically predisposed children did not find a causal relationship between childhood vaccination and T1DM.

Immunologic Mechanisms of Islet β-Cell Destruction

Self-Antigen Targets.   Given that the β cells are being gradually destroyed, presumably by a mechanism initiated by autoimmune T cells, is it important to determine the nature of the autoantigens stimulating this reaction?

Potential self- antigens, including insulin itself, GAD, or islet cell antigen ICA, are expressed on the β cells, especially when they are stimulated to express MHC class II antigen or increase their expression of class I. Based on the facts that insulin peptide expression in the thymus is important for negative selection and that insulin-specific autoantibodies occur in prediabetic individuals (see below), it is likely that insulin itself or a peptide derived from insulin (presented in the context of MHC class I and/or class II) is the target of the autoimmune attack. However, keep in mind that other antigens are released and become targets of the autoimmune attack (epitope spreading) in the course of tissue injury.

Cytotoxic Mechanism(s) Causing Islet Cell Destruction.   Assuming that we have in fact identified the probable initial autoantigen(s) in T1DM, what type of immune response elicited by this antigen(s) causes the tissue (islet cell) injury?

Unfortunately, there is only a scant amount of data available from human studies since the early lesions of T1DM leading to islet cell destruction are rarely visualized or sampled. However, in the rare instances in which the human pancreas has been examined early in the course of T1DM, a lymphocytic infiltrate surrounding the islets and death or necrosis of islet cells have been observed. The cells in such infiltrates consist of a mixture of CD4$^+$ and CD8$^+$ T cells, supporting the idea that a T cell-mediated process involving both CD4$^+$ T cells and CD8$^+$ T cells develops into a cytotoxic process that results in β-cell destruction.

Studies of NOD mice, the most commonly studied mouse model of spontaneous T1DM, support and expand on the human studies. T cell infiltration of the islets has been shown to precede disease in NOD mice; in addition, the infiltrating T cells can transfer disease to unaffected animals. Furthermore, it has been found that the infiltrating T cells are specific for islet cell–associated antigens (insulin, GAD, and ICA) and that CD8$^+$ cytotoxic T cells specific for insulin peptide have the capacity to selectively destroy β cells.

In the above scenario of β-cell destruction, β cells display antigens that are activators (as well as the subsequent targets) of reactive T cells, so the β cells are functioning as APCs. However, an APC of this kind, that is, a "non-professional" APC, would ordinarily fail to activate T cells recognizing an autoantigen (for which it usually has low affinity) for two reasons: (1) The "APC" lacks sufficient expression of MHC antigens and (2) it does not initially express costimulatory molecules that would provide a "second signal" to the T cell. This is where a viral infectious agent may play a role in triggering disease. One possibility is that a β cell infected with a virus could present a processed viral antigen to T cells that then produce interferon-γ (IFN-γ). IFN-γ then enhances MHC expression by the β cell, thereby facilitating the presentation of self-antigen to autoreactive T cells. This possibility is supported by studies in mice showing that expression of a transgene that encodes a viral antigen under an insulin promoter (that is thus preferentially expressed in the β cell) can lead to β-cell activation of T cells specific for the virus. This is then followed by β-cell destruction by the activated T cells if the mice are infected with the virus from which the transgenic viral antigen is derived. In effect, the viral infection of the β cells transforms them into more potent APCs that can open the door to activation of and destruction by autoreactive cells.

Another possibility is that the triggering virus does not infect the β cell but nevertheless activates virus-reactive T cells that cross-react with the islet cell self-antigens. Such activation of cross-reactive T cells by the β cells occurs (despite the poor antigen-presenting capability of the β cells) because the virus-reactive cells are intrinsically robust T cells that are more easily activated than self-reactive T cells. The cross-reactive T cells then produce cytokines that enhance islet cell MHC expression, allowing T cells recognizing the self-antigens to be activated and continue the β-cell destruction even when the infectious agent has been eliminated. The common denominator of both of these scenarios is that an exogenous infection can lead to production of cytokines in the pancreas, which causes β cells to exhibit increased MHC antigen expression; the infection thus converts the β cell into a more potent activator of self-reactive T cells. In T1DM the expression of MHC class II antigens is in fact detectable on β cells, indicating that they have probably been exposed to inflammatory cytokines from some source.

As indicated above, the cell ultimately responsible for β-cell destruction in T1DM is the CD8$^+$ T cell. What properties of this cell allow it to fulfill this function?

The ability to destroy cells infected with viruses make the CD8$^+$ CTL the body's chief adaptive immune responders to *viral pathogens. In addition, these cells are part of the body's immune surveillance mechanism; they kill neoplastic cells that express cancer antigens. The innate immune system also exerts these functions through natural killer cells, but in contrast to CD8⁺ CTL, natural killer cells are antigen nonspecific.*

The activation of a CD8⁺ CTL occurs when its TCR recognizes a specific antigen on the surface of an APC in the context of an MHC class I molecule. Such activation also requires a second signal, provided by CD80 (B7) and/or another costimulatory molecule on the surface of the APC, that binds to CD28 on the surface of the T cell. In the absence of this second signal, the antigen will induce anergy (unresponsiveness) rather than activation. Cytokines secreted by various cells also enhance CTL activation and expansion. These include IL-2 produced by the CD8⁺ T cell itself after initial activation and by CD4⁺ T cells that are being stimulated in the same area and IL-15 produced by the APC. Finally, CD4⁺ T cells may also participate in the activation of CD8⁺ CTL by reacting with a related antigen (in the context of MHC class II) on the APC surface and then expressing CD40L (see Case 4), a costimulatory molecule that interacts with CD40 on the surface of the APC to induce the up-regulation of CD80. In this way (and in the production of cytokines; see below), CD4⁺ T cells may contribute to tissue injury in T1DM. (Fig 16.2)

Once properly signaled, intrinsic and extrinsic controls decrease the activity of CD8⁺ T cells and turn off the CTL response. These include the increased expression of CTLA-4 on CD8⁺ T cells. CTLA-4, an inhibitory receptor for CD80

with higher affinity for CD80 than CD28, counters CD28 signaling and thus reduces the magnitude of the second stimulatory signal needed for the CD8⁺ T-cell response. CD8⁺ CTLs are also negatively regulated by regulatory T (T_{reg}) cells, such as Foxp3⁺ CD25⁺ "natural regulatory T cells" that are produced in the thymus or induced in the peripheral lymphoid system by transforming growth factor β_1 (TGF-β_1). In the NOD mouse model of T1DM, it has been observed that diabetes supervenes when T_{reg} cells decline in number and function; thus, investigators have proposed that the diabetes is actually due to a T_{reg} cell defect in this model. As discussed below, induction of T_{reg} cells is now a strategy for the prevention of T1DM.

There are several means by which activated CD8⁺ T cells cause target cell destruction (Fig. 16.3). Activated CD8⁺ T cells lyse target cells expressing the peptide recognized by their TCR; the T cells bind to the target cells and release preformed cytotoxic proteins stored in granules. This process initially involves polarization of the cytotoxic granules to the area of contact with the target cell followed by release of their contents (perforin, granzyme, granulysin, and the proteoglycan serglycin). Perforin helps release the cytotoxic enzymes into the target cell cytoplasm, leading to the induction of apoptosis (programmed cell death). An important feature of this cytotoxic program is that it avoids both innocent bystander killing and retrograde killing of the CTL itself.

A second mechanism, which involves cell–cell contact, is via the Fas–FasL pathway. The CTL may use FasL (CD178) on its surface to engage Fas (CD95) on a target cell and

Activation of CD8⁺ cytotoxic T cells

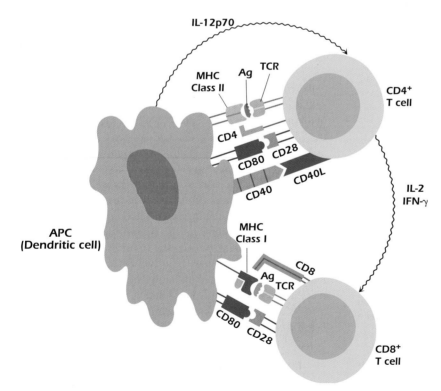

◉ Figure 16.2. CD4⁺ T cells facilitate CD8⁺ T-cell development. APCs produce cytokines following CD40/CD40L-mediated interactions with CD4⁺ T cells. These cytokines then induce CD4⁺ T cells to produce IL-2 and IFN-γ and up-regulate costimulatory molecules that facilitate CD8⁺ T-cell activation.

Mechanism 1

Mechanism 2

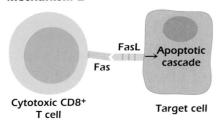

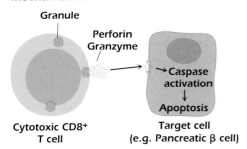 Figure 16.3. Cytotoxic CD8$^+$ T cells kill targets via two mechanisms: (1) cytotoxic granules are injected into the target; (2) cell–cell contact occurs allowing activation of Fas–FasL death pathway.

activate its death domain, thereby initiating apoptosis in that cell (see Case 6).

Three cytokines produced by CTLs [IFN-γ, lymphotoxin (LT) α, and TNF-α] enhance their cytotoxic capability. IFN-γ has direct antiviral activity through its ability to activate macrophages; however, it also increases cellular expression of MHC class I antigen, which affects the cell's ability to display peptide and serve as a CTL target. LT-α and TNF-α, both members of the TNF family, also activate macrophages but can directly initiate apoptosis of a target cell by binding its TNF receptor I (TNFR1) and activating this receptor's death domain. These potent cytokines are often expressed in membrane-bound form to control untoward effects on neighboring nontarget cells. Since apoptosis is the main mechanism of destroying the target cell, there is minimal inflammatory response generated in response to induced cell lysis: The remains of apoptotic cells are neatly removed by phagocytic cells and degraded; in contrast, the debris of necrotic cells elicits more indiscriminate inflammatory responses.

The involvement of locally produced cytokines in causing β-cell production may thus come from the CTL and/or from macrophages (TNF and IL-1) activated by autoreactive T cells. It seems likely that after the initial event both contribute to ongoing cell damage.

In addition to the cell-mediated immune destruction detailed above, autoantibodies may also participate in target cell destruction. Autoantibodies with specificity for islet cell autoantigens may be a cause of the destruction of β cells

in T1DM. This possibility is supported by the fact that these antibodies can be detected in the serum of patients with T1DM, and documentation of their presence has some ability to predict the future onset of disease in genetically susceptible disease-free relatives of T1DM patients. However, it seems equally likely that these antibodies are a consequence of the release of new self-antigens subsequent to β cellular damage; they may participate in ongoing damage as a secondary mechanism, if at all.

TREATMENT OF T1DM

What Treatment Options Exist for Individuals with T1DM?

In contrast to many other autoimmune diseases, the treatment of T1DM is directed exclusively at replacing the missing insulin, rather than at modulating the immune response. The Diabetes Control and Complications Trial (DCCT) was the first large, multicenter, randomized trial to document that intensive insulin treatment markedly reduces the microvascular complications associated with T1DM, including retinopathy, nephropathy, and neuropathy. Although only children above the age of 13 years were included in the study, the results of this and other trials are so convincing that most endocrinologists feel strongly that achieving excellent glycemia control is an important treatment goal, even in young children. Such control can be accomplished with multiple daily injections (MDIs), preferably using the combination of long- and short-acting insulin, or through the use of an insulin pump. The advantages of using continuous subcutaneous insulin infusion (CSII) via an insulin pump include the following: (1) the ability to adjust insulin doses in the early morning hours to counter growth hormone effects during puberty: (2) the precision of administering small doses, especially in young children; and (3) the ease of matching dosage to activity level, for example, decreasing basal infusion rates during athletic activity and using an extended bolus for a fatty meal. Furthermore, it has been shown that when compared with MDI, the use of CSII may result in a decreased number of hypoglycemic events and improved hemoglobin A$_1$C levels; in addition, CSII does not result in complications such as development of DKA that occur frequently with MDI. In any case, the goal of insulin replacement therapy is to keep blood glucose levels in the nondiabetic range (80–120 mg/dL) and hemoglobin A$_1$C at less than 7.0%.

Recently, experimental therapies such as islet cell transplantation have been tested in adult patients with long-standing diabetes and have shown that such therapy can result in at least temporary insulin independence. However, there are side effects from the required immunosuppressive therapy needed to prevent rejection of the transplanted tissue. Other experimental strategies for the treatment of patients with T1DM, such as the induction of endogenous islet regeneration and immunomodulation, are on the horizon.

Can We Predict and Prevent T1DM?

Very large primary prevention trials, such as the Diabetes Prevention Trial—Type 1 Diabetes (DPT-1, 104,000 individuals screened) and the European Nicotinamide Diabetes Trial (ENDIT, >30,000 individuals screened), have shown that the development of diabetes can be predicted with some accuracy. However, neither of these large trials succeeded in preventing the onset of the disease. Administration of oral or subcutaneous insulin (to induce immunologic tolerance to insulin) or nicotinamide to prediabetic individuals was unsuccessful, although there is evidence for a delay in onset in a subset of individuals (see below). Prediction of diabetes was achieved via evaluation of patients for the presence of autoantibodies, their insulin response in an intravenous glucose tolerance test, and their HLA type. Since the mid-1980s, it has been known that the process of β-cell destruction can be arrested effectively with immunosuppressive drugs such as cyclosporine, but there are serious side effects to this course of action.

In a number of ongoing secondary prevention trials, immunomodulation and immunosuppression (involving agents other than cyclosporine) are being tested to determine their ability to prevent further β-cell loss soon after the onset of diabetes. The goal of such therapy is to induce tolerance to the target antigen.

As indicated above, one approach to the development of treatments that delay or prevent disease is to administer relevant antigens in a manner that leads to antigen-specific tolerance. This approach depends on two factors: (1) the identification and use of an antigen that is central to T1DM pathogenesis and (2) the ability to induce effective tolerance to that antigen. Current studies utilizing this approach involve the oral administration of insulin (or GAD), since these antigens are considered important autoantigens in T1DM; in addition, oral antigen administration has been shown in mouse studies to be an effective way of inducing antigen-specific B- and T-cell tolerance (see Cases 17 and 18). A current trial of this type is focused on specifically defined subsets of susceptible individuals. All subjects, who have near relatives with T1DM, undergo testing for autoantibodies to insulin, ICA, and GAD and are HLA typed; the pattern of their insulin response is then evaluated via an intravenous glucose tolerance test. Of particular interest here is the intermediate-risk category, those with a 25–50% risk of developing disease within five years. These patients have the nonprotective HLA type and are ICA and anti-insulin autoantibody positive but do not have loss of the first phase

of insulin response to glucose. Individuals under study are randomly assigned to groups subjected to a tolerizing regimen of daily oral insulin pills (or given a placebo) to determine whether this treatment prevents the onset of clinical DM. Similar studies are under consideration, including one in which recombinant GAD65 is the orally administered tolerizing antigen and another in which the antigen (insulin) is administered by a nasal route. Clearly, our ability to impact the incidence of T1DM depends on gaining an understanding of the pathogenesis and timing of the early events leading to DM as well as the induction of tolerance.

REFERENCES

Ahern JA, Boland EA, Doane R, Ahern JJ, Rose P, Vincent M, Tamborlane WV (2002): Insulin pump therapy in pediatrics: A therapeutic alternative to safely lower HbA1c levels across all age groups. *Pediatr Diabetes* 3:10–15.

Akerblom HK, Vaarala O, Hyöty H, Ilonen J, Knip M (2002): Environmental factors in the etiology of type 1 diabetes. *Am J Med Genet* 115:18–29.

Anjos S, Polychronakos C (2004): Mechanisms of genetic susceptibility to type 1 diabetes: Beyond HLA. *Mol Genet Metab* 81:187–195.

Brown TB (2004): Cerebral oedema in childhood diabetic ketoacidosis: Is treatment a factor? *Emerg Med J* 21:141–144.

Christen U, von Herrath MG (2004): Induction, acceleration or prevention of autoimmunity by molecular mimicry. *Mol Immunol* 40:1113–1120.

Diabetes Control and Complications Trial Research Group (1993): The effect of intensive treatment of diabetes on the development and progression of long-term complications in insulin-dependent diabetes mellitus. *N Engl J Med* 329:977–986.

Diabetes Prevention Trial—Type 1 Diabetes Study Group (2002): Effects of insulin in relatives of patients with type 1 diabetes mellitus. *N Engl J Med* 346:1685–1691.

Drucker DJ (2003): Glucagon-like peptides: Regulators of cell proliferation, differentiation, and apoptosis. *Mol Endocrinol* 17:161–171.

Gale EA, Bingley PJ, Emmett CL, Collier T, European Nicotinamide Diabetes Intervention Trial (ENDIT) (2004): A randomised controlled trial of intervention before the onset of type 1 diabetes. *Lancet* 363:925–931.

Hirshberg B, Rother KI, Digon BJ 3rd, Lee J, Gaglia JL, Hines K, Read EJ, Chang R, Wood BJ, Harlan DM (2003): Benefits and risks of solitary islet transplantation for type 1 diabetes using steroid-sparing immunosuppression: The National Institutes of Health experience. *Diabetes Care* 26:3288–3295.

Hviid A, Stellfeld M, Wohlfahrt J, Melbye M (2004): Childhood vaccination and type 1 diabetes. *N Engl J Med* 350:1398–1404.

Madsbad S (1983): Prevalence of residual B cell function and its metabolic consequences in Type 1 (insulin-dependent) diabetes. *Diabetologia* 24:141–147.

Roep BO (2003): The role of T-cells in the pathogenesis of Type 1 diabetes: From cause to cure. *Diabetologia* 46:305–321.

Rogers J (2003): An overview of the management of nocturnal enuresis in children. *Br J Nurs* 12:898–903.

Rother K, Schwenk W (1995): An unusual case of the nonketotic hyperglycemic syndrome during childhood. *Mayo Clin Proc* 70:62–65.

Rother KI (2007): Diabetes treatment—Bridging the divide. *N Engl J Med* 356:1299–1301.

Sadeharju K, Hämäläinen AM, Knip M, Lönnrot M, Koskela P, Virtanen SM, Ilonen J, Akerblom HK, Hyöty H, Finnish TRIGR Study Group (2003): Enterovirus infections as a risk factor for type 1 diabetes: Virus analyses in a dietary intervention trial. *Clin Exp Immunol* 132:271–277.

Steele C, Hagopian WA, Gitelman S, Masharani U, Cavaghan M, Rother KI, Donaldson D, Harlan DM, Bluestone J, Herold KC (2004): Insulin secretion in type 1 diabetes. *Diabetes* 53:426–433.

Steffes MW, Sibley S, Jackson M, Thomas W (2003): Beta-cell function and the development of diabetes-related complications in the diabetes control and complications trial. *Diabetes Care* 26:832–836.

Stiller CR, Dupré J, Gent M, Jenner MR, Keown PA, Laupacis A, Martell R, Rodger NW, von Graffenried B, Wolfe BM (1984): Effects of cyclosporine immunosuppression in insulin-dependent diabetes mellitus of recent onset. *Science* 223:1362–1367.

Sulli N, Shashaj B (2003): Continuous subcutaneous insulin infusion in children and adolescents with diabetes mellitus: Decreased HbA1c with low risk of hypoglycemia. *J Pediatr Endocrinol Metab* 16:393–399.

Svensson J, Carstensen B, Mølbak A, Christau B, Mortensen HB, Nerup J, Borch-Johnsen K (2002): Increased risk of childhood type 1 diabetes in children born after 1985. *Diabetes Care* 25:2197–2201.

Vardi P, Shehade N, Etzioni A, Herskovits T, Soloveizik L, Shmuel Z, Golan D, Barzilai D, Benderly A (1990): Stress hyperglycemia in childhood: A very high risk group for the development of type 1 diabetes. *J Pediatr* 117:75–77.

Von Herrath M, Sanda S, Herold K (2007): Type 1 diabetes as a relapsing-remitting disease? *Nature Rev Immunol* 7:988–994.

Weintrob N, Benzaquen H, Galatzer A, Shalitin S, Lazar L, Fayman G, Lilos P, Dickerman Z, Phillip M (2003): Comparison of continuous subcutaneous insulin infusion and multiple daily injection regimens in children with type 1 diabetes: A randomized open crossover trial. *Pediatrics* 112:559–564.

17

CELIAC DISEASE

WARREN STROBER

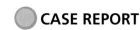 CASE REPORT

"Evan has diarrhea all the time and isn't growing."

Clinical History, Physical Exam and Initial Workup

An obviously distraught mother brings her three-year-old child, Evan, to you, his pediatrician, because he has been having severe diarrhea and does not seem to be growing. The mother states that the problem seems to have begun about 6 months before without any apparent precipitating event. At first she thought Evan had a viral gastrointestinal (GI) infection, but the diarrhea has persisted far too long for that to be the explanation. Upon questioning she states that the diarrhea did not start abruptly; rather it seemed to begin slowly and become progressively worse without Evan having any systemic (viral) symptoms or fever. As for other GI symptoms, his mother says that Evan does not complain of abdominal pain, but his abdomen seems to be bloated after meals. In addition, she has noticed that his stools are frequent and seem to be larger, more "oily" and have a more offensive smell than she was accustomed to seeing in her two older children when they were Evan's age; however, she has not noted any blood in the stools. His mother's greatest concern is that Evan is not outgrowing his clothes and has in fact lost weight. You inquire about the

types of foods in Evan's diet and learn that these consist of the usual "kid food," including cereals, spaghetti, chicken, and fish. Evan had not been breast fed and has been on cow's milk since well before the onset of symptoms.

Your physical examination of Evan reveals an irritable child without nasal congestion or skin rash. His abdomen is somewhat protuberant and tympanitic, but there are no areas of obvious tenderness and bowel sounds are normal. The extremities are negative except for slight ankle swelling (edema). Measurement of the child's weight and height reveals that he has fallen well below the 10th percentile in both. This is unexpected given Evan's previous growth curve and family history.

What is suggested by the history and physical examination?

This history of diarrhea without constitutional symptoms along with a physical examination documenting its persistent nature as evidenced by stunted growth makes you focus on the possible causes of persistent diarrhea and nutritional deficiency in infants and young children. Most acute infectious processes are ruled out by the history and physical findings. The possibility that Evan has a food allergy is also unlikely, since he would have more acute GI symptoms, possibly accompanied by pharyngeal edema or even anaphylactoid reactions immediately after food ingestion (see Case 11). In addition, food allergy would not be associated with evidence of malabsorption. The possibility

Immunology: Clinical Case Studies and Disease Pathophysiology, By Warren Strober and Susan R. S. Gottesman
Copyright © 2009 John Wiley & Sons, Inc.

that Evan has a form of inflammatory bowel disease is also unlikely in the absence of a history of abdominal pain or bloody stool and the lack of tenderness on the abdominal exam. It is possible that Evan has a food intolerance of some sort; the changes in the stool are suggestive of fat malabsorption that could be caused by villous atrophy. One type of food intolerance that must be strongly considered in this context is sensitivity to gluten protein, or celiac disease.

You decide to launch a two-pronged workup of Evan. The first prong will consist of general tests to verify the presence of malabsorption and its sequelae, nutritional deficiency. The second prong will consist of tests to determine the cause of the malabsorption, specifically the presence or absence of celiac disease. You decide to perform the workup in the hospital because the absorption studies require close patient monitoring.

The next day Evan is admitted to the general pediatric ward. To actuate the first prong of the plan, you order a complete blood count (CBC), routine electrolytes, and liver and kidney function chemistries. You also order blood tests for serum folate, iron, calcium, and vitamin D levels. For completeness, you order a sweat test to rule out the remote possibility that Evan has cystic fibrosis, a condition that very occasionally presents with GI symptoms in the absence of pulmonary symptoms.

What is the purpose of these studies?

The levels of essential nutrients can be abnormally low in the presence of malabsorption, and the types of nutrients which are deficient may give a hint to the underlying cause of disease. In addition, you want to assess the condition of the patient as a consequence of malnutrition. Although disease of relatively short duration is not associated with severe anemia or bone abnormalities, which usually occur in adults with long-standing illnesses, these possibilities should be examined and signs of mild anemia or bone disease addressed.

	Result	Reference Range
CBC:		
Hemoglobin (Hgb)	10 g/dL	11.2–16.5 g/dL
Hemocrit (Hct)	34%	35-49%
Mean Corpuscular Volume (MCV)	120 fL	80–100 fL
Mean Corpuscular Hemoglobin (MCH)	29 pg	27-31 pg
White Blood Cells (WBC)[a]	6,000/μL	4,800-10,800/μL
Platelets (PLT)	180,000/μL	130,000–400,000/μL

Chemistries:

Bicarbonate	17 meq/dL	18–25 meq/dL
Protein	5.5 gm/dL	6–8 gm/dL
Albumin	3.0 gm/dL	3.5–4.5 gm/dL
Vitamin B_{12}	300 pg/ml	200–600 pg/ml
Folate	4.0 ng/ml	5–20 ng/ml
Calcium	8.0 mg/dL	9–11 mg/dL
Serum Iron	100 μg/dL	70–180 μg/dL

[a]Some hypersegmented neutrophils.

All other chemistry tests are normal.
The sweat test is negative.

What is the interpretation of these laboratory results?

The hematocrit and hemoglobin are borderline low, indicating the presence of a mild anemia. Since the MCV is high and the folate level is low, the anemia appears to be a megaloblastic anemia due to folate deficiency; this is corroborated by the presence of hypersegmented granulocytes. Because the MCH and serum iron are normal, there is no evidence of iron deficiency anemia. The borderline low bicarbonate value probably reflects a mild metabolic acidosis due to the persistent diarrhea. The calcium level is slightly low, probably reflecting vitamin D deficiency; this could eventually affect bone density. The albumin level is also borderline low, reflecting protein deficiency; this is the probable cause of Evan's trace ankle edema since the latter results from decreased osmotic pressure in the blood vessels. These various deficiencies are consistent with the presence of a malabsorption syndrome.

To verify the presence of malabsorption, you order a D-xylose absorption test and a fat excretion study.

What are the D-xylose absorption test and fat excretion study designed to measure?

Both tests are designed to measure absorption in the duodenum and jejunum, the sites of absorption of most of our nutrients. Two different classes of molecules are chosen: sugar and fat. The D-xylose test measures the ability of the small intestines to absorb the simple sugar, xylose. D-xylose is a nonmetabolizable carbohydrate normally found as part of plant cell wall polysaccharide. The patient is administered a test dose by mouth, and the levels in the blood and urine are measured. It is normal in all but the most severely affected patients. The fat excretion study consists of measurement of the fat content of the stool over 72 h while the patient is on a defined fat intake.

The stool fat excretion study proves to be grossly abnormal (30% of fat intake secreted per day vs. normal value of <6% of intake secreted per day). The D-xylose test is inconclusive because of inadequate patient cooperation in taking the D-xylose.

The above tests establish the presence of malabsorption over an extended period of time resulting in the mild anemia and the reduced albumin level, but they do not identify celiac disease as the cause of these problems. Malabsorption, a general term for the defective absorption of nutrients, has numerous causes. Its consequences depend on which nutrients are involved and the length of time of occurrence. Malabsorption may be acute due to an infectious process or may begin gradually. In the latter, the gradual onset may be due to defective digestion or the inability to break down nutrients to an absorbable form (see Fig. 17.1 for normal intestinal villus structure). In an enzymatic defect, specific nutrients would not be metabolized and could not be absorbed. Lactose intolerance due to reduced or absent lactase levels is one common enzyme deficiency. Similarly, a defect in the intestinal epithelial cells themselves, such as mutated receptors, will prevent the active transport of specific nutrients from the intestinal lumen to the blood or lymphatics. Another possibility, a structural problem in the intestines, will cause more global nutritional deficiencies. Flattening of the intestinal villi or obstruction of the lacteals (the lymphatic vessels in the core of the villi) by tumor or infection will result in a decrease in the surface area for absorption. Segmental bowel removal via surgery

(which should be obvious to the treating physician) will also decrease the area available for absorption.

Specific Workup for Diagnosis of Celiac Disease

Your leading diagnosis for the underlying cause of the malabsorption is celiac disease, so you actuate the second prong of your plan, the performance of studies specific for this diagnosis.

What is celiac disease and why is that your leading diagnosis?

Celiac disease is an immune disorder (with certain autoimmune features) in which an immune response or lack of tolerance to gluten leads to chronic inflammation and a flattening or loss of intestinal villi (Fig. 17.2). The loss of surface area results in the malabsorption of all nutrients normally absorbed in that region of the intestines and subsequent malnutrition. Given the other causes of malabsorption, the gradual development of the diarrhea, the age of the patient, and the frequency of the disease in the population, celiac disease becomes the leading diagnosis to be considered.

Specific Antibody Tests. Because celiac disease is an immune disorder, you look for derangement of

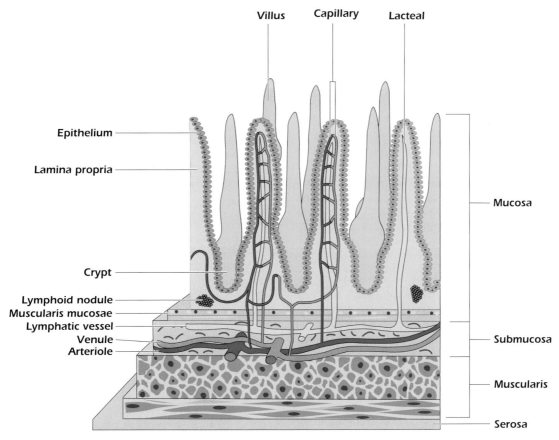

Figure 17.1. Schematic of normal villa.

the immune system, perhaps with evidence of a specific immune response to gluten or to intestinal wall structures that can cause the changes resulting in intestinal villous loss. Over the last two decades, several serologic tests have been developed based on the detection of antibodies that are specifically related to the disease process.

Antiendomesial Antibody Tests.   The endomysium is the layer of connective tissue that sheathes the muscle fibers, which is composed mostly of reticulin fibers. The fluorescent IgA antiendomesial antibody test examines the patient's serum for the presence of an (IgA) antibody that reacts in a reticular pattern with fibronectin and collagen fibrils in human umbilical cord tissue (hence its original designation "antireticular antibody"). Tissue is exposed to patient serum; binding of possible serum antibodies to tissue components is detected with a fluorescence-labeled antihuman IgA antibody. This test has excellent specificity and considerable sensitivity. In addition, since antiendomysial antibody titers correlate with the degree of villous atrophy, they can be used to assess the severity of disease and response to therapy. It should be noted, however, that a significant portion of patients with mild villous atrophy may yield negative test results, and results may be falsely positive in patients with liver disease or diabetes.

Recently, an update of the antiendomysial antibody test has been developed, an Enzyme-Linked Immunosorbent Assay (ELISA)–type test based on the fact that the endomysial antigen being detected in the tissue by endomysial antibody is tissue transglutaminase (tTG, see further discussion below). Because the ELISA is observer independent, unlike the fluorescent antiendomesial antibody test, it is more reproducible. Although this test is more sensitive, it may be somewhat less specific. In this newer diagnostic study, as in any ELISA, the purified antigen, in this case tTG2, is affixed to a plate by an anti-TG "capture" antibody and dilutions of patient serum to form a "sandwich" that is then detected with labeled antihuman IgA. The binding of the labeled anti-IgA is then quantitated using a densitometer, giving antibody titers (see Unit V).

Antigliadin Antibody Test.   A second diagnostic test for celiac disease is the IgA/IgG antigliadin antibody assay, also an ELISA-based assay. In this case the antibodies being detected are those specific for gliadin, the disease-inducing antigen. Gliadin is a constituent of gluten, a class of water-insoluble proteins in wheat and rye grains. This assay, which uses both labeled antihuman IgA and IgG, measures both IgA and IgG to gliadin. These tests are less sensitive and less specific than the antiendomesial/anti-TG tests. However, long-term positivity for IgA antigliadin is a reliable indicator of the presence of celiac disease; although the IgG antigliadin test

is quite nonspecific, it could be useful in celiac patients with concomitant IgA deficiency.

HLA Phenotyping.   A third test with high negative predictive value is based on the fact that celiac disease patients almost invariably have a particular human leucocyte antigen (HLA) type (i.e., a particular DQ2 or DQ8 HLA type; see discussion below). Because the lack of a celiac disease–associated HLA type almost definitely excludes the diagnosis, tissue typing can be useful. It should be noted, however, that the celiac disease–associated HLA type occurs quite frequently in normal individuals. Thus its presence does not necessarily indicate that a patient has celiac disease.

Evan's IgA endomysial antibody and IgA antigliadin antibody tests results prove to be positive. Evan's HLA type is the allotype found in celiac disease. At this point you make a presumptive diagnosis of celiac disease.

Morphologic Evidence of Celiac Disease: Biopsy.   You decide to confirm the diagnosis by ordering an intestinal biopsy and contact a pediatric gastroenterologist to perform this procedure. Several days later an intestinal biopsy is obtained from the duodenum by endoscopy.

Before the advent of the reliable antibody tests, multiple duodenal biopsies to establish the presence of the characteristic intestinal lesion and its response to therapy (gluten exclusion) were the standard of care in celiac disease. Today it is considered sufficient to perform one biopsy and then employ antibody tests posttherapy (after initiation of a gluten-free diet) to establish the diet's efficacy. Some believe that even one biopsy is not necessary if the clinical history is typical, the serologic tests are strongly positive, and the patient responds promptly to a gluten-free diet. However, biopsy offers unequivocal evidence for the disease, provides a baseline with which to evaluate the patient if and when disease reoccurs (if the patient fails to adhere to gluten exclusion), and may occasionally help rule out alternative diagnoses (such as the presence of immunodeficiency).

The biopsy is usually obtained with standard endoscopy, although it is desirable to biopsy the distal duodenum.

What are the microscopic features diagnostic of celiac disease?

Although celiac disease is associated with certain macroscopic endoscopic features, it is the microscopic pattern that is diagnostic. This pattern consists of villous atrophy associated with elongated intestinal crypts due to crypt hyperplasia (Fig. 17.2). The lamina propria, the loose connective tissue immediately under the epithelial surface, contains large numbers of plasma cells and T cells. In addition, there are increased numbers of intraepithelial lymphocytes (IEL) located above the basement membrane

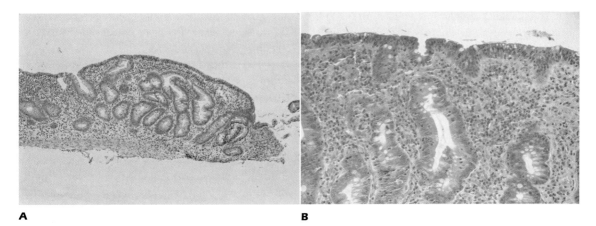

Figure 17.2. Severe intestinal villous atrophy in celiac disease. Note increased numbers of intraepithelial cells located in epithelial cell layer and dense infiltration of lymphocytes and plasma cells in lamina propria. **(A)** Low power **(B)** High power.

and between the intestinal epithelial cells. Several of these histologic features are more diagnostic of celiac disease than others. A completely "flat" intestinal mucosa (totally devoid of villi) is really seen only in celiac disease, not in other enteropathies. In addition, the mucosa in celiac disease is characterized by crypt hyperplasia, but in common variable immunodeficiency (CVID) or HIV infection (see Cases 5 and 9), it is characterized by aregenerative crypts. Finally, celiac disease is associated with plasma cell infiltration that is absent in the lesion associated with CVID, a disease marked by failure of B cells to undergo terminal differentiation to isotype-switched plasma cells. A marked increase in the number of IEL occurs in both celiac disease and CVID, so it is therefore not a distinguishing diagnostic feature.

The above description of the lesion in celiac disease is representative of full-blown, severe disease. In actuality patients display a spectrum of abnormalities ranging from an early lesion characterized by increased numbers of intraepithelial lymphocytes to moderate lesions in which crypt lengthening is also seen and, finally, to more advanced lesions associated with various degrees of villous atrophy as described above.

The biopsy report available several days later indicates severe villous atrophy, increased numbers of intraepithelial lymphoid cells, and a plasma cell infiltration of the lamina propria. With the diagnosis of celiac disease definitively established, the patient is put on a strict gluten-free diet.

You provide Evan's mother with several brochures and websites that provide extensive information as to how to achieve a diet that is completely gluten-free along with contact information for a celiac disease support group that supplies dietary guidance and other useful information. Finally, you inform Evan's mother that celiac disease is a lifelong condition and that Evan will have to be on the diet for the rest of his life. In later years, Evan may be free of symptoms with only partial adherence to the diet. However, this can lead to subclinical villous atrophy, a silent abnormality

associated with an increased risk for the development of intestinal neoplasm (particularly lymphoma).

Follow-Up Visit and Result of Treatment

Evan and his mother return after he has been on a gluten-free diet for two months. At this point his mother reports a substantial weight gain and growth spurt and the disappearance of the fatty stools. Other indicators of dietary deficiency are returning to normal levels: The hemoglobin and albumin levels have increased to normal values. A year later you note that Evan has regained a normal position on the growth curve, and a repeat antiendomesial antibody assay is now negative. This test will be repeated at appropriate intervals to monitor Evan's adherence to the diet.

DIFFERENTIAL DIAGNOSIS OF CELIAC DISEASE

In children, the chief alternative diagnosis to celiac disease is intolerance to a food component other than gluten. The most common is milk intolerance, a condition that leads to a similar clinical course and histologic abnormality. However, milk intolerance manifests itself soon after the introduction of milk, and the patient responds to a milk-free diet rather than a gluten-free diet. Another important distinction is that milk intolerance in infants is a transient condition, probably caused by immaturity of the mucosal immune response; thus, many milk-intolerant patients can ultimately have a normal (milk-inclusive) diet without GI consequences. Finally, in milk intolerance, the various serologic tests specific for gluten sensitivity are negative.

Other alternative diagnoses to consider when confronting a patient with symptoms of celiac disease are various immunodeficiency states such as CVID, IgA deficiency, and HIV infection. In two primary immuno-deficiencies, CVID and IgA deficiency, villous atrophy and malabsorption not sensitive to gluten exclusion may occur due to an autoimmune process. These diseases are identified by tests that show low immunoglobulin levels. IgA deficiency can occur along with celiac disease; in such cases, the diagnosis is established clinically by the response of the disease to a gluten-free diet. In the acquired immunodeficiency due to HIV infection, the diagnosis is made by the low $CD4^+$ T-cell levels, HIV antibody positivity, and the occurrence of opportunistic infections. In addition, there are subtle differences between the histologic HIV picture and the portrait of celiac disease, as mentioned above. Other causes of malabsorption and villous atrophy are graft-versus-host disease, radiation therapy, and GI lymphoma, all conditions that are easily distinguished from celiac disease on clinical grounds. Finally, in rare cases of eosinophilic gastroenteropathy or frank autoimmune enteropathy, an autoimmune response to self-antigens on epithelial cells is the cause of villous atrophy. In the former case, the GI mucosa is heavily infiltrated with eosinophils and there is *eosinophilia* (high eosinophil count in the peripheral blood). In frank autoimmune enteropathy, villous atrophy is present in the absence of positive serologic findings and responsiveness to a gluten-free diet; in many instances this is a diagnosis of exclusion.

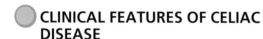

CLINICAL FEATURES OF CELIAC DISEASE

General Manifestations

Celiac disease can occur in several different clinical forms. *Active celiac disease*, such as in Evan's case, presents with frank GI symptoms; these patients generally have involvement of the more distal regions of the small intestine. *"Silent" celiac disease*, a second clinical form, is not associated with GI symptoms but makes its presence felt by the appearance of relatively subtle clinical abnormalities associated with nutritional deficiency, such as reduced bone density and anemia; bowel involvement is limited to the upper small intestine. A third form of celiac disease, known as *"latent" celiac disease*, is not associated with any discernible clinical abnormalities because the GI disease is not sufficient to cause either diarrhea or significant malabsorptions. These patients are discovered mainly through serologic testing, such as testing for the presence of anti-TG antibodies, of "at risk" individuals (family members of symptomatic patients) and random populations. This group constitutes the submerged part of the celiac disease iceberg that makes celiac disease one of the most commonly occurring genetically transmitted diseases.

Although celiac disease may occur in young children, as in Evan's case, the peak age of diagnosis is actually in the third and fourth decades of life. However, even in these late cases the disease may have been present in a latent form since an early age. For unknown reasons, females predominate over males by about 3:1. The onset of symptomatic celiac disease may be either gradual or abrupt; in the latter case, its first appearance may coincide with infection or some other precipitating event. While young children usually present with diarrhea, a wide variety of other symptoms may herald disease, particularly in older patients with long-standing disease. These include various manifestations of *chronic nutritional deficiency* such as short stature, delayed puberty, digital clubbing, apthous stomatitis (oral mucosal ulcers), and glossitis (inflammation of the tongue). In addition, for the same basic reason, the patient may exhibit one or more of the various skin, hematologic, musculoskeletal, neurologic, and reproductive abnormalities listed in Table 17.1.

In contrast to the numerous other nutritional deficiencies encountered in celiac disease, vitamin B_{12} deficiency is rare. Deficiencies in levels of vitamin B_{12} occur when there are abnormalities of intrinsic factor secretion in the stomach or abnormalities of B_{12} intrinsic factor absorption in the terminal ileum, areas of the GI tract rarely affected by celiac disease.

Celiac disease may also manifest mainly (if not entirely) as a skin condition known as *dermatitis herpetiformis*, a pruritic (itchy), vesicular (small blister) skin disease. It occurs mostly on the extensor surfaces of the limb joints but is not limited to these regions; it can occur on the trunk and other areas of the body as well. Histologically, dermatitis herpetiformis is characterized by granular IgA deposited, along with complement, in the basement membrane zone subjacent to the vesicles. The pathologic process is closely related to that of celiac disease. This is evidenced by the association of

TABLE 17.1. Manifestations of Nutritional Deficiency in Celiac Disease

Children	Growth failure
	Anemia: folate deficiency; Fe deficiency
	Neurologic symptoms: ? fat-soluble vitamin deficiency
	Hypoproteinemia: edema
Adults	Anemia
	Osteopenia: vitamin D deficiency
	Infertility
	Neurologic symptoms: periphery neuropathy; ataxia
	Hypoproteinemia: edema

dermatitis herpetiformis with HLA antigens identical to those involved in celiac disease and the skin disease clears when the patients follow a strict gluten-free diet. In addition, the skin IgA deposits contain an antibody that reacts to epidermal TG similar to the one found in patients with celiac disease (see below). Patients with dermatitis herpetiformis usually have subclinical villous atrophy indistinguishable from that occurring in mild to moderate celiac disease. Dermatitis herpetiformis can also be a minor feature of the clinical syndrome dominated by GI disease.

Long-Term Consequences of Celiac Disease

Malignancy. It has been recognized for many years that long-standing celiac disease, that is, celiac disease present for three to six decades, is not infrequently associated with the development of GI malignancy. In most cases, the malignancy is an intestinal lymphoma that appears to originate from the expanded population of intraepithelial lymphocytes. As noted below, this cell population is under the control of IL-15, so it seems likely that the chronic proliferative impulse of IL-15 ultimately gives rise to the cellular mutational "hits" necessary for the development of lymphoma (see also Case 24). Long-term epidemiologic study of celiac disease indicates that control of disease with a gluten-free diet greatly decreases or even eliminates the cancer risk. This is not unexpected; in the absence of the gliadin peptide–mediated inflammation, there is absence of the IL-15-driven proliferation necessary for the mutational risk.

Refractory Disease. Another manifestation of long-standing and untreated celiac disease is a condition known as refractory celiac disease (or "refractory sprue"). In this condition, the patient no longer responds to a gluten-free diet and continues to have severe villous atrophy and malabsorption in spite of the diet. In addition, the patient continues to be at risk for the development of malignancy, which is indeed a frequent outcome. The pathogenesis of refractory celiac disease is not understood, but it implies that the pathologic process leading to celiac disease may sometimes become independent of the presence of gluten in the diet.

Other Autoimmune Syndromes. As mentioned, patients with celiac disease frequently have autoimmune manifestations, including both the formation of autoantibodies and the presence of other autoimmune diseases. The most commonly occurring autoantibody is the aforementioned antiendomysial antibody. The reason that this antigen is a target for immune response in celiac disease is unclear. One factor may be that gliadin peptides form complexes with tTG2 that lead to the appearance of conformational tTG2 antigens not previously seen by the patient's

immune system—hence the usefulness of the test for antibody to tTG2 as a diagnostic tool. Antibodies against other organ-specific antigens also occur and include self-antigens present in the thyroid, adrenal, and islet cell tissues.

In many patients, autoantibodies are accompanied by frank autoimmune disease. Thus, celiac disease patients are prone to a number of other diseases, including insulin-dependent diabetes mellitus, autoimmune thyroiditis, IgA deficiency, Sjogren's syndrome, primary biliary cirrhosis, IgA nephropathy, and idiopathic pulmonary hemosiderosis. The basis of the association of celiac disease with autoimmunity is poorly understood but is at least partially related to the fact that the MHC haplotypes associated with celiac disease are also associated with other autoimmune states; thus, there may be genes that predispose patients to respond to self-antigens.

ORAL TOLERANCE AND NORMAL MUCOSAL IMMUNITY

Few sites in the body are as bombarded by foreign antigens as the GI tract. These include not only antigens derived from the foods we eat but also the antigens associated with the commensal bacteria that reside in the bowel lumen. The mucosal immune system has developed mechanisms to deal with this potential antigen onslaught collectively known as "oral tolerance." Oral tolerance allows the mucosal immune system to become unresponsive to these antigens while preserving its ability to respond to antigens associated with mucosal pathogens. One possible mechanism is the deletion of T cells in the thymus that react to mucosal antigens; this involves the entry of mucosal antigens and their subsequent presentation to developing T cells by thymic stromal and dendritic cells (see Case 3). Another mechanism relates to the propensity of the mucosal immune system to respond to mucosal antigens with the induction of regulatory T (T_{reg}) cells, which down-regulate responses to these antigens. Activation of such regulatory cells requires antigen–TCR (T-cell receptor) engagement, but the activation and proliferation of CD4$^+$ and CD8$^+$ T cells are inhibited in a nonspecific manner, probably through the production of transforming growth factor (TGF)-β. Both of these tolerance-inducing mechanisms occur simultaneously, with the deletion mechanism dominating when high levels of antigen are present, and the regulatory T-cell mechanism dominating with low levels of antigen.

Oral tolerance resulting from T_{reg} cells is a process that is mediated by at least two types of T_{reg} cells. One type is the so-called "natural" T_{reg} cell, identified by its expression of high levels of surface CD25 as well as an intracellular protein known as Foxp3. The latter is a transcription factor with an as-yet-unknown relationship to the suppressor function of the cell. Natural T_{reg} cells, which have specificity for self-antigens, develop in the thymus utilizing a poorly understood process that allows T cells with such specificity to escape negative selection. Such thymic development may occur when mucosal antigens find their way into the thymus after entering the circulation from the GI tract. Following their generation in the thymus, T_{reg} cells with mucosal antigen specificity may traffic back to the mucosal area and expand upon recognition of mucosal antigens at this site. T_{reg} cells with specificity for mucosal antigens may also develop in the mucosa itself from naive non-T_{reg} CD4$^+$ cells under the influence of TGF-β_1 and retinoic acid produced by a subset of dendritic cells. However, in combination with IL-6 (rather than retinoic acid) produced by the same type of dendritic cell, TGF-β_1 induces T_H17 effector cells, which are T helper cells that produce IL-17 (a proinflammatory cytokine). Thus, T_{reg} cell and effector cell induction have a reciprocal relationship.

A second type of regulatory cell participating in the mechanism of oral tolerance is called a Tr-1 T_{reg} cell. These cells are generated exclusively in the periphery (rather than centrally in the thymus) and are induced at these sites by dendritic cells producing IL-10 and/or interferon (IFN)-α. In the mucosa, these dendritic cells are likely to be distinct from those inducing natural T_{reg} cells, both in location and cytokine production. Tr-1 cells are more likely induced in relation to exogenous antigens than self-antigens, but this is not always the case. The separate participation of natural T_{reg} and Tr-1 T_{reg} cells in oral tolerance is not fully understood.

PATHOPHYSIOLOGY OF CELIAC DISEASE

Celiac disease is most essentially a type of food hypersensitivity resulting from an abnormal immune response to gliadin, an ingested protein antigen. Thus, from the point of view of oral tolerance, celiac disease represents a condition in which the normal mechanism of tolerance is not sufficient to prevent a response to a common food antigen. Whether this is due to an overwhelming effector cell response or to an impaired regulatory cell response is unclear. As will become apparent from the discussion below, some evidence for both of these pathologic mechanisms has been found.

Genetic Factors Underlying Celiac Disease

One important factor underlying the pathologic effector T-cell response to gluten in celiac disease is the very strong association of the latter with particular MHC (HLA) alleles. This association is based on the fact that the MHC alleles associated with disease (DQ2 or DQ8 alleles) are the MHC molecules preferentially utilized by dendritic cells to present gluten peptides to CD4$^+$ T cells and thus to induce effector T-cell responses to these antigens. Therefore, celiac disease patients have a built-in,

genetically determined mechanism for mounting responses to gluten peptides that may overwhelm normal mucosal tolerance mechanisms.

Initial studies in the early 1970s showed that 80–85% of celiac patients express the MHC class I allele HLA-B8 (vs. 25% of controls); later studies showed that various MHC class II alleles, such as HLA-DR3, DR5, DPB1, and DQ2, were also overexpressed. This association with a limited number of HLA alleles is best explained by the concept of *linkage disequilibrium*: Distinct alleles at different loci in a particular genetic region tend to be inherited together at a greater incidence than predicted by their individual frequencies. The reason for linkage disequilibrium is not completely understood, but it is widely assumed that the various sets of alleles inherited together provide some sort of selective advantage. In any case, it is now evident that celiac disease is associated with "an extended MHC haplotype" containing multiple HLA alleles rather than with a single MHC allele.

The strongest association of celiac disease is with HLA-DQ alleles; it is now well established that over 95% of celiac patients express either DQ2 consisting of the $DQ\alpha1*0501$ and $D\beta*0201$ alleles encoded by genes on the same chromosome (in cis) or DQ8 consisting of the $D\alpha1*0501$ and $D\beta1*0202$ alleles encoded on opposite chromosomes (in trans) (Fig. 17.3). In the former instance, the genes involved in expression of DQ2 are in linkage disequilibrium with the HLA-DR3 allele, and those associated with expression of DQ8 exhibit linkage disequilibrium with the HLA-DR5 or HLA-DR7 alleles.

Although the association of celiac disease with HLA genes is unusually strong, it does not account for the entire genetic background of celiac disease; the very same HLA alleles associated with celiac disease occur in normal people, and unaffected individuals actually constitute the majority of those with this HLA type. In addition, twin studies suggest that MHC genes contribute no more than 30% of the genetic background of the disease. One non-MHC susceptibility region has been identified in the long arm of chromosome 5 (5q31–33); this locus contains a number of immunologically relevant genes, including genes encoding T_H2 cytokines, the lipopolysaccharide receptor, CD14, and *TIM*, a gene involved in the control of T-cell differentiation (see case 12).

Characteristics of Gluten Peptide Antigen Causing Disease

The specific peptides that induce activation are derived from various gluten proteins as a result of their breakdown by digestive enzymes. They include peptides derived from α and γ gliadins as well as glutinins and are somewhat heterogeneous, although all are rich in proline and glutamine and resistant to further digestion. While these peptides are

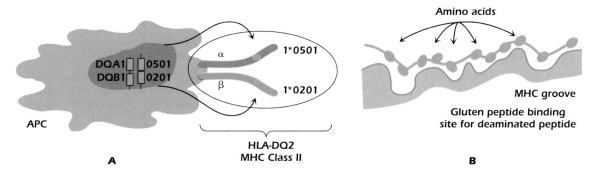

Figure 17.3. MHC alleles in celiac disease. (A) DQ2 alleles found in the majority of patients with celiac disease; these alleles are in linkage disequilibrium with HLA-B8 and HLA-DR3. (B) amino acids in a deaminated gluten peptide bind to the "groove" of the DQ2 MHC α and β chains.

usually derived from wheat proteins, they can be derived from rye or barley proteins as well.

Most of the gluten peptides arising from intestinal degradation do not stimulate immune reactions in their native form, since these peptides lack the negative charge that favors binding to HLA-DQ2 and HLA-DQ8. To obtain such binding ability, they must usually undergo glutamine deamination by TG2, an enzyme expressed on the brush border of epithelial cells or as an extracellular protein in the subepithelial region of the lamina propria. TG2 targets sites on peptides favoring the formation of negatively charged peptides. Since such sites exist on a large variety of peptides derived from various cereal proteins, TG2-mediated deamination results in a large repertoire of peptides that can bind to celiac-associated HLA molecules.

Since gluten peptides must be deaminated by TG2 to induce an immunologic response, attention has focused on the regulation of TG2 as a possible trigger for celiac disease. Indeed, TG2 synthesis is induced by inflammatory cytokines such as IL-6, suggesting that the onset of symptoms following an infection is due to cytokine-induced TG2 synthesis. However, this does not explain why this causes the loss of tolerance to deaminated gluten peptides in these individuals. In addition, the fact that antibodies directed at TG2 are the best serologic marker of the disease is somewhat puzzling, since TG2 is a self-antigen. One explanation is that in reacting with gluten, TG2 changes its physical state and reveals hidden antigenic sites not ordinarily present.

Upon activation by gluten peptides, T cells in the lamina propria produce the T_H1 cytokine IFN-γ. However, in celiac disease this T_H1 response is not driven by IL-12, the "master" T_H1 cytokine, as in the usual T_H1-type inflammation; instead it is driven by IFN-α and IL-18. The origin and significance of this difference are not fully understood, although one outcome may be the lack of granulomatous inflammation in celiac disease, a response that is characteristic of other T_H1 mucosal inflammations. Although the genetically determined T_H1 response to gluten peptides is

a major immunologic feature of celiac disease, it is unclear how this response actually results in its major pathologic feature, namely, the villous atrophy. Thus, while the T_H1 response leads to up-regulation of matrix metalloproteins and other substances that mediate tissue damage, these factors do not lead to villous atrophy in other T_H1 inflammations.

Epithelial Cell Factors Contributing to Celiac Disease

Recent studies have focused on the fact that celiac disease is characterized by the presence of large numbers of IELs and that interactions between these lymphocytes and epithelial cells play an important role in disease pathogenesis, even though CD4+ T cells reactive to gluten peptides are not present.

An important new finding in the study of this "above basement membrane" aspect of celiac disease is the elevation of epithelial cell IL-15 secretion. IL-15 is a cytokine that is known to induce IEL activation and proliferation; indeed, its overexpression in mice leads to the expansion of CD8+ T cells in the intestine and an immunopathologic picture resembling celiac disease. In addition, under the influence of IL-15, CD8+ IELs express the natural killer (NK) receptor NKG2D, and epithelial cells express the ligand for this receptor, the MHC class I–like molecule known as MIC. Thus, IL-15 induces IELs to become cytotoxic cells which attack epithelial cell via an antigen-non specific mechanism. Since the epithelial cells of celiac patients express increased amounts of MIC, and isolated IELs kill MIC-bearing target cells, it is likely that recognition of MIC-bearing cells by cytotoxic IELs is a major pathologic mechanism in celiac disease (Fig. 17.4).

However, the above scenario leaves open the question of the factors leading to increased IL-15 expression. One answer comes from the observation that certain gluten peptides distinct from those that bind HLA-DQ molecules trigger dendritic cells in the lamina propria or epithelial cells to produce IL-15; in addition, these peptides trigger epithelial cells to express MIC. This implies that celiac patients have a second, two-pronged genetic abnormality that involves (1) the ability of gliadin to bind and activate cells via a totally unknown receptor and (2) the ability to induce a particular cytokine via that interaction. At the moment the molecular basis of these putative capabilities is unknown.

Current View of Celiac Disease Pathogenesis

In summary of the immunopathogenesis of celiac disease, one can say that there is now sound evidence that at least two gliadin peptide–specific mechanisms are necessary for disease expression. One involves the presentation of gliadin peptides by lamina propria dendritic cells to CD4$^+$ T cells in the context of a specific set of inherited MHC molecules. This results in CD4$^+$ T-cell activation and the release of inflammatory cytokines. A second mechanism involves gliadin peptide–induced production of IL-15 by IELs, epithelial cells, and possibly dendritic cells, which results in cytotoxic IEL with the capacity to attack epithelial cells. Both of these pathologic processes can contribute to villous atrophy and malabsorption, although it is the IL-15/IEL centered mechanism that leads to the complete villous flattening so characteristic of celiac disease. It seems likely that these separate disease mechanisms engage in cross-talk that enables or intensifies their respective effects. IL-15 may be the linking factor since there is

recent evidence that IL-15 suppresses TGF-β_1 signaling, the major inhibitory cytokine produced by some of the negative regulatory T cells that mediate mucosal tolerance. Thus, the excess secretion of IL-15 may permit an ongoing T-cell response to gliadin peptides that is central to the pathogenesis of celiac disease. Another possibility is that epithelial cells interacting with gluten peptides express molecules (such as MIC and HLA-E) that are recognized by NK receptors on certain subpopulations of IEL and thus induce the latter to become cytotoxic for the epithelial cells (Fig. 17.4). This possible mechanism is favored by the secretion by epithelial cells of high levels of IL-15, a cytokine that activates IEL and up-regulates NK receptors.

TREATMENT OF CELIAC DISEASE

As already mentioned, a gluten-free diet is the mainstay of treatment of celiac disease and usually produces excellent results. The exceptions include very long standing cases in which there is irreversible damage to the mucosa and refractory celiac disease, which is unaffected by a gluten-free diet. While it may seem difficult to remove gluten from the diet, it can be done if the patient (or parent of the patient) is sufficiently motivated to carefully identify hidden sources of gluten in prepared foods and to find acceptable substitutes for gluten-containing foods. Although ingestion of gluten does not necessarily lead to symptomatology in the patient

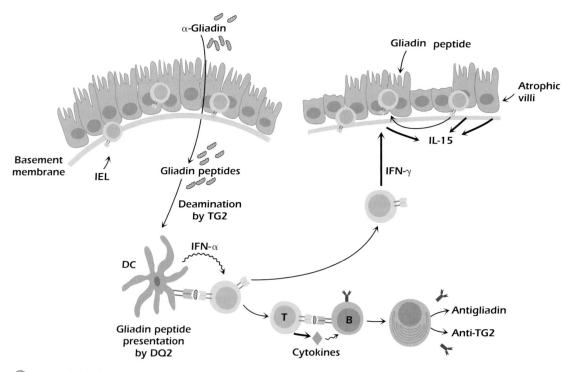

Figure 17.4. Immunologic mechanisms underlying celiac disease. Gluten peptides induce T-cell cytokine production in the lamina propria and activate epithelial cells to produce IL-15. These two processes act in tandem to stimulate intraepithelial cell cytotoxicity of epithelial cells.

who has been on a prolonged and strict gluten-free diet, it is not wise to encourage lapses in adherence to the diet, since this can lead to subclinical disease and increase the risk of the development of malignancy.

Nondietary approaches to the treatment of celiac disease are the subject of ongoing research efforts, but their effectiveness is as yet unproven. These include the use of agents to inactivate transglutaminase, agents to inhibit IL-15 or other aspects of the innate responses, and agents that block the gliadin peptide–specific T-cell response.

REFERENCES

Di Sabatino A, Pickard KM, Gordon LN, Salvati V, Mazzarella G, Beattie RM, Vossenkaemper A, Rovedatti L, Leakey NA, Croft NM, Troncone R, Coraszza GR, Stagg AJ, Monteleone G, MacDonald TT (2007): Evidence for the role of interferon-alpha production by dendritic cells in the T_H1 response in celiac disease. *Gastroenterology* 133:1175–1187.

Faria AM, Weiner HL (2006): Oral tolerance: Therapeutic implications for autoimmune diseases. *Clin Dev Immunol* 13:143–157.

Ferguson A, McClure JP, Townley RR (1976): Intraepithelial lymphocyte counts in small intestinal biopsies from children with diarrhea. *Acta Paediatr Scand* 65:541–546.

Gianfrani C, Levings MK, Sartirana C, Mazzarella G, Barba G, Zanzi D, Camarca A, Taquinto G, Giardullo N, Auricchio S, Troncone R, Roncarolo MG (2006): Gliadin-specific type 1 regulatory T cells from the intestinal mucosa of treated celiac patients inhibit pathogenic T cells. *J Immunol* 177:4178–4186.

Greco L, Babron MC, Corazza GR, Percopo S, Sica R, Clot F, Fulchignoni-Lataud MC, Zavattari P, Momigliano-Richiardi P, Casari G, Gasparini P, Tosi R, Mantovani V, De Virgiliis S, Iacono G, D'Alfonso A, Selinger-Leneman H, Lemainque A, Serre JL, Clerget-Darpoux F (2001): Existence of a genetic risk factor on chromosome 5q in Italian celiac disease families. *Ann Hum Genet* 65:35.

Green PH, Fleischauer AT, Bhagat G, Goyal R, Jabri B, Neugat AI (2003): Risk of malignancy in patients with celiac disease. *Am J Med* 115:191–195.

Green PH, Jabri B (2006): Celiac disease. *Annu Rev Med* 57:207–221.

Holmes GK, Prior P, Lane MR, Pope D, Allan RN (1989): Malignancy in coeliac disease—Effect of a gluten free diet. *Gut* 30:333–338.

Jabri B, Sollid L (2006): Mechanisms of disease: Immunopathogenesis of celiac disease. *Nature Clin Pract* 3:516–525.

Kárpáti S (2004): Dermatitis herpetiformis: Close to unraveling a disease. *J Dermatol Sci* 34:83–90.

Louka AS, Sollid LM (2003): HLA in coeliac disease: Unravelling the complex genetics of a complex disorder. *Tissue Antigens* 61:105–117.

Maiuri L, Ciacci C, Ricciardelli I, Vacca L, Raia V, Auricchio S, Picard J, Osman M, Quaratino S, Londei M (2003): Association between innate response to gliadin and activation of pathogenic T cells in celiac disease. *Lancet* 362:30–37.

Marsh MN (1992): Gluten, major histocompatibility complex, and the small intestine. A molecular and immunobiologic approach to the spectrum of gluten sensitivity ("celiac sprue"). *Gastroenterology* 102:330–354.

Mention JJ, Ben Ahmed M, Bègue B, Barbe U, Verkarre V, Asnafi V, Columbel JF, Cugnenc PH, Ruemmele FM, McIntyre E, Brousse N, Cellier C, Cerf-Bensussan N (2003): Interleukin 15: A key to disrupted intraepithelial lymphocyte homeostasis and lymphogenesis in celiac disease. *Gastroenterology* 125:730–745.

Meresse B, Curran SA, Ciszewski C, Orbelyan G, Setty M, Bhagat G, Lee L, Tretiakova M, Semrad C, Kistner E, Winchester RJ, Braud V, Lanier LL, Geraghty DE, Green PH, Guandalini S, Jabri B (2006): Reprogramming of CTL into natural killer-like cells in celiac disease. *J Exp Med* 203:1343–1355.

Molberg O, Mcadam SN, Körner R, Quarsten H, Kristiansen C, Madsen L, Fugger L, Scott H, Norén O, Roespstorff P, Lundin KE, Sjöstrom H, Sollid LM (1998): Tissue transglutaminase selectively modifies gliadin peptides that are recognized by gut-derived T cells in celiac disease. *Nature Med* 4:713–717.

Roberts A, Lee L, Schwarz E, Groh V, Spies T, Ebert EC, Jabri B (2001): NKG2D receptors induced by IL-15 costimulate CD28-negative effector CTL in the tissue microenvironment. *J Immunol* 167:5527–5530.

Rostom A, Dube C, Cranney A, Saloojee N, Sy R, Garritty C, Sampson M, Zhang L, Yazdi F, Mamaladze V, Pan I, MacNeil J, Mack D, Patel D, Moher D (2005): The diagnostic accuracy of serologic tests for celiac disease: A systemic review. *Gastroenterology* 128:S38–46.

Sardy M, Karpati S, Merk, B, Paulsson M, Smyth N (2002): Epidermal transglutaminase (TGase 3) is the autoantigen in dermatitis herpetiformis. *J Exp Med* 195:747–757.

Shan L, Qiao SW, Arentz-Hansen H, Molberg Ø, Gray GM, Sollid IM, Khosia C (2005): Identification and analysis of multivalent proteolytically resistant peptides from gluten: Implications for celiac sprue. *J Proteome Res* 4:1732–1741.

Sollid LM, Molberg O, McAdam S, Lundin KE (1997): Autoantibodies in celiac disease: Tissue transglutaminase—Guilt by association? *Gut* 41:851–852.

Sun CM, Hall JA, Blank RB, Bouladoux N, Oukka M, Mora JR, Belkaid Y (2007): Small intestine lamina propria dendritic cells promote *de novo* generation of Foxp3T reg cells via retinoic acid. *J Exp Med* 204:1775–1785.

Wan YY, Flavell RA (2007): Regulatory T cells, transforming growth factor-beta, and immune suppression. *Proc Am Thorac Soc* 4:271–276.

18

INFLAMMATORY BOWEL DISEASE

PETER MANNON*

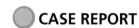 **CASE REPORT**

"In the last few months I've had increasing stomach cramps and now I see blood in my stool."

History and Initial Evaluation

Jason, a 21-year-old college student living at his school dormitory, comes to you, his primary care physician, with the above chief complaint. He states that about six months ago he noticed the onset of abdominal cramping pain around his belly button (umbilicus). It was most evident one to two hours after large meals and once was associated with vomiting, which relieved the pain. Three months ago, Jason noticed that he was losing weight and felt unusually fatigued; in addition, on several occasions he seemed to have a fever, but this was not associated with symptoms of a cold. Four weeks ago Jason became really concerned when he noticed that his stools were looser and more frequent and sometimes had blood in them. Somewhat frightened by the latter, he called his parents, who asked him to return home for medical evaluation.

On review of his systems, Jason reveals that the abdominal symptoms described above have been accompanied by

*With contributions from Warren Strober and Susan R. S. Gottesman

joint stiffness and some pain in his hands, wrists, hips, and ankles. On physical examination you note that Jason looks fairly well, if a bit underweight for his height. Abdominal examination reveals tenderness in both lower quadrants, especially on the right side, but the abdomen is soft, has normal bowel sounds, is free of palpable masses, and displays no liver or spleen enlargement. Rectal examination shows two large skin tags at the anal verge but no evidence of hemorrhoids, anal canal tenderness, or draining *fistulae* (abnormal connections between two structures). Other physical findings include three aphthous ulcers (canker sores) on the oral mucosa and mild clubbing of the fingers; however, the joints show no evidence of synovitis, loss of range of motion, or tenderness.

What is the differential diagnosis of bloody diarrhea?

Frank blood in the stool (ranging in color from maroon to brick red to bright red) suggests a source of bleeding in the lower gastrointestinal (GI) tract (small and large intestines, rectum). Although upper GI bleeding usually presents with dark tarry stools, blood may be seen as a result of very brisk bleeding from ulcers in the stomach or small bowel due to peptic ulcer disease, Meckel's diverticulum, or vascular lesions. In these settings, diarrhea does not necessarily occur; when it does, it is most likely related to the cathartic effect of the intraluminal blood itself and not to another underlying process. Such brisk bleeding would be unlikely to continue over a six-month period without the need for urgent medical intervention.

*Lower GI bleeding can result from inflammatory disease of the bowel or have noninflammatory causes. Noninflammatory causes include hemorrhoids, fissure-in-ano, diverticulosis, arteriovenous malformations or telangiectasia, eroded large polyps, or carcinomas in the distal bowel. Inflammatory causes of bloody diarrhea include enteric infections due to bacteria (such as toxin-mediated Clostridium difficile colitis), parasites, or viruses [such as cytomegalovirus (CMV) colitis]. In addition, one of the **inflammatory bowel diseases (IBDs)**, such as ulcerative colitis or Crohn's disease, may cause bloody diarrhea; and IBD that can occur in immunodeficiency states (such as chronic granulomatous disease, common variable immunodeficiency disease; see Case 5) or, rarely, in association with ischemic colitis due to bowel infarction. When bloody diarrhea occurs in the setting of inflammation, it is typically accompanied by the presence of polymorphonuclear cells in the stool, which is evident either as an obvious purulent exudate (as in dysentery) or as a covert finding noted on microscopic examination.*

Evidence from the patient's history, such as age, concomitant medical conditions, associated pain [epigastric, anorectal (tenesmus)], food/travel/contact/drug exposure history, presence of specific symptoms (proctitis, jaundice, fever), and duration of symptoms, can help determine the cause of bloody diarrhea. As noted above, the six-month history tends to rule out rapid and large bleeding episodes and some of the infectious causes (particularly some bacterial causes) of bloody diarrhea.

You order a complete blood count (CBC), erythrocyte sedimentation rate (ESR), and C-reactive protein (CRP) level and ask for a stool specimen to be sent for microscopic examination and culture.

Results of Blood Work.
The CBC reveals a mildly elevated white blood cell count (11,900 cells/μL, reference range 4800–10,800 cells/μL) without an increase in immature forms as well as a microcytic anemia (Hgb 9.1 g/dL, reference range 13.5–16 g/dL; mean corpuscular volume (MCV) 78 fL, reference range 85–98 fL), and an increased platelet cell count (630,000/μL, reference range 130,000–400,000/μL). The ESR is markedly elevated at 65 mm/h (reference range 0–30 mm/h) and the CRP is also increased.

How do you interpret these results?

The elevated white blood cell count, platelets, ESR, and CRP are all consistent with the presence of inflammation. The absence of immature white blood cell forms suggests that there is no current infection. Jason's significant anemia, which is microcytic (small size of red blood cells), is indicative of iron deficiency and suggests that there has been

blood loss for an extended period, which has depleted his iron stores.

Results of Stool Examination.
The microscopic examination reveals the presence of white blood cells, indicating that an inflammation is present. However, a search for the presence of ova or parasites proves negative, as does stool culture to determine the presence of an enteric bacterial pathogen (enterohemorrhagic *Escherichia coli, Salmonella, Shigella, Campylobacter jejuni*); in addition, a test for the presence of *C. difficile* toxin proves negative.

With evidence supporting an inflammatory state but no sign of a causative bowel infection, you entertain the possibility that Jason has a form of IBD, such as Crohn's disease or ulcerative colitis. Recognizing that the diagnosis and subsequent treatment of this disease will probably require special expertise, you refer Jason to a gastroenterologist for further workup.

Jason's Diagnostic Workup: Colonoscopy and Biopsy of Large Bowel

The next day Jason is seen by a gastroenterologist, who reviews the history and laboratory findings and performs another physical examination. He also comes to the conclusion that Jason's course suggests IBD.

What are the diagnostic features of IBD that lead the gastroenterologist to this conclusion?

The diagnosis of IBD should be entertained in patients who have persistent GI symptoms such as diarrhea, hematochezia (blood in the stool), and abdominal pain/cramps, particularly when these occur in a relatively young individual and are associated with unexplained constitutional symptoms such as fever, fatigue, and weight loss. The latter symptoms, while nonspecific, are in reality unmistakable clues that serious inflammation may be present. The index of suspicion is further increased when the patient also complains of certain extraintestinal symptoms such as arthritis, uveitis, fatigue, or unusual skin rashes such as erythema nodosum (inflammation of the subcutaneous fat that presents with small red painful nodules) and pyoderma gangrenosum (reddish nodules that become ulcerative lesions, usually on the legs); these extraintestinal symptoms are also hallmarks of this disease complex.

Crohn's disease and ulcerative colitis are the most common members of a diverse group of "idiopathic" IBDs, a disease category that also includes lymphocytic enteritis, collagenous enteritis/colitis, eosinophilic gastroenteritis, and autoimmune enteritis. While Crohn's disease and ulcerative colitis are related to each other both etiologically and genetically, they have very distinct immunopathologic bases and manifest different clinical patterns. Accordingly, they respond differently to the various drug and surgical treatments now available.

Assuming that Jason has inflammatory bowel disease, what criteria can the gastroenterologist use to distinguish Crohn's disease from its "sister" inflammatory bowel disease, ulcerative colitis?

Because both groups of patients experience clinical symptoms of abdominal pain, diarrhea, rectal bleeding, fever, and lethargy, other features (endoscopic, radiographic, and histologic) are used to distinguish Crohn's disease from ulcerative colitis. First, the **distribution of inflammation** *is considered.* **Crohn's disease** *can involve virtually any part of the digestive tract, from the mouth to the anus, although colonic inflammation alone or in combination with small bowel inflammation is the most frequently observed pattern. Thus, the distribution of inflamed bowel in the patient group as a whole is small bowel involvement (usually the terminal ileum) alone in 30% of patients, colonic involvement alone in 30% of patients, and involvement of both areas (usually terminal ileum, adjacent ascending colon, and not infrequently the rectum) in 40% of patients.* **Ulcerative colitis***, in contrast, is marked by inflammation limited to the rectum and colon. In virtually all cases this takes the form of involvement of the rectum alone (proctitis) or involvement of the rectum and various lengths of contiguous colon, extending in a retrograde fashion. Thus, the distribution of inflamed bowel in the ulcerative colitis patient group as a whole is rectum alone in 30% of patients, rectum and left colon to splenic flexure in 50% of patients, and the entire rectum and colon (so-called universal colitis) in 20% of patients. Occasionally, the colonic inflammation can extend across the ileocecal valve to involve a short segment of the terminal ileum ("backwash ileitis"), but it does not affect the rest of the small bowel.*

Second, the **continuity and character** *of the areas of inflammation and the effects of inflammation over time are taken into consideration. Crohn's disease manifests as a discontinuous inflammation giving rise to endoscopic findings of affected inflamed (red, swollen, friable) mucosa and, at times, ulcerated areas alternating with unaffected normal appearing areas ("skip areas") of bowel resulting in a "cobblestone-like" mucosal appearance. In contrast, ulcerative colitis is marked by continuous inflammation devoid of skip areas (Fig. 18.1).*

*The distribution of the inflammation in the bowel wall also distinguishes the two entities. Endoscopic biopsy samples only the superficial layer of the mucosa, generally to the muscularis mucosa, making histologic assessment difficult. However, Crohn's disease is marked by intense cellular infiltration involving the full thickness of the bowel wall. As a result, a removed segment of bowel involved by Crohn's disease characteristically has a "garden hose" appearance; on opening lengthwise, the bowel does not lie flat (Fig. 18.2). Over time, this thickening can lead to narrowing of the bowel lumen (strictures), giving rise to obstructive symptoms (vomiting, postprandial abdominal pain, constipation). Such obstruction accompanied by full-thickness inflammation leads to the formation of fistulae [inflammatory tracts connecting the diseased gut lumen to another part of the intestine (**enteroenteric fistula**), to the*

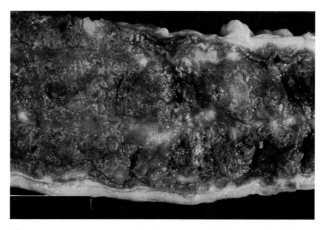

Figure 18.1. Section of large intestine (opened longitudinally) with ulcerative colitis illustrating the continuous nature of the ulceration and the flatness of the colon wall.

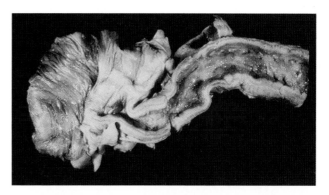

Figure 18.2. Section of small intestine and cecum with Crohn's disease illustrating the thickening of the intestinal wall. Notice that the bowel does not lay flat upon opening.

*bladder (**enterovesicular fistula**), to the skin (**enterocutaneous fistula**), and from the rectum to the perineum (**perianal fistula**)]. Alternatively, the obstruction and inflammation lead to intra-abdominal abscess formation accompanied by localized pain and systemic symptoms.*

In contrast, inflammation caused by ulcerative colitis tends to be superficial (above the muscularis mucosa). For this reason, bowel narrowing is rare, and ulcerative colitis is a nonfistulizing disease. Opening and examination of a segment of colon will reveal a flat piece of bowel with a continuous ulcerated hemorrhagic surface, sometimes punctuated by pseudopolyps (see Figs. 18.1 and 18.3). These pseudopolyps are relatively uninvolved areas of mucosa that are raised above the surrounding ulcerated areas and look like polyps. The involvement of the rectum typically produces proctitis symptoms (rectal urgency, feelings of incomplete evacuation, frequent bowel movements).

In summary, the endoscopic appearance of ulcerative colitis is inflammation involving the rectum and various lengths of colon extending proximally toward the cecum,

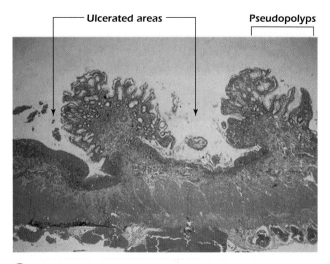

Figure 18.3. Low-power microscopic picture of ulcerative colitis showing pseudopolyps. These can be seen on gross examination as well.

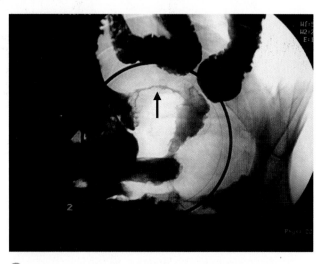

Figure 18.4. Barium X ray of a small bowel demonstrating a "string sign" in the terminal ileum resulting from luminal narrowing characteristic of Crohn's disease. This narrowing gives rise to the clinical symptoms of obstruction.

*depending on the extent of disease. Crohn's disease shows discontinuous involvement, possibly accompanied by narrowing of the lumen. Radiologic examinations [barium studies, computerized tomography (CT) scans, and magnetic resonance imaging (MRI) studies] are more useful in Crohn's disease than in ulcerative colitis, particularly to investigate disease in the small intestine. A double-contrast study using a barium swallow combined with gas can demonstrate the narrowing of the intestines (**string sign**; see Fig. 18.4), cobblestone appearance of the surface, fistulae formation (with the barium tracking along the connections), and discontinuous involvement characteristic of Crohn's disease. In ulcerative colitis, a barium enema with air contrast may be used to delineate the extent of disease in the*

colon, but endoscopic examination is just as useful and allows biopsy sampling. Although radiologic examination can supply information that help support the differential diagnosis of IBD, it is perhaps more useful for investigating the complications of established disease than as a primary diagnostic measure. This is most apparent when investigating obstructive-type abdominal pain (especially in bowel areas beyond the reach of endoscopes such as the mid-small bowel), when looking for infectious complications (such as abscess formation following bowel perforation), and when confirming the track of perianal fistulae or internal fistulae.

Finally, histologic features may help distinguish the inflammation present in Crohn's disease from that of ulcerative colitis; however, there are no histologic features on biopsy (as mentioned above, the biopsy being superficial only) that strictly distinguish the two diseases. A confluent inflammatory infiltrate in the lamina propria with a predominance of activity in the areas closest to the epithelial surface is supportive of ulcerative colitis (Fig. 18.5). On the other hand, noncaseating granulomas and a patchy, deep, and focal inflammatory cell infiltrate are supportive of Crohn's disease (Fig. 18.6). However, because granulomas are more likely to be found in the deeper areas or draining lymph nodes, they are found only infrequently in biopsy samples. These relatively distinct features are mixed with those common to both Crohn's disease and ulcerative colitis: distortion of the crypt architecture, an indication of the chronicity of inflammation, infiltration of the lamina propria with lymphocytes, macrophages and plasma cells (an indication of chronic inflammation), and the presence of polymorphonuclear cells (an indication of acute inflammation). The polymorphonuclear cells can infiltrate the crypt epithelium (cryptitis) or collect in the crypt lumen (crypt abscess). Because the limitations of histologic

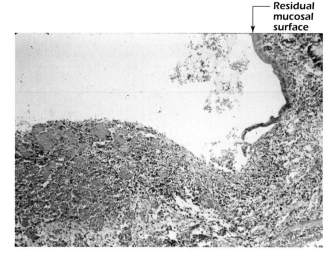

Figure 18.5. Microscopic picture of a large bowel wall characteristic of ulcerative colitis illustrating base of large ulcer, superficial underlying cellular infiltration, and exudation of cells into the bowel lumen.

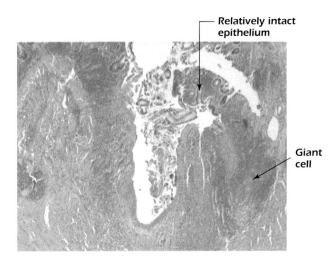

Figure 18.6. Microscopic picture of inflammation in Crohn's disease illustrating part of the full-thickness inflammation and granulomas containing giant cells. Example of small area of relatively intact surface epithelium is denoted with arrow.

distinction on mucosal biopsy are significant, they are not as useful in differentiating Crohn's disease from ulcerative colitis unless well-formed granulomata are present.

In recent years attempts have been made to distinguish Crohn's disease from ulcerative colitis by the presence of certain serologic markers. This has been only partially successful; the markers so far identified are present predominantly but not exclusively in one or the other disease. For instance, 70% of ulcerative colitis patients have high titer antibodies to p-ANCA (pericytoplasmic antineutrophil cytoplasmic antibody); 20% of Crohn's disease patients have low titers. On the other hand, many patients with Crohn's disease have high titer antibodies to OmpC (anti–outer membrane protein C) and ASCA (anti–Saccharomyces cerevisiae); although much less common, these antibodies can also occur in ulcerative colitis.

The above criteria allow assignment of a diagnosis of Crohn's disease or ulcerative colitis with some certainty to 90–95% of patients. The remaining 5–10% of cases (which necessarily involve only the colon because ulcerative colitis is strictly limited to this organ) are referred to as **indiscriminate colitis**. *Because the basic biologic behavior of the two diseases is intrinsically different, continued observation over time will often reveal the true nature of a patient's inflammation.*

Based on Jason's symptoms and physical examination, the gastroenterologist favors the diagnosis of Crohn's disease rather than ulcerative colitis, mainly because obstructive-type abdominal pain has dominated the clinical picture, and proctitis and rectal symptoms have not occurred (rectal urgency and sense of incomplete evacuation). In addition, anal skin tags are present (occur more frequently in Crohn's disease), and there is evidence

of oral mucosal involvement. However, he recognizes that in order to arrive at a definitive diagnosis, he will have to make a direct visual inspection of the colon and obtain biopsies. Accordingly, one week later, after following a bowel-cleansing protocol, Jason undergoes colonoscopy in an outpatient endoscopy suite.

This procedure reveals a bowel inflammation marked by the presence of scattered ulcerations in the rectum and sigmoid colon and patchy erythema in the transverse and ascending colon; in addition, it shows multiple ulcerations in the cecum up to and including the ileocecal valve (Fig. 18.7). When the colonoscope is inserted into the terminal ileum, it reveals the presence of a reddened, edematous, friable mucosa in this small bowel area. Biopsies are taken from the inflamed areas, normal appearing intervening mucosa, and sites of ulcers. On subsequent histologic examination, the biopsies show the presence of a severe infiltration of mucosa with mononuclear cells extending down to the level of the muscularis mucosa (see Fig. 18.6). The crypt architecture is distorted by shortening and branching, and some crypt spaces are filled with polymorphonuclear cells (crypt abscesses). In scattered areas, there are granulomatous whorls with associated multinucleated giant cells that show no evidence of necrosis. These endoscopic and biopsy findings are fully compatible with the diagnosis of Crohn's disease and lead the gastroenterologist to settle on this diagnosis.

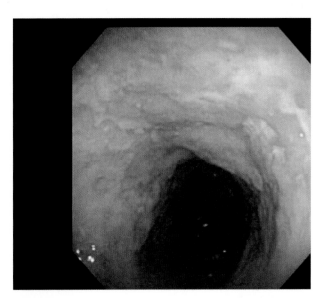

Figure 18.7. Endoscopic appearance of the descending colon in a patient with active Crohn's disease. Note the white-based ulceration, reddened patches, and some near-normal areas interspersed.

Jason's Subsequent Clinical Course and Treatment

The gastroenterologist communicates his findings to you, as Jason's primary care doctor; together you decide that you should speak to Jason and his family but that the gastroenterologist is best equipped to manage Jason at this time of active disease. Accordingly, you explain the results and describe the disease to the family, emphasizing that, although this is a lifelong condition, many individuals experience long periods of quiescence. The most important steps are to get the disease under control now so that no complications (such as fistulae) develop and then to maintain a lifestyle that does not provoke recurrent symptoms.

The gastroenterologist then initiates treatment for Crohn's disease by placing Jason on a mild anti-inflammatory agent called mesalamine (5-aminosalicylic acid). After taking this drug for two weeks, Jason has some improvement in his symptoms, but postprandial abdominal pain and intermittent bloody diarrhea persist. The gastroenterologist then decides to treat the inflammation more definitively with a short course of high doses of corticosteroids (prednisone by mouth) in addition to the mesalamine. Jason obtains complete resolution of his symptoms after about one week. The gastroenterologist then gradually reduces Jason's steroid dose over three months, and he remains symptom free on mesalamine alone. During this time, a barium study of his small bowel is performed which shows a narrowed area in the distal ileum; however, no additional treatment is instituted because Jason does not report any obstructive symptoms.

Unfortunately, eight months after discontinuing the steroids, the abdominal pain and diarrhea return, again associated with intermittent fever and fatigue. At this point the gastroenterologist once again finds abdominal tenderness on examination and performs a repeat colonoscopy that shows active inflammation of the colon, including some areas that had previously been unaffected. The gastroenterologist reinstitutes corticosteroid treatment and again sees rapid clinical improvement. This time, however, he adds azathioprine (6-mercaptopurine derivative) to the treatment regimen and continues with this therapy even after the corticosteroids have been tapered. Jason reports feeling well while taking azathioprine and mesalamine at his most recent visit, 12 months after discontinuing the corticosteroids.

CLINICAL FEATURES OF CROHN'S DISEASE AND ULCERATIVE COLITIS

Crohn's Disease

Jason's history and clinical course illustrate several points about Crohn's disease. First, because the disease often starts with mild and intermittent symptoms, patients often do not

seek medical care immediately; even if they do, they may (reasonably) not be investigated for the presence of IBD. Second, because Crohn's disease is an autoimmune disease, it is associated with other manifestations of a deranged immune system, such as migratory polyarthritis and erythema nodosum. Third, other symptoms are manifested over time as a result of the diarrhea and associated blood loss. Jason's iron deficiency anemia (which contributed to his fatigue) was the result of persistent low level of blood loss due to disease involvement of his colon. With extensive small bowel involvement, nutritional deficiencies as a result of malabsorption may also be recognized, including protein-losing enteropathy, vitamin B_{12} deficiency, or malabsorption of bile salts resulting in fat and vitamin deficiencies and wasting.

Like Jason, a large proportion of patients with aggressive Crohn's disease have a relapsing disease pattern that requires repeated courses of high-intensity anti-inflammatory medical treatment despite attempts to prevent exacerbations with chronic immunosuppressants such as azathioprine. These flare-ups are sometimes associated with physical or emotional stress—hence the doctor's advice about lifestyle choices. The recurrent bouts of inflammation are serious because they can lead to irreversible complications such as obstruction, the formation of fistulae, and even perforation. In fact, 60% of patients require surgical treatment 10 years after diagnosis, and nearly 80% of patients go "under the knife" by the time 20 years have passed. The general approach is to try to prevent relapses and complications and therefore avoid surgery, since the disease can involve any area of the GI tract and surgery is not curative. This can be contrasted with the surgical approach to ulcerative colitis (see below), highlighting the importance of distinguishing between these entities. Treatment of Crohn's disease has two goals: (1) rapid improvement of symptoms and (2) maintenance of remission. Mesalamine, corticosteroids, and even antibiotics help induce remission, and azathioprine is effective for remission maintenance. Most recently, an antibody directed against the inflammatory cytokine tumor necrosis factor α (called anti-TNF-α) has been effective in inducing remission and can also be helpful in maintaining remission in some patients for up to one year.

An additional long-term complication of active Crohn's disease is the increased incidence of cancer of the GI tract. The risk is increased five to six times over that experienced by the general population; this is significant but markedly below the increase in risk seen in ulcerative colitis (see below).

Ulcerative Colitis

As already discussed, the clinical presentation of ulcerative colitis is similar to Crohn's disease, both usually present with bloody diarrhea that is sometimes accompanied by abdominal pain. Although iron deficiency anemia may occur due to blood loss, malabsorption syndromes are not seen in ulcerative colitis since the small intestines are not affected. This disease also has a relapsing–remitting course with flare-ups sometimes precipitated by stress or *C. difficile* overgrowth. A serious complication more frequent in ulcerative colitis although still quite rare is toxic megacolon. This is a condition believed to be the result of the inflammatory involvement of the neural plexus in the bowel wall which is marked by the termination of all bowel movement, dilatation of the colon, gangrenous change, and the possibility of bowel rupture (a potentially lethal event).

A more common complication is the marked increase in colonic carcinoma. Those with a history of disease of 10 years or more that involves the entire colon have a 20 to 30-fold increase in the incidence of cancer. Screening these patients, normally done in the general population by removing any identified colon polyps, is challenging in those who are riddled with "pseudopolyps."

Since ulcerative colitis is limited to the colon, a patient with poorly controlled disease can, in the extreme, be treated with removal of the colon. This, of course, has its own set of difficulties, but in addition to dealing with the inflammation, it obviates the threat of colonic carcinoma.

THE PATHOGENESIS OF INFLAMMATORY BOWEL DISEASE

Immunopathologic Basis of Disease

As indicated above, Crohn's disease and ulcerative colitis are two very different clinical entities; however, there is clear evidence that they are related genetically and immunopathologically. This is perhaps best illustrated by certain multiplex families with many family members with IBD, in which some individuals have Crohn's disease and others have ulcerative colitis. In addition, some patients manifest an indeterminate colitis that cannot be clearly defined as either. Lastly, some emerging disease susceptibility genes are shared by both Crohn's and ulcerative colitis. These genetic/epidemiologic and clinical observations make it apparent that the two diseases are merely different manifestations of the same basic pathophysiology. It is therefore appropriate to begin our discussion by considering the basic underlying factors that are common to these two forms of the disease.

IBD: Autoimmune Disease Caused by "Auto-antigens" in Nonpathogenic Mucosal Microflora.

In recent years, the dominant view of the immunopathogenesis of IBD is that both Crohn's disease and ulcerative colitis are due to an excessive and/or unregulated immune

response to antigens present in the intestinal microflora. This is inferred from experiments showing that T cells from IBD patients proliferate and secrete inflammatory cytokines when exposed to antigens from their own intestinal microflora, but not when exposed to antigens from the microflora of other individuals, whereas T cells from healthy controls respond to antigens from neither of these bacterial sources (Fig. 18.8). The etiologic role of the microflora antigens is also supported by the study of numerous mouse models of mucosal inflammation which resemble IBD both pathologically and immunologically. In some models, the mucosal inflammation develops spontaneously because of the presence of a genetic defect, such as an IL-2 or IL-10 deficiency. In other models inflammation is induced by exposing the mouse per rectum to a **haptenating agent** (a compound that reacts with and adds chemical groups to proteins to render them immunogenic), such as trinitrobenzene sulfonic acid (TNBS), which can react with endogenous (self) proteins. In both types of mouse models, the inflammation either does not develop or is highly attenuated if the mouse is maintained under germ-free conditions. The colitis induced by exposure to TNBS (TNBS colitis) is particularly instructive because it only occurs if TNBS is delivered in the presence of ethanol; the ethanol is necessary to break the mucosal epithelial barrier and allow exposure of mucosal tissues to the bacterial microflora. In addition, the colitis only occurs in mouse strains that are genetically programmed to respond to components of the microflora, such as lipopolysaccharide (LPS), with high levels of IL-12 secretion. Thus, you could say that the induction of TNBS colitis requires an initial event in which the mucosal immune system is hyperresponding to the bacterial microflora with the production of IL-12; this sets the stage for a response to a particular antigen [TNP (trinitrophenyl)-substituted proteins], which causes the colitis.

The third and perhaps most powerful reason to believe that IBD represents an abnormal immune response to antigens in the intestinal microflora comes from the recent discovery that about 15% of patients with Crohn's disease have a homozygous mutation in the gene *CARD15* on chromosome 16 that encodes a protein known as NOD2. NOD2 is an intracellular sensor of muramyl dipeptide (MDP), a component of a ubiquitous glycoprotein (peptidoglycan) present in the cell walls of both Gram-positive and Gram-negative bacteria. Recent studies of NOD2-deficient mice provide insight into how a NOD2 mutation can lead to mucosal inflammation. In normal mice, peptidoglycan delivers a powerful signal to cells via the cell surface Toll-like receptor (TLR) 2 that leads to the activation of nuclear factor (NF)-κB, the transcription factor involved in the induction of inflammatory cytokines such as IL-12 and IL-18. Peptidoglycan also delivers a second signal to cells via NOD2. NOD2 is activated by

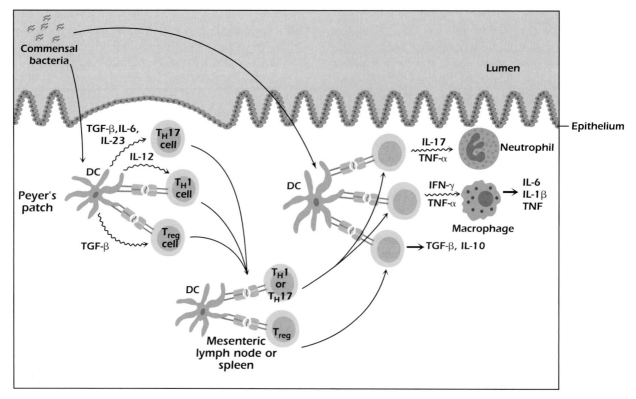

⬤ Figure 18.8. The dysregulated T_H1/T_H17 mucosal immune response underlying Crohn's disease. Antigens associated with the commensal microflora of the gut are taken up by dendritic cells in the Peyer's patches or lamina propria and presented to T cells. The latter cells then develop into T_H17 or T_H1 effector cells under the influence of the appropriate cytokines and migrate first to the draining lymph node and then to the lamina propria. At the latter site they produce inflammatory cytokines such as IL-17, IFN-γ, and TNF-α, which mediate tissue damage either directly or by acting on macrophages or neutrophils. This type of inflammatory response arises from a genetically determined defect in mucosal effector cell development or from deficient regulatory T-cell responses, which occur in parallel with the effector cell response.

MDP, which is released from peptidoglycan after the glycoprotein is taken up and degraded by intracellular enzymes. In normal mice, the NOD2 signal resulting from MDP activation mitigates the TLR2 signal from peptidoglycan, resulting in far less NF-κB activation and IL-12 production. In the absence of NOD2 or in the presence of a mutation in NOD2, such modulation does not occur and the mouse produces increased amounts of IL-12 in response to peptidoglycan and perhaps other TLR ligands. In human terms, on the basis of the above analysis of NOD2 function, patients with Crohn's disease who have a mutation in NOD2 are assumed to be unable to modulate peptidoglycan signaling, so they produce increased amounts of IL-12 upon exposure to their own microflora. This sets the stage for the T_H1 response causing Crohn's disease. As in the TNBS colitis model discussed above, where there is a tendency to hyperrespond to bacteria microflora, Crohn's disease patients may be similarly responding to as-yet-undefined antigens rather than to TNP-substituted proteins. Thus, the NOD2 mutation is in effect a gain-of-function mutation, which allows one to directly link immune hyperresponsiveness to a human genetic defect.

Effector versus Regulatory Cell Defects in IBD.
So far in the discussion of hyperresponsiveness to mucosal microflora we have focused on the possibility of an excessive "effector cell" response as the cause of IBD. Indeed, within the universe of mouse models of mucosal inflammation, TNBS colitis occurs only in strains that mount increased responses to mucosal constituents. In addition, colitis is seen in mice that (1) overexpress molecular components of the T_H1 pathway such as Stat4, (2) have cells that respond to antigens in the autologous microflora, and (3) have cells that can transfer colitis to immunodeficient recipients. Perhaps more importantly, in patients with IBD and NOD2 mutations, the genetic defect leads to effector cells that produce too much IL-12 and IFN-γ and thus sustain the inflammatory response.

However, IBD secondary to increased effector cell responses is only one side of the coin. On the flip side, IBD may be associated with a normal response to microflora antigens but a defect in the cellular mechanisms of the mucosal immune system that ordinarily down-regulate these responses and keep them in check. In this situation, even normal responses would be sufficient to give rise to inflammation.

Mucosal immune responses are somewhat unique in that they are governed by a phenomenon known as oral tolerance or oral unresponsiveness. Simply put, **oral tolerance** is the result of complex cellular mechanisms that prevent reactions by the mucosal immune system to the myriad of harmless antigens in the mucosal environment that would otherwise divert the system from productive host defense responses (and make our enjoyment of food impossible!). Host defense responses are elicited only because pathogenic organisms express mucosal adjuvants that overcome oral tolerance along with the virulence factors necessary for colonization and invasion. (The best studied example of such virulence is cholera toxin, a substance that both allows cholera to enter epithelial cells and primes the mucosal immune system for potent B- and T-cell responses.)

Two broad types of processes are thought to induce oral tolerance. One is a deletional process; oral antigens entering the mucosal immune system are followed by the silencing or frank elimination of naive T cells that could conceivably interact with these antigens. This **deletional tolerance** is thought to occur mainly in relation to the introduction of high antigen doses, since only large amounts of antigen could successfully eliminate the available clones. The second process thought to induce tolerance involves the induction of **regulatory cells** that suppress responses to mucosal antigens. This mechanism first became evident in cell transfer studies; it was shown that feeding an antigen to one animal led to the development of intestinal cells that could then render a second animal unresponsive to that fed antigen. Later it was shown that the intestinal cells transferring the tolerance were CD4$^+$ T cells and that the suppression was antigen nonspecific; in other words, the cells exhibited bystander suppression of responses to antigens other than the fed antigen. In addition, suppressor cell–mediated oral tolerance was elicited when mice were fed low doses of antigen; it is thought that this mechanism complements the deletional mechanism by suppressing responses of cells that inevitably escape the deletional process.

What are the characteristics of regulatory cells that maintain immune homeostasis?

The nature of the regulatory cells that prevent inflammation in the GI mucosa (and elsewhere) is still the subject of ongoing research. The roles of several populations of regulatory or suppressor T cells in maintaining oral tolerance have been identified. One cell type in particular, regulatory T (T_{reg}), cells have been discussed in relation to other autoimmune diseases (see Cases 14 and 15 and the introduction to this unit). These regulatory cells are so-called "natural" suppressor cells that bear certain surface markers such as CD25, GITR, CTLA-4, and most importantly a unique transcription factor known as Foxp3, a member of the forkhead family of transcription factors. Most T_{reg} cells originate in the thymus; it is here that they are educated to recognize self-antigens. However, there is recent evidence that T_{reg} cells can be induced in the peripheral tissues as well under the influence of transforming growth factor (TGF)-β.

How can T_{reg} cells be generated against microbial antigens as if these antigens were autoantigens?

Two possible scenarios for the presence of these regulatory cells in the mucosa arise from their different possible sites of origin. In one scenario, the T_{reg} cells are generated in the thymus as a result of exposure to antigens associated with the intestinal microflora that somehow gained access to the internal milieu. These cells then migrate to the intestine, where they reencounter the same antigens and are expanded, particularly when the epithelial barrier is breached during an inflammation. In this scenario, the regulatory cells of oral tolerance are a subset of regulatory cells that govern general responses to self-antigens; their prominence in the mucosal immune system arises from the fact that the mucosal tissues are exposed to bacterial antigens with the capacity to act as self-antigens and gain access to the thymus.

A second scenario is supported by recent data showing that a certain subset of mucosal dendritic cells (CD103$^+$ DC) have a special propensity to induce Foxp3 regulatory T cells locally by virtue of their ability to synthesize TGF-β and retinoic acid. Since these cells bear a surface antigen that allows them to bind to mucosal epithelial cells (CD103), it has been proposed that they gain this inductive capacity by exposure to epithelial cell factors and to vitamin A, a component of the food stream and a precursor of retinoic acid. In this scenario, the regulatory cells are generated locally in the gut mucosa rather than in the thymus.

Regardless of origin, mucosal suppressor cells mediating oral tolerance are antigen nonspecific; once specifically activated via their T-cell receptors (TCRs), they suppress responses elicited by any antigen. This lack of specificity arises from the fact that they act via suppressor cytokines or substances that are totally antigen nonspecific. TGF-β is the most important suppressor cytokine; mice with defective receptors for TGF-β are not protected from inflammation of the colon by administration of suppressor T cells. Suppressor T cells have been shown to both secrete TGF-β and express TGF-β on their cell surface. Furthermore, anti-TGF-β can abrogate oral tolerance, by blocking either the effector function of suppressor cells or their expansion.

Oral tolerance may be mediated by several other types of regulatory cells, including so-called Tr-1 cells that are induced by antigen stimulation in the presence of IL-10 and produce IL-10 as their regulatory cytokine. In addition, recent studies have shown that cells that bear surface TGF-β but do not express either Foxp3 or IL-10 have a role in maintaining oral tolerance.

The possible relationship of oral tolerance to IBD is evident from the study of the animal models of mucosal inflammation. In the study of TNBS colitis, it has been shown that feeding TNBS to mice at the time of colitis induction by TNBS administration per rectum prevents colitis due to the induction of TGF-β-producing suppressor T cells in the lamina propria. Similarly, in a number of other models it has been observed that impaired suppressor T-cell development or function allows the induction of colitis. The best studied of these is the cell transfer model using as recipients, immunodeficient mice that lack all T-cell development; these can be either SCID mice or RAG-2 deficient mice (see Case 2). These animals are repleted with either naive (CD45RB^{hi}) T cells or a combination of naive and memory (CD45RB^{lo}) T cells. Only mice given naive T cells develop colitis; mice receiving both naive and mature T cells remain colitis-free. The naive T-cell populations lack suppressor T cells, while memory T cells contain a subpopulation of regulatory T cells. This regulatory T-cell population acts via TGF-β since administration of anti-TGF-β to the mice blocks the protective function of the memory cells. It has also recently been documented that mice characterized by a defect in their ability to respond to TGF-β signaling cannot be protected by transfer of regulatory cells. However, IL-10 is also involved in some way in the protective effect of the suppressor cells in the memory T-cell population since anti-IL-10 antibodies also abrogate the T cell's protective function. Finally, it has been shown that administration of suppressor T cells after inflammation has been already established can be effective. This opens the door to the possible treatment of IBD by provision of regulatory cells.

The above data, showing the relation of regulatory cells to colitis in mice, establish that the lack of regulatory cells or impairment in their function can, theoretically at least, lead to mucosal inflammation. What, then, is the evidence we have that these cells account for disease in patients with IBD? The answer is that no convincing data have yet emerged showing that patients with IBD are truly deficient in the number or activity of local regulatory cells in the mucosal area. In perhaps the best study in which this has been explored in patients with Crohn's disease, it was found that inflamed mucosa contained increased numbers of suppressor cells as compared to control mucosa, albeit the numbers were lower than those in the mucosa from patients with another type of inflammation. Thus, the jury is still out on the question of whether IBD can be due to an underlying regulatory T-cell defect.

Pathophysiology of Inflammatory Bowel Disease

Regardless of whether the inflammation in IBD is initiated by an overactive effector T cell or a regulatory T-cell defect, it has become apparent that the inflammation is ultimately mediated by differentiated T cells with characteristic patterns of cytokine secretion. In Crohn's disease, there is strong evidence that the T cells involved are T_H1 and T_H17 T cells (see Case 15 for a description of T_H subset differentiation). In ulcerative colitis, the contributing T cells are T_H2-like natural killer T (NKT) cells.

Crohn's Disease. The data supporting a T_H1/T_H17 T-cell-mediated process in Crohn's disease are particularly compelling. First, dendritic cells in lesional tissues produce "master" cytokines that are known to induce T_H1/T_H17 responses such as IL-12p70 and IL-23, respectively (Fig. 18.8 and 18.9). Second, T cells in lesional tissues produce transcription factors such as Stat4, T-bet, and RORγt that are necessary for T_H1/T_H17 cytokine synthesis, providing evidence that these master cytokines are signaling T cells. Third, T cells taken from lesional tissues produce high levels of T_H1 cytokines (such as IFN-γ and TNF-α) and T_H17 cytokines (such as IL-17A, IL-17F, and IL-22), but there is no evidence that the T cells produce increased amounts of T_H2 cytokines. Third and most importantly, treatment of patients with the monoclonal antibody anti-IL-12p40, which targets the common chain of IL12p70 and IL-23 and thus affects both T_H1 and T_H2 T-cell induction, has been remarkably effective in preliminary studies in humans.

The prevalence of T_H1/T_H17 is responsible for the character of the inflammation in Crohn's disease (see Fig. 18.8). As noted in the chapter on multiple sclerosis (Chapter 15), T_H1/T_H17 T-cell-mediated lesions resemble delayed-type hypersensitivity reactions; both are characterized by an influx of macrophages and the development of granulomatous lesions. In addition, perhaps because of the T_H17 cells, often there is also neutrophilic infiltrate in the lamina propria or associated with the crypt epithelium (cryptitis) or crypt lumen (crypt abscesses) in Crohn's disease. Overall, the T_H1/T_H17 inflammation leads to a lesion densely infiltrated with inflammatory cells. In the earlier stages of disease this results in a thickened bowel wall; in later stages it leads to intestinal narrowing and obstruction and fistula or abscess formation. While the inflammation causes some damage to the overlying epithelium and scattered ulcerations, the lesion is not dominated by epithelial cell pathology as in ulcerative colitis. Finally, it is important to note that the T cells and macrophages in the Crohn's disease lesion release multiple inflammatory cytokines and substances that act as proximal mediators of tissue damage. These include TNF-α, IL-1β, IL-6, reactive oxygen species, prostaglandins, and matrix metalloproteinases.

In recent years, some controversy has arisen regarding the relative importance of the T_H1 response and the T_H17 response in the pathogenesis of Crohn's disease. In initial studies of murine models of colitis and humans with

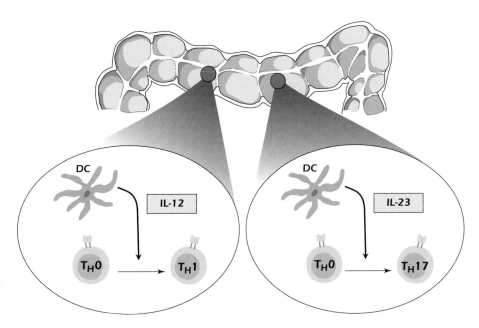

⬤ Figure 18.9. Crohn's disease is a composite of T_H1 and T_H17 inflammation.

Crohn's disease (which were conducted before the discovery of IL-23 and IL-17), IL-12 and IFN-γ were considered the major drivers of inflammation in this disease. However, more recent murine studies, in which either the T_H1 or the T_H17 response was eliminated, showed that the T_H17 response appeared to be more important in some models; in other models, the T_H1 response appeared more important. This difference may be related to the chronicity of the inflammation. T_H17 predominance seems associated with more chronic disease and is documented in experiments of cell transfer colitis; T_H1 predominance is seen in more acute disease models such as TNBS colitis. In humans with Crohn's disease, there is evidence that both responses occur simultaneously; it is therefore possible that the Crohn's lesion is a composite of acute and chronic inflammation. However, only studies of patients treated with agents that selectively target either the T_H1 or the T_H17 response will determine which is more important.

Ulcerative Colitis. T_H1 cytokines are not elevated in ulcerative colitis and the cellular infiltrate does not have the granulomatous character characteristic of T_H1 responses. So is this form of IBD a T_H2 T-cell-mediated disease? The answer to that question is no, since IL-4, usually the defining cytokine of T_H2 responses, is also not elevated. The presence of a T_H2 response is supported only by the fact that ulcerative colitis is accompanied by a moderately increased IL-5 level and is marked by the presence of autoantibodies such as p-ANCA. Recently, the situation was clarified with studies that began with an analysis of oxazolone colitis in mice; this model, which bears a histologic similarity to ulcerative colitis, is induced by intrarectal administration of a haptenating agent (oxazolone) that is structurally unrelated to TNBS. This analysis revealed that oxazolone colitis starts as a T_H2,

IL-4-dependent inflammation but rapidly evolves into one that depends on IL-13 produced not by conventional CD4$^+$ T cells but rather by NKT cells (Fig. 18.10). This finding in a mouse model suggested that ulcerative colitis might be due to a similar process. In fact, in human patients ulcerative colitis was also associated with an elevated production of IL-13 by NKT cells. Moreover, these NKT cells were cytotoxic to epithelial cells, particularly when stimulated by IL-13. Although IL-13 and NKT cells are associated with ulcerative colitis, it is too early to say that they necessarily cause this disease. As in the case of Crohn's disease, proof of causation of tissue damage depends on the demonstration that a therapy specifically affecting this atypical T_H2 process ameliorates the disease. The origin of the NKT-cell response in ulcerative colitis is poorly understood.

What are NKT cells?

NKT cells are distinct from T cells in that they express cell surface marker proteins more commonly found on NK cells. Another difference is that they respond to narrowly defined glycoprotein antigens that are presented in the context of an MHC class I–like molecule known as CD1d. NKT cells recognize microbial antigens and cross-reacting self-antigens. They are considered part of the innate immune system producing cytokines early in the immune response and reacting to antigens released from dying cells.

On this basis it is possible that the recognition by NKT cells of activated epithelial cells expressing CD1d and releasing antigens is the key initiating step in the pathologic process that culminates in clinical ulcerative colitis. Gut epithelial cells can induce NKT cell to produce IL-13; this in turn leads to epithelial cell injury and ulceration. The rupture of the epithelial barrier then leads to further

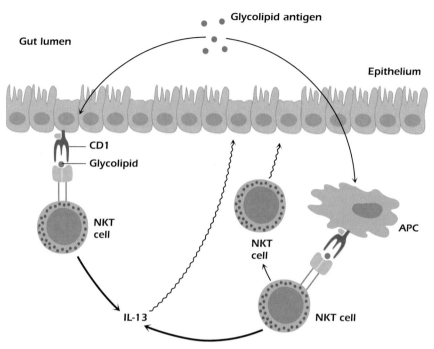

Figure 18.10. Dysregulated mucosal immune response underlying ulcerative colitis. Antigens (probably glycolipid antigens) associated with the commensal microflora of the gut are presented to NKT cells by epithelial cells via CD1d. The NKT cells then produce IL-13, a cytokine that has direct injurious effects on epithelial cells. Alternatively, the NKT cells stimulated by IL-13 kill epithelial cells via their inherent cytotoxic function. In either case, epithelial cells are the targets of immune injury, and the pathologic process results in ulceration.

NKT-cell stimulation via positive feedback of the pathologic process. However, this attractive hypothesis does not take into account the factors that lead up to epithelial stimulation of NKT cells and will obviously require further elaboration.

As in Crohn's disease, the immune mechanism underlying ulcerative colitis dictates the immunopathology. Thus, as indicated above, the cellular mechanism causing tissue damage in ulcerative colitis is focused on the epithelial layer and is directly responsible for the superficial, ulcerative nature of the disease. Since this pathologic process leads to chronic epithelial cell death and healing, it requires repeated cycles of epithelial cell regeneration, creating a situation in which the epithelial cells are at increased risk of undergoing malignant transformation. This is believed to contribute to the very high risk for the development of colon cancer in patients with long-standing, pan-colonic ulcerative colitis, a risk far greater than for the development of colon cancer in normal individuals or even in patients with Crohn's disease.

Role of Epithelial Barrier Function and Innate Immunity in IBD.
Two other somewhat interrelated factors that contribute to normal integrity of the GI tract and mucosal immune system are factors in the pathogenesis of

IBD: (1) the ability of the epithelium to function as a barrier against the entry of mucosal microflora or their component antigens and (2) the ability of mucosal cells (both epithelial cells and underlying antigen-presenting cells) to respond to ligands from bacteria and viruses via TLRs (and other recognition molecules) as part of the innate immune system.

The epithelial layer is an important physical barrier separating the antigen-rich colonic contents from the immune cells in the lamina propria. This is the first line of defense against the development of IBD; mice in which the barrier has been compromised by expression of an inhibitor of N-cadherin (a component of the epithelial cell tight junction) develop mucosal inflammation. In addition, as already discussed, disruption of the barrier function by ethanol is necessary for the development of TNBS colitis in mice. In addition to serving as a passive barrier, the epithelial cells may participate actively in the innate immune system. Because epithelial cells express TLRs and other sensors of the microbial environment that bind bacterial/viral molecules, they stimulate production of cytokines, chemokines, and other modulators of the immune response. These host defense elements include relatively low molecular weight proteins called defensins; these molecules are secreted into the intestinal crypts and regulate the microbial colonization of these areas.

Defects in cytokine, chemokine, and defensin secretion may contribute to the initiation of chronic inflammation in IBD.

The epithelial cells, dendritic cells, macrophages, NK cells, and NKT cells of the innate immune system can induce an inflammatory response by interaction with microbial components. For example, the NOD2 mutations in Crohn's disease discussed above result in excessive IL-12 responses to peptidoglycan and thus a mucosal milieu that is primed for inappropriate response to other mucosal antigens. It is possible or even likely that other yet to be discovered genetic defects occurring in IBD also involve the innate immune response, especially signaling via the TLRs.

Genetic Factors in IBD

Family and twin studies first provided unequivocal evidence that susceptibility to IBD is at least partially inherited. Later, genomewide scans of patient populations and multiplex families led to the identification of several chromosomal disease susceptibility regions that contain a (usually unidentified) disease gene within the region. Progress toward identifying actual disease genes has recently been made through studies of the association of single-nucleotide polymorphisms (SNPs) with disease. The discovery that IBD is characterized by multiple chromosomal susceptibility regions and is associated with multiple SNPs strongly suggests that it is a genetically heterogeneous disease caused by multiple combinations of gene abnormalities, with each conferring only a low, albeit important, risk for disease development. The *CARD15* gene in the IBD-1 susceptibility region on chromosome 16 is an exception to this rule; it confers a high risk for the development of Crohn's disease, although even this mutation probably requires the presence of other mutations/polymorphisms to confer disease. About 15% of Caucasian patients with Crohn's disease bear a *CARD15* gene mutation on both chromosomes, compared to 1 in 500 normal individuals. As already discussed above, *CARD15* encodes the intracytoplasmic protein NOD2 that recognizes and is activated by MDP, a component of the bacterial cell wall. In addition to the evidence that *CARD15* mutations cause increased production of inflammatory cytokines in response to innate immune stimuli such as TLR ligands, there is evidence that the mutations may result in decreased production of epithelial cell defensin and cause changes in bacterial concentrations in the small intestinal crypts. Other genes thought to contain mutations/polymorphisms leading to IBD include *MDR-1* (Chr7), *OCTN1/2* (Chr5), and *DLG5* (Chr10) (genes involved in epithelial cell transport function) and *ATG16L1* (Chr12) (a gene involved in cellular autophagy). On the flip side of the coin, a polymorphism in the gene encoding the receptor for IL-23 has been associated with resistance to the development of Crohn's disease. This polymorphism is particularly interesting in view of the proposed role of IL-23 in the immune mechanism underlying the disease.

 ## TREATMENT OF INFLAMMATORY BOWEL DISEASE

The evolution of medical treatment for Crohn's disease and ulcerative colitis has advanced with better understanding of the underlying immune mechanisms. There are two considerations in the approach to treatment of IBD: (1) inducing a good response and (2) maintaining that response over the long term. Conventional treatments include corticosteroids and newer agents directed against the inflammatory cytokine TNF-α which induce beneficial effects in days to weeks. Immunosuppressants such as azathioprine and anti-TNF-α drugs can then maintain the response over months to years. Traditional approaches to the acute inhibition of inflammation involving the use of corticosteroids (to inhibit T-cell proliferation and decrease cytotoxic functions of lymphocytes, inhibit monocyte cytokine production, and interfere with trafficking of immune cells to sites of inflammation) have been successful. However, given the chronic, relapsing nature of Crohn's disease, the failure of corticosteroids to reliably maintain remission, and the management of steroid side effects (including Cushinoid appearance, osteoporosis, glucose intolerance, and cataracts), development of new therapies is crucial.

Although mesalamine compounds have demonstrated clinical efficacy in relatively mild cases of ulcerative colitis, convincing data of effectiveness remain to be seen in Crohn's disease. The mechanism of action of salicylate-based drugs is not entirely clear. One possibility is that they act primarily by inhibiting the lipoxygenase pathway and leukotriene production; this in turn interferes with the trafficking and function of polymorphonuclear cells, important inflammatory effectors in all forms of IBD. These compounds may also act as scavengers of cytotoxic free radicals.

A second line of agents appropriate for maintaining the response to initial therapy or adding to suboptimal responses to initial drugs consists of the various agents that directly affect immune function. Azathioprine (6-mercaptopurine), the major player, has recently been shown to act not as a blunt inhibitor of cellular proliferation but rather by blocking an intracellular pathway that prevents apoptosis of memory effector T cells; thus, the drug helps to decrease the number of active T cells that survive at sites of inflammation. Other drugs in this category (methotrexate, cyclosporin, mycophenylate mofetil) act as anti-inflammatory agents by largely unknown mechanisms but have been used in Crohn's disease with varying degrees of success. Even antibiotics (ciprofloxacin, metronidazole) can improve mild to moderate symptoms in Crohn's disease and can help close perianal fistulae, presumably by decreasing luminal bacterial counts (and antigenic load).

Most recently a new class of "biologic" agents has appeared for the treatment of severe IBD inflammation. These "attack" the inflammation at various points of the pathways that mediate the disease. One such agent already in use is anti-TNF-α, an anticytokine that not only neutralizes a major effector cytokine, especially of T_H1/T_H17 responses, but also has probable apoptotic effects on antigen-presenting cells. Anti-TNF-α is initially effective in about 50–60% of patients but unfortunately becomes less effective with repeated administration in the majority of patients. Interestingly, anti-TNF-α drugs are also effective in ulcerative colitis, likely because TNF-α is an important common inflammatory cytokine located "downstream" in the inflammatory cascade in both diseases. Other anticytokines target the "master" cytokines of the inflammatory response in IBD: anti-IL-12, anti-IL-23, or anti-IL-12p40 in Crohn's disease or anti-IL-13 in ulcerative colitis. As discussed in Case 15, IL-12 and IL-23 are heterodimeric molecules that share a common chain (IL-12p40); thus, an anti-IL-12p40 targets both T_H1 and T_H17 responses. Such an antibody has undergone preliminary testing in Crohn's disease and has proven to be quite effective. Other antibodies that target only the T_H17 response, such as anti-IL-17, are currently being evaluated.

Yet another biologic approach to therapy of IBD is based on the possibility that the disease may be due to inadequate suppression of the mucosal immune response by regulatory T cells. Here the aim of therapy is to augment the regulatory T-cell response and to overcome the effector T-cell response whether or not the adequacy of regulatory T cells is the prime cause of the disease.

This is only a sampling of the host of additional approaches to biologic therapy of IBD. Newly acquired knowledge about the pathogenesis of IBD, increased awareness of the possible points of "attack," and novel targets for future drug development all hold promise for patients with these difficult diseases.

REFERENCES

Duchmann R, Herman E, Mayet W, Ewe K, Buschenfelde KM (1995): Tolerance exists towards resident intestinal flora but is broken in active inflammatory bowel disease (IBD). *Clin Exp Immunol* 102:448–455.

Elson C, Cong Y (2002): Understanding immune-microbial homeostasis in intestine. *Immunol Res* 26:87–94.

Faria AM, Weiner HL (2005): Oral tolerance. *Immunol Rev* 206:232–259.

Hugot J, Chamaillard M, Zouali H, Lesage S, Cézard JP, Belaiche J, Almer S, Tysk C, O'Morain CA, Gassull M, Binder V, Finkel Y, Cortot A, Modigliani R, Laurent-Puig P, Gower-Rousseau C, Macry J, Colombel JF, Sahbatou M, Thomas G (2001): Association of NOD2 leucine-rich repeat variants with susceptibility to Crohn's disease. *Nature* 411:599–603.

Mannon P, Fuss I, Mayer L, Elson C, Sandborn W, Present D, Dolin B, Goodman N, Groden C, Hornung R, Quezado M, Neurath MF, Salfeld J, Veldman GM, Schwertschlag U, Strober W for the Anti–IL-12 Crohn's Disease Study Group (2004): Anti-interleukin-12 antibody for active Crohn's disease. *New Engl J Med* 351:2069–2079.

Mowat AM (2003): Anatomical basis of tolerance and immunity to intestinal antigens. *Nature Rev Immunol* 3:331–341.

Ogura Y, Bonen D, Inohara N, Nicolae DL, Chen FF, Ramos R, Britton H, Moran T, Karaliuskas R, Duerr RH, Achkar JP, Brant SR, Bayless TM, Kirschner BS, Hanaue SB, Nuñez G, Cho JH (2001): A frameshift mutation in NOD2 associated with susceptibility to Crohn's disease. *Nature* 411:603–606.

Podolsky D (2002): Inflammatory bowel disease. *New Engl J Med* 347:417–429.

Strober W, Fuss IJ, Mannon PJ (2007): The fundamental basis of inflammatory bowel disease. *J Clin Invest* 117:514–521.

Strober W, Murray P, Kitani A, Watanabe T (2006): Signaling pathways and molecular interactions of NOD1 and NOD2. *Nat Rev Immunol* 6:9–20.

Yen D, Cheung J, Scheerens H, Poulet F, McClanahan T, McKenzie B, Kleinschek M, Owyang A, Mattson J, Blumenschein W, Murphy E, Sathe M, Cua DJ, Kastelein RA, Rennick D (2006): IL-23 is essential for T cell-mediated colitis and promotes inflammation via IL-17 and IL-6. *J Clin Invest* 116:1310–1316.

19

PSORIASIS

BRUCE STROBER*

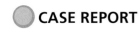

CASE REPORT

"I have a new rash."

Presentation and Initial Workup

Robert, a 28-year-old investment banker, calls to tell you that about four weeks ago he noticed the onset of a persistent "skin rash" consisting of areas of redness that have gradually developed into itchy, red, and scaly plaques. At first the rash was only present on his elbows, knees, and scalp, but a little later it also appeared as discrete lesions on his lower back, abdomen, and both legs. Because he thought it was an allergic reaction and would clear up on its own, he was at first reluctant to interrupt his busy schedule to seek medical help. Now he realizes that the rash lesions are gradually enlarging and getting "thicker"; they do not seem to be receding at all. As a result he is quite concerned and wants an appointment with you, his dermatologist.

In your office, Robert recounts the above history and, when questioned, remembers that three to four months before the onset of this skin problem he had a mild "flu" characterized by a fever of 101.2°F, myalgias (muscle aches), headache, sore throat, and cough. After

five days this illness resolved, but two to three days later droplet-sized erythematous (red) papules (small, well-circumscribed solid elevations) appeared on his trunk and extremities. This earlier rash resolved over the next six to eight weeks and he was free of skin symptoms for several months until the onset of the present skin problem. He denies constitutional symptoms at this time, stating that, aside from the rash, he feels quite well.

Your physical exam of Robert reveals that he has symmetric, erythematous, hyperkeratotic scaling plaques over the extensor surfaces of his upper and lower extremities, his lower back and abdomen, and focally within his scalp (Fig. 19.1). Approximately 25% of his body surface area is involved. The removal of the thick overlying scale from one of the plaques causes pinpoint bleeding. The oral and rectal mucosa are not involved, but the glans penis has a discrete 1 cm erythematous, slightly scaly plaque. The remainder of the exam is normal.

What is the differential diagnosis of a symmetric, scaly rash over the trunk and extremities?

*Symmetric cutaneous eruptions manifested as scaly patches and plaques result from the thickening of the epidermis (**acanthosis**). Usually, a thickened epidermis implies an increase in epidermal cell division. The differential*

*With contributions from Warren Strober and Susan R. S. Gottesman

Immunology: Clinical Case Studies and Disease Pathophysiology, By Warren Strober and Susan R. S. Gottesman
Copyright © 2009 John Wiley & Sons, Inc.

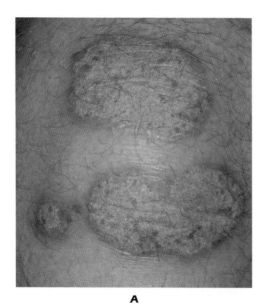

A

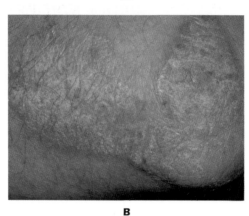

B

Figure 19.1. Appearance of typical psoriatic plaques characterizing chronic plaque psoriasis (psoriasis vulgaris): **(A)** plaque on thigh; **(B)** plaque on elbow.

diagnosis of such lesions includes inflammatory dermatoses such as psoriasis, pityriasis rubra pilaris, pityriasis rosea, lichen planus, and secondary syphilis. Of these dermatoses, psoriasis is the most common and occurs in the pattern seen in this patient, that is, on the extensor surfaces, scalp, and genital region. Pityriasis rubra pilaris is usually marked by reddish orange lesions that begin around hair follicles and subsequently coalesce into large patches. Pityriasis rosea begins with a solitary patch (the "herald patch") that is larger than the subsequently developing patches and papules, which are often distributed in a "Christmas tree" pattern on the trunk. Lichen planus is also pruritic (itchy) but usually occurs on either the distal areas of the extremities (wrist and shins, commonly) or on the oral or genital mucosa. Secondary syphilis can mimic many other diseases but develops weeks after a primary syphilic chancre on the genitals. This primary lesion, however, may go undetected by the patient and therefore the lack of a history of a genital lesion does not rule it out.

How does the physical examination and history help you with Robert's diagnosis?

*Considerations of the differential diagnosis leads you to believe that the rash is due to a common form of psoriasis known as chronic plaque psoriasis or psoriasis vulgaris. You are supported in this diagnosis by the observation of bleeding after removal of scale from one of the plaques. This is called the "**Auspitz sign**"and is highly characteristic of psoriasis.*

Robert's history is also consistent with psoriasis. In the months prior to the onset of his current skin lesions, he had a flulike illness followed by a papular eruption that subsequently disappeared. This first episode is characteristic of guttate psoriasis, a form of usually transient psoriasis that is frequently associated with a preceding infection. (See description of guttate psoriasis below). In about 20% of patients with guttate psoriasis the guttate papules develop into full-blown psoriatic plaques; in another 20–30%, the papules disappear and plaque-forming psoriasis appears later, as in Robert's case. Furthermore, the majority of individuals who experience recurrent gluttate psoriasis are likely to develop plaque-forming psoriasis.

In Robert's case and in most cases of chronic plaque psoriasis, the clinical presentation is sufficient for diagnosis; you do not need laboratory tests or histopathologic analysis of the lesions. Nevertheless, to confirm the diagnosis, you perform a skin biopsy and send a blood test for RPR (rapid plasma reagin) for antiphospholipid antibodies to rule out syphilis.

Confident in your diagnosis, you discuss treatment options for Robert pending the test results. You inform Robert that mild cases of psoriasis can be treated with topical medications, such as topical corticosteroids, analogues of vitamins A and D, tars, anthralin, and newer drugs such as the topical immunomodulators. In Robert's case, the widespread nature of his disease makes the daily application of topical medications too cumbersome and thus unrealistic. Therefore you discuss phototherapy [ultraviolet (UV) irradiation] or therapies that are taken systemically, such as methotrexate and cyclosporine; if these drugs fail to control his disease, injectable biologic agents such as alefacept, etanercept, or efalizumab can be administered (see further discussion below).

Robert elects to use topical medications until the diagnosis is confirmed and to discuss the other systemic treatment options with his family.

Definitive Diagnosis

The next day the RPR comes back negative; five days later the biopsy report comes back with the diagnosis of psoriasis.

What are the histopathologic features found in a biopsy of a psoriatic lesion?

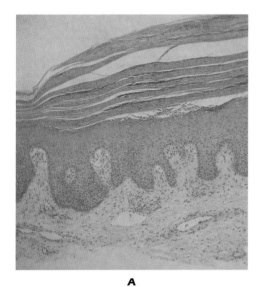

A

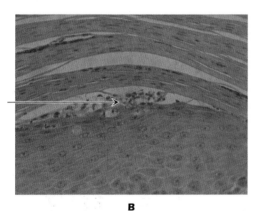

B

Figure 19.2. Histopathology of a psoriasis plaque in chronic plaque psoriasis: (**A**) low power, 10X; (**B**) high power, 40X; hematoxylin and eosin. Note the collections of neutrophils within the parakeratotic scale (arrow).

Histopathologically (see Fig. 19.2), the lesion of psoriasis displays the following primary features: (1) keratinocyte hyperplasia characterized by thickening of the epidermis (acanthosis) and downward expansion of the rete pegs that may be associated with multiple overlying layers of keratin or scale (parakeratosis) and loss of the highest layer of the epidermis (the granular layer); (2) acute and chronic inflammation characterized by infiltration of the superficial layer of the epidermis by neutrophils as well as infiltration of the dermis by lymphocytes, monocytes, and dendritic cells; and (3) numerous ectatic (dilated or distended) blood vessels scattered in the upper layers of the dermis (telangiectasia within the papillary tips).

Robert's Treatment Plan

Robert ultimately decides that UV phototherapy, while safe and effective, will not fit into his busy lifestyle. He found

that with his extensive skin involvement, the topical medications were indeed too problematic to use effectively. Thus, you elect to start methotrexate at a conservative dose. This dose can be increased monthly to improve efficacy. Robert understands that he cannot drink alcohol while taking methotrexate and that he must concomitantly take folic acid every day to reduce the risk of toxicity and negative side effects, such as nausea. He must not try to conceive a baby during therapy and for three months after he stops taking it. Finally, you ask him to come into the office every six to eight weeks for monitoring of any adverse effects of the drug, including myelosuppression, pulmonary toxicity, and hepatotoxicity. In the long term, a liver biopsy might be necessary to ensure that no liver damage is occurring.

NORMAL STIMULATION AND RESPONSE OF T CELLS TO ANTIGENS AND SUPERANTIGENS

As discussed more fully below, the immunopathogenesis of psoriasis involves the activation of T cells by antigens and superantigens. Before we launch into a discussion of the details, we will review the major immunologic events that are normally involved in such activation.

Mechanisms Involved in T Cell Recognition of Antigens

The physiologic stimulation of all T cells is through an antigen-specific T-cell receptor (TCR) that recognizes peptide derived from antigen when it is presented to the T cell in the context of a major histocompatibility complex (MHC) molecule on the surface of an antigen-presenting cell (APC). MHC class II molecules present antigen to $CD4^+$ T cells. The peptides associated with MHC class II are relatively long, at least 13 amino acids in length, and are derived by degradation of *exogenous* (from outside the cell) antigen in the endosomes of the APC. The MHC class II molecule is made up of two chains, an α chain and a β chain; each chain has two domains. The peptides lie in the groove created by the juxtaposition of these chains and are noncovalently bound to the α_1 and β_1 domains of the molecules. This groove is open ended so that peptides of various lengths (as long as 30 amino acids) may be accommodated; since binding is not highly specific, a single MHC molecule can present a wide variety of peptides. The MHC class II genes are polygenic, adding to the variety of antigens an individual can display. (Individuals can express six to eight different MHC class II molecules.) There is also considerable polymorphism of the MHC class II genes within the population.

A similar situation applies to antigen-specific stimulation of $CD8^+$ T cells, except that the peptides are recognized in the context of MHC class I molecules. In addition, the peptides presented by class I are derived mostly from endogenous antigens (i.e., antigens arising within the cells, such as viral antigens). MHC class I is composed of an α chain, which has three domains, and a smaller invariant chain, β_2-microglobulin. The α_1 and α_2 domains form the peptide-binding groove. Since this groove is not open at the end, the class I molecules are more restrictive and can only accommodate peptides 8–11 amino acids long.

The TCR is made up of an α-glycoprotein chain and a β-glycoprotein chain (different from the α and β chains of the MHC molecule); each of these has a variable (V) and a constant (C) region, much like the immunoglobulin molecule. In recognizing the peptide complexed to an MHC molecule, the Vα and Vβ domains of the TCR come into contact with both the peptide antigen and the MHC chains. However, this interaction is generally too weak to result in T-cell stimulation. For T cells to be stimulated, the coreceptor molecule, CD4 or CD8 must migrate within the plane of the membrane to interact with MHC class II or MHC class I, respectively, and thus increase the stability of TCR binding. The CD4 molecule is a single glycoprotein chain that binds to an invariant site on the Class II β chain. The CD8 molecule is a dimer that binds to the nonpolymorphic α_3 domain of class I. Additional interactions between other accessory molecules and their ligands (i.e., CD40 and CD40L) further strengthen the signal to the T cell.

Stimulation by Superantigen

Superantigens are molecules that are able to stimulate a large percentage of the T-cell population (hence the name superantigen) without engaging the TCR as described above for antigens. Specifically, superantigens bind to the outside portion of the Vβ domain of the TCR and to the outside portion of the α_1 or β_1 chain of MHC class II, thus bringing the APC and T cell together. Since the portion of the Vβ region of the bound TCR is derived from the germline-encoded segments of the molecule, this binding occurs in all cells with TCRs belonging to a particular Vβ family. In humans, over 20 Vβ families have been identified; one type of superantigen can react with 2–3 Vβ families, resulting in stimulation of 2–30% of an individual's T cells. This is in sharp contrast to normal antigens, which stimulate only 1 in 10^4 to 1 in 10^6 T cells. The superantigens identified thus far are derived from pathogens, bacteria or viruses, and function as intact proteins without processing in APCs. Another important difference between antigens and superantigens is that superantigens induce proliferation of both CD4$^+$ and CD8$^+$ T cells without the help of accessory molecules. However, because of this property, superantigen-stimulated T cells will die by apoptosis unless they are rescued by recognition of and stimulation by conventional antigens and costimulatory survival signals.

What do you think might be the consequence of stimulating such a large proportion of T cells?

Stimulation of large numbers of CD4$^+$ and CD8$^+$ cells results in the massive release of cytokines, particularly interleukin-2 (IL-2), tumor necrosis factor β (TNF-β), and interferon-γ (IFN-γ), and can thus cause host toxicity, skin sloughing, and even death. Staphylococcal enterotoxin (SE) and toxic shock syndrome toxin [(TSST-1), both derived from Staphylococcus aureus)], as well as streptococcal superantigen (SSA), and streptococcal pyrogenic exotoxins (SPE) are examples of particularly potent superantigens. Staphylococcal enterotoxins are a common cause of severe food poisoning. TSST-1 causes toxic shock syndrome, a condition characterized by capillary leak, hypotension, an erythrematous rash, and desquamation of the skin, all the result of the massive cytokine release. Mycobacteria and rhabdoviruses also give rise to superantigens.

Evolutionary Benefit of Superantigen Stimulation

How does the microorganism benefit from stimulation of such a massive number of T cells?

Stimulation by superantigens may lead to T-cell proliferation as discussed above, but it may also lead to T-cell death or anergy. For those superantigens that cause toxicity, the stimulation causes T-cell death or anergy following cytokine release and this favors the survival of the microorganism.

● THE IMMUNOPATHOGENESIS OF PSORIASIS

Armed with the knowledge of normal T-cell stimulation by antigens and superantigens, you are now in a better position to learn about the immune mechanisms underlying psoriasis.

Psoriasis is due to an immune dysregulation within the skin characterized by the appearance of cutaneous T cells producing IFN-γ and IL-17 (T_H1/T_H17-type cytokines), which are probably responding to self-antigen in the skin. This in turn leads to the induction of an inflammatory milieu that accelerates keratinocyte proliferation and the development of epidermal hyperplasia (acanthosis), angiogenesis leading to increased skin vascularization, and the inflammatory cellular infiltrate that are the hallmarks of the psoriatic lesion (as noted above).

The inciting event that results in these T cell-mediated events and the development of psoriasis is thought to be an encounter with an antigen during an infection. However, only one organism, the β-hemolytic streptococcus (in groups A, C, and G), has been shown to have a psoriogenic propensity. Whether or not other organisms also have this propensity remains to be determined. In addition, the ability to link any type of infection with the onset of disease is limited by the fact that, in many patients, the infection is asymptomatic or results in only minor symptoms. The pathogen causing the infection is likely to have been completely eliminated by the time of onset of the autoimmune disease.

In psoriasis initiated by an infection with β-hemolytic streptococci, the following hypothesis concerning the pathogenesis has been proposed: Individuals susceptible to psoriasis on genetic grounds respond to a superantigen associated with this organism, streptococcal exotoxin, with the activation of many different T-cell populations (T-cell clones), including those recognizing streptococcal antigens that may cross-react with self-antigens present in the skin. The latter, self-antigen-cross-reactive T-cell subpopulation is then further expanded by a conventional antigen, possibly derived from streptococcal M protein (also associated with the initiating organism), which contains a number of polypeptide sequences similar to antigenic components normally present in the skin or occurring during skin inflammation. Further stimulation by conventional antigen thus leads to expansion of T-cell populations that are capable of mediating the self-sustaining autoimmune skin inflammation of psoriasis. These inciting events all occur within the tonsils and associated lymph nodes. In summary, the effector cells that cause psoriasis are generated in the lymphoid tissues as a result of a "double hit": The first consists of streptococcal superantigen activation of T cells and the second consists of the specific activation and expansion of those T-cell clones within the superantigen-stimulated population that recognize conventional streptococcal epitopes that mimic the body's naturally occurring keratin (Fig. 19.3).

Certain forms of psoriasis are associated with pharyngeal infection with β-hemolytic streptococci; in patients with these forms of psoriasis, the tonsils and their draining lymph nodes contain a markedly increased frequency of T-cell clones that are reactive to peptides sharing extensive amino acid sequences with peptides in streptococcal M proteins. Since these M proteins also share amino acid sequences with peptides in skin keratins, especially those keratins that are up-regulated in psoriasis lesions, the M proteins are in effect inducing the development of self-reactive T cells. Finally, peripheral and (especially) lesional T cells of such psoriatic patients display increased use of $V\beta_2$ and $V\beta_{17}$ TCR chains, chains associated with streptococcal superantigen stimulation.

How can an infection in the tonsils lead to autoimmunity in the skin?

It has been reported that streptococcal exotoxin induces T-cell expression of cutaneous lymphocyte-associated antigen (CLA), an integrin that facilitates the homing of lymphocytes to the skin. Thus, it is possible that streptococcal infection in the tonsils (and draining lymph nodes) leads to the expansion of skin-homing T cells in these organs with the potential of reacting to antigens in the skin.

This may explain the marked improvement in psoriasis sometimes noted after tonsillectomy.

This model of psoriasis development corresponds most closely to **guttate psoriasis**, the transient form that occurred in Robert, which often precedes chronic plaque psoriasis. This form of psoriasis is the one most clearly related to streptococcal infection and to the T-cell findings ensuing from such infection. Whether it also explains the more common and severe chronic plaque psoriasis characterizing Robert's later course requires further study, including clarification of the specificity of the T cells in these lesions. Note, however, that the circulating T cells responding to peptides found in M proteins and keratin were all obtained from patients with chronic plaque-forming psoriasis; thus, this model may indeed apply to this form of psoriasis.

Another question is whether infectious agents other than streptococcus can cause plaque-forming psoriasis. It seems likely that other infectious organisms capable of producing superantigens would also have the ability to stimulate cells that cross-react with skin antigens, but further studies will be necessary to answer this question.

The Cellular Interactions Resulting in Psoriasis

With the above discussion of the potential inciting event, the sequence of cellular events that may result in psoriatic skin lesion can now be described. As shown in Figure 19.3, T cells reactive with skin antigens (presumably originating in the oropharynx: tonsils and associated lymph nodes) first enter the skin from the circulation and react to antigens expressed by keratinocytes. This leads to initial keratinocyte damage and release of antigen(s), which sets up the secondary immune response that perpetuates the psoriatic inflammation (Fig. 19.4).

In this secondary response, immature APCs (Langerhans cells in the epidermis or dendritic cells in the dermis) capture released antigen and subsequently migrate through afferent lymphatics to a local, skin-draining lymph node (Fig. 19.4). Here, the now mature APCs present the keratinocyte antigens to additional T cells whose receptors recognize this antigen in the context of MHC on the cell surface and thus induce further keratinocyte-reactive CD4$^+$ and CD8$^+$ T-cell activation and expansion. However, expansion also requires costimulation by other cell surface proteins found on the surfaces of the APC and the T cell. These costimulatory interactions include those between intercellular adhesion molecule 1 (ICAM-1) and leukocyte function-associated antigen 1 (LFA-1), LFA-3 and CD2, and CD80/CD86 and CD28. Tolerance for self-keratinocyte antigens is now broken.

In the next step, the activated T cells stimulated in this way express CD40 ligand (CD40L), a costimulatory molecule that "back stimulates" the APCs to produce cytokines that, in turn, induce differentiation of CD4$^+$

**Overview of Sensitization of CD8⁺ T cells
in Tonsil and Elicitation of Psoriasis**

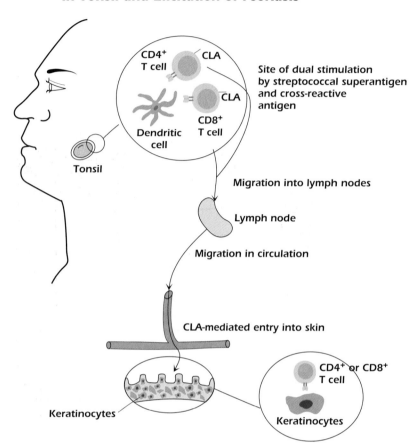

Figure 19.3. Development of autoimmune CD4⁺ and CD8⁺ T cells in tonsils induced by streptococcal superantigen and cross-reactive antigens. T cells migrate to the skin where they induce initial release of keratinocyte antigens.

T cells into the T_H1 and T_H17 T cells, the immediate effector cells of the inflammatory response. These APC cytokines include IL-12 and IL-23, related molecules consisting of a common p40 chain linked to a p35 chain in the case of IL-12 and linked to a p19 chain in the case of IL-23. IL-12 supports T_H1 cells that produce IFN-γ and TNF-α, and IL-23 induces T_H17 cells that produce IL-17, TNF-α, and IL-6. It is likely that both T_H1 and T_H17 T-cell cytokines are necessary for the full-blown psoriatic inflammation, although recent work has suggested that the T_H17 cytokines are more important.

The clonally expanded and activated T_H1 and T_H17 T cells, which are now capable of acting as memory/effector cells, leave the lymph node and circulate freely throughout the body. However, as a result of stimulation by dendritic cells derived from the skin, it is possible that the T cells are induced to express CLA, allowing these cells to home back to the skin. Entry of these cells into the skin also requires other interactions, including those involving integrins [such as LFA-1 and ICAM-1 and VLA-4 and vascular cell adhesion molecule 1 (VCAM-1)] and those between various chemokines released by endothelial cells, monocytes, dendritic cells, and keratinocytes in the inflamed skin

and chemokine receptors on circulating T cells. For this reason, only a small percentage of activated, circulating T cells enter *uninflamed* skin. Following reentry into the skin, the T cells that reencounter the same (or similar) activating antigen release T_H1 cytokines that, in turn, stimulate the production of numerous other cytokines and chemokines by resident cells within the skin, including keratinocytes. This has a multiplier effect leading to infiltration of additional activated T cells and other inflammatory cells, including neutrophils. Finally, while both CD4⁺ and CD8⁺ T cells are induced by inciting superantigens in psoriasis, the role of CD4⁺ may be to provide a cellular and cytokine milieu that supports the activation of CD8⁺ T cells; the CD8⁺ cells are the actual effector cells of the disease. This possibility is supported by the fact that CD4⁺ T cells are found mainly in the dermis of lesions where they are in close contact with dendritic cells, whereas CD8⁺ T cells are more commonly encountered in the epidermis in contact with keratinocytes. In addition, it is the CD8⁺ T cells that manifest the oligoclonality indicative of reactivity to a limited set of autoantigens as well as the capability of recognizing autoepitopes in the context of HLA-Cw6, an allele that occurs in greater than 60% of patients.

Elicitation of Psoriatic Lesions

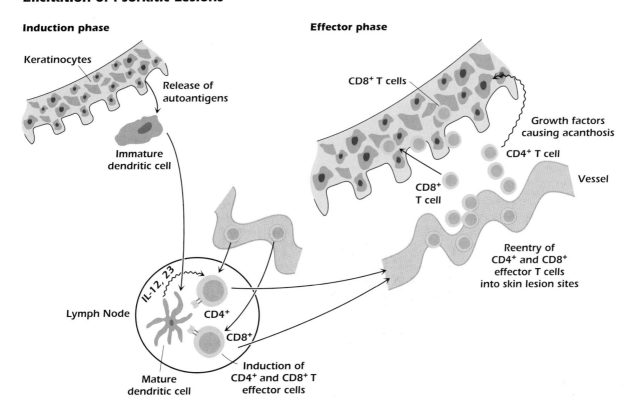

Figure 19.4. Induction of inflammation in the psoriatic skin. Antigens are taken up and processed by skin APCs which then migrate to draining nodes. At the latter site the APCs induce the activation of CD4$^+$ and CD8$^+$ effector cells which migrate back to the skin where they mediate psoriatic inflammation via T$_H$1/T$_H$17 responses and cell mediated cytotoxicity.

The formation of a psoriatic plaque requires the continued presence of activated T cells and their persistent expression of plaque-inducing cytokines or cell surface factors that form a "cytokine network" facilitating the psoriatic lesion. Thus, by the release of specific cytokines acting as growth factors or by cell-to-cell interactions, activated T cells that are in intradermal sites trigger the hyperproliferation of keratinocytes. Subsequently, other cytokines produced by stimulated nonlymphoid cells in the skin contribute to the psoriatic lesion. These include keratinocyte-derived IL-8, which functions as a chemotactic factor attracting neutrophils, and vascular endothelial growth factor (VEGF), which induces the proliferation of the dermal vasculature. [Neutrophils may not be essential to the psoriatic process as they are not found in the typical psoriatic lesions that develop in the severe combined immunodeficiency disease (SCID) xeno-transplant mouse models.] Finally, a psoriatic plaque might function as a secondary lymphoid tissue in which APCs can present the relevant antigen to infiltrating naive T cells, further perpetuating an unchecked process of T-cell activation.

The immunopathologic processes described above also occur within the joints and at the insertion of ligaments and tendons into bone. As a result, 20–30%

of patients with psoriasis will experience psoriatic arthritis during their lifetime. The pathophysiology of psoriatic arthritis closely parallels that of psoriasis involving the skin. However, instead of acting upon keratinocytes, infiltrating T cells influence the proliferation of and cytokine release by synoviocytes and osteoclasts. The end result can be a destructive inflammation of the joints, ligaments, and tendons; the joint inflammation can lead to significant disability in some patients.

GENETIC FACTORS IN PSORIASIS

That psoriasis is in part genetically determined was first clearly established by the concordance of about 60% in monozygotic twins. More recently, genome-wide scans in which microsatellite markers were correlated with the presence of disease in multiplex families led to the identification of at least six different susceptibility regions (PSOR1–6) in psoriasis, some of which overlap with regions identified in other autoimmune diseases, such as rheumatoid arthritis and asthma. Probably the most important genetic determinant, one that may account for 30–50% of genetic susceptibility to psoriasis, is found in the PSOR1 region on chromosome 6 (p21) corresponding to part of a 200-kb locus in the MHC region that contains the *HLA-B* and *HLA-C* genes. It has long been known that psoriasis is strongly associated with *HLA-Cw6*. The *HLA-Cw*0602* allele occurs in approximately 65% of patients versus only 10–15% of control individuals; in addition, individuals homozygous for this allele are $2\frac{1}{2}$ times more likely to develop the disease than individuals heterozygous for this allele. Despite this association, it is still not clear that the *HLA-Cw*0602* allele is actually the "disease gene" in psoriasis. This gene could be associated with the disease because it is in strong linkage disequilibrium with another gene in the MHC region; in fact, genes other than MHC have been proposed as candidate genes in the PSORS1 locus. However, the studies mentioned above support the idea that this HLA allele is a disease gene, since it is possible that this MHC class I molecule could be necessary to present psoriasis-associated antigens to CD8$^+$ T cells.

Other psoriasis susceptibility loci have been confirmed, including one on chromosome 17 (q24–q25); candidate genes known to be present in this locus are proteins involved in T cell antigen-presenting interactions that could therefore influence the development of self-reactive T cells. Thus, genes outside the MHC complex might also be factors in psoriasis susceptibility.

The strong evidence of genetic predisposition underlines the fact that the common infection(s) thought to induce psoriasis must fall upon a fertile genetic soil to actually produce disease. Thus, while it is generally accepted that certain superantigens and antigens play a key role in the pathogenesis of psoriasis, it is now abundantly clear that these must interact with cells having certain genetically determined properties.

CLINICAL FEATURES AND COURSE OF PSORIASIS

The initial lesions of psoriasis often make their appearance after an upper respiratory tract infection, but this is not always the case; some patients can recall no preceding infectious episode. Primary HIV infection can be one of the initiating infections and can lead to a florid presentation that is difficult to treat. The natural history of psoriasis following the initial symptoms is one of unpredictable exacerbations and remissions; the latter only rarely lead to complete and/or long-lasting freedom from disease. After the initial presentation, the disease settles down into a chronic, bothersome condition that varies in intensity depending on levels of stress, time of year (with the colder months associated with worsening flares), and the presence or absence of concomitant infections. Specific drugs, including lithium and β blockers, and withdrawal of systemic corticosteroids,

may cause exacerbations. The effect of diet is not well confirmed, but some patients see immediate worsening following alcohol intake.

There are many different types of psoriasis. ***Chronic plaque psoriasis*** (psoriasis vulgaris), one of the types affecting Robert, is the most common form and is marked by thick, erythematous plaques with overlying scale. The scale can be very adherent and may bleed if removed (Auspitz sign). The plaques of psoriasis can appear anywhere on the body, including the trunk, extremities, genitals, intergluteal cleft, scalp, and face. However, the most commonly affected areas are the elbows, knees, lower back, and scalp.

Another form of psoriasis is ***pustular psoriasis*** (of Von Zumbusch). This consists of an acute generalized eruption of sterile pustules that may be accompanied by fever, lymphocytosis, hypocalcemia, and hypoalbuminemia. If pustular psoriasis is limited to the hands and fingers, it is called acrodermatitis continua of Hallopeau; when it occurs on only the palms and soles, it is called pustulosis palmaris et plantaris. Pustular psoriasis also appears during pregnancy, when it is referred to as pustular psoriasis of pregnancy or "impetigo herpetiformis."

Two other forms of psoriasis are ***guttate psoriasis*** and ***erythrodermic psoriasis***. Guttate psoriasis, a form that also occurred in Robert's case, is characterized by small psoriatic papules and plaques (0.5–1.5 cm) distributed diffusely over the trunk and proximal extremities. As discussed above, streptococcal infection (i.e., streptococcal pharyngitis) often precedes this form of psoriasis, which commonly occurs in children and adolescents. Erythrodermic psoriasis is characterized by large erythematous patches (involving greater than two-thirds of the body surface area) without much overlying scale. Both the plaque and pustular variants of psoriasis may progress to this more severe form of the disease, which may be difficult to distinguish from other skin conditions that lead to generalized erythroderma, such as atopic dermatitis and cutaneous T-cell lymphoma.

Psoriasis may be associated with both nail disease (onychodystrophy) and arthritis. Nail disease involving both the fingernails and toenails is a prominent feature of patients with psoriasis; it occurs in 50% of all patients and 90% of patients with concomitant arthritis. The features of nail psoriasis include pitting, distal onycholysis, subungual hyperkeratosis, oil spots, and subungual hemorrhage. The arthritis associated with psoriasis is usually marked by involvement of a few asymmetric joints, including the sacroiliac joint. The pathologic lesion is similar to that found in rheumatoid arthritis, but the patient is seronegative for rheumatoid factor. Importantly, rapid joint destruction is quite common in psoriatic arthritis.

Psoriasis may be related to ***Reiter's syndrome***, a postinfectious disease constellation usually defined by the presence of urethritis, conjunctivitis, and arthritis. However,

Reiter's syndrome may also be associated with skin lesions on the penis (balanitis circinata) and the palms and soles (keratoderma blenorrhagicum); in addition, significant onychodystrophy occurs in some patients. Because these skin lesions resemble psoriasis at the histopathologic level, some investigators believe that Reiter's syndrome is a variant presentation of psoriasis with psoriatic arthritis.

Psoriasis is associated with other systemic diseases. As already mentioned, psoriatic arthritis occurs in 20–30% of patients with psoriasis. Psoriatic arthritis usually presents years after the first presentation of skin disease. It is rare for a patient to have psoriatic arthritis without cutaneous lesions, and the diagnosis may be made solely on clinical features, family history, and the presence of nail changes. The frequency of inflammatory bowel disease is higher in patients with psoriasis, and many patients with psoriatic arthritis have asymptomatic bowel inflammation. Hypertension, obesity, and diabetes mellitus are also more common in psoriatic patients. There is no clear increased risk of malignancy in patients with psoriasis. Yet patients who have undergone long-term treatment with ultraviolet phototherapy (PUVA) are at increased risk for both nonmelanoma skin cancers and melanoma. In contrast to patients with atopic eczema, patients with psoriasis very rarely get superimposed infections in their skin lesions.

 TREATMENT OF PSORIASIS

The treatment of psoriasis depends on disease severity and may involve topically applied drugs, locally injected intralesional corticosteroids, UV radiation to the entire body, or systemic (oral, parenteral, or injectable) agents. The overriding goal of all treatments is to suppress or eliminate the CD4$^+$ and/or CD8$^+$ T cells that dominate the immune response leading to plaque formation.

Patients with limited disease have plaques that cover less than 5% of their body surface area (BSA; note that the palm of the hand equals 1% of BSA). These patients have *mild* psoriasis that requires only topical, locally applied therapies including topical corticosteroids, which can act nonspecifically to suppress inflammation. However, if they are overused, topical corticosteroids can induce undesirable local side effects such as epidermal atrophy, increased telangiectases, bruising, and striae. Further, continuous use of topical corticosteroids can result in a diminished response (tachyphylaxis). Topical analogues of vitamin D (calcipotriene) regulate keratinocyte proliferation and differentiation and inhibit T-cell activation. Topical immunomodulators such as pimecrolimus or tacrolimus also block T-cell activation and are very effective at controlling psoriasis on the face and in the *intertriginous* areas (areas between skin folds). Finally, local injection of a corticosteroid or cyclosporine into the involved dermis is highly effective in the treatment of stubborn plaques.

For those patients with moderate to severe psoriasis who cannot afford the time commitment of UV phototherapy, systemic agents given orally or via injection are the most practical approach. Conventional systemic therapies, such as methotrexate and cyclosporin, target the inflammatory cells of psoriasis. Methotrexate specifically inhibits the synthesis of purine nucleotides and thus cell division and preferentially acts on lymphoid cells. However, it has recently been reported that the skin-homing molecules CLA and E-selectin, which are markedly down-regulated during methotrexate treatment, are up-regulated after this therapy is discontinued, coinciding with relapses. Methotrexate also treats psoriatic arthritis (unlike topical therapies and UV phototherapy). Because patients receiving methotrexate are at risk for hepatic, pulmonary, and hematologic toxicity, they must be monitored closely. Cyclosporin, which inhibits IL-2 production and thus directly inhibits T-cell activation, is extremely effective for psoriasis but is associated with renal toxicity and hypertension and is usually not suitable for long-term treatment. Oral retinoids such as acitretin are derivatives of vitamin A; they inhibit epithelial cell proliferation, inducing cell differentiation and inhibiting inflammation. Retinoids are rarely effective alone, but results are excellent when they are used in combination with UV phototherapy; the dose of ultraviolet light needed for clearance of lesions is reduced significantly.

The newer, biologic therapies are systemic agents that make use of recombinant DNA technology to create novel proteins that target the various pathophysiologic steps in psoriasis. Alefacept is a receptor fusion protein that contains the LFA-3 domain (found naturally on APCs) which binds specifically to CD2 (present in high density on memory effector T cells). Alefacept selectively binds to activated T cells that express higher amounts of CD2 on their surfaces than resting (naive) T cells. Consequently, alefacept improves psoriasis by inducing a granzyme-mediated apoptosis of the memory effector T cells that comprise the core T_H1/T_H17 response. Etanercept is a soluble version of the receptor for TNF-α, binds to free TNF-α, and thus inhibits this cytokine's ability to promote inflammation in the skin and the joints. Efalizumab is a monoclonal antibody directed against CD11a, a component of LFA-1. In binding to LFA-1, efalizumab blocks the ability of activated T cells to exit the vasculature of the skin and thus inhibits T-cell trafficking to psoriatic plaques. Finally, anti-IL-12p40 is an antibody that neutralizes both IL-12 and IL-23 and thus blocks the activity of the major dendritic cell cytokines that drive the inflammation of psoriasis. Recent clinical studies suggest that this agent may be particularly effective in the control of psoriasis.

In practice, phototherapy, topical agents, and systemic agents are often combined to augment clinical response, depending on the needs of the patient and his or her ability to tolerate the various modalities. Regardless, psoriasis is a lifelong illness without a cure. Therefore, patients must endure the chronic use of effective suppressive therapies that hopefully require a minimal alteration in lifestyle and carry a small risk of toxicity.

REFERENCES

Baker BS, Swain AF, Valdimarsson H, Fry L (1984): T-cell subpopulations in the blood and skin of patients with psorasis. *Br J Dermatol* 110:37–44.

Bowcock AM (2005): The genetics of psoriasis and autoimmunity. *Annu Rev Genomics Hum Genet* 6:93–122.

Bowcock AM, Krueger JG (2005): Getting under the skin: The immunopathogenesis of psoriasis. *Nat Rev Immunol* 5:699–711.

Brandrup F, Holm N, Grunnet N, Henningsen K, Hansen HE (1982): Psoriasis in monozygotic twins: Variation in expression in individuals with identical constitution. *Acta Derm Venerol* 62:229–236.

Gudjonsson JE, Johnston A, Sigmundsdottir H, Valdimarsson H (2004): Immunopathogenic mechanisms in psoriasis. *Clin Exp Immunol* 135:1–8.

Gudjonsson JE, Karason A, Antonsdottir A, Runarsdottir EH, Hauksson VB, Upmanyu R, Gulcher J, Stefansson K, Valdimarsson H (2003): Psoriasis patients who are homozygous for the HLA-Cw*0602 allele have a 2.5-fold increased risk of developing psoriasis compared with Cw6 heterozygotes. *Br J Dermatol* 148:233–235.

Gudjonsson JE, Thorarinsson AM, Sigurgeirsson B, Kristinsson KG, Valdimarsson H (2003): Streptococcal throat infections and exacerbation of chronic plague psoriasis: A prospective study. *Br J Dermatol* 149:530–534.

Johnston A, Gudjonsson JE, Sigmundsdottir H, Love TJ, Valdimarsson H (2004): Peripheral blood T-cell responses to keratin peptides that share sequences with streptococcal M proteins are largely restricted to skin-homing CD8(+) T cells. *Clin Exp Immunol* 138:83–93.

Lee E, Trepicchio WL, Oestreicher JL, Pittman D, Wang F, Chamian F, Dhodapkar M, Krueger JG (2004): Increased expression of interleukin 23 p19 and p40 in lesional skin of patients with psoriasis vulgaris. *J Exp Med* 199:125–130.

Leung DY, Travers JB, Giorno R, Norris DA, Skinner R, Aelion J, Kazemi LV, Kim MH, Trumble AE, Kotb M, Schlievert PM (1995): Evidence for a streptococcal superantigen-driven process in acute guttate psoriasis. *J Clin Invest* 96:2106–2112.

Lewish HN, Baker BS, Bokth S, Powels AV, Valdimarsson H, Fry L (1993): Restricted T-cell receptor Vbeta gene usage in the skin of patients with guttate and chronic plague psoriasis. *Br J Dermatol* 129:514–520.

Lin WJ, Norris DA, Achziger M, Kotzin BL, Tomkinson B (2001): Oligoclonal expansion of intraepidermal T cells in psoriasis skin lesions. *J Invest Dermatol* 117:1546–1553.

Nussbaum R, Krueger JG (2002): Treatment of inflammatory dermatoses with novel biologic agents: A primer. *Adv Dermatol* 18:45–89.

Prinz JC, Gross B, Vollmer S, Trommler P, Strobel I, Meurer M, Plewig G (1994): T-cell clones from psoriasis skin lesions can promote keratinocyte proliferation *in vitro* via secreted products. *Eur J Immunol* 24:593–598.

Sigmundsdottir H, Gudjonsson JE, Valdimarsson H (2003): Interleukin-12 alone can not enhance the expression of the cutaneous lymphocyte associated antigen (CLA) by superantigen-stimualted T lymphocytes. *Clin Exp Immunol* 132:430–435.

Sigmundsdottir H, Johnston A, Gudjonsson JE, Bjarnason B, Valdimarsson H (2004): Methotrexate markedly reduces the expression of vascular E-selectin, cutaneous lymphocyte-associated antigen and the numbers of mononuclear leucocytes in psoriatic skin. *Exp Dermatol* 13:426–434.

Telfer NR, Chalmers RJ, Whale K, Colman G (1992): The role of streptococcal infection in the initiation of guttate psoriasis. *Arch Dermatol* 128:39–42.

Valdimarsson H, Baker BS, Jonsdottir I, Powles A, Fry L (1995): Psoriasis: A T-cell-mediated autoimmune disease induced by streptococcal superantigens? *Immunol Today* 16:145–149.

Vollmer S, Menssen A, Prinz JC (2001): Dominant lesional T-cell receptor rearrangements persist in relapsing psoriasis but are absent from nonlesional skin: Evidence for a stable antigen-specific pathogenic T-cell response in psoriasis vulgaris. *J Invest Dermatol* 117:1296–1301.

Yawalkar N, Karlen S, Hunger R, Brand CU, Braathen LR (1998): Expression of interleukin-12 is increased in psoriatic skin. *J Invest Dermatol* 116:1053–1057.

20

IgA NEPHROPATHY AND KIDNEY TRANSPLANTATION

ROSLYN B. MANNON*

 CASE REPORT: PART I

"I see blood in my urine."

Clinical History and Initial Evaluation

Olivia, your 23-year-old patient, comes to see you after noticing blood in her urine. She states that about one month ago she developed "cold" symptoms with a cough, runny nose, sore throat, and fever (all upper respiratory symptoms). She did not seek medical attention because she is an elementary school teacher and many of her students were similarly ill; even now several children in her class are being treated for streptococcal throat infections. Four days into her illness, her urine appeared dark in color. She increased her fluid intake, but the color of her urine did not change. She also noted some back pain and took acetaminophen without relief. Because her urine still appears abnormal and her cold symptoms have persisted, she comes to your office for further advice. Other than the mild upper respiratory complaints and urine color, Olivia reports no additional symptoms; in particular she has had no shortness of breath, chills, weight loss, or night sweats. She has no difficulty urinating and no pain on urination and denies using any medications except the acetaminophen or ibuprofen for her fever.

*With contributions from Warren Strober and Susan R. S. Gottesman

You review her previous medical history both by referring to your records and by talking to Olivia. She says that she has been in good health and active all of her life; in fact, in both high school and college she ran track on the school teams. When asked about similar episodes, Olivia initially denies any but does remember that about six years ago, at a routine sports physical, protein was detected in her urine. She was told that this was due to dehydration, and the doctor cleared her for participation. She has no history of kidney stones, urinary tract infections, or kidney infections.

On physical exam, Olivia appears well with only some nasal congestion and rhinitis. Her blood pressure is elevated at 135/80 (normal limit about 120/70). Her heart rate is slightly elevated at 88/min (normal limit 60–80/min). Her temperature is 37.5°C. Her sclerae are clear and her tympanic membranes show no erythema (redness). Her oropharynx shows tonsillar enlargement and injection without exudates (pus). There are some small (<1 cm) anterior cervical lymph nodes. Lungs are clear to auscultation. Abdominal exam reveals no hepatomegaly (liver enlargement). There is no tenderness at the costovertebral angle (CVA) (tested by "punching" that region of the back). The extremities show no edema (swelling) and there is no rash.

You obtain basic laboratory studies, including a complete blood count (CBC), chemistries, and urine analysis.

Immunology: Clinical Case Studies and Disease Pathophysiology, By Warren Strober and Susan R. S. Gottesman
Copyright © 2009 John Wiley & Sons, Inc.

The urine is evaluated immediately in your office by dipping a reagent strip ("dipstick") into the sample. The reading shows 2+ blood and 2+ protein (reference values: negative), with no glucose or ketones. You decide to look at a "spun urine" yourself. (A *spun urine* is a urine sample that has been centrifuged to obtain a concentrated precipitate free of liquid for microscopic examination.) There are 5–10 white blood cells (WBCs) per high-power field, 10–15 red blood cells (RBCs) per high-power field, and granular casts. The RBCs do not look round and even but are distorted in shape. Finally, careful examination of the slide reveals two red cell casts (Fig. 20.1).

CBC and chemistry tests are sent as stat tests to the neighboring hospital laboratory. Results come back within the hour, while you still have Olivia waiting in your office. CBC results are within normal limits, with no evidence of anemia or increased WBCs. Chemistries reveal an albumin level of 2.9 g/dL (reference range 3.2–5.5 g/dL), a total protein level of 5.2 g/dL (reference range 5.5–9 g/dL), a blood urea nitrogen (BUN) of 12 mg/dL (reference range 10–20 mg/dL), and a creatinine of 1.0 mg/dL (reference range 0.5–1.1 mg/dL), giving a BUN–creatinine ratio of 12:1 (reference range 10:1–20:1).

What is the significance of the abnormal urine sample results?

Olivia's urine specimen shows a number of abnormalities, including levels of protein, blood, and white cells. Protein in the urine (proteinuria) is detected by reagent indicator strips. The strips are scored as follows: trace: 5–20 mg/dL, 1+: 30 mg/dL, 2+: 100 mg/dL, 3+: 300 mg/dL, and 4+: 2000 mg/dL. Protein detection by this method is more specific for albumin than for other proteins and may not detect immunoglobulin light chains, as can occur in plasma cell proliferations. If the urine is dilute, then the protein level detected may be falsely low. Similarly, concentrated

specimens may yield falsely high protein levels. Thus, for a reliable quantitative assessment of proteinuria, a 24-h urine collection should be obtained. While proteinuria most frequently occurs because of glomerular injury, it may also occur because of renal tubular damage. The proteins excreted due to glomerular disease are generally larger, since an intact glomerular membrane normally does not permit passage of proteins >50 kDa. A urine protein electrophoresis can distinguish among albumin, globulins, and light chains, but sizing of urinary proteins requires gel electrophoresis.

*RBCs may enter the urine ("hematuria") from anywhere in the urinary tract. A few RBCs (two or three per high-power field) are considered normal, but any more than that indicates abnormality. RBCs that result from kidney problems are **dysmorphic** (show blebbing, membrane folding, and vesicle formation), but those from the collecting system maintain their usual biconcave appearance. The high number and distorted shape of the red cells in Olivia's urine indicate that they may be gaining entry into the filtrate from within the kidney itself.*

WBCs in the urine ("pyuria") may be present under normal circumstances but should not exceed one to five per high-power microscopic field. The presence of additional WBCs can indicate urinary tract infection as well as interstitial inflammation or glomerular inflammation.

Several types of casts may be detected in the precipitate of a urine sample. These casts can appear similar to coarsely granular casts indicative of degenerated cells and are nonspecific in nature. Red cell casts (Fig. 20.1) contain only red cells, which may appear dysmorphic within the cast. The presence of red cell casts is indicative of glomerular disease and requires urgent attention. They are often associated with other urinary abnormalities such as proteinuria, hematuria, and pyuria, as in Olivia's case.

Based on the fact that Olivia's urine contains RBCs, casts (especially red cell casts), and elevated protein levels, you strongly suspect that she has kidney disease and you refer her to a nephrologist. You arrange for her to see the specialist the following afternoon; in the meantime you order a 24-h urine for protein and creatinine levels. You instruct Olivia to go to the lab for the container and to collect her urine for the next 24 h. When she returns the collection to the lab, she is instructed to wait for the results and bring them with her to the nephrologist's office.

The Diagnosis

The next day the lab calls you to report that the 24-hour urine specimen from Olivia contains 2.4 g of total protein (reference range <150 mg/day) and 1150 mg of creatinine (reference range 500–2000 mg/day). The calculated creatinine clearance is 80 ml/min (reference range 88–128 ml/min).

What additional information have you gathered from the 24-h urine results?

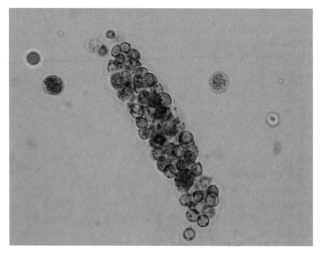

Figure 20.1. Sedi-stained urine sample demonstrating a red cell cast. (Photograph courtesy of Dr. James Balow.)

This level of protein excretion is abnormal. Although you knew this from the initial random urine sample, these results not only confirm the first set of data on Olivia but also quantitate the level of protein excretion. While not in the nephrotic syndrome range (see below), it is quite elevated. As noted above, proteinuria may be due to tubular or glomerular damage. One way to differentiate between the two is to evaluate the urine protein by electrophoresis and determine the level of albumin excretion, a marker of glomerular damage.

Creatinine, a waste product of muscle metabolism, is freely filtered and excreted by the kidney. It is not reabsorbed and is only minimally secreted. The urine creatinine is compared to the level in the blood to arrive at a creatinine clearance rate. This is used to estimate the glomerular filtration rate (GFR) or volume of blood filtered through the kidney per unit time. As such it is dependent on kidney function but is also influenced by blood flow.

The 24-h urine protein level confirms that Olivia has nephritic rather than nephrotic syndrome as suggested by her clinical manifestations.

What are the definitions of these two syndromes?

Nephrotic syndrome and nephritic syndrome are two of several types of glomerular syndromes which are categorized on the basis of laboratory and clinical findings. Any one of a number of etiologies can be the cause of either of these two glomerular dysfunctions. **Nephrotic syndrome** *is defined by >3.5 g/day of proteinuria, severe edema, hypoalbuminemia (presumably due to loss through the urine), hyperlipidemia, and lipiduria. It indicates severe glomerular damage.* **Nephritic syndrome** *is characterized by an acute onset of hematuria, mild to moderate proteinuria (<3.5 g/day), and hypertension. Olivia's presenting symptoms, history, physical examination, and laboratory data are all consistent with nephritic syndrome.*

You make a tentative diagnosis of glomerulonephritis. Later that day, the nephrologist calls, having just seen Olivia and reviewed her lab data, and concurs with your diagnosis.

What is glomerulonephritis and what are its possible causes?

Glomerulonephritis *refers to a specific type of renal disease. It presents with albuminuria and RBCs and/or inflammatory cells in the urine. There are a number of primary causes as well as several secondary causes of glomerulonephritis. Diseases in which the glomerulonephritis is primary include those that originate from and are centered in the kidney, whereas diseases in which the glomerulitis is secondary include generalized diseases that involve a number of organs, including the kidney. Key features of each allows you to narrow the list down to a relatively few possible causes, based on Olivia's history and physical examination (Table 20.1). For example, you would not consider diabetic nephropathy, because there is no history or evidence of diabetes mellitus. Among the primary causes under*

TABLE 20.1. Differential Diagnosis of Glomerular Disease with Nonnephrotic Range Proteinuria and Hematuria under Consideration for Olivia

Diseases Limited to Kidney	Systemic Diseases
IgA nephropathy	Systemic lupus erythematosus
Focal segmental glomerulonephritis	Postinfectious disease
	Poststreptococcal
Membranoproliferative disease	Endocarditis
Mesangioproliferative disease	Goodpasture's disease
	Vasculitis
	Wegener's granulomatosis
	Microscopic polyangiitis

consideration in this case, IgA nephropathy is first on the list because of its high frequency. In addition, several secondary causes must be considered in this context, including lupus nephritis and other **crescenteric diseases** *(diseases associated with the formation of glomerular infiltrates shaped like crescents) such as Wegener's granulomatosis, Goodpasture's disease, or a postinfectious glomerular disease such as poststreptococcal glomerulonephritis. You can distinguish among these possibilities by renal biopsy and serologic testing. The presence of elevated levels of antistreptolysin antibody (ASO) titers in the serum would suggest poststreptococcal glomerulonephritis; elevated anti-double-stranded DNA antibody titers as well as elevated C3 and C4 complement levels would point to lupus nephritis. Elevated ANCA (antinuclear antibody) would point to Wegener's granulomatosis, and anti–glomerular basement membrane (anti-GBM) antibody would indicate Goodpasture's disease. Finally, it is important to check the patient's hepatitis B and C status by serologic testing to rule out glomerular disease consequent to liver infection (see Vasculitidies, case 13).*

Definitive Diagnosis and Etiology of Renal Disease: IgA Nephropathy

To verify the diagnosis of glomerulonephritis and to distinguish among the causes of this disease, the nephrologist arranges for a needle biopsy of the kidney to be performed under ultrasound guidance and has Olivia's blood drawn for several serologic tests. The tissue from the renal biopsy is preserved for routine histologic examination, fluorescent antibody studies, and electron microscopy to assist in the differential diagnosis. The following results are available after several days.

Kidney

- Light microscopy of hematoxylin and eosin (H&E)–stained biopsy tissue shows normal glomeruli with

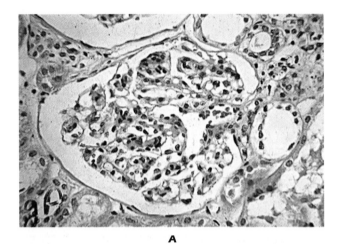

A

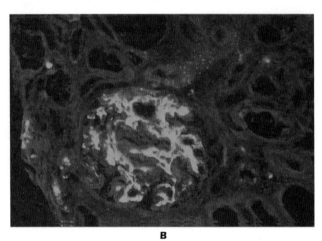

B

Figure 20.2. (A) Light microscopy of glomerulus consistent with IgA nephropathy. Diffuse mesangial proliferation with hypercellularity is present (200X). (B) Immunofluorescence staining of a kidney demonstrating IgA staining (green fluorescence) within the mesangium (200X). (Photomicrographs courtesy of Dr. Sharda Sabnis, AFIP.)

minimal hypercellularity (Fig. 20.2A). There are no crescents within the glomeruli. The interstitial areas, tubules, and vessels also appear normal. According to the report, 12 glomeruli were present in the sample, allowing an adequate evaluation.

- Fluorescent microscopic examination of the biopsy tissue stained with labeled antibodies demonstrates diffuse deposition of IgA antibody within the mesangial areas (cells and matrix supporting the glomerular tuft) (Fig. 20.2B) as well as deposition of complement component C3. There is no deposition of IgM, IgG, or C1q.

- Electron microscopy supports the diagnosis of IgA nephropathy; there is focal thinning of the GBMs and electron-dense deposits in the mesangium.

Serological Tests

- Anti-double-stranded DNA, ASO, ANCA, anti-GBM antibodies and tests for hepatic viral titers are returned as negative.

The diagnosis of IgA nephropathy is now established based on clinical, laboratory, and biopsy results.

Therapy

You and the nephrologist begin treating Olivia with an angiotensin-converting enzyme (ACE) inhibitor called lisinopril at 10 mg/day to control her blood pressure (see below). Although her blood pressure improves to 125/72, Olivia's proteinuria persists at 1.5 g/day. As a result, you refer her back to the nephrologist, who starts Olivia on intravenous and oral steroid therapy according to a recommended regimen.

CLINICAL FEATURES AND MONITORING OF IgA NEPHROPATHY

IgA nephropathy is a kidney disease characterized by proteinuria, hematuria, and progressive renal failure. It is one of the most common causes of glomerulonephritis and tends to have an onset in young adulthood (second and third decades of life). Early in the disease, there may be no symptoms, so the patient may be unaware that he or she is ill. At this point the disease is detected only if the patient is subjected to routine medical screening for an unrelated reason. More often, however, clinical manifestations such as those noted by Olivia occur, which raise sufficient concern to prompt a visit to a physician. The most common symptom, occurring in about 50% cases, is gross hematuria with or without associated flank pain. Many (but not all) patients with this type of presentation can relate the onset of these symptoms to an upper respiratory infection. At the other end of the presentation spectrum, approximately 10% of patients present with advanced renal disease characterized by severe proteinuria, edema, and renal failure. This latter patient group illustrates the fact that IgA nephropathy can be a rapidly progressive and potentially fatal disease.

Diagnostic procedures to verify the presence of IgA nephropathy should be undertaken as soon as possible, as early detection and early treatment can lead to possible prevention of progression to renal failure. As in Olivia's case, diagnosis starts with urinalysis; the presence and characteristics of various formed elements in the urine not only can indicate whether urinary tract disease is present but also can help distinguish between upper and lower urinary tract disease. Thus, the presence of RBCs that are *dysmorphic* (exhibiting variations in shape, size, and hemoglobin content) and the presence of red or white cell casts are indicative of glomerular disease rather than lower urinary tract disease. Detection of proteinuria is a key early finding that can be accomplished with a simple urine dipstick indicator. However, this method may not detect low (but nevertheless significant) levels of protein excretion; a 24-h urine collection more reliably quantitates protein loss. This collection can also be used to calculate a creatinine clearance and GFR. These simple and readily available tests also allow early prediction of the outcome of the renal disease. A poor outcome is predicted by persistent microscopic hematuria, 24-h protein excretion of >1 g, and impaired renal function at the time of diagnosis as indicated by the creatinine clearance. In addition, the presence of glomerular crescents in the renal biopsy is a poor prognostic sign.

A more critical indicator of prognosis, particularly when blood pressure is normalized by medication, is urine protein excretion. For example, at one year of follow-up, the risk of developing end-stage renal disease is 60% with protein of >3 g/day, 25% for 1.5–3.0 g/day, 13% for 0.5–1.5 g/day, and 0% with <0.5 g/day. Some investigators suggest that early biopsy is also merited; they believe that biopsy findings of mild glomerular changes and tubulointerstitial disease can predict poor outcome independent of serum and urine studies.

Of course, regardless of the underlying cause, renal insufficiency is accompanied by the clinical manifestations of poor fluid management (edema) and blood pressure control; as it progresses, there is secondary hyperparathyroidism with resultant bone changes and decreased erythropoietin production leading to anemia.

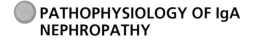

PATHOPHYSIOLOGY OF IgA NEPHROPATHY

The etiology of IgA nephropathy remains uncertain. A strong environmental effect is likely given the association of the onset of disease with upper respiratory infection. However, such infection is followed by renal disease in only a small minority of individuals, so it is clear that a genetic predisposition must also be present. This possibility is supported by reports of familial case clustering and by the association of the disease with polymorphisms in the ACE gene and in selectin genes. A susceptibility locus on chromosome 6q22–23 has also been described.

The initiating effect of upper respiratory infection suggests the presence of an abnormality of mucosal immunity, perhaps one characterized by an excessive IgA response that ultimately leads to IgA deposition in the kidney. Support for this possibility comes from a mouse model of IgA nephropathy, known as the hyper-IgA (HIGA) mouse, which manifests abnormally increased numbers of surface IgA (sIgA)–expressing B cells in the

lamina propria, decreased IgA secretion into the bowel lumen, and (most importantly) renal deposition of IgA. A similar abnormality exists in human IgA nephropathy compared to normal individuals: patients with this disease have an increase in the percentage of circulating $\gamma\delta$ T cells that is associated with higher levels of sIgA B cells and higher serum IgA concentrations. In addition, peripheral cells from patients with IgA nephropathy exhibit increased IgA production when cultured and stimulated *in vitro*, an increase that is reduced by removal of the $\gamma\delta$ T cells. The $\gamma\delta$ T cells are T cells that express the alternative T-cell receptor (TCR). $\gamma\delta$ (the majority of peripheral T cells express the $\alpha\beta$ TCR) $\gamma\delta$ T cells traffic preferentially to skin, lung, and intestinal sites and interact with CD1 of the major histocompatibility complex (MHC). The mechanism by which $\delta\gamma$ T cells affect IgA B-cell development is unclear, but these studies suggest that IgA nephropathy in humans is indeed associated with or even due to excessive IgA production. Unfortunately, this compelling concept is not backed up by evidence of excessive *in vivo* IgA responses. An elevated memory IgA response following oral immunization with recall antigens or following nasal administration of common vaccine antigens is not seen in IgA nephropathy patients. Therefore, the concept that a basic abnormality in the *magnitude* of the mucosal IgA response (possibly as a result of $\gamma\delta$ T-cell abnormality) underlies IgA nephropathy must be considered unproven at the present time.

Another theory of IgA nephropathy is that it is due to an intrinsic defect in the *structure* of IgA, which leads to abnormalities in its distribution. It is based on evidence that in IgA nephropathy the IgA1 subclass is characterized by a defect in glycosylation, which causes a deficiency in hinge region sialic acid. As a result, the IgA1 has a tendency to aggregate and form polymers with an increased affinity for the mesangium of the kidney. Alternatively, the sialic acid deficiency causes impairment in the mechanism that normally allows clearance of IgA antibody–antigen complexes in the liver. Thus the increase in these IgA forms favors IgA deposition in the kidney. The fact that IgA nephropathy only rarely occurs in other disease states with elevated IgA levels, such as IgA producing plasma cell myeloma or HIV infection, can be explained by assuming that it is not high levels of IgA *per se* that causes disease but rather an altered form of circulating IgA. This concept of disease pathogenesis is convincing, yet it does not explain why IgA nephropathy usually does not occur very early in life, as one would expect with the presence of a structural IgA lesion that can be presumed to have existed from birth.

The IgA deposited in the kidney in IgA nephropathy is unlikely to be part of an IgA complex with a specific antigen since no specific antigen has been consistently detected in patient sera or kidney biopsy specimens. On the other hand, aggregates of IgA (or IgA–antigen complexes not containing a specific antigen) and fibronectin are found in the circulation of patients with considerable frequency. Indirect evidence that these IgA–fibronectin aggregates play a role in the kidney deposition of IgA comes from two observations: (1) Fibronectin binds avidly to an anti-inflammatory molecule known as uteroglobin that under normal circumstances prevents IgA–fibronectin complex formation and (2) mice with a targeted deletion of the uteroglobin gene develop a disease similar to human IgA nephropathy. Thus, the picture that emerges is that the IgA in IgA nephropathy forms immune complexes with an abnormal tendency to associate with fibronectin (in spite of normal levels of uteroglobin), and that these form deposits in the kidney. In any case, some have suggested that IgA–fibronectin complexes can be used as serologic markers for IgA nephropathy and related diseases characterized by IgA deposition in the kidney (such as Henoch–Schonlein purpura).

Once deposited in the kidney, IgA complexes initiate a robust inflammatory response that results in the severe renal injury characteristic of IgA nephropathy. IgA does not itself activate complement and is generally considered an anti-inflammatory immunoglobulin. However, upon deposition in the kidney, IgA binds another protein, mannan-binding protein (MBP), which does activate complement (see Case 8); thus, IgA nephropathy is somewhat paradoxically characterized by complement-mediated damage. Because the deposition of MBP in the kidney is uniquely related to its affinity for IgA, this protein is not detected in other glomerular diseases, such as lupus nephritis.

In addition to MBP, a variety of cytokines and growth factors have also been associated with the development and progression of IgA nephropathy. These include interleukin-6 (IL-6), tumor necrosis factor (TNF)-α, platelet-derived growth factor and its receptor, and transforming growth factor (TGF)-β (which is fibrosis inducing). In some cases, the serum or urinary levels of these factors have been used to monitor disease activity. The presence of these factors may be due to the induction of a mixed T_H1/T_H2 immune response to tubular epithelial cells and cells in the glomerulus, which express high levels of CD80 and CD86, respectively, and thus act as antigen-presenting cells (APCs). In fact, the level of expression of these two costimulatory proteins is correlated with the extent of loss of renal function in patients with the disease. The nature of the antigen or antigens being presented by these surrogate APCs is not yet known.

TREATMENT OF IgA NEPHROPATHY

Appropriate treatment of patients with IgA nephropathy depends on the extent of the disease. For those with mild disease at presentation (urine proteins of <0.5 g/day, mild hematuria, and mild histologic features on renal biopsy), management of blood pressure to <125/75 with ACE

inhibitors or angiotensin receptor blockers (ARBs) is all that is required. In some instances, combining ACE inhibitors with ARBs can result in reductions in blood pressure and proteinuria better than those achieved with individual therapy alone. In patients with more substantial proteinuria at presentation (>2 g/day proteinuria and/or biopsies with more advanced pathology), treatment with ACE inhibitors and/or ARBs is also initiated, with the goals of reducing proteinuria to <1.0 g/day and maintaining normal blood pressure. If substantial proteinuria persists, oral corticosteroid therapy with pulse intravenous corticosteroids is instituted. At least three to six months of continuous steroid treatment is usually necessary for any benefit to occur. Finally, in cases of more aggressive disease (declining renal function and glomerular crescent changes), additional immunosuppressive therapies have been used, including administration of cyclophosphamide, mycophenolate mofetil, and azathioprine. At present, there are no large, randomized trials underway to determine which combination of agents is most effective.

Another treatment option is the administration of omega-3 fatty acids ("fish oil"), but it is not at all clear that this is beneficial. Some studies suggest that this therapy slows the pace of disease in those patients with continued renal deterioration in spite of treatment with ACE inhibitor/ARB and steroid therapy. However, other studies suggest that there is no significant benefit (or detriment) to this form of therapy.

 ## CASE REPORT: PART 2

Olivia Returns

About two years later, Olivia returns to your office with nausea, vomiting, and headache. Olivia admits that she has only intermittently seen the nephrologist and has stopped taking some of her medications. Specifically, she stopped the steroid therapy because it made her gain weight, develop acne, and worsened her blood pressure. The nephrologist had also placed her on fish oil therapy, but Olivia stopped it because "it made me smell as stinky as a fish!" She has continued to take the lisinopril. According to your records, her last creatinine was 1.5 mg/dL.

On exam, Olivia's blood pressure is 160/100 and she has gained 20 kg (44 lbs) since she was last weighed in your office. Her fundi show flat discs. Her lungs are clear, and she has a soft systolic heart murmur. There is 2^+ pitting edema extending to the knees. You urgently send chemistries and urine analysis with microscopic evaluation. Her serum creatinine comes back as 10.0 mg/dL with a BUN of 68 mg/dL. Her albumin is now 2.3 with a protein of 4.5 and she is also mildly anemic. Her urine shows 3^+ protein, many RBCs, but no red cell casts. A renal ultrasound study shows no obstruction.

These findings indicate that Olivia has had progressive renal deterioration, is uremic, and unfortunately now has *end-stage renal disease (ESRD)*. You send her back to the nephrologist. She agrees with your assessment and does not feel that additional diagnostic steps (such as a renal biopsy) are necessary to confirm the diagnosis, so she arranges for Olivia to be dialyzed.

What is uremia?

Uremia is a clinical syndrome that is the consequence of electrolyte, fluid, and metabolic imbalances that result from renal failure. Nausea, vomiting, anorexia, and mental status changes are among the presenting symptoms. It is believed to be the result of multiple toxins and imbalances rather than one specific element. It must be corrected with a degree of urgency.

Treatment Recommendations for ESRD Secondary to IgA Nephropathy: Dialysis versus Transplantation

Olivia is now in renal failure and requires treatment to replace kidney function.

What are the treatment options for ESRD?

Quite simply, in renal failure the function of the kidney must be replaced so that toxic waste products can be removed from the body. This is achieved by one of two methods: dialysis (hemodialysis or peritoneal dialysis) or kidney transplantation.

Kidney transplantation is the preferred mode of therapy for many patients with IgA nephropathy, since patient and graft survival after transplantation for this renal disease is similar to if not better than that of other glomerular diseases. In particular, transplantation is associated with a 10-year patient survival rate of 93% and 10-year graft survival rate of 75%. However, this generally favorable picture is counterbalanced by the fact that IgA nephropathy recurs within the transplanted kidney at a rate of 30–50%, reflecting the fact that this is fundamentally a systemic disease in which the kidney is merely a target organ. The risk of recurrence is highest in younger patients and in those recipients with higher serum creatinine or proteinuria 6 months posttransplant. It has been debated whether the graft source alters recurrence rate; some investigators have demonstrated higher recurrence rates in recipients of grafts from living related donors, but this is not a consistent finding. Although these recurrence rates are high, they are not high enough to contraindicate transplantation as a treatment for IgA nephropathy; as noted above, the survival rates posttransplantation are quite favorable. In addition, these recurrence rates do not yet reflect the possibly favorable impact of the newer immunosuppressive strategies now used to prevent graft rejection.

After discussing her options, Olivia decides to be evaluated for renal transplantation. She is sent to a local transplant center for assessment of her suitability as a recipient based on her medical and psychosocial status. Despite her history of noncompliance to prescribed therapy, Olivia is placed on a waiting list for cadaveric kidney transplantation. In addition, the center evaluators suggest that she approach family members to be potential donors.

Considerations of Kidney Transplantation in the United States

Approximately 50,000 individuals are currently awaiting kidney transplantation in the United States; this number is increasing with the growing recognition of ESRD and with the improvement in transplantation success rate. Because only about 9000 cadaveric kidneys become available each year, along with 7500 kidneys from living donors, a large (and growing) number of patients must wait years for transplantation. Cadaveric donors must be free of systemic diseases such as malignancies and infections and must have renal function as close to normal as possible at the time of death. Living donors must have normal blood pressure, the absence of kidney stones or other structural abnormalities of the kidneys, and, of course, a willingness to donate. Finally, donors and recipients are matched by ABO blood type, since severe, hyperacute rejection can occur with an ABO mismatch. (Blood-type compatibility is determined by standard blood bank procedures employing panels of red cells of known specificity, which determine whether the recipient has IgM antibodies for donor blood-type antigens.) Recently, protocols to "desensitize" recipients in cases of ABO mismatch are being used in some transplant centers. Of course, since this procedure must precede transplant by several weeks, it is only done with living donations.

The main predictor of the success of kidney transplantation is the donor source. Kidneys from living donors, whether related or unrelated to the recipient, have better survivals than kidneys from deceased donors. The potency of immunosuppressive agents has facilitated transplantation substantially over the past 40 years. However, maximizing outcome depends on the suitability of donor and recipient pairing with respect to tissue type, or the match between the human leukocyte antigens (HLAs) of the donor and recipient. HLA delineation is done at a special tissue-typing laboratory. The most clinically relevant of these antigens are the class I (A and B) and class II DR antigens. Each parent contributes half of his or her HLA genes (the set on each chromosome) to each child, so each child is typically haploidentical (matching the set or haplotype on one chromosome) to each parent. Each individual has six antigens inherited from his or her parents in the HLA regions being tested. On a purely statistical basis, siblings are 25% HLA identical ("0 mismatched"), 50% haploidentical, and 25% nonidentical (100% mismatched). Because HLA-identical grafts have excellent short- and long-term survival, it is best to select a living donor with a matched HLA type. Kidneys from haploidentical and nonidentical donors have progressively lower survival rates. As these genetic regions are highly polymorphous within the population, a matching HLA type would be unlikely to be found in a cadaver kidney. Other factors affecting graft and patient outcomes include the race of the recipient (African Americans and native Americans have worse outcomes than Caucasians), rejection episodes in the first year posttransplantation (predict reduced long-term graft survival), age of both recipient and donor (survival declines with age of both donors and recipients), length of time between removal of the kidney from the donor and its transplantation into the recipient (higher rates of long-term graft loss occur with donor organs subjected to cold ischemia for >24 h), and degree of prior sensitization of the recipient (see below). This last factor in particular will determine how the immunosuppression regimen should be tailored to the individual.

After Olivia is placed on the waiting list, additional information is gathered to provide as much data as possible regarding the suitability of a potential match. Assessment of donor and recipient tissue type provides a "theoretical" assessment of the outcome, but compatibility is also evaluated in a more direct and immediate manner. The sensitization of the recipient to antigens from potential donors is evaluated. The recipient may have a preexisting immune response due to sensitization as the result of pregnancy, blood transfusion, or prior transplantation. Before a specific donor is identified, a general idea of the patient's degree of sensitization and identification of particularly strong preexisting antibodies is evaluated on a population basis. The reactivity of antibodies in the recipient's sera is measured against a pool or panel of HLA antigens representing those found in the potential donor population; this is referred to as the patient's panel-reactive antibody (PRA) level. PRA level can be measured using several different *in vitro* tests. The complement-dependent cytotoxicity (CDC) assay uses a panel of target lymphocytes, usually T cells, patient serum, and complement; cell lysis occurs if specific antibodies are present. This test predominantly measures antibodies against class I HLA. Alternatively, solid-phase immunoassays are used. These include an ELISA (enzyme-linked immunosorbant assay)–based test using microtiter plates coated with purified soluble HLA antigens of both class I and class II. After incubation with patient serum, bound antibody is detected with a tagged antihuman IgG antibody, the reaction is developed using a colorimetric substrate, and the light absorbance is read. Another test employs labeled bead particles coated with HLA antigens are employed as targets; reactivity against them can be read using a flow cytometer or a luminex technology. These solid-phase immunoassays are used to arrive at a "calculated" PRA and have the advantage of allowing identification of the specific reactivity of the antibodies present in the patient's serum. All of the assays can be used to establish antibody titers through serial dilutions of the serum.

Living Kidney Donation

The information regarding cadaver kidney donations is relayed to Olivia. When her family members learn that she may have a five-year wait for a cadaveric organ and that the outcome is better with a living donor, her brother volunteers to serve as a kidney donor.

Upon evaluation, the transplant team learns that Olivia and her brother are matched by blood type and are HLA haploidentical. Her brother is healthy and consequently is considered a reasonable donor.

Once the actual potential donor is identified, recipient antibody status specific for the HLA of the donor at hand is assessed by a test called a "cross match." This can be accomplished using adaptations of some of the same technologies described above to arrive at the PRA, but now the donor's lymphocytes are used as the target. Donor cells [which can be peripheral lymphocytes, splenocytes, or lymphocytes from lymph nodes (the latter two in the case of a deceased donor)] are mixed with recipient serum at various dilutions; the outcome is assessed in the CDC test (CDC cross-match) or by using the flow cytometer (flow cross-match). In the flow cross-match, the presence of anti-HLA class I (antibodies reacting against both the T and B cells) versus the presence of anti-HLA class II (antibodies reacting against the B cells only) can be estimated; the presence of antibody to donor cells is measured following the addition of fluorescent-tagged antihuman antibody for detection of bound antibody and fluorescent-stained anti-CD3 (T-cell antigen) or anti-CD20 (B-cell antigen). More recently, single antigen beads matching the donor HLA type and using luminex technology have been employed to evaluate recipient serum for specific antibodies. These assays have different levels of sensitivity. A positive cross-match indicates that the recipient has preformed antibody against one or more donor antigens and that immediate or hyperacute rejection may occur, resulting in immediate graft failure. Because it is the least sensitive and predominantly measures class I, a positive CDC is most likely to predict hyperacute rejection. These practical tests of compatibility help a transplant team decide whether a donor organ is appropriate, determine the advisable immunosuppressive regimen, and (in the case of living donors) ascertain whether desensitization by plasmapheresis should be attempted. For more on plasmapheresis, see Case 14.

Transplant and Early Follow-Up

A CDC cross-match between Olivia and her brother is negative, as is the final flow cross-match. That is, Olivia lacks circulating antibodies that react with her brother's cells within the sensitivity of these assays. The transplant is scheduled, and immunosuppression is begun three days prior to the transplant. Because Olivia is receiving a haploidentical kidney, the transplant team decides on an immunosuppressive regimen consisting of daclizumab (anti-CD25 antibody), prednisone, mycophenolate mofetil, and tacrolimus. The surgeries for both donor and recipient are uncomplicated. A laparoscopic procedure is used to remove the kidney from her brother, and he returns home after two days in the hospital. By postoperative day 3, Olivia's serum creatinine is 0.9 mg/dL, indicating that the transplanted kidney is working well. She remains free of infection and is discharged home on a regimen of immunosuppressive therapy.

The Necessity of Immunosuppressive Therapy: Mechanisms of Graft Rejection

Following transplantation of either partially or completely mismatched tissue, foreign donor histocompatibility antigens are detected by recipient T cells through a process called *allorecognition* (Fig. 20.3). Since the frequency of alloreactive T cells is relatively high (they comprise about 2% of peripheral T cells), the response to mismatched tissue is usually quite strong. Allorecognition occurs via one of two pathways. In *direct allorecognition*, recipient T cells recognize components of foreign MHC as if this complex were similar to ordinary exogenous non-MHC antigens being presented by self-MHC. In this pathway, cytotoxic CD8$^+$ T cells become activated and are the primary destructive arm of the rejection response. In *indirect allorecognition*, recipient T cells recognize processed foreign MHC peptides in the context of self-MHC antigens. In this pathway CD4$^+$ T cells become activated as in the pathway utilized by the immune system for recognition of ordinary exogenous antigens. The activated CD4$^+$ T cells become effector cells that help in the development of delayed-type hypersensitivity, antibody

production, and cell-mediated cytotoxicity reactions to the foreign MHC antigens. Indirect allorecognition is critical to acute rejection responses and may perpetuate responses leading to chronic graft rejection.

T-cell activation requires at least two signals. The first signal is delivered through the TCR/CD3 complex recognizing antigen associated with MHC molecules; this signal is anchored by CD4 in the case of class II (Fig. 20.4) or CD8 and class I MHC molecules (see Case 3). The second signal is antigen independent and is delivered through costimulatory molecules. The primary costimulatory molecules are CD28, which binds B7 (CD80 and CD86) on APCs, and CD154 (CD40L), which binds CD40. Costimulatory signals have been viewed as "positive" in their contribution to activation, but a number of newer "negative" costimulatory signals have been identified as inhibiting activation. These are actively being studied as potential regulators of the immune response. Once the T cell is activated, IL-2 is transcribed, translated, and secreted; it then stimulates the production and excretion of other activating cytokines. The engagement of these cytokines with their receptors, which could be considered a third activation signal, sets the stage for cell division and maturation.

While the main cellular element involved in rejection is the T cell, the rejection response also involves B cells, NK cells, and macrophages. These cells amplify the T-cell rejection response via their release of cytokines and chemokines and the production of antibodies.

Rejection responses to foreign tissue can take four different forms:

- *Hyperacute rejection* occurs minutes to hours after implantation and reperfusion of the graft and is due to preformed anti-donor antibodies. These antibodies deposit on the endothelium of the graft, leading to complement activation, thrombosis, and graft ischemia.

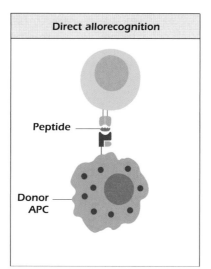
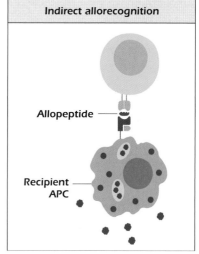

Figure 20.3. Direct versus indirect allorecognition of foreign antigens.

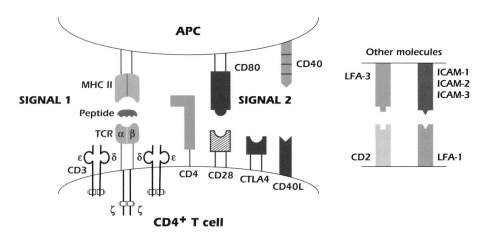

Figure 20.4. T-cell activation requires two signals. A number of costimulatory molecules have been described as "positive" facilitators of the immune response. Negative costimulatory molecules include B7-CTLA4.

- *Accelerated acute rejection* occurs a few days after implantation, typically in presensitized individuals. It is mediated by both cellular and antibody effector responses.

- *Acute rejection* typically occurs days to weeks after transplantation but also occurs much later, after years of apparently successful engraftment. Although acute rejection is most frequently due to cell-mediated injury, it can also be mediated by antibodies. In this type of rejection, T cells stimulated by IL-2 and IFN-γ cause organ injury via cytotoxic responses mediated by release of granzyme B and perforin (see Diabetes mellitus Case 16). In addition, the T cell releases chemokines that cause the influx of other injurious cells. The acute rejection response can be associated with localized graft tenderness as well as systemic manifestations consisting of chills, myalgias, and fever. If this response is not brought under control, it results in irreversible graft injury and, ultimately, graft loss.

- *Chronic allograft rejection* is the most common cause of late kidney graft failure. This form of rejection occurs months to years after transplantation and is a chronic process characterized by progressive fibrosis of the graft associated with a gradual decline in renal function and increasing proteinuria. Chronic allograft rejection is due to both antigen-dependent and antigen-independent inflammatory processes. Despite the potency of current immunosuppressive regimens, chronic allograft rejection continues to plague kidney transplantation, even while short-term graft survivals have shown significant improvement.

Immunosuppressive Therapies

As already noted, immunosuppression regimens used to prevent transplant rejection have improved dramatically over the past decade. Such regimens typically consist of a cocktail of agents that attack the immune response on a number of levels, such as glucocorticoids, an antimetabolite such as mycophenolate mofetil or azathioprine, and a calcineurin inhibitor (CNI) such as tacrolimus or cyclosporin. In addition, patients at high risk for rejection are usually given some form of *induction therapy* (initial, short-term administration of immunosuppressive agents that precedes more long-term immunosuppression) consisting of a monoclonal or polyclonal antibody that attenuates a basic immunologic mechanism involved in the rejection process. Because glucocorticoids inhibit both T-cell and macrophage function by their adverse effects on cytokine production, they are useful in both the treatment of acute rejection and amelioration of chronic rejection. However, long-term glucocorticoid therapy is fraught with many undesirable side effects, including increased susceptibility to infection, hyperlipidemia, hypertension, glucose intolerance, and psychological effects such as mania and psychosis (see Case 15). In addition, these agents invariably cause bone loss and may result in osteoporosis and avascular necrosis.

CNIs, notably cyclosporin A and tacrolimus, are immunosuppressive agents that have dramatically improved transplantation outcomes since their introduction some 20 years ago. Cyclosporin A and tacrolimus act by first binding to cytoplasmic proteins known as cyclophilin and FK-binding protein, respectively; the resultant complexes bind to and inhibit calcineurin, a molecule that normally dephosphorylates the nuclear factor of activated T cells (NFAT). Inhibition of calcineurin results in the lack of NFAT translocation to the nucleus and thus impaired transcription of the genes for the cytokines, IL-2, interferon (IFN)-γ, IL-4, and TNF-α. CNIs also induce expression of TGF-β, which has a positive anti-inflammatory effect but also is profibrotic (an undesirable effect). Although

CNIs have dramatically improved graft survival over the past two decades, their use is not without significant side effects. These include hypertension, hirsutism, glucose intolerance and overt diabetes, hyperlipidemia, neurotoxicity manifested by tremor, and nephrotoxicity. The nephrotoxicity consists of both acute effects that lead to functional alterations in GFR and renal blood flow and chronic effects causing tubular atrophy, interstitial fibrosis, and arteriolar hyalinosis. Since these side effects are dose related, the trough levels of CNIs must be monitored carefully so they do not exceed therapeutic target levels.

Antimetabolite agents are the third component of the triumvirate of antitransplant rejection therapies. Because they act by interfering with some aspect of DNA/RNA synthesis, they affect cell growth; this has a great impact on hematopoietic cells because of their normally high rates of turnover. Azathioprine, one of the oldest antimetabolite agents, is a purine analogue related to 6-mercaptopurine; when incorporated into DNA, it inhibits RNA transcription and translation. Azathioprine thus depresses bone marrow production of cells capable of mediating rejection. Not surprisingly, however, it also causes hematologic side effects, notably thrombocytopenia, leukopenia, and anemia. In addition, it can cause cholestatic hepatitis. Mycophenolate mofetil (MMF), a more recently developed antimetabolite, has largely replaced azathioprine in clinical practice because it is more effective at reducing acute rejection rates when used with steroids and cyclosporine and is associated with improved long-term graft survival rates. MMF is an inhibitor of inosine monophosphate dehydrogenase (IMPDH), an enzyme critical to de novo purine biosynthesis. The absence of guanosine nucleotides has a selective effect on B- and T-lymphocyte proliferation; lymphocytes depend on de novo purine synthesis more than other hematopoietic cells. The clinical effect is a reduction in cytotoxic T-cell function and antibody formation. Side effects of MMF include anemia, thrombocytopenia, and leukopenia. In addition, the use of high doses may cause gastrointestinal toxicity and diarrhea.

Sirolimus is an antimetabolite with a unique mechanism of action. This agent binds FK-binding protein but, in contrast to the tacrolimus/FK-binding protein complex, the sirolimus/FK-binding protein complex inhibits the target of rapamycin (TOR) protein, a regulatory kinase that is critical to cell proliferation. In recent trials, sirolimus (used in place of azathioprine or placebo), in combination with steroids and cyclosporine, was effective in reducing acute rejection rates, graft, and patient loss. However, while sirolimus does not have nephrotoxicity, it is a bone marrow depressant and causes leukopenia, anemia, and thrombocytopenia. In addition, it quite commonly causes hyperlipidemia, particularly hypertriglyceridemia, and has been associated with decreased wound healing as well as prolongation of acute tubular necrosis following cold ischemic injury. Thus, like CNIs, sirolimus doses must be monitored by careful measurement of trough drug levels.

As mentioned above, many transplant centers utilize induction therapy in addition to the above immunosuppressive agents. The most widely used is monoclonal anti-CD25 (anti-IL-2R) antibody therapy, an agent that binds to and blocks the IL-2 receptor, thus disrupting signal 3. Induction therapy using either basiliximab or daclizumab, two antibodies of about equal efficacy, has had a significant effect on reducing acute rejection rates in the United States and abroad. Both of these antibodies are "humanized" murine antibodies; only the antibody-binding site of daclizumab is derived from the mouse and only the variable region of basiliximab is of murine origin. Thus, antibody responses (human antimouse) to these agents are minimal and both drugs are relatively free of any significant side effects. Recent antirejection strategies utilizing daclizumab in combination with MMF/tacrolimus in children have proven to be effective; this suggests that steroid usage can be eliminated in some cases.

Other types of induction therapy include the use of anti-CD3 monoclonal antibody (OKT3, Muromonab) or anti–thymocyte globulin (ATG) in recipients at high risk of acute rejection or in cases of steroid-resistant acute rejection. OKT3 is a murine monoclonal antibody that binds human CD3 molecules resulting in opsonization and removal of the T cells from the circulation. In some patients, T cell activation may occur and lead to a cytokine release syndrome marked by fever, chills, and rigors as well as a capillary leak syndrome resulting in pulmonary edema. Other negative effects include transient nephrotoxicity due to hemodynamic changes, aseptic meningitis, increased susceptibility to viral infections [especially cytomegalovirus (CMV) infection], and increased risk of posttransplant B-cell lymphoma due to Epstein–Barr virus. Since OKT3 is a murine antibody, its use is also limited by the development of antimurine antibodies; however, a humanized antibody is currently under study.

ATG is an antibody prepared by immunizing rabbits with thymus tissue obtained from patients who have undergone therapeutic thymectomy. It thus consists of antibodies against a number of T-cell surface molecules (including CD3, CD4, CD8, HLA class I, and CD28) and results in rapid depletion of lymphocytes due to cell lysis or clearance by the reticuloendothelial system. As in the case of OKT3 administration, use of ATG results in symptoms from cytokine release as well as increased risk for opportunistic infections. In addition, ATG commonly causes leukopenia and thrombocytopenia, which usually limits the doses that can be used. As with other types of induction therapy, ATG is being used to improve the outcome of transplantation in high-risk patients, to manage rejection in steroid-resistant patients, or to avoid the use of steroids and other immunosuppressants altogether.

Early Follow-Up

Six weeks after surgery Olivia is seen in the transplant clinic for follow-up evaluation. She is without complaints on a regimen of prednisone, mycophenolate, tacrolimus, a multivitamin, valgangciclovir and bactrim. [The latter two drugs are administered to prevent opportunistic infections (see Case 9)]. On examination, her blood pressure is excellent (115/62), she is afebrile, and her incision has healed. However, her laboratory studies show a serum creatinine of 1.5 mg/dL, BUN of 26 mg/dL, and Hgb of 10.5 mg/dL; urinalysis reveals 1+ protein, 1–5 WBC, 1–5 RBC, occasional granular casts, and tubular epithelial cells. Trough (lowest) tacrolimus level is 6.0 ng/ml.

The serum creatinine has increased compared to the immediate post-operative period. What is the differential diagnosis of a rising creatinine?

> *The differential diagnosis of an elevation in serum creatinine a short time after transplantation is not extensive. Leading the list of possibilities is (1) acute rejection, due most commonly to acute cellular rejection or more occasionally to a humoral (antibody) response against donor MHC antigens (chronic rejection as a cause would be most unusual); (2) tacrolimus or cyclosporine toxicity marked either by alterations of intraglomerular hemodynamics or, in rare instances, by direct endothelial damage and resultant thrombotic microangiopathy; (3) acute tubular necrosis (ATN), more commonly seen in the early posttransplant period in recipients of cadaveric grafts having been subjected to prolonged periods of cold ischemia and more likely in recipients with an intercurrent illness resulting in intravascular volume depletion and/or hemodynamic alterations; (4) urinary tract obstruction; (5) infection within the graft, usually due to bacterial infection of the urinary tract system or to recently recognized BK polyoma virus infection has been seen and is an important cause of graft failure; or (6) recurrent glomerulonephritis, particularly in patients with glomerulopathies known to recur after transplantation.*

Deciding among these diagnostic possibilities requires careful evaluation of the patient's clinical presentation as well as his or her urinary and other laboratory findings. In the past, fever, chills, and graft tenderness were associated with acute rejection; with today's more potent immunotherapy, these signs and symptoms can be absent. On the other hand, urinary abnormalities continue to provide important diagnostic clues. Significant proteinuria can be a sign of antibody-mediated acute rejection (but it also occurs in chronic rejection). The presence of red and white cells occurs in both acute cellular rejection and ATN; the presence of granular and pigmented casts is more specifically linked to the presence of ATN.

Laboratory tests to evaluate a rising creatinine in the immediate posttransplant period include measurement of trough levels of the immunosuppressive drugs to determine if the drugs are being taken as prescribed or if the doses prescribed are too high. In addition, renal ultrasound can determine the possibility of urinary tract obstruction and provide measurement of indices of vascular resistance. These measurements, made by Doppler ultrasound evaluation of blood flow to the kidney, have been reported to be diagnostic of acute rejection. However, high levels of resistance (>0.9) can be associated not only with acute rejection but also with ATN and drug toxicity. Thus, the most important and most revealing test, as in the initial diagnostic period, is a renal biopsy.

In initial studies of her high creatinine level, Olivia undergoes renal ultrasound, which reveals that urinary obstruction is not present. A renal biopsy performed under ultrasound guidance demonstrates mild inflammation of the glomeruli and moderate interstitial inflammation, including infiltration of cells adjacent to tubules within the cortex (Fig. 20.5). There are no vascular changes and no interstitial fibrosis or evidence of thrombotic microangiopathy. Imunohistochemical stains show no evidence of C4d deposition or HLA-DR expression that would suggest antibody mediated rejection. These pathologic findings are compatible with acute cell-medicated rejection of moderate intensity. Additional studies focused on antibody rejection reveal a repeat negative CDC and flow cross-match against her brother's cells. Thus the rejection process is cell mediated in origin.

The transplant team discusses the situation with Olivia. At this point she admits that she has been skipping some MMF and tacrolimus doses (which may explain her relatively low trough level). The transplant team advises and

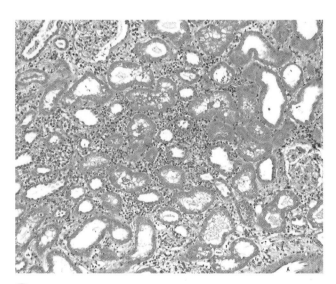

Figure 20.5. H&E-stained section of a human kidney transplant demonstrating histologic features of acute cellular rejection. There is diffuse interstitial inflammation and infiltration of tubular epithelial cells ("tubulitis"). (Photomicrograph courtesy of Dr. David Kleiner, NCI.) (200X).

Olivia agrees with institution of anti–rejection therapy consisting of solumedrol for three days rapidly tapered to 20 mg of oral prednisone daily. As expected, her tacrolimus level rises to 12 ng/mL, and her dose is maintained. She is discharged after five days with a serum creatinine of 1.2 mg/dL. She is then closely followed at weekly intervals for the next four weeks with stable serum creatinine.

Epilogue of Case

One year after transplant, Olivia returns to your office for follow-up. Her blood pressure is well controlled and her serum creatinine is 1.3 mg/dL. She is delighted with her outcome and has returned to work after almost nine months of therapy. She also appears compliant with her medications.

REFERENCES

Ballardie FW (2007): Quantitative appraisal of treatment options for IgA nephropathy. *J Am Soc Nephrol* 18:2806–2809.

Barratt J, Smith AC, Molyneux K, Feehally J (2007): Immunopathogenesis of IgAN. *Semin Immunopathol* 29:427–443.

Donadio JV, Grande JP (2002): IgA nephropathy. *New Engl J Med* 347:738–748.

Galla JH (1995): IgA nephropathy. *Kidney Int* 47:377–387.

Girlanda R, Mannon RB, Kirk AD (2007): Diagnostic tools for monitoring kidney transplant recipients. *Semin Nephrol* 27:462–478.

Glassock RJ (1999): The treatment of IgA nephropathy: Status at the end of the millenium. *J Nephrol* 12:288–296.

Halloran PF (2004): Immunosuppressive drugs for kidney transplantation. *New Engl J Med* 351:2715–2729.

Julian BA, Wyatt RJ, Matousovic K, Moldoveanu Z, Mestecky J, Novak J (2007): IgA nephropathy: A clinical overview. *Contrib Nephrol* 157:19–26.

Larsen CP, Knechtle SJ, Adams A, Pearson T, Kirk AD (2006): A new look at blockade of T-cell costimulation: A therapeutic strategy for long-term maintenance immunosuppression. *Am J Transplant* 6:876–883.

Meier-Kriesche HU, Schold JD, Srinivas TR, Kaplan B (2004): Lack of improvement in renal allograft survival despite a marked decrease in acute rejection rates over the most recent era. *Am J Transplant* 4:378–383.

Ponticelli C, Traversi L, Feliciani A, Cesana BM, Banfi G, Tarantino A (2001): Kidney transplantation in patients with IgA mesangial glomerulonephritis. *Kidney Int* 60:1948–1954.

Wada J, Sugiyama H, Makino H (2003): Pathogenesis of IgA nephropathy. *Semin Nephrol* 23:556–563.

21

RHEUMATOID ARTHRITIS

BARBARA MITTLEMAN*

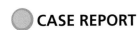 **CASE REPORT**

"I feel achy and my hands are stiff."

History and Initial Evaluation

Mary, a 45-year-old woman, comes to you, her primary care physician, with complaints of not feeling well. She says that she is feeling generally weak and tired, has had some weight loss, and finds doing her job as an office secretary increasingly difficult. She initially attributed this to stress at work, but as time passed and she realized that it had been going on for over six months, she thought it was too long a time to merely be work stress. Mary decided to finally come in for a checkup because she is now also having trouble typing due to stiffness in her fingers, which is interfering with her ability to work. When you question her further, Mary indicates that she feels stiff all over when she wakes up in the morning and has difficulty fixing breakfast because of the stiffness in her hands; in fact, in the morning she cannot even make a complete fist. The problems typing are also worse in the morning and improve a little by afternoon. As you go through a review of her systems, Mary admits to having dry eyes and dry mouth but denies hair loss, oral or nasal ulcers, skin rash, or any cardiovascular, respiratory, gastrointestinal, or genitourinary symptoms. She has had no

change in her regular menstrual cycles. Her husband is well and her two children are away in college and doing fine. She has had no recent contact with small children, nor has she traveled recently. When asked about family history, she says that a maternal aunt had "crooked fingers" but does not know her diagnosis.

While taking Mary's history you make several general observations about her physical status. You note that she is walking slowly and looks uncomfortable as she bears weight on her feet. She is well groomed but her business attire clashes with the fact that she is wearing tennis shoes. In addition, it is quite obvious that her hands are visibly swollen. On physical examination, you note that Mary's weight is 5 lbs lower than her weight on a previous visit for a routine checkup and that the former weight had been appropriate for her height. She is a little surprised at your request to measure her height, which in fact has not changed. Mary has tenderness and swelling (possibly due to inflammation of the joint synovial lining) in both ankles and wrists and in all her metacarpophalangeal (knuckle) and proximal interphalangeal joints. There is no skin rash, and you cannot palpate any subcutaneous nodules. The rest of her physical examination, including her thyroid exam, is normal. Mary's history and physical examination lead you to believe that she has some form of arthritis. In trying to determine which form might be present, you consider

*With contributions from Warren Strober and Susan R. S. Gottesman

Immunology: Clinical Case Studies and Disease Pathophysiology, By Warren Strober and Susan R. S. Gottesman
Copyright © 2009 John Wiley & Sons, Inc.

Mary's recent history and pattern of joint involvement and how that would enter the differential diagnoses.

What are the subtypes of arthritis and how does Mary's history and physical exam help you to distinguish among them?

*Arthritis may be broadly subdivided into inflammatory and noninflammatory types. In general, **noninflammatory arthritis** is exacerbated by exercise and improves with rest; the most common types of **inflammatory arthritis** are worse in the morning and improve during the day, a temporal pattern that Mary has described. There are many different causes of inflammatory arthritis; it is important to distinguish among their etiologies for the purposes of prognosis and treatment. In addition, although osteoarthritis (see below) is the most common type of noninflammatory arthritis, it may develop an inflammatory component and needs to be part of your differential diagnosis.*

Pattern recognition is important in the diagnosis of arthritis type. Key questions include the mode of onset of the illness, the number of affected joints, the symmetry of involvement, the distribution (axial or appendicular), and evidence of major organ involvement or an association with a metabolic disorder.

*• Mode of onset: Acute onset arthropathies include infectious arthritis, reactive arthritis, crystal-induced arthritis, and palindromic rheumatism. **Infectious** or **septic arthritis** with an acute onset may be caused by virtually any blood-borne bacteria. The most frequent bacterial organisms involved are* Staphylococcus aureus *in adults and* Neisseria gonorrhoeae *in young adults. Viral illnesses such as parvovirus B19, rubella, and hepatitis B may also present with acute-onset arthritis; however, in this case the joint disease may be a consequence of immune complex deposition rather than direct infection. **Reactive arthritis** is a general term for acute nonpurulent (non-pus-forming) arthritis that arises as a complication of an infection elsewhere in the body, usually enteric or urogenital; it was originally described as presenting in association with conjunctivitis and urethritis. **Crystal-induced arthritis** is commonly caused by uric acid crystals (gout) or calcium pyrophosphate crystals (pseudogout) in the joints, but other types of crystals can also be present; this form of arthritis is often associated with an underlying metabolic disorder. **Palindromic arthritis** is a rare inflammatory arthritis in which the patient suffers painful episodes of joint inflammation without clear cause and with no residual impairment between attacks. In rare instances, rheumatoid arthritis (RA) or psoriatic arthritis may also present with an explosive onset and therefore masquerade as an acute arthritis; thus, acute onset of arthritis does not rule out these diagnoses.*

Insidious-onset arthropathies include RA; juvenile idiopathic arthritis (JIA); osteoarthritis; infectious arthritis associated with slow-growing agents such as mycobacteria, spirochetes (syphilis and Lyme disease), and fungal organisms; hypertrophic osteoarthropathy (characterized by clubbing of fingers and usually associated with pulmonary disease); neuropathic arthropathy (bone and joint changes

secondary to loss of sensation); and psoriatic arthritis (see Case 19).

*• Number and distribution of affected joints: RA is the classic example of a symmetric polyarthritis involving small joints and, to a lesser extent, larger joints; psoriatic arthritis, polyarticular gout, reactive arthritis and osteoarthritis present in an asymmetric fashion and/or preferentially involve large joints. However, parvovirus B19–associated arthritis and erosive osteoarthritis can resemble RA in their presentations, making these forms difficult to distinguish from seronegative RA (RA without autoantibodies). Because axial involvement arthritis dominates in the **spondyloarthropathies** (arthritis involving the spine), either alone or in combination with peripheral joint arthritis, it can thus be confused with RA. This is especially true because the cervical spine is commonly involved in RA as well as in polyarticular and systemic-onset JIA and **Still's disease** (arthritis associated with spiking fevers and rash, more commonly seen with JIA).*

***Osteoarthritis,** the most common type of arthritis, is a degenerative joint disease in which "wear and tear" of the joint leads to erosion of the cartilage followed by damage to underlying bone. As such, it is associated with age, increased weight, prior injury to joint, and/or repetitive trauma. Although not an inflammatory-type arthritis, there can be secondary inflammatory changes that can make distinction from other causes of arthritis difficult. It should be noted, however, that osteoarthritis is limited to the musculoskeletal system; the presence of disease in other organ systems points towards a systemic connective tissue disease.*

• Constitutional symptoms: These include fatigue, weight loss, and generalized body aches, which occur in systemic illnesses including endocrine abnormalities such as hypothyroidism, malignancies, and connective tissue diseases like RA and systemic lupus erythematosus (SLE; see Chapter 22). The combination of an insidious onset of peripheral symmetric polyarthritis involving small joints with associated constitutional symptoms makes the diagnosis of RA likely in Mary's case but does not exclude other underlying systemic illnesses.

On the basis of Mary's morning stiffness and symmetric arthritis involving the small joints, you conclude that the most likely diagnosis is rheumatoid arthritis. However, you order a number of diagnostic tests to confirm this clinical diagnosis. These consist of radiographic studies of her hands, wrists, and hips, a bone density scan, and various blood studies. The latter include a complete blood count (CBC), chemistries including liver function tests, thyroid function, muscle enzymes, markers of inflammation, and autoantibody studies, keeping in mind the differential diagnosis of inflammatory arthritis. You explain to Mary that no one test is diagnostic and that it is important to determine the underlying cause for her arthritic symptoms for both prognosis and treatment. A return appointment is scheduled in one week; in the interim you prescribe a nonsteroidal anti-inflammatory drug (NSAID) for some relief of symptoms.

Definitive Diagnosis

The results of the studies you ordered are as follows:

	Result	Reference Range
CBC		
Hemoglobin	10.3 mg/dL	12.5–15 mg/dL
Mean corpuscular volume	93 fL	88–99 fL
White blood cell count	Normal	
Platelets	540,000/μL	130,000–400,000/μL
Chemistry panel	Normal	
Thyroid-stimulating hormone, T3 and T4	Normal	
Muscle enzymes	Not elevated	
Hepatitis B and C serology	Negative	
Erythrocyte sedimentation rate (ESR)	60 mm/h	0–30 mm/h
C-reactive protein (CRP)	2.4 mg/dL	<0.5 mg/dL
Rheumatoid factor (RF)	385 IU/mL	<20 IU/mL
Anticyclic citrullinated peptide (CCP) antibodies	125 IU/mL	(<20 IU/mL)
Antinuclear antibody (ANA)	1:80, speckled pattern	Negative
Anti–Sjögren's syndrome (SS) A antibody	58 EU	<19 EU
Anti–SSB antibody	Negative	Negative

Radiographs of Mary's wrists and hands show periarticular osteopenia without evidence of erosions or joint space narrowing. Bone density scan is normal.

How do you interpret the laboratory and radiographic data?

The findings of an elevated ESR and CRP along with an elevated platelet count substantiate your diagnosis of a systemic inflammatory disorder. Mild anemia, which in Mary's case is normochromic, normocytic (normal red cell hemoglobin content and size), is not uncommon in chronic illnesses. The lack of white blood cell elevation suggests that her inflammation is not due to an infectious process. In

addition, chronic infection with hepatitis B or C has been specifically ruled out by negative serologies and normal liver function tests. Other pertinent negatives include lack of evidence of muscle injury, thyroid dysfunction, or other metabolic disorders.

The autoantibody studies support your diagnosis of an underlying autoimmune disease. Although many of these autoantibodies bear the name of a specific disease entity (such as anti–Sjögren's syndrome A antibody), in reality they are not disease specific; they must be interpreted in aggregate and along with the clinical picture (see below). On the basis of the clinical picture and laboratory and radiographic data, you conclude that Mary has seropositive (autoantibodies present) RA with clinical and antibody evidence of associated Sjögren's syndrome, an autoimmune disease of the lacrimal and salivary glands, which occurs in isolation or in association with other autoimmune diseases (RA most commonly).

Treatment Plan

When Mary returns for her next appointment you inform her that she has RA and explain at length the nature of this illness and its treatment. You emphasize that, although RA is a chronic disease, powerful medications are available to control its destructive effects. You also tell her that the optimal treatment of RA requires special expertise and that you would like to defer definitive treatment until she is under the care of a rheumatologist colleague. You advise her to continue taking the NSAID until she sees the rheumatologist; in anticipation of a recommendation for therapy with a tumor necrosis factor α (TNF-α) inhibitor, you place a tuberculin skin test with a purified protein derivative (PPD) (which is read as negative in 48 h).

The following week, Mary is seen by the rheumatologist, who reviews the results of the studies you have conducted. She concurs with your diagnosis and counsels Mary that, in order to avoid joint destruction, it will be best to take an aggressive approach to her still early arthritis, particularly because she is positive for RF and anti-CCP antibodies, both predictive of persistent and severe disease. Consequently, the doctor continues the NSAID medication and initiates treatment with methotrexate, one of the disease-modifying antirheumatic drugs (DMARD), along with anti-TNF-α, an effective biologic therapy. She also prescribes artificial tears for the symptomatic management of Mary's dry eyes and advises Mary to exercise as much as possible.

CLINICAL FEATURES AND DIAGNOSIS OF RA

RA is a chronic inflammatory disease that affects almost 1% of the world population. The majority of patients are female, with a female-to-male ratio of 3:1. The peak age of onset is in the fourth and fifth decades, but RA may affect

TABLE 21.1. 1988 Revised American Rheumatism Association Criteria for Classification of Rheumatoid Arthritis

Criterion	Definition
1. Morning stiffness	Morning stiffness in and around joints lasting at least 1 h before maximal improvement
2. Arthritis of three or more joint areas	At least three joint areas simultaneously having soft tissue swelling or fluid (not bony overgrowth alone) observed by physician; 14 possible joint areas are (right or left) PIP, MCP, wrist, elbow, knee, ankle, and MTP joints
3. Arthritis of hand joints	At least one joint area swollen as above in wrist, MCP, or PIP joint
4. Symmetric arthritis	Simultaneous involvement of same joint areas (as in criterion 2) on both sides of body (bilateral involvement of PIP, MCP, or MTP joints is acceptable without absolute symmetry)
5. Rheumatoid nodules	Subcutaneous nodules over bony prominences or extensor surfaces or in juxta-articular regions observed by physician
6. Serum rheumatoid factor	Demonstration of abnormal amounts of serum "rheumatoid factor" by any method that has been positive in less than 5% of normal control subjects
7. Radiographic changes	Changes typical of RA on PA hand and wrist radiographs, which must include erosions or unequivocal bony decalcification localized to or most marked adjacent to the involved joints (osteoarthritis changes alone do not qualify)

Note: For classification purposes, a patient is said to have RA if he or she has satisfied at least four of the seven criteria. Criteria 1–4 must be present for at least six weeks. Patients with two clinical diagnoses are not excluded. Designation as classic, definite, or probable rheumatoid arthritis is not to be made.
Abbreviations: MCP, metacarpophalangeal; MTP, metatarsophalangeal; PA, posteroanterior; PIP, proximal interphalangeal; RA, rheumatoid arthritis.

any age group. The presence of at least four of the seven classification criteria used by the American Rheumatism Association, for a period of six weeks or more has a high sensitivity (92%) and specificity (89%) for RA (Table 21.1).

While the diagnosis of RA relies on the presence of joint abnormalities, it is important to realize that RA is a systemic disease with extra-articular manifestations. These include (1) skin involvement such as rheumatoid nodules (included in the classification criteria) and vasculitis; (2) ocular involvement such as keratoconjuctivitis sicca (as seen in Sjögren's syndrome) and scleritis; (3) pulmonary involvement such as interstitial pneumonitis, pleuritis, and pulmonary nodules; (4) renal involvement such as amyloidosis (deposition of amyloid proteins) and interstitial nephritis; (5) hepatic involvement marked by elevated transaminases; and (6) hematologic abnormalities such as anemia. In addition, RA is associated with a variety of neurologic manifestations, including peripheral entrapment neuropathies due to local synovitis, mononeuritis multiplex resulting from rheumatoid vasculitis involving the vasa nervorum, central neurologic sequelae of atlantoaxial subluxation (erosion of the odontoid process or inflammation of the transverse ligament causing posterior slippage of the odontoid process), basilar invagination (upward impingement of the odontoid process), and subaxial subluxation (at any level). Finally, a unique feature of RA is its association with splenomegaly and leukopenia, a triad known as **Felty's syndrome**. The latter occurs in seropositive, erosive, long-standing RA patients with rheumatoid nodules and the *HLA-DRB$_1$0401* allele (see below). Felty's syndrome is also associated with a high incidence of hepatic abnormalities and increased susceptibility to lymphoid malignancies.

Laboratory features in RA (Table 21.2) are consistent with an acute-phase response; specifically the elevated ESR and CRP. Typically, the acute-phase reactants correlate with disease activity, but this can vary from patient to patient. RA patients may also demonstrate thrombocytosis (increased platelets), hypergammaglobulinemia (high circulating globulins, usually immunoglobulin), eosinophilia (high peripheral blood eosinophil count), and hypocomplementemia (low complement components), usually in the setting of more severe arthritis and extra-articular disease. The cause of anemia in RA is multifactorial; impaired iron utilization, chronic inflammation, reduced erythropoietin, bone marrow effects of the proinflammatory cytokines [TNF-α, interleukin (IL) 1β, and IL-6], and medications all play a role. Synovial fluid analysis from affected joints will reveal a translucent inflammatory fluid with low viscosity, 2000–50,000 white blood cells per milliliter, and negative cultures.

RF, a serologic marker included in the classification criteria (Table 21.1), is an autoantibody (IgM is the one currently measured) against the Fc portion of IgG. It is found in >80% of patients with RA and is associated with a more severe disease spectrum. However, it is also present in about 5% of the healthy population and in patients with other rheumatologic diseases, including Sjögren's syndrome, mixed connective tissue disease, inflammatory myositis, mixed cryoglobulinemia, and SLE. In addition, it can be seen in nonrheumatologic conditions such as infections with the hepatitis B and C viruses, subacute bacterial endocarditis, sarcoidosis, asbestosis, primary biliary cirrhosis, and malignancy. As mentioned above, the presence of RF has a prognostic value in RA

TABLE 21.2. Expected Alterations in Laboratory Test Results in Rheumatoid Arthritis

Slight leukocytosis with normal differential white blood cell (WBC) count[a]

Thrombocytosis[a]

Slight anemia (hemoglobin 10 g/dL), normochromic and either normocytic or microcytic[a]

Normal urinalysis[a]

ESR of 30 mm/h or more (Westergren method) and C-reactive protein (CRP) level of more than 0.7 pg/mL[a]

Normal renal, hepatic, and metabolic function[a]

Normal serum uric acid level (before initiation of salicylate therapy)

Positive RF test and negative antinuclear antibody test (Negative test for RF in serum found in up to 30% of patients early in illness;
   in seropositive patients and in some of these "seronegative" patients there will be a positive test for anticyclic citrullinated peptides)[a]

Elevated levels of α_2- and α_1-globulins

Normal or elevated serum complement level

"Typical" arthrocentesis obtained when obvious fluid is present in early RA reveals the following[b]:

- The joint fluid is straw colored and slightly cloudy and contains many flecks of fibrin.
- A clot forms in fluid left standing at room temperature.
- There are 5000–25,000 WBC/μL present and at least 50% of these are polymorphonuclear leukocytes.
- Some large polymorphonuclear leukocytes with granules staining positively for immunoglobulins (IgG and IgM) and complement C3 can often be found; no crystals are present.
- Complement C4 and C2 levels are depressed, but the C3 level can be normal.
- IgG in synovial fluid may approach serum concentrations.
- The synovial fluid glucose level is usually normal but can be depressed, occasionally to less than 25 mg/dL.
- Cultures are negative.

[a]Essential tests.
[b]Routinely, the cell count and differential, along with culture and examination for crystals, are the only essential tests on synovial fluid in this clinical situation.

patients; it predicts worse disease, more extra-articular manifestations, and more erosions compared to patients without this marker (seronegative RA).

The diagnostic power of RF positivity is limited by its lack of specificity for RA, as discussed above. However, another antibody associated with RA, known as anti-CCP, has great specificity for RA and has in fact been shown to substitute for RF as a diagnostic marker in this disease, especially when present at moderate to high levels. This antibody is called anti-CCP because it recognizes a citrullinated peptide derived from fillagrin, a protein associated with keratin filaments. High levels of anti-CCP antibodies also have prognostic value since this antibody can be present in the blood years before the first symptom of RA develops. In addition, several studies have also suggested that the presence of anti-CCP antibody predicts more aggressive disease.

RA is also characterized by the presence of ANA, a group of antibodies against nucleus-associated proteins and nucleic acids (see the immunopathogenesis section of this chapter). These antibodies and their pattern of reactivity can be detected in the patient's serum by incubating it with commercially prepared cells affixed to slides and then adding a fluorescent-tagged antihuman antibody that reacts with ANA bound to the cell. The pattern of binding

to the cell nucleus, which is visualized with a fluorescent microscope, loosely correlates with the target of the autoantibodies (see Case 22). Although more commonly seen in SLE and mixed connective tissue disease, ANA can be positive in RA as well as other autoimmune diseases: JIA, Sjögren's syndrome, scleroderma, polymyositis, and dermatomyositis. However, low-titer ANA may also be found in healthy individuals (albeit at a low frequency) and in patients with nonrheumatologic diseases, including chronic infections [infectious mononucleosis, tuberculosis (TB), and subacute bacterial endocarditis], Hashimoto's thyroiditis, autoimmune hepatitis, primary autoimmune cholangitis, and primary pulmonary hypertension. Specific ANAs known as anti-SSA/Ro and anti-SSB/La antibodies are present in patients with primary Sjögren's syndrome (75% are positive), while anti-SSA/Ro antibody alone can be found in patients with secondary Sjögren's syndrome associated with RA (10–15%). As in Mary's case, SS autoantibodies, among the large group of ANA with specificity against ribonucleoproteins, give rise to a speckled nuclear pattern on the immunofluorescent assay.

Radiographic features of RA are unique and help both in the diagnosis of the disease and in guiding its therapy. The progression of pathologic joint change in RA is captured by scoring systems for use in the setting of clinical trials, such as the Larsen classification as defined below; however numerical scoring is generally not used in clinical practice. Magnetic resonance imaging (MRI) is useful in assessing changes in early RA by revealing the presence of periarticular soft tissue swelling followed by periarticular osteopenia (grade 1 in the Larsen classification) and, later, by the appearance of marginal joint erosions (grade 2). With progression of the disease, changes can be seen on conventional radiographs and include increasing destruction of articular cartilage, joint space loss, and the formation of a synovial pannus (grade 3). Then, with further progression, significant deformities of the involved bones occur, including flexion/extension deformities and ulnar deviation of the phalanges (grade 4). Finally, severe mutilating arthritis supervenes and is marked by destruction of all the joint surfaces, ankylosis, and complete loss of motion (grade 5).

IMMUNOPATHOGENESIS OF RA

General Considerations

While the precise etiopathogenesis of RA remains a mystery, there is little doubt that it is an autoimmune disease driven by the interplay of genetic and environmental factors. The brunt of the inflammation is focused on the joints. At these sites autoimmune inflammation is associated with the proliferation and activation of synoviocytes and chondrocytes that, when unchecked, result in joint destruction. The basis of the autoimmunity in RA involves the same processes that lead to this abnormality in other organ-specific and systemic autoimmunities (see the introduction to this unit). Thus, it should not be surprising that many of the autoimmune mechanisms involved in RA are similar to those of other autoimmune diseases, such as SLE. However, because the autoantigens involved in RA are largely unique, inflammation is channeled into the joints.

Genetic Susceptibility: The Role of HLA-DR.
Initial studies involving analysis of family incidence data indicated that RA is to some extent genetically determined. More recently, analysis of concordance rates in monozygotic twins versus dizygotic twins showed that genetic factors account for fully 60% of the "variation in liability to disease." One such genetic factor was discovered in the 1970s with the observation that the human leukocyte antigen (HLA)-DR4 occurred in about 70% of RA patients compared to 30% of controls. Later studies refining this observation showed that RA was most highly associated with the DR4 β chains *DRB*0401*, *DRB*0404*, *DRB*0101*, and *DRB*1402*. These studies established that an allele in the major histocompatibility complex (MHC) had a genetic influence on RA. However, the occurrence of these MHC alleles in normal individuals

indicates that this MHC gene is not sufficient to cause RA. In addition, HLA-DR4 is not associated with RA in Native American patients and, at best, has a weak association with RA in African-American patients, indicating that HLA-DR4 is not a necessary cause of RA. Thus, the HLA-DR4 alleles are, at most, susceptibility factors that operate in cooperation with a number of other genetic factors to result in RA.

Since CD4$^+$ T cells respond to antigen in the context of MHC class II molecules, the link between MHC class II genes and RA may occur as a result of the T-cell response to autoantigen(s) involved in the etiology of RA (see Case 16). In support of this idea, RA severity and extra-articular manifestations are associated with a particular HLA-DR β-chain epitope, called the shared epitope because it is found on the β chain of DR1, DR6, and DR10 as well as on DR4. However, this simple explanation of the role of HLA-DR4 in the pathogenesis of RA does not fit well with the fact that this HLA allele (in combination with HLA-DR3) is also associated with susceptibility to the development of type 1 diabetes mellitus, an autoimmune disease with a nonoverlapping set of autoantibodies. Thus, it is possible that HLA-DR4 is not specific for the antigens involved in RA; in fact, it may be involved in the immune response to a number of autoantigens in various autoimmune diseases.

Very recently a "genome-wide" search for single-nucleotide polymorphisms (SNPs) associated with RA showed that a polymorphism in the gene encoding Stat4 was strongly associated with both RA and SLE. The expression of Stat4, a transcription factor, in T helper cells, leads to a gene expression program resulting in the production of interferon (IFN) γ (Fig. 21.1). Again, this polymorphism represents a susceptibility rather than a single gene mutation necessary and sufficient for either of these diseases. However, the finding that the same SNP was associated with both RA and SLE suggests a relationship between these two diseases and, by extension, that both these diseases are due in part to underlying T-cell abnormalities.

Environmental Influences.
While the idea that infectious agents are a cause of RA is not tenable on the basis of modern methods of detecting the presence of infection, it is still possible that these agents act as triggers of RA. The idea here is that an infection, not necessarily involving joint tissue, induces an immune response that then allows the initiation of a self-sustaining autoimmune reaction in genetically susceptible individuals. Commonly implicated pathogens include Epstein–Barr virus, parvovirus, retroviruses, mycoplasma, rubella, mycobacteria, and bacterial cell wall components. Similar or identical infectious triggers could also initiate other autoimmune diseases, such as multiple sclerosis and diabetes mellitus, but in each case

the autoimmunity induced would depend on the presence of preexisting genetic factors (see Cases 15 and 16, respectively).

Experimental Models of RA. In recent years important insights into the pathogenesis of RA has come from the study of animal models. We will use a short discussion of several of these models to set the stage for a description of the immunologic findings in the human disease.

The most widely studied experimental model of RA is known as ***collagen-induced arthritis (CIA)***, an arthritis induced in mice by injection of type II collagen with adjuvant (a nonspecific stimulus of the immune response). The joint inflammation that ensues several weeks later bears a striking resemblance to that seen in human joints involved by RA. In this model, collagen-specific T-helper cells that have been induced by dendritic cells presenting the antigen (collagen) can transfer disease to naive (unimmunized) animals, suggesting that the arthritis is a CD4$^+$ T-cell-mediated inflammation. Initially, this T-cell-mediated inflammation was thought to be a T_H1-mediated event marked by IL-12p70 induction of IFN-γ-producing cells from T_H0 cells (see Fig. 21.1 and the T-cell cytokine section below). However, it has been shown more recently that the more important T-cell response is a T_H17-mediated event in which IL-17-producing cells are the main effectors. This response requires IL-23 dependent differentiation of T_H0 cells to T_H17 cells, rather than IL-12p70.

Collagen-specific antibodies are also generated in the CIA mouse model. These antibodies are mainly of the IgG2 subclass, a complement-fixing antibody isotype (see Case 4 for a discussion of antibody isotype functions). Complement activation, a process that generates fragments (such as C3a and C5a) with chemoattractant properties, results in the influx of acute inflammatory cells into the joint site and thus may be a factor initiating joint destruction in this model. Although collagen-specific immunity (both antibody and T-cell mediated) indicates that collagen is an important autoantigen in this model, anticollagen autoantibodies are not a prominent feature of human RA. Nevertheless, the model is still useful for the study of RA because similar mechanisms may obtain in the human disease in relation to other autoantigens. In addition, the mechanisms of tissue injury may be similar, providing a valid model for the testing of prospective therapeutic agents.

A second experimental model of RA is created by implanting SCID (severe combined immunodeficiency) mice with human synovial tissue or enzymatically dispersed human synovial cells along with cartilage explants. Synoviocytes from RA patients (but not those from control individuals) invade the cartilage explants and create pannuslike formations that resemble those seen in the joints of RA patients (see below). These formations occur even with dispersed synovial cells in the absence of accompanying donor (human) lymphocytes or macrophages. Since diseased tissue is being transplanted, the early inciting events of arthritis have been bypassed and are thus not elucidated in this model. Nevertheless, the ***SCID transplant model*** suggests that joint destruction may

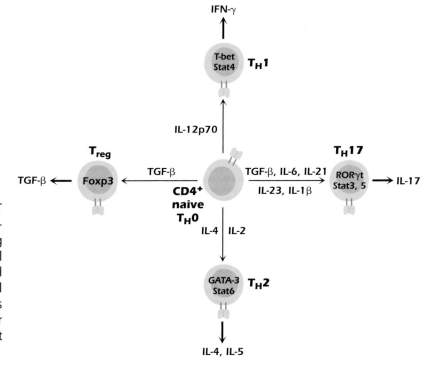

Figure 21.1. T-cell differentiation. Naive T cells can undergo four pathways of differentiation depending on the mixture of inducing cytokines in the local enviroment. T_H1 T-cell development requires IL-12p70 and T_H2 T-cell development requires IL-4. T_H17 and T_{reg} cell development both require TGF-β, but T_H17 cells require, in addition, a complex array of other factors, some of which inhibit T_{reg} development (IL-6).

proceed independently of infiltrating inflammatory cells and may be solely dependent on resident synoviocytes and chondrocytes once the inflammation has been initiated.

In a third mouse model of arthritis, a spontaneously appearing arthritis in *K/BxN mice*, the inflammation is due to an autoantibody. K/BxN mice are a cross (F1 generation) between K/B mice that bear a T-cell receptor transgene specific for a bovine ribonuclease peptide and NOD (autoimmunity prone nonobese diabetes) mice, and they develop autoantibodies to glucose-6-phosphate (G6P) isomerase and arthritis. The pathogenic role of autoantibodies in this model is shown by the fact that the disease is transferred to naive recipients with sera or with the anti-G6P isomerase antibodies and not with cells. In addition, tissue injury is a complement-dependent process requiring local deposition of C3 components. Macrophages attracted to the joint site, presumably by complement components and chemokines, ultimately play a major role in bringing about joint destruction. While this model is of considerable theoretical interest, it should be noted that anti-G6P isomerase antibodies are not found in human RA.

Taken together, these models provide strong evidence that an arthritis similar to RA can be induced by CD4$^+$ T cells executing a T$_H$17-mediated inflammation or by antibodies mediating inflammation through a complement-dependent process. In addition, they suggest that after the disease is initiated, the inflammation can be continued in the absence of T cells.

Immune Effectors in Human RA

Autoantibodies. The underlying immune mechanisms leading to the elaboration of autoantibodies in autoimmune diseases is discussed in the chapter on the quintessential antibody-mediated autoimmunity, SLE (see Case 22). These same immune mechanisms apply to the occurrence of autoantibodies in RA; however, in this case it is not clear that these antibodies are necessary for the development of RA.

As will be discussed below, some autoantibodies occurring in RA, in particular RF and anti-CCP antibodies, are produced within the inflamed joint, so they have the potential to mediate damage at this critical location. Anti-CCP antibodies are detectable in the serum well in advance of clinically apparent joint disease, suggesting that they cannot mediate tissue injury by themselves but may participate in such injury in the presence of other immune effectors. In addition to the above disease-specific autoantibodies, RA patients not infrequently synthesize autoantibodies associated with other autoimmune diseases. These include ANA, seen in approximately 25–30% of RA patients, and SS-A, seen in RA patients with concomitant Sjögren's syndrome.

Rheumatoid Factor. RF is produced in large amounts by the rheumatoid synovial tissue, and immune

complexes containing RF have been found in RA synovium and on the surface layers of cartilage. RF can fix and activate complement through the classical pathway, thereby initiating tissue injury through the elaboration of proinflammatory mediators, and chemotaxis and activation of a variety of effector cells capable of causing tissue injury (see Case 8 for a detailed discussion of complement pathways).

Studies have shown that the RF produced in patients with RA differs from that found in healthy individuals or in those with *paraproteins* (monoclonal immunoglobulins). The RF produced in RA binds to the Fc portion of IgG with greater avidity than RF paraproteins, presumably because cells producing RF in RA have undergone affinity mutation during an antigen-driven T-cell-dependent process.

The Cellular Response in RA. A large number of cells populate the RA joint and play a role in the development and progression of RA. The activity of specific cell populations and the nature of their interactions with one another remain active fields of research. The following is a summary of cells seen in the diseased joint with descriptions of some features that may clarify their roles:

The Synovial Cells. The hallmarks of RA—immune activation, infiltration of mononuclear cells and intimal lining hyperplasia—are seen primarily in the synovial tissue (Fig. 21.2). In a normal joint, the synovial intimal layer is 1–2 cell layers thick, but in joints affected by RA this may increase to as many as 4–10 cellular layers. The normal synovial lining contains equal numbers of type A and B synoviocytes. Type A synoviocytes are macrophage-like bone-marrow-derived cells with macrophage surface markers (CD14, CD68, Fc receptor); type B synoviocytes are fibroblast-like cells that express proteins such as vascular cell adhesion molecule 1 (VCAM-1), CD55, cadherin 11, and the proteoglycan synthesis enzyme [uridine diphosphoglucose dehydrogenase (UDPGD)]. Both types of cells are increased in RA, but type A cells are disproportionately increased.

- *Synovial T Cells.* Synovial T lymphocytes in chronic RA may form structures resembling the architecture of a lymph node or may be part of a more diffuse lymphoid infiltrate. The T cells constitute more than 50% of the cells found in the RA synovium; the majority of these are CD4$^+$ T cells. They are in immediate contact with B cells and dendritic cells; these three cell types sometimes form germinal center–like aggregations within the synovial tissue.
  RA synovial CD4$^+$ T cells exhibit high surface expression of the activation markers HLA-DR and CD27 and can provide help to B cells, thereby driving antibody production. Synovial T cells also express CD40L and CD28, which interact with CD40 and CD80/CD86,

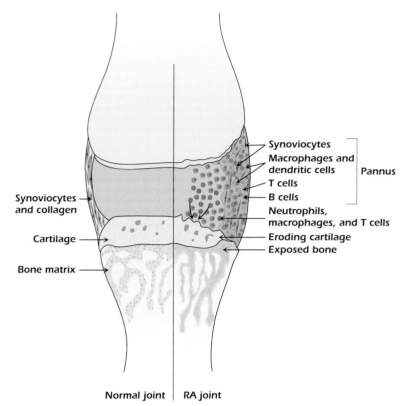

Normal joint ｜ RA joint

Synoviocytes
Macrophages and dendritic cells
T cells
B cells
Pannus

Neutrophils, macrophages, and T cells
Eroding cartilage
Exposed bone

Synoviocytes and collagen

Cartilage

Bone matrix

Figure 21.2. Pannus formation. Inflammatory cells secrete cytokines and other mediators, which lead to the formation of a thickened synovium infiltrated with inflammatory cells known as a pannus. This is accompanied by cartilage destruction and bone resorption. The pannus ultimately becomes locally invasive at the interface of the cartilage and bone, causing "marginal erosions" characteristic of RA.

respectively, on antigen-presenting cells; this leads to activation of both interacting cells and robust production of inflammatory cytokines.

The RA synovial T cells also express receptors for specific chemokines, such as CCR5, the receptor for macrophage inhibitory protein (MIP) 1α and β, and CXCR4, the receptor for stromal cell–derived factor 1. Synovial T cells stimulated by chemokines in turn stimulate macrophages, which then produce TNF-α through activation of the nuclear factor (NF) κB transcription factor pathway. Thus, the synovial T cells may contribute to joint inflammation by providing help for B-cell antibody production and/or cytokine production. This scenario of joint inflammation favors the view that effector T cells, rather than regulatory (suppressor) CD4$^+$ T cells (T$_{reg}$ cells), predominate in the diseased joint, probably because the effector T cells have overwhelmed the ability of T$_{reg}$ cells to control the autoimmune response.

- *Synovial B Cells.* The synovial B cells and terminally differentiated plasma cells are important components of RA inflammation; however, as mentioned above, it is not clear that pathogenic antibodies are a necessary component of such inflammation. Discrete lymphoid follicles are found in the sublining of the RA synovium. These aggregates are composed of the usual constituents: plasma cells, B cells, T cells, and follicular dendritic cells. The B cells express the pan-B-cell markers CD19 and CD20 as well as the proliferation marker Ki67 and the receptor for B-lymphocyte stimulator (BlyS), a member of the TNF superfamily that has been found to be an important regulator of B-cell differentiation. Besides producing RF, the B cells in the synovium are the source of other autoantibodies, such as anti–type II collagen antibodies and anti-CCP antibodies.

- *Other Cells in RA Synovium.* In addition to T cells and B cells, the synovium in RA contains a number of other cells that participate in the inflammatory process. These include *dendritic cells*, highly efficient synovial antigen-presenting cells (APCs) that constitute up to 5% of the synovial fluid mononuclear cells; *macrophages/monocytes*, potent effector cells that have a pivotal role in the initiation of tissue injury, mostly through secretion of soluble mediators, particularly TNF-α and IL-1 (see below); *mast cells*, effector cells that are located at the sites of cartilage erosion and correlate with a more intense clinical synovitis; *nurse-like cells* that stimulate the expression of class II MHC proteins and CD40 on the B cells (making the B cells more efficient APCs for T cells) and produce cytokines such as IL-6, IL-8, and granulocyte–macrophage colony-stimulating factor (GM-CSF); and, finally, *natural killer (NK) cells* that may produce cytokines that stimulate B cells to produce RF.

Cellular Composition of the Effusion. Although it is only rarely identified in the synovial tissue, the *neutrophil* is the most common cell type in the inflamed joint effusion. Neutrophils mediate tissue damage by elaboration of reactive oxygen species (superoxide radicals, hydrogen peroxide), nitric oxide, and proteolytic enzymes. *T cells* and *macrophages/monocytes* constitute the remaining cells seen on examination of fluid removed from an involved joint.

Soluble Mediators: Cytokines, Chemokines, and Growth Factors.

As suggested above, soluble factors such as cytokines, chemokines, and growth factors play critical roles in the pathogenesis of RA, as both key signaling molecules and agents of tissue damage. We will begin by considering the role of cytokines in RA (Fig. 21.3).

Cytokines are proteins that function as paracrine hormones, inducing cellular activation, movement, altered expression of surface molecules, and/or change in cell phenotype or function. They may be effective as soluble or membrane-bound molecules.

T-Cell Cytokines. CD4$^+$ T helper cells are divided into subsets depending on the cytokines they produce (see Case 15 and Fig. 21.1). T_H0 cells (naive T cells) are capable of differentiating into one of four T_H subsets, each with distinct functions in the immune response: T_H1, T_H2, T_H17, and T_{reg} cells. T_H1 cells are primary producers of IFN-γ and IL-2 but not IL-4, IL-5, or IL-13. The T_H2 cells have the complementary profile, producing IL-4, IL-5, and IL-13 but not IFN-γ or IL-2. T_H17 cells are the primary producers of IL-17 and IL-22 but make relatively little IFN-γ. T_{reg} cells produce TGF-β and have a negative regulatory

or immunosuppressive effect. TNF-α, GM-CSF, IL-3, and IL-10 are produced by both T_H1 and T_H2 cells as well as by non-T cells.

The cytokines secreted by cells in the inflamed joints of RA patients demonstrate a T_H1/T_H17 bias, with detectable IFN-γ, IL-2, and IL-17 in both synovial tissue and fluid but not IL-4 and IL-5 (Fig. 21.3). However, these T-cell cytokines are present in low amounts in the inflamed tissue relative to other cytokines, presumably because macrophages and fibroblasts rather than T cells seem to be the main cytokine-producing cells in RA. This does not mean that T-cell cytokines do not play a key pathogenic role; in the CIA model, disease does not occur in the absence of IL-23 (and, by extension, IL-17). It may be that the IL-17 produced by T cells is the communication link between the T cells and nonlymphoid cells, stimulating the latter to produce a host of cytokines that are the proximal causes of RA inflammation. In support of this idea, IL-17 activates neutrophils and monocytes; perhaps most pertinent to the discussion of RA, IL-17 (possibly in synergy with IL−1β and TNF-α) activates synovial fibroblasts to produce chemokines, prostaglandins, and matrix metalloproteinases (MMPs).

Macrophage and Fibroblast Cytokines. After an initiating signal, such as that emanating from T cells described above, macrophages migrate into the synovium, markedly increase in number, and produce large quantities of cytokines. The major proinflammatory cytokines produced by macrophages and fibroblasts in RA synovium include the IL-1 family, TNF-α, IL-6, IL-15, various CSFs, chemokines, and growth factors.

Development of Inflammation in RA

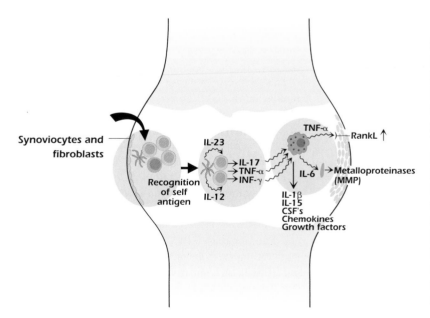

Figure 21.3. Cells and cytokines involved in RA inflammation of joint. The inflammation is initiated by the entry of autoreactive T cells and B cells into the joint. The T cells are activated by antigen-presenting dendritic cells or other "nonprofessional" presenting cells and then produce T_H1 and T_H17 cytokines. The latter then activate macrophages, which produce a host of inflammatory cytokines and chemokines. The cytokines and chemokines cause the entry of other inflammatory cells such as neutrophils. Some of these cytokines act on synoviocytes and fibroblasts to induce the production of additional mediators that bring about tissue destruction. Activated T cells also help B cells produce antibodies that mediate inflammation by binding to Fc receptors on macrophages and by complement activation.

- **The IL-1 Family.** The IL-1 family includes IL-1α, IL-1β, IL-18, and IL-1Ra (the natural receptor antagonist of IL-1). IL-1α and IL−1β are major proinflammatory cytokines contributing to the amplification of the inflammatory response of RA and leading to eventual tissue destruction. High levels of IL-1 have been found in RA joints in both human and animal studies. Within the joint, IL-1 induces fibroblast proliferation and increases the production of IL-6, IL-8, GM-CSF, and prostaglandins. It also induces up-regulation of adhesion molecules on type B synoviocytes and endothelial cells and enhances bone resorption, thereby contributing to the ingress of cells to the joint and the clinically observed osteopenia. Circulating IL-1 also contributes to fatigue and other systemic symptoms as a result of its direct action in the central nervous system (CNS).

- **TNF-α.** TNF-α has many properties similar to IL-1, including its ability to induce the production of other cytokines, the expression of adhesion molecules and the proliferation of synoviocytes. It also stimulates collagenases, MMPs, and prostaglandins, specifically PGE2, thereby contributing to the enzymatic breakdown of joint matrix. TNF-α induces bone resorption and inhibits bone formation, and TNF blockade has shown significant bone-protective effects in humans. Circulating TNF-α also contributes to fatigue and systemic symptoms, particularly cachexia (wasting syndrome).

- **IL-6.** An IL-1 inducible cytokine, IL-6 has a number of important roles: It drives immunoglobulin synthesis by B cells, assists in the differentiation of T cells, and induces the release of acute-phase reactants by the liver. IL-6 may collaborate with TGF-β to induce the differentiation of T_H17 cells, favoring their induction over T_{reg} cells. There is a good correlation between the acute-phase reactants (CRP, haptoglobin, fibrinogen) and serum IL-6 activity in patients with RA. Circulating IL-6 also contributes to fatigue and systemic symptoms.

- **IL-15.** IL-15 is an inducer of T-cell proliferation, especially CD8 T cells, and may be the main growth-factor-type cytokine for synovial T cells. It induces TNF-α production by the macrophages via a T-cell contact mechanism.

- **Colony-Stimulating Factors.** GM-CSF is a macrophage activator leading to IL-1 secretion, HLA-DR expression, regulation of neutrophil function, and tumoricidal activity.

- **Chemokines.** Chemokines are a group of chemoattractant proteins that bring cells to sites of inflammation via their interactions with adhesion molecules on the cells. The receptors are named based on their cysteine residues or nonconserved amino acids between the residues (C–C or C–X–C). Many chemokines are secreted by the RA synovium [including IL-8, MIP-1α and MIP-1β, macrophage chemoattractant protein 1 (MCP-1 CCL2) and RANTES (CCL5)]. Such chemokines, especially IL-8, are responsible for the presence of neutrophils in the inflamed joint.

- **Growth Factors.** Platelet-derived growth factor (PDGF) and fibroblast growth factors (FGFs) have proinflammatory effects in the RA synovium. They stimulate fibroblast overgrowth and angiogenesis (blood vessel formation) and induce the migration of monocytes and macrophages.

Joint Damage and Destruction

The inflammatory cells and the substances they release initiate the joint destruction that is characteristic of unchecked RA. While the mechanisms involved in this process are many, they can be grouped into several categories as discussed below.

The Demand for Oxygen: Ischemia and Angiogenesis.
The inflammation and proliferation of the RA synovium is accompanied by new blood vessel formation. Nevertheless, local tissue ischemia and low oxygen tension of the synovial fluid develop because the neovascularization does not keep pace with the increase in tissue mass. Pressure exerted by the increased synovial bulk and effusion causes obliteration of the capillary flow, leading to cycles of ischemia-reperfusion injury in the joint.

Tissue hypoxia is itself a contributor to injury through its ability to stimulate the production of angiogenic factors such as vascular endothelial growth factor (VEGF); VEGF, in turn, induces the expression of matrix-degrading collagenases. In addition, angiogenic factors such as IL-8, TNF-α, and FGF may themselves cause tissue injury; pretreatment of mice with angiostatic compounds causes attenuation of CIA arthritis, and introduction of these compounds during the course of the disease causes regression of the pathology in both the CIA and SCID models of RA.

Cartilage Destruction and Pannus Formation.
Cartilage is composed of chondrocytes and extracellular matrix (ECM). The major components of the ECM are type II collagen and aggrecan (a large aggregating proteoglycan). Aggrecan fills in the meshwork created by collagen and binds covalently to chondroitin sulfate and keratin sulfate. Chondrocytes both produce and break down these ECM components.

Cartilage destruction in RA is the result of both mechanical forces and enzymatic reactions. Depletion of proteoglycans occurs early in RA synovitis, probably due to the effects of hypoxia, oxygen free radicals, and cytokines (such as IL−1β) acting on chondrocytes; the chondrocytes in turn produce proteolytic enzymes, MMPs, and cathepsins. MMPs are a group of zinc-containing enzymes that includes collagenase-1 and -3, stromelysin-1 (MMP-3), and the aggrecanases. Cathepsins (B, L, and K) are lysosomal cysteine proteases. The interaction of these enzymes with cartilage leads to its mechanical weakening and tendency to fragmentation, with eventual loss of structural integrity. The chondrocytes also both express and interact with RANTES, leading to the production and secretion of MMP-3 and additional chemokines that, in turn, attract other inflammatory cells to the area and cause further cartilage damage.

The proliferating synovium containing synoviocytes, fibroblasts, inflammatory cells, and so on, is referred to as a *pannus*; this structure becomes locally invasive at the interface of weakened cartilage and bone and causes the marginal erosions characteristic of RA (see Fig. 21.2).

Bone Destruction: The RANK Ligand System.

Bone resorption in RA is driven by RANKL [Receptor Activator of NF-κB Ligand (Fig. 21.4)]. RANKL is produced by activated T cells and type B synoviocytes and is activated on osteoclast precursor cells that express RANK. Such activation occurs via soluble RANKL or by contact with cells expressing surface RANKL; it causes elaboration of MMPs and cathepsins, leading to bone resorption. A naturally occurring soluble decoy receptor, osteoprotegerin (OPG), antagonizes the RANK–RANKL system by binding to RANK and blocking RANKL activation. All three substances (RANK, RANKL, and OPG) are found in RA synovium, but the ratio of RANKL to OPG is much higher than normal, leading to net bone destruction.

Summary of RA Immunopathology

The initiating event of RA is most likely the antigen-driven induction of effector T cells that, under normal circumstances, would be self-limiting and harmless. However, a proinflammatory cascade is induced in the genetically susceptible host, which leads to the recruitment and local proliferation of inflammatory cells such as those described above. This, in turn, induces chondrocytes and synovial

cells to release chemokines and destructive enzymes, resulting in the degeneration of articular cartilage and the resorption of periarticular bone. Antibodies may play a role in this process by forming local immune complexes that activate complement, leading to further inflammation by cell activation via Fc receptors and cell recruitment via complement fragments. If not interrupted by endogenous counterregulatory forces or by treatment, the result is self-amplifying, and chronic inflammation of the joint that inevitably leads to deformity and destruction of this structure.

TREATMENT OF RA

The management of RA has changed dramatically in the last decade due to introduction of targeted biologic therapies that address key components of the inflammatory process. Early diagnosis and aggressive treatment are now the preferred approach, with clinical trials showing tremendous benefit not only in symptom relief but also in slowing the pace of structural damage that leads to permanent joint deformity and disabilities. This represents a change from earlier regimens, which were designed solely for symptom control. New forms of biologic therapy that might lead to even further control of the disease are also being introduced. To assess such therapies in clinical trials, the seven clinical and laboratory measures of RA (Table 21.1) established by the American College of Rheumatology (ACR) are used to create semiquantitative measures of efficacy. The mainstays of RA treatment include NSAIDs, disease-modifying antirheumatic drugs, corticosteroids, and biologic therapies.

Nonsteroidal Anti-Inflammatory Drugs

NSAIDs are often the first-line agents prescribed at symptom onset, before the patient even sees a rheumatologist. They produce good subjective symptom responses, especially in early arthritis. A number of compounds are available in this class and their selection and dose depend on the particular needs of individual patients; however, agents that are long-acting are generally preferred. Some patients

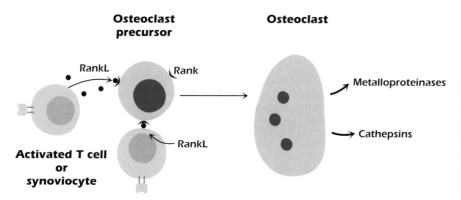

Figure 21.4. Induction of osteoclasts. Activated T cells and synoviocytes produce RANKL, an inducer of osteoclasts. Osteoclasts produce mediators, such as cathepsins and MMPs, that are responsible for cartilage destruction and bone resorption.

at risk for gastrointestinal bleeding require concomitant gastroprotective agents, and all patients require monitoring for hepatotoxicity, nephrotoxicity, hypertension, and edema.

Disease-Modifying Antirheumatic Drugs (DMARD)

Agents referred to under the acronym DMARD are the next line of therapy for RA. This is a heterogeneous group of drugs, including methotrexate, sulfasalazine, hydroxychloroquine, gold salts, D-penicillamine, and, more recently, lefluriomide, with varied and often poorly understood modes of action. Methotrexate interferes with DNA synthesis by inhibiting the enzyme required for regeneration of folate cofactors involved in methylation of DNA bases; it targets rapidly dividing cells such as inflammatory cells. Sulfasalazine, a combination of salicyclic acid and sulfonamide, inhibits neutrophil responses and oxygen free-radical production. Hydroxychloroquine is an antimalarial agent that may inhibit antigen presentation and the induction of T helper cells. Lefluriomide limits T- and B-cell proliferation by targeting a limiting enzyme in the pyrimidine nucleotide synthesis pathway of these cells. D-penicillamine reduces RF titers and immune complex formation by an unknown mechanism. Gold salts remove toxic metabolites and inhibit collagenase activity. Given that these agents attack different components contributing to RA, combination therapy with a DMARD is an acceptable current strategy, but efficacy must be evaluated in the individual patient. Studies with anti-TNF agents have commonly been conducted with methotrexate as the anchor drug (see below). One study has shown benefit with a combination of three DMARDs (methotrexate, sulfasalazine, and hydroxychloroquine); the clinical improvement paralleled that seen with anti-TNF therapies. The use of these agents require careful monitoring that depends on their particular toxicities. For instance, use of methotrexate requires monitoring for hepatic toxicity and gold salts require monitoring for renal toxicity.

Corticosteroids

Corticosteroids are potent anti-inflammatory drugs suppressing proinflammatory cytokines as well as cyclo-oxygenase-2. However, the extensive and serious side effects associated with long-term use remain an important limiting factor in the use of steroids to treat RA and other chronic autoimmune diseases (see Case 14). A few studies have shown slowing of radiographic progression when steroids were used in combination with a DMARD. This is counterbalanced by the sustained bone density loss associated with steroid administration, which persists even after steroid treatment has stopped; in addition, systemic side effects include hyperglycemia, hypertension, cardiovascular disease, cataracts, weight gain, and dermatologic changes. Steroids are currently used mainly as a bridging therapy while waiting for a prescribed DMARD to exert its effect. Intra-articular steroid administration is commonly used as adjunctive therapy to suppress synovitis when only one or a few joints exhibit symptoms of a flare.

Biologic Therapies

TNF-α Inhibitors. The three agents currently approved in the category of "biologic therapy" include infliximab, a *chimeric* (mouse–human combination) monoclonal antibody against TNF-α; etanercept, a soluble TNF receptor blocker; and adalumimab, a fully humanized monoclonal antibody to TNF-α. The anti-TNF-α agents have shown significant benefit in clinical trials in terms of symptomatic improvement, improvement in objective signs of inflammation, and radiographic changes. Using the ACR criteria for grading response discussed above, these responses have been on the order of approximately 60% for ACR20, 40% for ACR50, and 20% for ACR70. Furthermore, anti-TNF therapy is associated with a reduction in the progression of erosions as measured by radiography. A recent clinical trial, the BeST study, has shown persistently good clinical responses in patients initially treated with a combination of methotrexate and anti-TNF therapy, even following discontinuation of the anti-TNF medication.

Caution should be used in administering anti-TNF medications. All patients should be screened with a PPD before starting therapy as was done in Mary's case; if the result is positive, prophylactic treatment is required to prevent reactivation of latent TB. The reactivation of TB can occur because of the powerful suppression of T cell–macrophage interactions caused by anti-TNF agents. With infliximab, there is a chance of developing human antichimeric antibodies (HACA; see Case 25), which may limit the usefulness of the agent; concurrent methotrexate treatment is recommended to prevent HACA development, as methotrexate has more generalized immunosuppressive activity. A recent meta-analysis also showed an increased risk of malignancy (pooled odds ratio 3.3) and infection (pooled odds ratio 2.0) in patients treated with anti-TNF agents.

Interleukin-1β Inhibition. Anakinra is a recombinant human IL-1 receptor antagonist available as a daily subcutaneous injection. Clinical trials have shown modest improvement in clinical symptoms and modest decreases in the rate of joint destruction as measured radiographically. Anakinra may be more effective in combination with methotrexate, but it should not be combined with the anti-TNF medications because a higher risk of infections has been reported with this combination.

Newer Immunomodulators. Three newer immunomodulators include CTLA4-Ig, rituximab, and IL-6 blockers.

Cytotoxic T-Lymphocyte-Associated Antigen 4–Immunoglobulin (CTLA4–Ig). Abatacept is a selective T-cell costimulation modulator that binds to the CD80/CD86 ligands on APCs and blocks their ability to stimulate the proliferation and activation of T cells. It has been approved for treatment in RA patients, and recent studies have shown efficacy in patients who have not responded to anti-TNF therapy.

Rituximab. An anti-CD20 monoclonal antibody initially approved for the treatment of B-cell lymphoma, rituximab has now been approved for the treatment of RA patients who have failed to respond to TNF inhibition. This reagent results in the killing of mature B cells and reduces antibody production, particularly of the autoantibodies. Rituximab has been shown to have efficacy in combination with methotrexate or corticosteroids.

Interleukin-6 Blockade. Toclizumab, a humanized anti-IL6 receptor blocker that binds to both the soluble and membrane-bound receptor, has shown benefit with statistically significant ACR50 and ACR70 responses.

REFERENCES

Cho YG, Cho ML, Min SY, Kim HY (2007): Type II collagen autoimmunity in a mouse model of human rheumatoid arthritis. *Autoimmunity Rev* 7:65–70.

Girbal-Neuhauser E, Durieux JJ, Arnaud M, Dalbon P, Sebbag M, Vincent C, Simon M, Senshu T, Masson-Bessière C, Jolivet-Reynaud C, Jolivet M, Serre G (1999): The epitopes targeted by the rheumatoid arthritis-associated antifilaggrin autoantibodies are posttranslationally generated on various sites of (pro)filaggrin by deimination of arginine residues. *J Immunol* 162:585–594.

Kouskoff V, Korganow AS, Duchatelle V, Degott C, Benoist C, Mathis D (1996): Organ-specific disease provoked by systemic autoimmunity. *Cell* 87:811–822.

McInnes IB, Schett G (2007): Cytokines in the pathogenesis of rheumatoid arthritis. *Nature Rev Immunol* 7:429–442.

Monach P, Hattori K, Huang H, Hyatt E, Morse J, Nguyen L, Oritz-Lopez A, Wu HJ, Mathis D, Benoist C (2007a): The K/BxN mouse model of inflammatory arthritis: Theory and practice. *Methods Mol Med* 136:269–282.

Monach PA, Verschoor A, Jacobs JP, Carroll MC, Wagers AJ, Benoist C, Mathis D (2007b): Circulating C3 is necessary and sufficient for induction of autoantibody-mediated arthritis in a mouse model. *Arthritis Rheum* 56:2968–2974.

Nigrovic PA, Binstadt BA, Monach PA, Johnsen A, Gurish M, Iwakura Y, Benoist C, Mathis D, Lee DM (2007): Mast cells contribute to initiation of autoantibody-mediated arthritis via IL-1. *Proc Natl Acad Sci USA* 104:2325–2330.

Schellekens GA, de Jong BA, van den Hoogen FH, van de Putte LB, van Venrooij WJ (1998): Citrulline is an essential constituent of antigenic determinants recognized by arthritis-specific autoantibodies. *J Clin Invest* 101:273–281.

22

SYSTEMIC LUPUS ERYTHEMATOSUS

KEITH HULL and GABOR ILLEI*

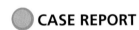

CASE REPORT

"I feel tired, my joints hurt, and I have a rash."

History and Initial Evaluation

Jessica, a 22-year-old student, comes to see you, her internist, because over the last three or four months she has been feeling increasingly tired. Initially, she thought that this was due to stress, but over the last month she has developed a rash on her face and neck and has pain in her hands. Upon questioning, she also reports joint stiffness in the mornings and recurrent painless sores in her mouth.

On physical examination you note that Jessica is slightly hypertensive (blood pressure 150/95). In addition, she has three small ulcers in her mouth and has skin rashes, the latter consisting of an erythematous, indurated rash on her checks and bridge of her nose (malar rash) that spares the nasolabial folds and a second erythematous rash with small circumscribed elevations and discoloration (papulomacular) on the sun-exposed areas of her neck and upper chest. Finally, she also has evidence of bilateral swelling and stiffness in her metacarpophalangeal (MCP) joints that is consistent with arthritis.

*With contributions from Warren Strober and Susan R. S. Gottesman

What is your initial diagnostic impression?

*You realize immediately that this patient is presenting with many of the classical symptoms associated with a relatively uncommon but very distinctive disease, **systemic lupus erythematosus (SLE)**. These symptoms include (1) the "butterfly" rash, an erythematous indurated rash involving the malar areas but sparing the nasolabial fold (Fig. 22.1); (2) the rash on sun-exposed areas (due to photosensitivity, one of the hallmarks of SLE); (3) painless oral ulcers; (4) evidence of arthritis in her hands; and (5) hypertension (in SLE high blood pressure frequently results from a lupus-associated renal disease called **lupus nephritis**, which can be asymptomatic early in the disease).*

You order a complete blood count (CBC), serum chemistries, urinalysis with microscopic evaluation, spot urine protein/creatinine ratio, an "autoantibody panel" to determine the titers of a number of autoantibodies [including antinuclear antibody (ANA), anti double-stranded DNA (dsDNA), anti-Smith (Sm), anti-SS (Sjögren's syndrome)A, and anti-SSB antibodies], and complement C3 and C4 levels. Her preliminary urinalysis, done immediately in your office by dipping a reagent stick ("dipstick"), shows 2+ protein and mild hematuria (red cells in urine). It will be several days to a week before the

Immunology: Clinical Case Studies and Disease Pathophysiology, By Warren Strober and Susan R. S. Gottesman
Copyright © 2009 John Wiley & Sons, Inc.

283

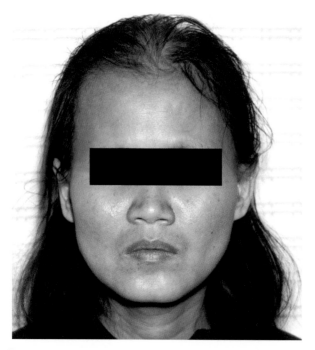

Figure 22.1. Malar rash and alopecia. Characteristic erythematous, indurated malar rash and diffuse alopecia in a lupus patient.

rest of the results are in. Because you suspect that Jessica has SLE and evidence of renal disease (loss of protein in urine, hypertension), you start her on a relatively low dose of the steroid prednisone, ask her to come back in 7–10 days, and direct her to submit a 24-h urine collection before she returns so that you can evaluate her renal function more accurately.

Several days after Jessica's initial visit, the results of her laboratory studies become available. In addition to mild leukopenia (decreased white blood cells) and anemia, they reveal the following results:

	Results	Reference Range
Albumin	3.1 mg/dL	3.5–4.5 mg/dL
Blood urea nitrogen (BUN)	12 mg/dL	<20 mg/dL
Serum creatinine	0.9 mg/dL	0.8–1.4 mg/dL
Liver enzymes	Normal	
Spot protein/creatinine ratio	0.9	<0.15
ANA	5.2 EU	<1.0 EU
Anti-dsDNA	67 EU	<25 EU
Sm antibodies	Positive	Negative
SSa antibodies	Positive	Negative
C3 and C4	Low–normal	

What is your interpretation of the autoantibody and complement results?

The most characteristic autoantibodies produced in SLE are targeted at components of the cell nucleus: the DNA, RNA, and protein–nucleic acid complexes (Table 22.1). If visualized using prepared normal target cells, certain characteristic patterns of staining will appear within the nucleus. Homogeneous or diffuse nuclear staining is seen for antibodies directed against chromatin or histones; rim or peripheral nuclear staining is visible for dsDNA; a speckled pattern appears for non-DNA nuclear constituents including ribonucleoprotein; and nucleolar staining is seen for nucleolar RNA. These nuclear antigens are frequently concentrated in surface blebs of patient cells undergoing apoptosis, suggesting an explanation for their preferential immunogenicity. Jessica's antibodies against the Sm antigen and dsDNA represent two subsets of ANA antibodies specific for SLE. Anti-Sm antibody titers remain relatively constant and do not necessarily relate to disease activity, but serum titers of dsDNA antibodies tend to vary with disease activity, especially in relation to the severity of the kidney disease (glomerulonephritis). This association may reflect the tendency of anti-dsDNA antibodies to form immune complexes and to fix complement, both of which can lead to tissue damage in the kidney. Decreased levels of complement components indicate increased complement consumption (utilization), another feature of SLE. In addition to the ANA antibodies, numerous additional autoantibodies that are not specific for the disease exist in SLE patients. Cell surface proteins of red blood cells, platelets, and leukocytes may also be targeted by autoantibodies in SLE, resulting in the clinical entities of hemolytic anemia, idiopathic thrombocytopenic purpura (ITP due to antiplatelet antibodies), and antineutrophil antibody-mediated neutropenia. To complete the discussion of antibodies in SLE, it should be noted that they frequently have antibodies to phospholipid components of cell membranes. These include anticardiolipin antibody, lupus anticoagulant, and/or anti-β_2 glycoprotein and account for the tendency of lupus patients to form clots (to be in a hypercoagulable state) and/or to bleed.

In spite of the documented presence of ANA autoantibodies in Jessica and their prevalence in SLE (in over 95% of patients), you recall that the presence of ANA alone does not guarantee a diagnosis of SLE or any other underlying autoimmune disease for that matter. It is but one of a constellation of signs and symptoms needed to make the proper diagnosis (see below). Thus, you consider SLE a working diagnosis rather than a definitive one at this point.

Progression of Disease and Definitive Diagnosis

When Jessica returns one week after her first visit, she reports some improvement in her arthritis, but you find that she is more hypertensive (165/98 Hg/mm) and that she has

TABLE 22.1. Autoantibodies in SLE

Antibody	Antibody Target	Specificity for SLE	Frequency (%)	Clinical Association
ANA	Various nuclear antigens	+	>95	Nonspecific
Anti-dsDNA	Double-stranded DNA	+++	60–90	Diagnostic SLE marker; nephritis
Antihistones	Histone proteins (H1, H5, H2A, H2B, H3, and H4)	++	50–70	Drug-induced lupus
SS-A (Ro)	Ribonucleoproteins (Ro52 and Ro60)	+	20–60	Subacute cutaneous lupus erythematosus (SCLE), neonatal lupus, Sjögren's syndrome
SS-B (La)	Ribonucleoproteins (La)	+	15–40	Congenital heart block in neonatal lupus, Sjögren's syndrome
Anti-Sm	U1, U2, U4/6, and U5 spliceosome particles	+++	10–30	Diagnostic SLE marker; no specific clinical association
Anti-RNP	U1 spliceosome particle	++	10–30	Raynaud's disease, musculoskeletal disease, mixed connective tissue disease
Anticardiolipin	β_2-glycoprotein I, various phospholipids, and protein–phospholipid complexes	−	10–30	Thrombosis, fetal loss, thrombocytopenia

gained 8 lbs. She also has bilateral pitting edema (swelling due to fluid accumulation) up to her midcalf. Microscopic urinalysis continues to show hematuria with dysmorphic red blood cells, now with granular and red blood cell casts. Her protein–creatinine ratio is 2.7 and the 24-h urine collection shows a total protein of 2.9 g/day.

What is the significance of these findings?

The proteinuria, dysmorphic red blood cells, and red cell casts are diagnostic of glomerular disease with the amount of protein loss being in the nephritic, rather than the nephrotic, range (<3.5 g/day; see Case 20 for a detailed discussion of renal disease). The combination of hypertension, proteinuria, and nephritic sediment (hematuria and cellular casts) is characteristic of proliferative lupus nephritis and establishes that Jessica does have lupus nephritis (Table 22.2). A kidney biopsy is usually obtained at this point to classify the histologic type

of nephritis and to determine its activity and chronicity. This information has important prognostic significance and is the major determinant of optimal treatment.

The evidence of nephritis in the context of the other features of Jessica's case now convinces you that she does indeed have SLE and you conclude that optimal treatment for her is best provided by an experienced rheumatologist. You therefore refer her to a rheumatologist colleague and he sees Jessica the next day. After reviewing her course and performing a physical examination, he agrees that she needs a kidney biopsy and promptly arranges for one to be performed. However, he feels that treatment with high-dose steroids should be started immediately, since Jessica's symptoms have worsened significantly in the short time since her initial visit. The rheumatologist therefore increases her prednisone dose to 60 mg/day

TABLE 22.2. Clinical Characteristics of Proliferative and Membranous Lupus Nephritis

Characteristic	Proliferative	Membranous
Early signs/symptoms	Frequently asymptomatic	Frequently asymptomatic
Hypertension	Common	Less common
Proteinuria	Variable	Nephrotic range
Urinary sediment	Nephritic (hematuria, cellular casts)	Nephrotic (oval fat bodies)
Loss of renal function	Uniform, if untreated can be rapid	Variable slow progression
Elevated anti-dsDNA levels and/or hypocomplementemia	Common marker of disease activity	Less common

Note: There may be a significant overlap of the features of proliferative and membranous lupus nephritis, and they may coexist. A kidney biopsy is needed to establish definite histologic type. Mixed membranous and proliferative pattern is associated with a worse prognosis.

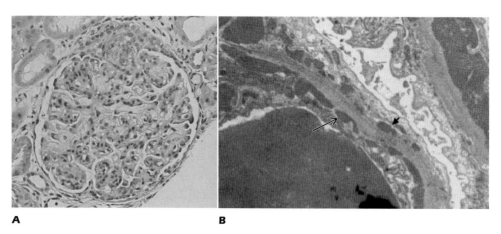

A   **B**

Figure 22.2. **(A)** Hematoxylin–eosin stain of kidney biopsy. Representative glomerulus demonstrating mesangial expansion and cellular proliferation leading to loss of capillary loops. The intense pink staining indicates probable heavy immune complex deposition. There is an early cellular crescent at the top of the figure. **(B)** Electron microscopy shows subendothelial (long arrow) and subepithelial (short arrow) immune complex deposition.

(1 mg/kg), starts her on a diuretic for the purpose of increasing her fluid excretion and decreasing her blood pressure, adds other antihypertensive therapy, and, because of the side effects of steroids, initiates bone protective treatment.

Two days later a biopsy of the right kidney is performed as an outpatient procedure without incident. According to the pathology report, on light microscopy (Fig. 22.2A), the biopsy shows that more than 50% of the glomeruli (7/12) display mesangial expansion and cellular proliferation. In addition, the glomeruli exhibit uniform thickening of the capillary loops as well as occasional *cellular crescents* (proliferations in the Bowman's space of the glomerulus that infringe upon the glomerular structure) and wire loop lesions, but no glomerular sclerosis. Finally, there is a moderately dense lymphocytic infiltrate in the interstitium but no interstitial fibrosis and no tubular atrophy. Electron microscopy (Fig. 22.2B) shows heavy

immune complex deposition in the mesangium and on both the subepithelial and subendothelial sides of the capillary basement membrane. A few tubuloreticular bodies are also noted. The histologic diagnosis is diffuse proliferative and membranous lupus nephritis [World Health Organization (WHO) classes IV and V; Table 22.3].

What conclusions does the rheumatologist draw from these biopsy findings?

The biopsy findings confirm the clinical diagnosis of lupus nephritis and show that Jessica's renal disease consists of a mixed proliferative and membranous lupus nephritis. The light microscopy reveals a high degree of disease activity (cellular proliferation, cellular crescents, and interstitial inflammation) but no signs of irreversible, chronic changes, such as glomerular sclerosis, interstitial fibrosis, or tubular atrophy. The wire-loop lesion indicates heavy immune complex deposition. The presence of a mixed membranous and proliferative lesion suggested by the thickened capillary loops is confirmed on electron microscopy. ***In proliferative***

TABLE 22.3. WHO Classification and Histologic Features of Lupus Nephritis

WHO Class	Histologic Characteristics
I	Normal histology
II	Mesangial expansion with cell or matrix; preservation of mostly intact capillary loops; mesangial immune deposits
III	Proliferative, necrotizing, or sclerosing lesions affecting less than 50% of glomeruli; compromised capillary loop lumens by leukocyte infiltration, endocapillary proliferation, and endothelial cell swelling and proliferation; subendothelial immune deposits
IV	Same as in class III but affecting more than 50% of glomeruli; loss of capillary space is the hallmark
V	Generalized basement membrane thickening; subepithelial and/or intramembranous immune deposits[a]
VI	Widespread sclerosis of glomeruli without any sign of active inflammation.

[a]Mixed membranous (class V) and proliferative (class III or class IV) patterns exist and represent a group with worse prognosis and should be treated as proliferative lupus nephritis.

*lupus nephritis electron-dense deposits (presumably immune complexes) are seen on the endothelial side of the glomerular basement membrane (subendothelial deposits); in **membranous lupus nephritis** they are subepithelial or intramembranous. The subendothelial immune complex deposits suggest very active disease. **Immunofluorescence studies** (staining of tissue with fluorescent-labeled antibodies) are not necessary in most cases since the diagnosis of immune-mediated glomerulonephritis is not in question. However, they are generally more readily (and more rapidly) available than electron microscopy. In Jessica's case, such a study would show a "full-house" picture, with accumulation of immunoglobulins (IgG, IgM, IgA) and complement components (C3 and C1q) along the glomerular basement membrane and the mesangium.*

The kidney biopsy provides an excellent snapshot of the central pathogenic event in SLE, the deposition of immune complexes in a target organ (in this case the kidney), and the subsequent initiation of complement-mediated inflammation (see Case 8). Immune complex deposition in the kidney may be seen in other autoimmune diseases and in chronic infections. Such deposition will lead to a proinflammatory cytokine milieu; if untreated, it will result in irreversible organ damage.

Further Clinical Course and Treatment

Jessica is started on monthly intravenous pulse cyclophosphamide and monthly pulse methylprednisolone. At the same time, her daily prednisone is tapered to a low-dose alternate-day regimen and she is started on plaquenil (hydroxychloroquine) to deal with extrarenal symptoms (see Case 21). Jessica has a good initial response to this regimen: The proteinuria disappears, her urinary sediment clears, and her arthritic symptoms improve. After six months of treatment she is switched to maintenance therapy, consisting of quarterly cyclophosphamide pulses. She continues to take plaquenil to prevent a flare of her extrarenal symptoms. The plan is to treat her with quarterly cyclophosphamide pulses for one year after she has achieved renal remission. At this point both Jessica and her rheumatologist know that she will require long-term monitoring and repeat therapy if problems reemerge.

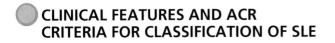

CLINICAL FEATURES AND ACR CRITERIA FOR CLASSIFICATION OF SLE

Lupus erythematosus (often referred to simply as "lupus") is a heterogeneous autoimmune disorder consisting of four different subtypes: SLE, chronic cutaneous lupus erythematosus (CLE or discoid lupus), subacute CLE, and drug-induced lupus. The prevalence of lupus in the United States is estimated to range from 15 to 51 cases per 100,000 persons; however, this estimate probably

underestimates the true prevalence. The incidence rates of SLE in the United States vary between 2 and 8 cases per 100,000 individuals each year. SLE affects females nine times more frequently than males and usually presents between the teens and 40s. In the United States, African-Americans, Hispanics, and Asians have a greater incidence of SLE than Caucasians. Generally, the onset of lupus at an earlier age is associated with a more severe disease course.

The most frequent presenting complaints of SLE include constitutional symptoms (such as fever, malaise, fatigue, anorexia, and weight loss) as well as symptoms involving the skin or joints; however, the disease may be diagnostically challenging, particularly in the absence of the skin rash. Read on for a discussion of the major clinical features of SLE.

Dermatologic Symptoms

Over 70% of SLE patients will have cutaneous findings sometime over the course of their disease. Skin manifestations can be classified as acute, subacute, or chronic. Acute lupus-related rashes can present in various ways; in the majority of cases, the rash makes its appearance following exposure to ultraviolet light or sunlight. The most characteristic acute rash associated with SLE is the so-called **malar** or **"butterfly" rash**, which involves the cheeks and bridge of the nose but spares the nasolabial folds (see Fig. 22.1). Acute rashes are associated with systemic manifestations and heal without scarring. **Subacute cutaneous lupus erythematosus (SCLE)**, associated with systemic lupus in 60% of cases, presents as a papulosquamous rash on exposed areas of the upper body or as an annular-polycyclic rash limited to the back and hands. The annular-polycyclic rash consists of annular lesions with central hypopigmentation, **telangiectasia** (small dilated superficial blood vessels), and a red scaly border. **Discoid lupus erythematosus**, the most common form of chronic cutaneous lupus, is usually not associated with systemic manifestations, and only 10–15% of patients with this form of lupus are positive for ANA. The lesions in discoid lupus have a characteristic appearance marked by follicular plugging and atrophy as well as signs of inflammation. They heal with hypopigmentation and/or scarring and can be disfiguring.

In addition to lupus-specific rashes, patients with SLE can present with a variety of nonspecific skin manifestations such as **Raynaud's phenomenon**, painful discolored digits (white to blue to red) following exposure to cold caused by vasoconstriction of digital blood vessels. Other important mucocutaneous manifestations include **aphthous ulcers** (painful mouth ulcers), alopecia (see Fig. 22.1), telangiectasias, pigment changes, palpable purpuras due to vasculitis, petechiae (small red spots due to tiny capillary hemorrhages) as the result of thrombocytopenia (low platelets), and urticaria (hives).

Musculoskeletal Symptoms

Bilateral, symmetric arthralgia and arthritis affecting the proximal interphalangeal joints, metacarpophalangeal joints, wrists, and knees, frequently associated with morning stiffness, are very common features of SLE and overlap in presentation with other underlying causes of arthritis, including rheumatoid arthritis. Although erosive arthritis is exceedingly rare, approximately 10% of SLE patients will develop deforming arthritis (*Jaccoud's arthropathy*) due to weakening of the soft tissue supporting the joint. SLE patients are also predisposed to osteoporosis and avascular necrosis, as a function of both the underlying disease and the concomitant corticosteroid therapy. Although myalgia is a common symptom, frank myositis is rare.

Cardiopulmonary Involvement

Patients with SLE have an increased risk of developing ischemic heart disease as a consequence of hypertension and accelerated arteriosclerosis. More specific for SLE are the sterile immune complex vegetations (**Libman–Sacks endocarditis**) that can develop on the valvular surfaces of the heart. These may break off, forming emboli and resulting in peripheral embolic phenomena. Pleuritis is the most common pulmonary manifestation of SLE; pulmonary complications such as acute lupus pneumonitis, pulmonary embolism, pulmonary hemorrhage, or alveolitis occur only rarely. Chronic pulmonary manifestations include interstitial fibrosis, pulmonary hypertension, and shrinking lung syndrome, a manifestation thought to result from chronic pleural scarring and diaphragmatic dysfunction or perhaps phrenic nerve dysfunction. Pleuritic chest pain in SLE patients can represent costochondritis, pleuritis, or pericarditis.

Hematologic Manifestations

The vast majority of patients with SLE will develop anemia during the course of their disease. This is most frequently anemia of chronic disease; however, in a minority of patients it is secondary to a sometimes life-threatening autoimmune hemolytic anemia that results from the effect of autoantibodies on erythrocytes. Formation of antilymphocyte and antineutrophil antibodies often results in leukopenia. Similarly, antiplatelet antibodies can cause thrombocytopenia. Occasionally, patients with SLE can develop life-threatening thrombotic thrombocytopenic purpura, a syndrome in which multiple blood clots (fibrin thrombi) form within small vessels throughout the body; it manifests as fever, neurologic impairment, microangiopathic hemolytic anemia (characterized by red blood cell fragments), renal impairment, and thrombocytopenia.

Renal Complications

The kidney is the most commonly involved major organ in SLE; clinically significant renal involvement is present in 50–60% of patients. Based on histology, renal involvement is classified into six groups by using WHO classifications that range from normal to the irreversible stage of glomerulosclerosis (Table 22.3). The most important classes are classes III and IV (focal and diffuse proliferative glomerulonephritis) and class V (membranous lupus nephritis). Proliferative and membranous lupus nephritis have distinct clinical presentations (see Table 22.2), but it is important to keep in mind that both evolving and mixed patterns exist. Determination of the exact histologic type through kidney biopsy can provide additional information about the activity and chronicity of the process, both of which have important therapeutic and prognostic significance.

Neuropsychiatric Symptoms

Neurologic symptoms are a not infrequent manifestation of SLE. Seizures account for about 25% of focal neurologic manifestations and can occur during periods of disease inactivity. In many cases (30%), a contributing cause for the seizure is not identified. Stroke accounts for another 20% of focal neurologic events and may result from a variety of causes including emboli, coagulopathy, atherosclerotic disease, and hypertension. Antiphospholipid antibodies, such as anticardiolipin antibodies and lupus anticoagulant, may play a significant role in the thrombotic events occurring in SLE. Acute inflammatory involvement of the brain and spine (cerebral vasculitis, cerebritis, transverse myelitis) are rare but ominous nonfocal neurologic manifestations of SLE. Infection should always be considered in the differential diagnosis of this complication, especially in patients on immunosuppressive therapy.

Behavioral changes represent at least one-third of neurologic manifestations occurring in SLE. Mood disorders, especially depression, are common among patients with lupus; neurocognitive defects occur as well.

Diagnostic Criteria

The diagnosis of SLE is made based on the constellation of clinical and laboratory findings presented above. In many cases, this diagnosis is difficult to make and/or delayed because of the heterogeneity of the disease and its evolution over time. The American College of Rheumatology (ACR) has established classification criteria for SLE clinical trials (Table 22.4). These require that a patient fulfill at least 4 of the 11 criteria listed. These criteria may be helpful, but it is important to remember that they were not created to establish the diagnosis. Some patients who clearly have lupus may fulfill only three of the ACR criteria but have other characteristic manifestations.

TABLE 22.4. ACR Classification Criteria for SLE

Manifestation	Definition
Malar rash	Fixed erythema, flat or raised, over malar eminences, tending to spare nasolabial folds
Discoid rash	Erythematous raised patches with adherent keratotic scaling and follicular plugging; atrophic scarring may occur in older lesions
Photosensitivity	Skin rash as a result of unusual reaction to sunlight, by patient history or physician observation
Oral ulcers	Oral or nasopharyngeal ulcerations, usually painless, observed by a physician
Arthritis	Nonerosive arthritis involving two or more peripheral joints, characterized by tenderness, swelling, or effusion
Serositis	Pleuritis—convincing history of pleuritic pain or rub heard by a physician or evidence of pleural effusion OR Pericarditis—documented by ECG or rub or evidence of pericardial effusion
Renal disorder	Persistent proteinuria greater than 0.5 g/day or greater than 3+ if quantitation not performed OR Cellular casts—red cell, hemoglobin, granular, tubular, or mixed
Neurologic disorder	Seizures—in absence of offending drugs or known metabolic derangements, e.g., uremia, ketoacidosis, or electrolyte imbalance OR Psychosis—in absence of offending drugs or known metabolic derangements, e.g., uremia, ketoacidosis, or electrolyte imbalance
Hematologic disorder	Hemolytic anemia—with reticulocytosis OR Leukopenia—less than 4000/μL total on two or more occasions OR Lymphopenia—less than 1500/μL on two or more occasions OR Thrombocytopenia—less than 100,000/μL in absence of offending drugs
Immunologic disorder	Anti-DNA: antibody to native DNA in abnormal titer OR Anti-Sm: presence of antibody to Sm nuclear antigen OR Positive finding of antiphospholipid antibodies based on (1) abnormal serum level of IgG or IgM anticardiolipin antibodies, (2) positive test result for lupus anticoagulant using a standard method, or (3) false-positive serologic test for syphilis known to be positive for at least 6 months and confirmed by *Treponema pallidum* immobilization or fluorescent treponemal antibody absorption test
Antinuclear antibodies	Abnormal titer of ANAs by immunofluorescence or an equivalent assay at any point in time in the absence of drugs known to be associated with "drug-induced lupus" syndrome

 THE IMMUNOPATHOGENESIS OF SLE

The immunopathogenesis of SLE is best considered as a breakdown in immunologic tolerance that leads to autoreactive effectors, primarily autoimmune antibodies. The common basis is an autoimmune attack; however, in contrast to other autoimmune diseases with restricted, often organ-specific targets, the autoantibodies in SLE are capable of attacking numerous cell types in the body. The autoantibodies cause pathology by a variety of mechanisms, depending on the organ affected and the involvement of secondary factors such as complement activation, immune complex deposition, and leukocyte infiltration. As you will learn shortly, much of the pathology is the result of immune complex deposition, which can affect numerous organs. All of these factors account for the extreme variability of this disease among individual patients, which makes diagnosis difficult and often necessitates care by numerous specialists.

General Influences on Susceptibility to SLE

Genetic Factors. The pathogenesis of SLE has a strong genetic component; there is a 24% concordance of disease between monozygotic twins, compared to only 2% between dizygotic twins. However, while single gene defects can lead to lupuslike conditions in animal models, the genetic influence in humans is clearly polygenic and different combinations of genes may lead to disease in different patients. The various genes involved may also result in the different manifestations of the disease. This is supported by extensive studies in mice with spontaneously developing lupus-like syndromes that show that different genetic loci are responsible for various aspects of SLE, such as the initial loss of tolerance, the amplification of the autoimmune process, and the severity and specificity of organ involvement.

Hormonal Influences. The striking female-to-male ratio of 9:1 in SLE suggests that sex hormones play a major role in the pathogenesis of lupus. This hypothesis is supported by the fact that the gender bias is most pronounced during the ages when women are hormonally cycling and is much smaller before puberty and after menopause, when estrogen levels are low. In addition, in many of the mouse strains that develop a lupuslike syndrome, the females show earlier and more severe disease than the males.

Environmental Factors. Immunologic abnormalities can be detected in both mice with lupuslike syndromes and humans with SLE well before the onset of clinical symptoms, suggesting that initiation of disease requires a triggering event. The trigger has not yet been clearly identified, but several environmental factors, including UV light, drugs, infections, and stress, are candidates because they are known to cause disease flares. UV light, a well-known trigger of SLE, causes inflammation and enhanced apoptosis of skin cells, creating an inflammatory milieu that promotes the exposure of nuclear autoantigens. Infectious agents, particularly viruses, can promote the onset of autoimmune manifestations by several mechanisms, including the induction of autoantibodies either by **molecular mimicry** (similarity of viral antigens to self-antigens) or by exposure of cryptic antigens. Although several viruses have been suggested as possible etiologic agents, no definitive link with any virus has been established to date.

Autoantibody Induction in SLE

Normal Mechanisms of B-Cell Anergy and Its Defective Induction in SLE. Growing evidence supports the idea that autoantibodies are generated by B-cell responses that are similar to normal immune responses directed at exogenous (foreign) antigens. Thus, cells producing autoantibodies (responses to self-antigens)

undergo normal immunoglobulin class switching (such as the switch from IgM to IgG), affinity maturation, and somatic mutation (see Case 4).

This leads to an important question: How do certain self-antigens subvert the normal B-cell differentiation pathway for the purpose of producing pathogenic autoantibodies? One part of the answer lies in understanding the mechanisms that normally prevent the emergence of autoreactive B cells. B cells are quite unlike T cells; they do not develop in a central lymphoid organ such as the thymus, where they could undergo an extensive selection process to weed out cells with self-specificity. Instead, B cells pass through a number of "checkpoints" at which the cell is signaled via the B-cell receptor (BCR) and is deleted or rendered permanently anergic if the signal arises from a self-antigen (Fig. 22.3). See Case 1 for a discussion of B-cell differentiation in the bone marrow and Case 5 for a description of how the immature B cell emerges from the bone marrow and must transit through several steps to become a mature but still naive B cell that can then enter the follicle when drawn in by its specific antigen. Those discussions however, did not deal with situations in which the continued survival of the B cell might not be desirable. The checkpoints to prevent the stimulation and continuation of autoreactive B cells take place first in the bone marrow, then in the periphery during the transition from immature B cell to mature naive B cell, and finally in the germinal center itself (Fig. 22.3).

The checkpoint in the bone marrow involves crosslinking of the BCR and elimination of autoreactive cells by: (1) "receptor editing," in which the B cell rearranges a new light chain to form a new BCR with different non-autoantigen specificity, or (2) deletion of the B cell. Additional checkpoints occur as B cells just emerging from the bone marrow pass through transitional stages (T1, T2, and T3) on the way to becoming mature naive B cells of the various types described below. In contrast to T2 B cells, which precede the mature B cells, it appears that T3 B cells may be permanently anergic B cells that do not give rise to mature B cells. Recent studies have shown that these anergic B cells are in fact autoreactive B cells that are induced to become anergic by BCR stimulation in the absence of costimulation; stimulation of T3 B cells results in anergy because it causes disruption in the BCR signaling complex. Estrogen can decrease BCR signaling at this stage and thereby decrease anergy induction; this may explain why SLE occurs at a far greater frequency in females than in males. In addition, costimulation of T3 B cells with CD40L or exposure of the B cell to the cytokine BAFF [B-cell activating factor belonging to the tumor necrosis factor (TNF) family] can rescue these cells from anergy; thus, stimulation of these normally anergic cells by extrinsic factors could lead to autoimmunity in SLE.

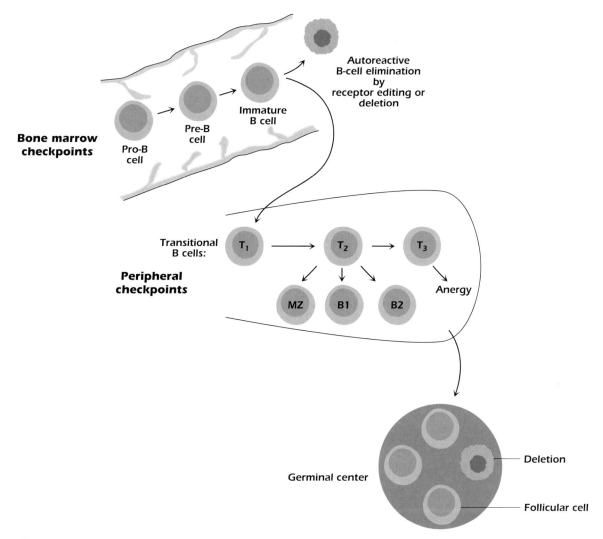

Figure 22.3. B cells can be deleted or induced into permanent anergy at many points during their development. In the bone marrow autoreactive cells undergo "receptor editing" or deletion. In the periphery they are deleted or anergized during various transitional stages ($T_1 \rightarrow T_3$). Alternatively, they become cells with low affinity for self-antgens (MZ B cells or B1 B cells) or B2 cells, the precursors of follicular B cells. Finally, if an autoreactive B cell persists to become a germinal center B cell, it can be deleted at this site as well.

Mature B cells consist of several subtypes: B1 B cells, B2 B cells, marginal zone B cells (MZ B cells), and mantle zone B cells. The relationship among these subsets and the timing of divergence during development have not been precisely delineated. B2 B cells are the "conventional" B cells; they enter the follicle forming the germinal center and respond to antigen and T-cell help with affinity maturation and isotype class switching (see Cases 4, 5, and 25). The mantle zone B cells surrounding the germinal center are primary follicle cells that are pushed to the outside when the germinal center forms. The B1 B cells and the MZ B cells occupy unique areas; B1 B cells are in the body cavities and MZ B cells are in the spleen, mucosal associated lymphoid tissue, and mesenteric lymph nodes

(see Case 24). Both B1 B cells and MZ B cells (but particularly the former) respond to antigen without T-cell help and with the production of IgM of limited diversity. MZ B cells of the spleen are especially important in our defense against pneumococcal pneumonia; their development in the spleen some time after birth explains the susceptibility of newborns to *Streptococcus pneumonia*. Both B1 and marginal zone B cells may be part of our more immediate response to infectious organisms before the B2 B cells can fully respond to stimulation. Because the antibodies they produce have more broad specificity than those produced by the B2 cells, they may cross-react with self-antigens.

In addition to producing IgM to combat infectious agents, B1 B cells are capable of producing nonpathogenic IgM autoantibodies. There is some evidence that in SLE such cells can enter the germinal center of lymph nodes and undergo somatic mutation to make pathogenic autoantibodies. Thus, the ability of the immune system to exclude B1 cells from germinal centers is another checkpoint that may be dysregulated in SLE. Another checkpoint involves MZ B cells. MZ B cells may diverge from those destined to be B2 B cells in one of the later transitional stages. There is evidence that they can arise in part from autoreactive B cells that escape deletion at a transitional stage and are then expanded by the cytokine BAFF. Studies of mouse models of SLE have shown that such cells can undergo class switching and somatic mutation to become producers of pathogenic autoantibodies under some circumstances; thus, the ability to prevent autoantibody production by MZ B cells is another checkpoint that may be disabled in SLE. A final checkpoint occurs in the germinal center, the main site of B-cell somatic mutation and class switching. It is known from mouse studies that a large proportion of the foreign antigen–driven B-cell maturation in the follicle results in cells with potential autoreactivity but that these cells undergo negative selection by an as-yet-unknown mechanism at the germinal center checkpoint. Since many of the autoantibodies in SLE display somatic mutation, it has been assumed that B cells producing these antibodies have escaped negative selection at the germinal center checkpoint. Recently it has been shown that an Fc receptor (FcγRIIb) present on B cells that binds IgG by its Fc fragment may provide negative signals to B cells in the germinal centers following binding of antigen–antibody complexes. Thus, the generation of autoantibodies in germinal centers in SLE may also result from reduced FcγRIIb function (see below).

Autoantigens.

Abnormalities of B-cell selection at the checkpoints described above can only be one aspect of the development of autoantibodies in SLE since these abnormalities would give rise to a large and unfocused array of autoantibodies, not the relatively restricted array that occurs in SLE. Thus, a second factor implicated in the development of autoantibodies in SLE is related to the nature of the autoantigens evoking these autoantibodies.

A majority of autoantigens in systemic autoimmune states are conserved intracellular molecules [such as nucleic acids, nucleotide binding proteins, or tRNA synthetase enzymes] that normally are not recognized by the immune system in a fashion that would evoke an immune response; instead, they are released in a way that ensures continued induction of anergy as long as the signaling of costimulatory molecules does not occur. However, these antigens often share structural similarities and are subject to certain apoptosis-related changes, such as nucleic acid cleavage, proteolysis, or protein modification. These features might promote increased recognition and processing by immunocompetent cells because they evoke interactions with pattern recognition receptors [PRRs; such as Toll-like receptors (TLRs)], which stimulate the cells through an innate immune mechanism. The TLRs are expressed on numerous cell types, including T cells, B cells, macrophages, dendritic cells, and epithelial cells, and recognize molecular patterns normally found in microorganisms. Activation of TLRs leads to a proinflammatory response and the up-regulation of costimulatory molecules. In addition, because a large number of autoantigens are concentrated in "apoptotic blebs" on the surface of cells undergoing apoptosis, they are more exposed to professional antigen-presenting cells (APCs) (cells whose main function is antigen presentation). Finally, some autoantigens are generated secondarily to immune-mediated tissue damage, such as that caused by cytotoxic T-cell-mediated granule-induced apoptosis. Here, again, the self-antigens are juxtaposed with immune elements and may facilitate ordinarily "forbidden" immune responses.

Cellular Interactions Leading to Autoantibody Production.

Starting with the exposure of self-antigens and the defects in B-cell anergy state, there are two possible mechanisms to explain autoantibody induction; one involves both T cells and B cells and the other only B cells. In the first mechanism, the locus of the autoimmune defect occurs in a T-cell subpopulation with the capacity to respond to a self-antigen because of an underlying (antigen-specific) defect in a central or peripheral tolerance mechanism (see the introduction to this unit III). In this scenario, the initial event is most likely the uptake of the autoantigen by an APC followed by presentation to and activation of a T cell. Because the latter requires up-regulation of costimulatory molecules on the surface of the APC (such as CD80 or CD86) to induce a robust T-cell response, it may involve autoantigens with an intrinsic capacity to stimulate the APCs, such as those stimulating through PRRs (see above). In the next step, the autoreactive T cells interact with B cells emerging from the bone marrow, which also encounter the autoantigen and present it to the self-antigen specific T cell. This interaction with the T cell provides the B cell with a second signal (via CD40L–CD40) and results in nonanergic, fully competent B cells able to produce autoantibodies. This mechanism is favored by the existence of several murine models of SLE in which T-cell abnormalities are found in association with B cells that produce autoantibodies. It is also supported by recent studies showing that T-cell production of the B-cell growth factor BAFF can induce B cells, particularly MZ B cells, to become active secretors of pathogenic autoantibodies.

The second proposed mechanism of autoantibody induction involves the B cells alone. Here, the normally anergic B cells with specificity for specific self-antigens are redirected from the anergic state by antigens that directly deliver a second signal to the B cell, such as the aforementioned antigens that stimulate cells through PRR. This mechanism is supported by recent studies showing that the anergic state of B cells can be reversed by both direct stimulation and interactions with T cells.

Antigen Presentation and Lymphocyte Response in SLE

The first proposed mechanism, in which T cells have a central role in stimulating autoreactive B cells, requires that the T cells themselves be stimulated by antigen. Activation of T cells by APCs requires presentation of antigen in the context of major histocompatibility complex (MHC) molecules to the T-cell receptor (TCR) (signal 1) as well as stimulation of the T cell via costimulatory molecules such as B7 (CD80 and CD86 on APCs) (signal 2). Ordinarily, self-antigens will not successfully induce activation of T cells and may even induce tolerance of T cells because these antigens are not able to induce expression of costimulatory molecules on the APCs. However, APCs can be activated to express costimulatory molecules by cytokines. Interferon (IFN) α, one of the strongest of such exogenous activators, is overproduced in SLE and may therefore be a key facilitator of responses to self-antigens in this disease. In addition, this cytokine is induced by known triggers of SLE flares, such as viruses and UV light; this may explain how such exogenous influences act as triggers. APCs can also be induced to express costimulatory molecules by TLR ligands. These ligands include DNA and RNA molecules, which are known to elicit autoantibody responses in SLE. There is also evidence that debris from apoptotic cells can stimulate a subpopulation of dendritic cells (DCs) to produce type I IFNs, which then induce DC maturation and activation of self-reactive T cells. Thus, it is possible that self-antigens in SLE do have the ability to induce T-cell responses. Finally, since B cells are also APCs, activation of B cells by cytokines and antigens may lead to T-cell stimulation of autoreactive B cells, as mentioned above in the discussion of autoantibodies.

Although the number of T cells in SLE patients is normal or decreased, they exhibit an activated phenotype, especially during active disease. Recent studies of the biochemical basis of this increased activation indicate that it is a complex phenomenon that may differ from patient to patient. One contributing abnormality is a "rewiring" of the TCR due to decreased CD3ζ expression and surrogate Syk and FcRγ chain expression. CD3ζ is one of the peptide chains of CD3 that transmits the signal into the cell when the TCR binds its specific antigen. This is accomplished via the ability of CD3ζ to be phosphorylated on its ITAM (immunoreceptor tyrosine-based activation motif). Syk, an intracellular tyrosine kinase, can activate ITAM on other CD3 peptide chains, compensating for CD3ζ chain loss. FcRγ, the γ chain of the high-affinity Fc receptor for IgE, is a member of the TCR ζ chain family. This

Fc chain may mediate signal transduction through Syk and thus also compensates for CD3ζ chain loss. Another abnormality found on the SLE T cell is a preclustering of *lipid rafts* (collections of signaling molecules in a localized region on the cell surface) and consequent exaggeration of Ca^{2+} responses, resulting in a reactive T-cell state. This abnormality also leads to increased expression of CD44, an adhesion molecule involved in T-cell migration. Finally, T cells in SLE patients exhibit decreased IL-2 production, perhaps because of dysregulation of the balance between the transcriptional activator CREB and the transcriptional repressor CREM. Maintenance of this balance depends partly on stress and hormones in the environment. CREM will decrease IL-2 production by binding to its promoter and thus decrease the T cell's ability to promote activation-induced cell death. In addition to its effect on IL-2 production, CREB also increases the expression of Foxp3, a transcription factor specific for negative regulatory T cells. This change in the balance between CREM and CREB has several consequences, including increased activation of B cells and alterations in the generation of regulatory T cells.

The end result of this collection of T-cell defects is that T cells in SLE display a lack of tolerance to self-antigens, are in an activated state, and can interact with B cells to prevent induction of anergy as suggested above. Evidence in support of this comes from extensive studies of various murine models of SLE as well as the fact that anti-DNA antibodies in SLE patients exhibit somatic mutations suggestive of T-cell-dependent affinity maturation (T-cell help). In addition, active SLE patients have a T-lymphocyte repertoire characterized by selective activation of particular T-cell subpopulations. Cell lines generated from T cells of SLE patients have been found to specifically help autologous B cells produce anti-dsDNA or antihistone antibodies (which are specifically reactive to nucleosome). Finally, the spontaneous T-cell activation may be due at least partially to altered suppressor T-cell function.

B cells also exhibit increased activation in SLE. However, in contrast to T cells, they exhibit an increased rate of proliferation that correlates with an increase in the spontaneous secretion of immunoglobulins, especially pathogenic IgG autoantibodies. There is evidence that this hyperresponsiveness is due to abnormalities in T-cell/B-cell interactions and excessive T-cell help. However, other abnormalities, such as increased IL-6 and IL-10 production and increased IL-6R expression on B cells, may also play roles in this process.

As alluded to above, B cells may act as efficient APCs for a variety of autoantigens and thus promote the breakdown of peripheral T-cell tolerance. In SLE such interactions are facilitated by the increased expression of CD40L (CD154), a costimulatory molecule that is transiently expressed on the surface of activated T cells as well as other activated hematopoietic cells that stimulate B cells (and other APCs) through CD40. Increased expression of CD40L may also be an important mechanism in SLE because, as discussed in Case 4, the CD40–CD40L interaction between B and T cells is necessary for germinal center formation and isotype switching of the immunoglobulin produced by the B cell. Thus, increased expression can lead to the perpetuation of the germinal center reactions that promote autoantibody production. Indeed, early clinical studies indicated that blocking the CD40/CD40L interactions led to disruption of germinal center reactions and may have clinical benefit. However, these clinical studies are presently on hold because they may cause thromboembolic side effects.

Cytokines play an important but still uncertain role in SLE. Traditionally, cytokines are characterized as T_H1- or T_H2-type cytokines and, accordingly, autoimmune diseases are grouped as T_H1- or T_H2-type diseases based on the dominance of one or the other cytokine group in the disease (see Case 15). With respect to such grouping, the literature on the role of cytokines in SLE is confusing and often contradictory. It thus seems likely that lupus cannot be characterized as either a type 1 or a type 2 disease and that cytokines arising from both T-cell pathways contribute to SLE in different ways. For instance, T_H1 T-cell production of IFN-γ may enhance costimulatory molecule expression on APCs, whereas T_H2 production of IL-4 and IL-6 may enhance B-cell expansion, both processes that are necessary for autoantibody production. As already mentioned above, attention has recently been drawn to the function of IFN-α in SLE, since mononuclear cells in SLE patients display evidence of IFN-dependent cell activation and treatment of hepatitis patients with IFN-α can cause SLE. IFN-α production in SLE is likely to arise by stimulation of APCs via their TLRs with DNA and RNA released from apoptotic cells or with DNA- and RNA-containing aggregates. The IFN-α then acts on the immune system to induce autoantibody formation, notably by inducing upstream activation of APCs and downstream activation of T cells. Some investigators believe that IFN-α secretion is so important that SLE can be ameliorated by treatment blocking this cytokine.

The Role of Complement in SLE

The complement system can be regarded as a double-edged sword with respect to SLE. On the one hand, it may protect against the development of SLE; on the other, it may play a key role in mediating local tissue damage. The protective function of complement is supported by the fact that homozygous deficiencies in any of the early complement components of the classical pathway are the strongest known susceptibility factors for the development of SLE symptoms in humans (see Case 8). Such susceptibility is highest for deficiencies of any of the C1 complex proteins or C4 (>80%) and drops significantly for C2 and

C3 (10%). In rare instances, deficiencies in components of the membrane attack complex (C5–9) can also lead to SLE symptoms. The mechanisms underlying this association are still poorly understood, but it is generally believed that complement deficiency favors the development of autoreactive B cells because of its association with impaired clearance of apoptotic cells and/or abnormal lymphocyte activation.

Once SLE is established, complement becomes a disease-enhancing factor in autoantibody-mediated tissue injury. Measures of complement activation parallel disease activity, and immune complexes at sites of tissue injury are associated with the various consequences of complement activation, including the presence of C3, C4, and other complement components; the release of the anaphylatoxins C3a and C5a; and the activation of the membrane attack complex.

Mechanisms of Tissue Injury Caused by Immune Complex Deposition: Role of Fc Receptors

Glomerular deposition of IgG anti-dsDNA immune complexes is thought to be responsible for most of the renal injury that occurs in SLE glomerulonephritis. These complexes are identified by the histological detection of anti-dsDNA antibodies in the glomeruli of patients with active glomerulonephritis, clinical studies demonstrating high concentrations of serum anti-dsDNA antibodies coinciding (or preceding) active glomerulonephritis, and enrichment of IgG anti-dsDNA antibodies in glomerular tissue relative to serum and other organs. As discussed above, tissue damage resulting from such deposition is caused by immune complex activation of the complement system. Another, and perhaps equally important, mechanism arises from the fact that the immune complexes activate effector cells (monocytes and macrophages), which express cell surface Fcγ receptors (receptors for IgG).

Three classes of Fcγ receptors are recognized. FcγRI is expressed on monocytes, macrophages, and a subset of dendritic cells and has a high affinity for monomeric IgG. The FcγRII family of receptors is expressed on the same cells but is of low affinity and interacts most effectively with multivalent IgG-opsonized particles and immune complexes as well as IgG bound to cell surfaces. FcγRIIIa and FcγRIIIb are encoded by two different genes; they differ in their affinities for ligand and in the cells that express them. FcγRIIIa has an intermediate affinity and is expressed on mononuclear phagocytes, mesangial cells, and natural killer (NK) cells. FcγRIIIb is expressed exclusively on neutrophils and eosinphils and demonstrates a low affinity for ligand. A unique aspect of the FcγRs is their heterogeneity; a conserved ligand-binding domain is associated with alternative intracytoplasmic signaling motifs. Depending on the motif, the effector cell is either activated (through FcγRI,

FcγRIIa, and FcγRIII) or inhibited (FcγRIIb). Activating and inhibitory FcγRs are coexpressed on effector cells; the ratio of signals from these opposing receptors is critical in setting the threshold for the inflammatory activity of immune complexes. Proinflammatory cytokines such as IFN-γ and TNF-α up-regulate FcγRIII and down-regulate FcγRIIb, resulting in a lowered threshold for immune complex stimulation. (Recall that in the discussion above we mentioned that reduced FcγRIIb expression on germinal center B cells leads to a defect in anergy induction by antigen–antibody complexes.) Recently, it was shown that C5a has a similar effect, providing an additional mechanism by which an activated complement system can contribute to local tissue damage (Fig. 22.4). Conversely, up-regulation of FcγRIIb by substances such as intravenous immunoglobulin (IVIG) raises the threshold for IC stimulation and suppresses the inflammatory response.

In addition to its effects on the kidney, immune complex deposition (with or without activation of inflammatory cells) contributes to arthritis, vasculitis, endocarditis, and some aspects of pulmonary and cardiac manifestations in SLE patients.

In summary, SLE is a complex systemic autoimmune disease dominated by the production of pathogenic autoantibodies. An emerging concept is that SLE may be due to a number of interactive abnormalities that give rise to somewhat different forms of disease in different patients. The core abnormality in SLE is a failure to maintain B cell tolerance and thus the emergence of B cells producing autoantibodies. Important factors underlying this defect in tolerance include intrinsic abnormalities of B cells leading to altered selection/deletion of autoreactive B cells at the various checkpoints, T-cell dysfunction leading to T cells that support and/or induce the autoreactive B cells, production of cytokines such as IFN-α that activate APCs and other cells, and the generation of cellular products such as DNA and RNA that activate cells via innate immune mechanisms and serve as antigen targets. Tissue injury in SLE is mainly the result of the deposition of immune complexes and the subsequent activation of complement and Fc receptor function. As shown in Figure 22.5, these defects self-amplify as a result of various positive-feedback loops.

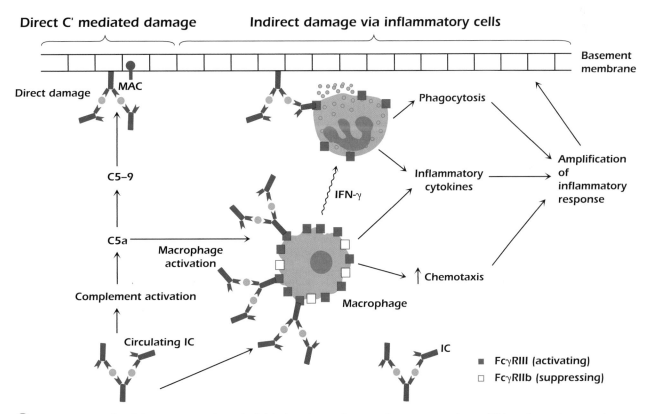

Figure 22.4. Role of immune complexes in initiating tissue damage. Immune complexes (ICs) activate the complement cascade, leading to the release of C5a and activation of the membrane attack complex (C5–9), which contributes to tissue damage directly. C5a also activates effector cells through the activator FcγRs. This leads to increased production of inflammatory cytokines and decreased expression of the inhibitory FcγRIIb resulting in further amplification of the inflammatory response, including activation of antigen-presenting cells, lymphocytes, neutrophils, and endothelial cells. This uncontrolled inflammatory process will eventually lead to tissue destruction and organ damage.

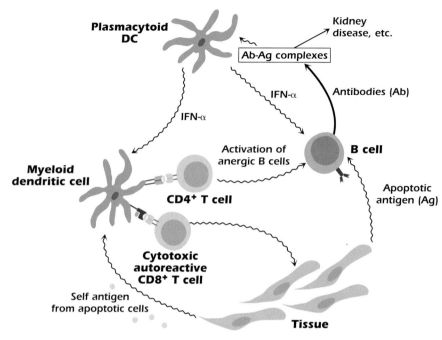

Figure 22.5. Possible feedback loops leading to tissue injury in SLE.

TREATMENT OF SLE

The treatment of SLE is best handled by a multidisciplinary team of physicians, each expert in specific aspects of this diverse disease. The challenge is to treat the underlying immune abnormalities as well as the various comorbid conditions and psychosocial problems that are also frequently present. Every lupus patient must be counseled on the damaging effects of sunlight and educated on sun avoidance and the appropriate use of sunscreens.

Treatment of Major Organ Involvement

The cornerstone of treatment of major organ SLE manifestations is corticosteroid therapy, which can be applied as high-dose daily treatment or as bolus intravenous therapy for one to three days. For most major organ manifestations that are not expected to completely resolve with a limited duration of corticosteroid therapy, an immunosuppressive agent is started at the same time. Based on the experience of treating severe lupus nephritis, cyclophosphamide is the traditional choice for the most severe manifestations, which include nephritis, pulmonary hemorrhage, and central nervous system (CNS) vasculitis. Cyclophosphamide can be given daily or as a monthly IV pulse therapy. The efficacy of the two approaches is similar, but monthly pulse cyclophosphamide is associated with fewer of the severe side effects of the daily regimen, which include hemorrhagic cystitis and bladder cancer. Pulse cyclophosphamide is effective in most patients but seems to be less affective in African-Americans. Because

cyclophosphamide is an alkylating agent that inhibits DNA replication, cyclophosphamide-induced infertility is common and of major concern. The risk of infertility increases with the cumulative dose and the age of the patient. Recently, several studies suggest that mycophenolate mofetil, an agent that inhibits guanosine nucleotide synthesis and immune cell proliferation, has no effect on fertility; this may be an alternative to cyclophosphamide in treating lupus nephritis. Both cyclophosphamide and mycophenolate mofetil are commonly used as immunosuppressive agents in transplant patients (see Case 20).

Treatment of Minor Manifestations of SLE

"Minor" manifestions of SLE (such as arthalgias, myalgias, and pleurisy) can often be managed by nonsteroidal anti-inflammatory drugs; rashes can be treated with topical corticosteroids. In addition, antimalarials such as hydroxychloroquine are good choices for arthritis, fatigue, and mucocutaneous manifestations that do not respond to topical treatments. More severe manifestations require systemic therapy with prednisone; dosing and length of treatment depend on the severity of the symptoms and the response to therapy. If the response is incomplete or steroids cannot be tapered in a short period of time, a steroid-sparing agent such as azathioprine or methotrexate should be added.

Novel Therapies

There are a number of novel, experimental approaches to the treatment of lupus nephritis. These include the use of biologic agents such as blocking cytokines or costimulatory molecules and the use of immunoablative chemotherapy with or without bone marrow transplantation in the hope that the regenerating immune system will not be autoimmune prone.

REFERENCES

Austin HA, Illei GG (2005): Membranous lupus nephritis. *Lupus* 14: 65–71.

Contreras G, Pardo V, Leclercq B, Lenz O, Tozman E, O'Nan P, Roth D (2004): Sequential therapies for proliferative lupus nephritis. *N Engl J Med* 350: 971–980.

Crispin JC, Kyttaris VC, Juang Y.-T, Tsokos GC (2007): Systemic lupus erythematosus: New molecular targets. *Ann Rheum Dis* 66: 65–69.

Crow MK, Kyriakos AK (2004): Interferon-α in systemic lupus erythematosus. *Curr Opin Rheumatol* 16: 541–547.

Davidson A, Aranow C (2006): Pathogenesis and treatment of systemic lupus erythematosus nephritis. *Curr Opin Rheumatol* 18: 468–475.

D'Cruz DP, Khamashta MA, Hughes GR (2007): Systemic lupus erythematosus. *Lancet* 369: 587–596.

Ginzler EM, Dooley MA, Aranow C, Kim MY, Buyon J, Merrill JT, Petri M, Gilkeson GS, Wallace DJ, Weisman MH, Appel GB (2005): Mycophenolate mofetil or intravenous cyclophosphamide for lupus nephritis. *N Engl J Med* 353: 2219–2228.

Gottlieb BS, Ilowite NT (2006): Systemic lupus erythematosus in children and adolescents. *Pediatr Rev* 27: 323–330.

Hochberg MC (1997): Updating the American College of Rheumatology revised criteria for the classification of systemic lupus erythematosus. *Arthritis Rheum* 40: 1725.

Houssiau FA, Vasconcelos C, D'Cruz D, Sebastiani GD, Garrido Ed Ede R, Danieli MG, Abramovicz D, Blockmans D, Mathieu A, Direskeneli H, Galeazzi M, Gül A, Levy Y, Petera P, Popovic R, Petrovic R, Sinico RA, Cattaneo R, Font J, Depresseux G, Cosyns JP, Cervera R (2002): Immunosuppressive therapy in lupus nephritis: The Euro-Lupus Nephritis Trial, a randomized trial of low-dose versus high-dose intravenous cyclophosphamide. *Arthritis Rheum* 46: 2121–2131.

Jacobi AM, Diamond B (2005): Balancing diversity and tolerance: Lessons from patients with systemic lupus erythematosus. *J Exp Med* 202: 341–344.

Krishman S, Warke VG, Nambiar MP, Tsokos GC, Farber DL (2003): The FcR gamma subunit and Syk kinase replace CD3 zeta-chain and ZAP-70 in the TCR signaling complex of human effector CD4 T-cells. *J Immunol* 170: 4189–4194.

Kurien BT, Scofield RH (2006): Autoantibody determination in the diagnosis of systemic lupus erythematosus. *Scand J Immunol* 64: 227–235.

Takada K, Illei GG, Boumpas DT (2001): Cyclophosphamide for the treatment of systemic lupus erythematosus. *Lupus* 10: 154–161.

Tan EM, Cohen AS, Fries JF, Masi AT, McShane DJ, Rothfield NF, Schaller JG, Talal N, Winchester RJ (1982): The 1982 revised criteria for the classification of systemic lupus erythematosus. *Arthritis Rheum* 25: 1271–1277.

23

SCLERODERMA

ATSUSHI KITANI*

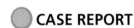 **CASE REPORT**

"In the last month I have noticed that my hands are puffy."

History and Initial Evaluation

You receive a call from a colleague, a primary care physician, asking if he can send his patient to see you, a rheumatologist, within the next few days. He briefly relates the patient's history and physical examination. Britney, a 42-year-old bank executive, came to see him with the complaint that in the last month her hands have become swollen, stiff, and mildly itchy. On physical examination he found that not only her fingers and hands but also her forearms and feet all exhibit some degree of swelling but that the swelling was firm and nonpitting (not depressible). He was starting the workup, but because he was confident that she had some form of connective tissue disease, he thought it advisable to involve you from the outset. You request some laboratory tests so that results will be ready when the patient arrives to see you.

At your first appointment with her, Britney relates the same set of complaints: Her hands are swollen, stiff, and

mildly itchy. When questioned about other limb symptoms, she recalls that about eight months ago, during the last winter season, she noticed that her fingers turned bluish white and became numb on exposure to cold air. Over the summer the same thing happened to the fingers she was using to hold a cold soft drink can. She has also had persistent aching pain in her wrists, ankles, and knees but has not noticed joint swelling.

Britney denies a history of headache, body/muscle pain or weakness, shortness of breath, swallowing difficulties, heartburn, or change in bowel habits. In addition, she denies any exposure to chemicals such as vinyl chloride, L-tryptophan, and organic solvents. She is not taking any medications except over-the-counter acetaminophen for occasional pain relief.

On physical examination you note that Britney has a generally healthy appearance and normal vital signs (her blood pressure is 120/70). She has a normal oral aperture and ability to protrude her tongue. Her heart and lungs are normal and her liver and spleen are not enlarged. However, examination of Britney's hands reveals diffuse, nonpitting swelling over her fingers and hands; in addition, the skin in these areas is shiny (exhibits *sclerodactyly*). Her forearms and feet also seem slightly swollen but her face is not swollen. Britney does not have digital pitting scars or *telangiectasia* (small dilated blood vessels near the skin surface).

*With contributions from Warren Strober and Susan R. S. Gottesman

---

Immunology: Clinical Case Studies and Disease Pathophysiology, By Warren Strober and Susan R. S. Gottesman
Copyright © 2009 John Wiley & Sons, Inc.

What are Britney's pertinent physical findings and history, and how does this direct your differential diagnosis and investigation?

*This history and physical examination suggest to you that Britney has early **scleroderma (Systemic sclerosis; SSc)**. The described reactions of her fingers on exposure to cold are known as **Raynaud's phenomenon**, a vascular perturbation that is often the initial symptom of the majority of patients with SSc. Typically, Raynaud's phenomenon consists of a well-demarcated triphasic color response occurring in one or more fingers; initially the finger(s) turn white (**pallor**) then blue (**cyanosis**) and, upon rewarming, red (**rubor**) (Fig. 23.1). These three distinct color phases, which may not be seen in all patients or with each episode, are brought on by cold exposure, vibration, or emotional stress. Pallor and/or cyanosis may be associated with coldness and numbness and rubor with throbbing pain. Raynaud's phenomenon is due to digital ischemia caused by abnormal regulation of local blood flow. In advanced cases of scleroderma it is associated with fixed structural abnormalities of the digital arteries and cutaneous arterioles such as intimal thickening and lumenal narrowing. Raynaud's phenomenon may also occur in other, nonautoimmune diseases in which blood flow to the digits is impaired upon exposure to cold. Most typically, it occurs in cold agglutinin disease (see Case 26); therefore, a plasma cell dyscrasia could be one of the differential diagnoses.*

The other prominent feature of Britney's history and physical examination is that the swelling of her extremities manifests as a nonpitting edema. Pitting edema, in which depression or indentation persists after pressure applied to the skin is released, can be caused by numerous systemic illnesses causing fluid accumulation, such as various types of heart, liver, and kidney diseases; however, in these cases the edema is most prevalent in dependent areas of the body, such as the feet and ankles. Localized edema may be caused by regional vascular problems. Nonpitting swelling raises the possibility of thyroid disease (myxedema), myositis

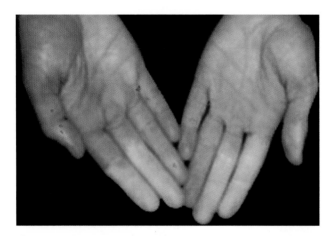

Figure 23.1. Raynaud's phenomenon. The white digits indicate the vasoconstriction of the digital arteries and the reduced blood flow to the fingers.

(inflammation of the muscles), and rare immune reactions to a variety of drugs and chemicals; the most prominent is a reaction to L-tryptophan.

The combination of Raynaud's phenomenon, the swollen fingers and hands, and the skin changes are strongly suggestive of the diagnosis of scleroderma; however, the other possibilities should be ruled out.

Britney gives you copies of her laboratory test results ordered by her primary care physician:

	Results	Reference Range
Complete blood count (CBC)		
Red blood cells (RBC)	$4.5 \times 10^6/\mu L$	$4.3 - 5.7 \times 10^6/\mu L$
Hematocrit (Hct)	35%	37–47%
White blood cells (WBC)	6800 /μL	4,500–11,000 /μL)
Differential count within reference limits		
Platelets (PLT)	425,000 /μL	150,000–450,000 /μL
Chemistries		
Blood urea nitrogen (BUN)	11 mg/dL	7–20 mg/dL
Creatinine	0.7 mg/dL	0.6–1.2 mg/dL
Protein	7.7 g/dL	6.0–8.0 g/dL
Albumin	4.0 g/dL	3.4–5.4 g/dL
Cholesterol	139 mg/dL	<200 mg/dL
Creatine kinase	130 U/L	30–135 U/L

Liver function tests: all within normal limits
Thyroid function tests: all within normal limits

Immunologic Parameters		
Complement component levels		
C3	108 mg/dL	85–175 mg/dL
C4	26 mg/dL	15–45 mg/dL
CH50[a]	194 U/ml	150–250 U/ml
Serum Immunoglobulin levels		
IgG	2420 mg/dL	640–1350 mg/dL
IgA	640 mg/dL	70–310 mg/dL
IgM	310 mg/dL	90–350 mg/dL
Antinuclear antibodies (ANA)	1:2560, speckled	<1:40

[a]Measurement of complement activity; see Case 8

The hand X-ray report is normal.

The above tests, combined with her physical examination, indicate normal cardiac, liver, and kidney function. They rule out a hematologic disease, plasma cell dyscrasia, and thyroid disease. The tests are positive for hypergammaglobulinemia (elevated immunoglobulin levels) and antinuclear antibody (ANA), consistent with one of the connective tissue autoimmune diseases, including scleroderma.

Of the connective tissue diseases, the history and physical examination is not supportive of systemic lupus erythematosus (SLE) or rheumatoid arthritis. The normal creatine kinase speaks against myositis (autoimmune diseases of muscle) and lack of elevated eosinophils rules out a drug reaction or eosinophilic fasciitis (see differential diagnosis section).

At this point you tell Britney that, pending further diagnostic studies, her condition is best classified as "undifferentiated connective tissue disease" with features of scleroderma. You explain that scleroderma is quite variable in its severity and she might have a mild case. Finally, you indicate she will require a number of blood tests and other procedures to establish the diagnosis and a baseline for possible visceral organ involvement. Meanwhile you prescribe celecoxib [a type of nonsteroidal anti-inflammatory drug (NSAID)] for her arthralgia and hydrocolloid duo-DERM for pruritis (itching). You advise her to dress warmly both on trunk and extremities in the coming cold season and to avoid smoking since the latter can cause vasocontriction and thus can precipitate a Raynaud's attack.

You have blood drawn for additional laboratory tests, including autoimmune serologies, and arrange for a chest X ray, pulmonary function tests, and a skin biopsy. You ask Britney to return in one week to see how she is faring on the medication.

Further Diagnostic Workup and Evaluation of Disease Activity

If scleroderma is strongly suspected at an early stage, as in Britney's case, what additional tests should be performed?

Basically, two types of studies need to be done, one to establish the diagnosis and another to determine the extent of disease and establish a baseline of disease activity. For diagnosis it is essential to obtain: (1) serologic studies to detect the presence of antibodies associated with scleroderma and for establishing the type of scleroderma present: anti-topoisomerase I (Scl-70), anti-centromere, anti-U1 RNP; and (2) a skin biopsy to detect the presence of skin fibrosis. In addition, nail-fold capillary microscopy can be performed. This consists of surface microscopy of the nail folds to detect the presence of vessel dilatation and areas of avascularity ("drop-out" areas).

To determine the extent of disease and to establish a baseline, the following tests are performed: (1) chest X ray to detect the presence of pulmonary fibrosis (basilar fibrosis is common); (2) pulmonary function tests including diffusion capacity of carbon monoxide; (3) hand X rays to rule out joint inflammation and to detect the presence of bone calcinosis (excess bone density); (4) electrocardiography and echocardiography to detect cardiac conduction defects and arrhythmia, pericardial disease, and cor pulmonale (right heart failure); and (5) barium swallow and cine-esophagograms to detect the presence of esophageal dysmotility. These latter tests can be performed over a period of several months to minimize disruption of the patient's schedule.

One week later, Britney returns to your office. She reports she has not had Raynaud's phenomenon episodes, possibly because she has taken your advice to avoid the cold.

The chest X-ray report is normal; there is no major lung fibrosis, no evidence of basilar fibrosis (sometimes seen in early scleroderma), and no evidence of arthritis. Bone density is normal. Additional studies of pulmonary function and skin biopsy are to be performed over the next few weeks.

Two weeks later, Britney returns to your office for further update of her workup. Pulmonary function tests show that her vital capacity (VC) is 85.8% of predicted normal value; relation of forced one-second expiratory volume to forced vital capacity (FEV1/FVC) is 88.7% (normal >80%); CO diffusion capacity (DL_{CO}) is 9.36 mL/min/mm Hg (normal 9–11); and (DL_{CO}/VA) is 61.9% (normal range <70%). These results indicate that Britney has a slight decrease in her diffusion capacity but has otherwise normal pulmonary function.

The autoantibody profile provides the following results:

Autoantibody Specificity	Result	Reference Range
Anti-Scl70/topoisomerase I	172 U	<24 U
Anti-centromere	5.0 U	<10 U
Anti-RNP	5.0 U	<15 U
Anti-SS-A/Ra	9.2 U	<10 U
Anti-SS-B/Lo	9.4 U	<10 U
Anti-DNA	10 IU/ml	<10 IU/ml

Indirect fluorescence staining of the HEp2 cell line with patient serum shows a speckled and nucleolar pattern (Fig. 23.2). (See Case 22 for autoantibody description and testing.)

What is the clinical significance of a positive Scl70 (topoisomerase I) antibody value as well as the meaning of the other serologies?

Listed in Table 23.1 are the various types of autoantibodies detected in scleroderma patients as well as the types of scleroderma with which they are associated (as discussed in detail below, scleroderma occurs in "limited" and "diffuse" forms). The antinuclear antibody is found in a wide variety of diffuse autoimmune disorders, but most of the other antibodies listed are specific for SSc. The exception is anti-PM/Scl, which is found in both SSc and myositis as well as in patients with overlap syndrome, which has features of both. As indicated, anti-topoisomerase (Scl70) is detected in only 25–40% of the diffuse type of SSc. Although these antibodies have specificity for SSc, it is apparent from this table that they each tend to occur in a limited number of patients.

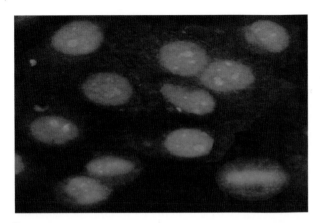

Figure 23.2. Indirect fluorescence staining of HEp2 cells with patient serum demonstrating anti-Scl-70 antibody positivity by fluorescence microscopy.

Antinuclear antibodies are detected by the staining of cultured laryngeal carcinoma cell line, HEp2 cells. Anti-topoisomerase I is associated with a mixed staining pattern. The latter consists of homogeneous staining (positive staining of chromosomes in mitosis), speckled staining (fine speckling of the interphase cells), and nucleolar staining (staining of the nucleoli of most cells). Anti-RNA polymerase III, anti-U3 RNP (fibrillin), anti-Th/To-RNP and anti-PM/Scl give antinucleolar patterns. These autoantibodies are more qualitatively and quantitatively assessed by application of Western blotting and enzyme-linked immunosorbent assay (ELISA) techniques (see unit V for detailed description of assays).

It should be noted that some of the SSc-specific autoantibodies are mutually exclusive: In one study anti-topoisomerase I and anti-centromere antibodies occurred together in only 0.52% of 5423 patients. The anti-Th/To antibodies identify a novel subset of SSc patients who have limited disease (see definition below), exhibit lung disease and renal crisis, and have a higher mortality rate than patients with anti-centromere antibodies. The association of these autoantibodies with particular clinical features of SSc suggests that (1) these clinical

features are associated with the generation of unique auto-antigen determinants, increases in autoantigen expression level, or changes in autoantigen subcellular localization or (2) these different autoantibodies have direct pathogenic effects that lead to particular patterns of tissue damage.

Definitive Diagnosis and Treatment Plan

The pathology report of Britney's skin biopsy states that the biopsied skin displays a thin epidermis, thickened bundles of collagen in the reticular dermis, and mild perivascular inflammatory infiltrates surrounding dermal blood vessels. These changes are fully consistent with and support the diagnosis of scleroderma.

This skin biopsy result, when added to the history of sclerotic skin changes, followed within one year by the onset of episodes of Raynaud's phenomena, reduced diffusion capacity in pulmonary function test, and positive anti-topoisomerase I antibody serology, tips the balance strongly in favor of a diagnosis of SSc. As shown in Table 23.2, scleroderma occurs as a limited or diffuse disease. On the basis of Britney's data, it appears that she falls into the diffuse disease category. You discuss this diagnosis with Britney and recommend that she enter the hospital to initiate pulse therapy with cyclophosphamide, an immunosuppressive agent.

Although no drug or treatment has currently proved effective in altering disease course in diffuse SSc, recent reports suggest that oral or intravenous cyclophosphamide plus prednisolone therapy tends to prevent the development of fibrosis and its complications in the early stages of this disease. You therefore treat Britney with cyclophosphamide (CYC) given as a 500-mg intravenous pulse. You plan to administer similar pulses at weeks 1 and 2 followed by monthly pulses for six months (to be repeated during each winter season). To reduce bladder toxicity, you administer mesna (to neutralize the urotoxic metabolites of cyclophosphamide, thus protecting the bladder) and provide adequate hydration. You also start Britney on prednisolone (a corticosteroid), 25 mg/day, planning to taper this dose by 5 mg every month. You also prescribe a sustained-release form of

TABLE 23.1. Autoantibody Profile of SSc

Autoantibody	Dominant Subsets[a]	Clinical Association
Antinuclear antibody	Diffuse and limited (>90% in both)	Nonspecific, numerous autoimmune diseases
Anti-topoisomerase I (Scl 70)	Diffuse (25–40%)	Pulmonary fibrosis, cardiac involvement
Anti-RNA polymerase III	Diffuse (25%)	Severe skin involvement, renal crisis
Anti-U3-RNP (fibrillarin)	Diffuse and limited (<10%)	Pulmonary hypertension, cardiac and muscle involvement
Anti-centromere	Limited (50–90%)	CREST syndrome
Anti-Th/To-RNP	Limited (15%)	Lung disease, renal crisis, small bowel involvement
Anti-PM/Scl	Overlap	Myositis

[a]Approximate percentages in dominant subsets.

TABLE 23.2. Features of Limited and Diffuse Scleroderma

Limited Scleroderma:	
Skin involvement	On distal limbs to elbows and knees and on face (95%)
Raynaud's phenomenon	Precedes skin disease by a year or longer (95%)
CREST syndrome	**C**alcinosis (45%), **R**aynaud's phenomenon, **E**sophageal hypomotility, **S**clerodactyly, **T**elangiectasia (80%)
Visceral involvement	Nonprogressive gastrointestinal, pulmonary fibrosis (35%), isolated pulmonary hypertension after 10–15 years (12%)
Prognosis	Good, except when associated with pulmonary hypertension; 5-year survival $\sim$ 90%, 10-year survival $\sim$ 75%
Diffuse Scleroderma:	
Skin involvement	Widespread, distal and proximal extremities, face, trunk (100%)
Raynaud's phenomenon	Onset within 1 year or at time of skin changes (90–95%)
Visceral involvement	Pulmonary fibrosis, can be progressive (35–59%); renal hypertensive crisis (15%); gastrointestinal, cardiac involvement, progressive
Prognosis	Poor: 5-year survival $\sim$ 70%, 10-year survival $\sim$ 55%

the calcium channel blocker nifedipine to reduce the occurrence of Raynaud's phenomenon. If this proves ineffective, you plan to try an angiotensin II antagonist (losartan) or a serotonin antagonist (ketanserin).

Britney's clinical course can be monitored by pulmonary function tests or, more conveniently, by following markers of pulmonary function, KL-6, and/or surfactant protein A and D levels. KL-6 is a mucin-like high-molecular-weight glycoprotein produced by alveolar type II pneumocytes and bronchiolar epithelial cells; surfactant proteins A and D (SP-A and SP-D) belong to the collectin subgroup of the C-type lectin superfamily and are produced by alveolar type II cells and Clara cells. These components are produced in excess in patients with scleroderma involving the lung. When Britney starts CYC treatment, her KL-6 level is 514 IU/ml (normal range <500 IU/ml), but this level decreases to below 200 IU/ml after six months on the CYC regimen in the winter season.

Differential Diagnosis of Scleroderma

The early symptoms of SSc—arthralgia, myalgia, Raynaud's phenomenon, and puffy hands—are common in other rheumatic diseases, such as SLE, polymyositis, rheumatoid arthritis, and mixed connective tissue disease. SLE can be distinguished from SSc by their differing autoantibody patterns (anti-double-stranded DNA in SLE, anti-Scl70 in SSc). In addition, SLE is associated with a characteristic facial skin rash (butterfly rash) and lack of sclerodermatous skin changes. Rheumatoid arthritis can be distinguished from SSc by its joint changes and characteristic serology (rheumatoid factor). Myositis and mixed connective tissue disease can be difficult to

distinguish from SSc during their early stages. However, even early on they can be distinguished from SSc by elevated serum levels of creatine phosphokinase (CPK) and aldolase arising from muscle damage.

Several other diseases are sometimes confused with SSc because they present with scleroderma-like skin features. One is **scleredema**, a condition characterized by edematous induration of the trunk, face, shoulders, and proximal extremities. However, scleredema occurs mainly in children, possibly following streptococcus infection, and resolves within a year. Eosinophilic fasciitis may also mimic SSc; it is characterized by eosinophilic and monocytic inflammation of the muscle fascia (lining around muscles) and circulating eosinophilia that is sometimes precipitated by strenuous physical exertion. Patients with eosinophilic fasciitis exhibit first diffuse swelling, stiffness, and tenderness of the arms and legs followed by induration of the skin and subcutaneous tissues. However, these patients are not subject to Raynaud's phenomena or visceral involvement. Finally, skin thickening of the fingers and hands also appears in association with type 2 diabetes mellitus, mycosis fungoides (a T-cell malignancy localizing to the skin), **amyloidosis** (a condition in which abnormal proteins called amyloid are deposited in various organs and tissues throughout the body), and scleromyxedema.

CLINICAL FEATURES OF LIMITED AND DIFFUSE SCLERODERMA

As mentioned above, SSc has two main clinical patterns, a "limited" pattern and a "diffuse" pattern. As shown in

Table 23.2, these patterns define relatively mild and relatively severe forms of SSc that appear to be due to two highly related, yet distinct pathologic processes associated with somewhat different patterns of autoantibody generation. In limited SSc, the skin manifestations are associated with a low (and late) incidence of visceral disease; the exception to this rule is the frequent occurrence of esophageal problems and the late occurrence of pulmonary hypertension. In contrast, in diffuse SSc the skin manifestations are associated with multiorgan visceral involvement early in the course of the disease. Another distinction between the two forms of scleroderma is that Raynaud's phenomenon tends to precede the skin disease by a considerable length of time in the limited disease but appears at the same time as the skin manifestations in the diffuse disease.

Recently, a third subset of patients with SSc has been identified. This category consists of patients with Raynaud's phenomena, nailfold capillary changes, and characteristic SSc-associated antibodies but no skin changes. Such patients may or may not later develop one of the forms of SSc described above.

The cutaneous manifestations of SSc begin with an edematous phase that progresses in stages to increasingly firm, thickened, and eventually indurated (hardened) skin; concomitantly, the skin becomes deeply pigmented. In patients with diffuse scleroderma, these skin changes become generalized, involving both distal and proximal extremities, followed in several years by involvement of the face and trunk. Tendon friction rubs, sclerodactyly, and digital pitting scars are frequently observed. Raynaud's phenomenon occurs in 95% of cases of both limited and diffuse SSc. Arthralgia or arthritis is present in more than half of scleroderma patients.

Approximately 90% of patients with both the limited and diffuse forms of SSc have symptoms of esophageal disease. Symptoms consist of heartburn, regurgitation, or dysphagia caused by the reduced tone of the gastroesophageal sphincter or by dilatation or dysmotility of the distal esophagus. In some patients dysmotility of the small and large bowel also occur; affected patients commonly complain of bloating, abdominal distension, and pain. Diminished peristalsis associated with dysmotility leads to bacterial overgrowth and can result in chronic diarrhea and malabsorption.

Pulmonary involvement occurs in at least two-thirds of SSc patients and is now the leading cause of mortality in this disease. The most common symptom of this complication is exertional dyspnea, often accompanied by a nonproductive cough. Lung injury is caused by two processes: (1) fibrosing alveolitis or (2) obliterative vasculopathy of the medium and small pulmonary vessels. Both interstitial fibrosis and pulmonary vascular disease are present to some degree in most patients; however, interstitial lung disease is more prominent in patients with diffuse SSc. Chest X ray and high-resolution computerized tomography (CT) scans demonstrate interstitial fibrosis predominantly of the lower lobes.

Cardiac features include pericarditis, heart failure, and varying degrees of conduction block; in addition, arrhythmias are observed in a minority (<10%) of patients with diffuse SSc.

Significant renal disease occurs in 10% of patients with diffuse SSc. Renal involvement is often associated with hypertension and mild to moderate proteinuria. Renal crisis mimics malignant hypertension caused by the activation of the renin–angiotensin system and can rapidly progress to renal failure.

PATHOPHYSIOLOGY OF SCLERODERMA

Genetic and Environmental Factors in SSc Pathogenesis

Although the concordance of SSc in monozygotic twins is low, the presence of genetic factors in this disease is indicated by the occurrence of clusters of familial cases and the presence of SSc-related autoantibodies in unaffected family members. This supposition has more recently been supported by the discovery that a single nucleotide polymorphism (SNP) in fibrillin-1 protein is strongly associated with SSc in a Native American tribe with a high prevalence of this disease. Fibrillin-1 is an extracellular matrix (ECM) protein that affects the activity of transforming growth factor (TGF)-β_1, a cytokine intimately linked to SSc pathogenesis (see further discussion below). In addition, SNPs in other molecules associated with the disease process have been found. While these findings provide solid evidence that genetic factors are involved in SSc pathogenesis, much more work is needed to define precisely how they contribute to disease susceptibility.

Environmental factors can also trigger the onset of scleroderma. Infection with cytomegalovirus has been proposed as a triggering event since scleroderma patients frequently manifest cytomegalovirus antibodies and viral proteins, which cross-react with proteins found on the surface of fibroblasts. Thus, SSc may be subject to autoantibody formation due to *molecular mimicry*; the body's response to the infectious agent subsequently causes an autoimmune response to a self-antigen (see Case 15 and introduction to this unit).

Immunopathology of SSc

The Role of T Cells and T_H2 Cytokines in SSc.
SSc is fundamentally an autoimmune state; its most distinctive feature is the presence of T cells and B cells that induce abnormalities of fibroblast collagen production and vascular injury. Thus, with respect to fibroblast function, it

has been shown that early SSc skin lesions are characterized by the presence of an inflammatory cell infiltrate adjacent to fibroblasts actively producing collagen. It is likely that cells within the infiltrate, particularly T cells, are driving this fibroblast activity. This view is supported by the fact that the T-cell populations present in such infiltrates have been shown to be oligoclonal (consisting of a limited number of clones of different specificities) and thus likely to be responding to a limited number of self-antigens. In addition, these T cells are predominantly CD4$^+$ T helper 2 (T$_H$2) T cells producing IL-4 and other T$_H$2 cytokines, that is, cytokines that have been implicated in the induction of factors that stimulate collagen production. (See Case 15 for a discussion of T$_H$ subsets.) Finally, it should be noted that B cells are also found in the inflammatory infiltrates associated with SSc lesions and that autoantibodies produced by such B cells have been shown to play a role in the excess fibroblast activity characterizing SSc (see further discussion below).

The Role of TGF-β_1 in SSc. The important pathologic link between T cells and SSc is implicit in the relation of T$_H$2 cytokines to collagen production. The inflammation-induced fibrosis has been shown to be a two-stage process. The first stage is the induction of IL-13Rα2 on the surface of macrophages. This occurs by the signaling of either IL-4 or IL-13 through IL-13Rα1 in conjunction with tumor necrosis factor (TNF) α, which signals through its own receptor (Fig. 23.3). In the second stage, IL-13 signals through the newly expressed IL-13Rα2 on the macrophages to induce the production of a central profibrotic factor, TGF-β_1, that then induces a number of downstream factors that are the proximal stimulators of collagen production. In particular, TGF-β_1 induces IGF-1 (insulin-like growth factor 1) and Egr-1 (early growth response 1) production; these three factors act together to stimulate fibroblasts to produce collagen. In SSc, TGF-β_1 is thought to induce connective tissue growth factor, which also plays a role in the fibrotic process.

The importance of TGF-β_1 production in the pathology of SSc is underscored by the fact that in several murine models TGF-β_1 signaling can be shown to play a key role in

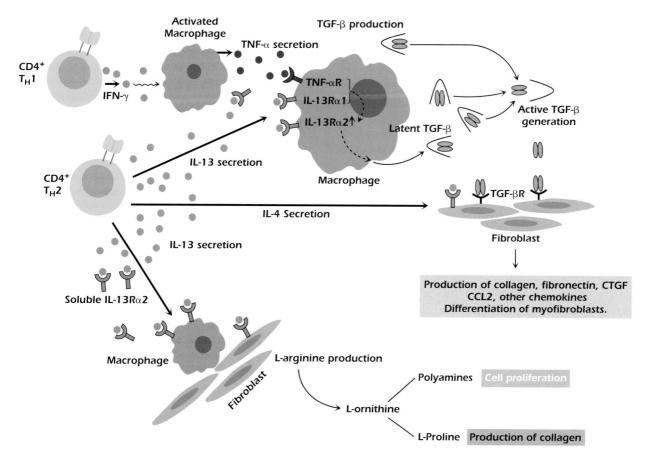

Figure 23.3. Roles of IL-13 and TGF-β in macrophage and fibroblast activation. The combination of TNF-α and IL-13 induces IL-13Rα2 expression and the IL-13 signals via this receptor to induce TGF-β. TGF-β promotes fibroblasts to produce collagen, fibronectin, and connective tissue growth factor (CTGF) and to differentiate into myofibroblasts. Fibroblasts also produce L-arginine that promotes their proliferation and collagen production.

dermal fibrosis. In one such model, scleroderma-like dermal fibrosis and abnormalities of ECM deposition are associated with the presence of fibroblasts bearing a constitutively active TGF-β_1 receptor. In addition, the scleroderma-like disease occurring in the tight-skinned mouse (Tsk-1 mouse) is associated with a genetic abnormality of the ECM-related protein called fibrillin. The fibrillin protein might influence TGF-β_1 function because it contains a domain similar to a protein that binds to latent TGF-β_1. It has been shown that such mice are less likely to develop fibrosis if they lack the ability to express the IL-4 receptor because IL-4 is one of the cytokine products characteristic of T_H2 cells. This latter piece of evidence in the mouse model supports the supposition that T_H2 and T_H2 cytokines are pivotal in triggering the human disease.

The Role of B Cells and Autoantibodies in SSc.

Autoantibodies present in SSc also play a role in the fibrotic process characterizing this disease. Indirect supporting evidence comes from the observation that the different clinical forms of SSc are associated with specific autoantibody patterns; this suggests that the antibodies determine some of the clinical manifestations. The titer of the autoantibody anti-Scl 70 (anti-topoisomerase) correlates with the clinical severity of SSc, and its epitopes correlate with the clinical manifestations. Anti-Scl 70 may form antigen–antibody complexes that then interact with tissue macrophages via Fc receptors; the macrophages in turn may release profibrotic factors such as TGF-β_1. Other autoantibodies associated with SSc that could play a role in the pathologic process include anti–matrix metalloprotease 1 (MMP-1) and anti-MMP-3, anti-fibrillin-1, anti-fibroblast antibody, and anti–platelet-derived growth factor (PDGF) receptor. These have been postulated to react with ECM proteins, the fibroblasts themselves, and platelets to either directly or indirectly propagate the fibrotic process (see also Case 21).

Intrinsic abnormalities of the B cells themselves have been identified in SSc, including B-cell hyperreactivity and overexpression of CD19, a B-cell-signaling molecule. This correlates with the fact that an important B-cell activation factor known as BAFF (B-cell activation factor of the TNF family) has been shown to be elevated in SSc and the extent of elevation correlates with the severity of the skin fibrosis.

The possible mechanism of autoantibody production and the roles of autoantibodies in the pathogenesis of SSc are summarized in Figure 23.4. The generation of antibodies to intracellular molecules suggests the possibility of stimulation by apoptotic cellular debris. This would be similar to mechanisms discussed in SLE (see Case 22).

The above findings suggest that B cells and B-cell products (such as autoantibodies) play a larger role in the pathogenesis of SSc than previously thought. However, it still remains possible that these abnormalities, while contributing to the pathologic process, are secondary to the T-cell abnormality and the pathologic role of TGF-β_1.

Effector Mechanisms in SSc

The Role of Fibroblasts.

Fibroblasts in SSc are not only the cellular source of the collagen that causes the characteristic fibrotic lesions but also the source of various chemokines that play an important role in the fibrotic reaction (Fig 23.3). One such chemokine is monocyte chemotactic protein (MCP) 1 [also known as chemokine (C–C motif) 2 (CCL2)] produced by SSc fibroblasts. This chemokine stimulates the production of collagen and MMP-1, a protein that regulates ECM turnover. In addition, CCL2 signaling via its receptor, CCR2, acts on myofibroblasts to induce their differentiation into collagen-producing fibroblasts. Finally, IL-4 triggers CCL2 production, which in turn may facilitate T_H2 T-cell differentiation; thus, CCL2 amplifies the T_H2-induced fibrotic process via TGF-β_1, as described above. Because many other chemokines have been detected in human SSc lesions, it is likely that these factors also contribute to the development of the SSc lesion.

Vascular Injury in SSc.

Vascular injury (such as Raynaud's phenomenon) is an early clinical feature of diffuse SSc and reflects a poorly understood disease-induced imbalance between vasoconstriction-controlling factors such as endothelins and vasodilatation-controlling factors such as nitric oxide (NO) and prostacyclin. Whatever the cause, the imbalance leads to tissue oxygen deprivation and a host of downstream events that mediate tissue injury, leukocyte infiltration, and thrombosis. One such event is increased microvascular permeability and subsequent exposure of platelets in the blood to tissue proteins; this leads to thrombosis as well as the release of PDGF, a factor that participates in the recruitment of fibroblasts and their differentiation into collagen-producing myofibroblasts. In this way, vascular injury is an important contributor to tissue fibrosis.

TREATMENT OF SCLERODERMA

It is not yet possible to treat SSc with agents that attack its underlying abnormalities and ameliorate the disease in its totality. However, varying success has been achieved with treatment directed toward specific manifestations of the disease. The most "global" type of therapy has consisted of immunosuppression with cyclophosphamide, a treatment reserved for patients with diffuse disease affecting vital organs. This approach, which obviously assumes that the disease is propagated primarily by an immune defect rather than a fibroblast defect, has been of proven value in SSc involving the lung. In current ongoing studies, high doses of cyclophosphamide are given in conjunction with other immunosuppressive approaches (anti–thymocyte globulin and gamma radiation followed by hematopoietic rescue by infusion of autologous stem cells). Other, more limited

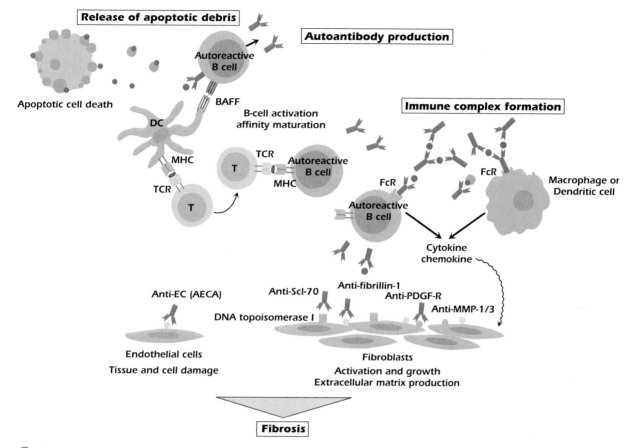

Figure 23.4. Potential roles of autoantibodies in SSc. Though the mechanism of autoantibody production is still unclear, it is suggested that cells undergoing apoptosis release debris that contain molecules which serve as autoantigens. Autoantibody production that ensues is likely similar in manner to that for foreign antigen. Immune complex formation then occurs with autoantigens and autoantibodies and these complexes bind to Fc receptors on macrophages or other cells to induce cytokine and chemokine production. DNA topoisomerase I is found to bind the surface of fibroblasts and then further binding of anti-Scl 70 to topoisomerase I induces fibroblast activation. Other autoantibodies also contribute to fibroblast activation and growth, ECM production, and vascular injury.

types of therapy aimed at specific aspects of SSc are listed below:

- **Skin Sclerosis.** A variety of agents including intravenous immunoglobulin administration, treatment with anti-B-cell monoclonal antibodies (anti-CD20), and TGF-β_1 inhibitors have been used.

- **Skin Ulcers.** This manifestation of the disease is the result of vascular abnormalities and has been treated with sildenafil (a vasodilator), endothelin receptor antagonists such as bosentan, and agents that stimulate fibroblast growth factor receptors to induce capillary-rich granulation tissue.

- **Lung.** After careful staging of the extent of pulmonary disease (alveolitis and interstitial fibrosis) and therefore the acquisition of markers of disease activity, this manifestation is usually treated with cyclophosphamide as indicated above. A recent double-blind study reported

definite, albeit modest improvement with this therapy. Pulmonary hypertension associated with lung problems has been treated with bosentan.

- **Fibrosis.** An impressive number of experimental antifibrotic therapies are currently being tested or will be tested in the near future based on our increasing knowledge of the pathogenesis of SSc. One such therapy of great theoretical promise is anti-TGF-β, since this molecule appears so central to the SSc pathologic process. Unfortunately, however, a recently reported multicenter, randomized, placebo-controlled phase I/II trial of recombinant human anti-TGF-β antibody therapy showed no evidence of efficacy in SSc. Other therapies that could be considered include recombinant soluble (decoy) IL-13α2 receptor, soluble type II TGF-β receptor, IL-10 (a cytokine that directly suppresses collagen synthesis in fibroblasts and has been found to be an effective treatment for liver fibrosis), endothelin-1 antagonist (bosentan), inhibitors for arginase-1, and matrix metalloproteases. Finally, anti-TNF-α agents such as eternacept are currently being tested since these agents have proven anti-inflammatory activity and may also act in SSc via their ability to inhibit IL-13α2 receptor-mediated signaling.

REFERENCES

Denton CP, Black CM, Abraham DJ (2006): Mechanisms and consequences of fibrosis in systemic sclerosis. *Natl Clin Pract Rheumatol* 2:134–144.

Denton CP, Merkel PA, Furst DE, Khanna D, Emery P, Hsu VM, Silliman N, Streisand J, Powell J, Akesson A, Coppock J, Hoogen F, Herrick A, Mayes MD, Veale D, Haas J, Ledbetter S, Korn JH, Black CM, Seibold JR, Cat-192 Study Group, Scleroderma Clinical Trials Consortium (2007): Recombinant human anti-transforming growth factor beta1 antibody therapy in systemic sclerosis: A multicenter, randomized, placebo-controlled phase I/II trial of CAT-192. *Arthritis Rheum* 56:323–333.

Fichtner-Feigl S, Strober W, Kawakami K, Puri RK, Kitani A (2006): IL-13 signaling through the IL-13alpha2 receptor is involved in induction of TGF-beta1 production and fibrosis. *Nat Med* 12:99–106.

Hasegawa M, Fujimoto M, Kikuchi K, Takehara K (1997a): Elevated serum levels of interleukin 4 (IL-4), IL-10, and IL-13 in patients with systemic sclerosis. *J Rheumatol* 24:328–332.

Hasegawa M, Fujimoto M, Kikuchi K, Takehara K (1997b): Elevated serum tumor necrosis factor-alpha levels in patients with systemic sclerosis: Association with pulmonary fibrosis. *J Rheumatol* 24:663–665.

Henness S, Wigley FM (2007): Current drug therapy for scleroderma and secondary Raynaud's phenomenon: Evidence-based review. *Curr Opin Rheumatol* 19:611–618.

Scala E, Pallotta S, Frezzolini A, Abeni D, Barbieri C, Sampogna F, De Pità O, Puddu P, Paganelli R, Russo G (2004): Cytokine and chemokine levels in systemic sclerosis: Relationship with cutaneous and internal organ involvement. *Clin Exp Immunol* 138:540–546.

Stephanie Gu Y, Kong J, Cheema GS, Keen CL, Wick G, Gershwin ME (2008): The immunobiology of systemic sclerosis. *Semin Arthritis Rheum*, in press.

Walker JG, Fritzler MJ (2007): Update on autoantibodies in systemic sclerosis. *Curr Opin Rheumatol* 19:580–591.

Wynn TA (2004): Fibrotic disease and the T(H)1/T(H)2 paradigm. *Nat Rev Immunol* 4:583–594.

Yanaba K, Hasegawa M, Takehara K, Sato S (2004): Comparative study of serum surfactant protein-D and KL-6 concentrations in patients with systemic sclerosis as markers for monitoring the activity of pulmonary fibrosis. *J Rheumatol* 31:1112–1120.

Unit IV

MALIGNANCIES OF THE LYMPHOID SYSTEM

INTRODUCTION: CLASSIFICATION OF LYMPHOID MALIGNANCIES

SUSAN R. S. GOTTESMAN

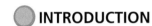

INTRODUCTION

The chapters in this unit are a sampling of lymphoid neoplasms. You might question why a detailed description of these diseases should go into a book on immunologic disorders. The first reason is that knowledge of immunology brings insights to the understanding of lymphoid neoplasms; conversely, knowledge of lymphoid neoplasms brings insights to the understanding of immunology. In recent years our steadily expanding knowledge of the immune system has allowed us to create a much more rational system of classifying neoplasias involving lymphoid cells. Thus, instead of relying only on the histology of lymphoid malignancies, we can now utilize the vast array of cellular markers and cellular products to define more precisely the type of cell that expands in the various lymphoid malignancies and we can use that information to better understand the behavior of these cell types in their guise as malignant cells. At the same time, the study of lymphoid malignancies has reflected back on our understanding of the development of normal lymphoid cells. In particular, the study of malignant cells has allowed us to derive hypotheses about the factors that control the normal immune response. For example, in the study of lymphoid neoplasms of the B-cell lineage, the various B-cell malignancies can be related directly to the differentiation and activation sequence of normal B cells. In addition, the identification of some of the molecular abnormalities involved in the malignant transformation of specific subtypes has provided us with a window through which we can view the genetic underpinnings of the immune response.

A second reason that an understanding of lymphoid neoplasms is important to immunology concerns the relationship between the normal immune response and the development of malignancy. We know that the incidence of lymphoid malignancies increases with any perturbation of the immune system, whether immunodeficiency or chronic antigenic stimulation by an exogenous or autoimmune stimulus. The association of neoplasia with immunodeficiency disease is hypothesized to be due to the lack of immune surveillance of aberrant cells and/or perhaps more accurately of cells transformed by oncogenic viruses, since many of the neoplasms presenting in the setting of immunodeficiency are virus associated. The increased incidence of neoplasia in the setting of chronic inflammation may result from increased cell proliferation (epithelial cells as well as lymphoid cells) and, particularly when the stimulation is of limited antigenic diversity, the tendency of the immune cells (especially B cells) to introduce errors into their genome in their normal process of refining their immune response.

Immunology: Clinical Case Studies and Disease Pathophysiology, By Warren Strober and Susan R. S. Gottesman
Copyright © 2009 John Wiley & Sons, Inc.

Thus, the normal immune response provides a detailed framework or platform upon which we can construct a better understanding of the series of cellular events that lead to neoplastic transformation.

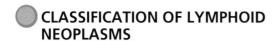

CLASSIFICATION OF LYMPHOID NEOPLASMS

Lymphoid neoplasms are categorized by (1) the specific cell type that is malignant and the stage of differentiation in which it is frozen or which accumulates (both of these often relating directly to a normal cell counterpart), (2) a genetic mutation if specific for that malignancy, and (3) clinical features of the disease or the neoplasm's pattern of organ involvement. This classification system, recommended by the World Health Organization (WHO) in 1996, reflects our greater understanding of the immune system and improved ability to specifically treat subtypes of this disease. Previous classification schemes were based primarily on either morphology of the malignant cell without regard to lineage or the clinical course of the disease. A condensed version of the WHO classification is as follows:

> B-cell neoplasms
>> Precursor B cell
>> Peripheral or Mature B cell
> T/Natural Killer (NK) cell neoplasms
>> Precursor T cell
>> Peripheral or Mature T/NK cell
> Hodgkin lymphoma

There are in fact almost 30 different kinds of lymphoid neoplasms; for an expanded list, see Table UIV.1.

In the WHO classification, the terms *leukemia* and *lymphoma* are often combined (leukemia/lymphoma) and attached to a single malignant designation. These terms denote clinical presentation: Leukemia presents with peripheral blood and/or bone marrow involvement, whereas lymphoma presents with a mass, either in lymphoid tissues such as lymph nodes or spleen or at extranodal sites. For some neoplasms, both presentations are common, so the distinction is artificial rather than biological. Because the WHO classification and recommended treatment are based on the malignant cell type rather than the presentation, leukemia/lymphoma designations are not separately indicated when diagnosing the disease. Only those neoplasms in which the vast majority of patients present with a circulating (leukemia) or solid (lymphoma) phase are these indicated as a leukemia or lymphoma.

A second notable feature of this classification scheme is that, whereas the mature B-cell neoplasms are divided into the malignant counterparts of the B-cell subsets discussed in preceding chapters such as follicular center B cells and

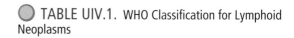

TABLE UIV.1. WHO Classification for Lymphoid Neoplasms

B-Cell Neoplasms

Precursor B lymphoblastic leukemia/lymphoma

  B lymphoblastic leukemia/lymphoma, NOS[a]

  B lymphoblastic with recurrent genetic abnormalities (7 types)

Mature B-cell neoplasms

  Chronic lymphocytic leukemia/small lymphocytic lymphoma

  B-cell prolymphocytic leukemia

  Follicular lymphoma

  Mantle cell lymphoma

  Extranodal marginal zone lymphoma of mucosa-associated lymphoid tissue (MALT) type

  Nodal marginal zone lymphoma

  Splenic marginal zone lymphoma

  Hairy cell leukemia

  Diffuse large B-cell lymphoma and subtypes: mediastinal, primary effusion, intravascular, HHV8-assoc., etc.

  Burkitt lymphoma

  Plasma cell myeloma/plasmacytoma

  Heavy chain diseases

  Lymphoplasmacytic lymphoma

  Lymphomatoid granulomatosis

  Posttransplant lymphoproliferative disorders

T/NK-Cell Neoplasms

Precursor T lymphoblastic leukemia/lymphoma

Mature T/NK-cell neoplasms (selected)

  T-cell prolymphocytic leukemia

  T-cell large granular lymphocytic leukemia

  NK cell leukemia

  Peripheral T-cell lymphoma (unspecified)

  Mycosis fungoides

  Sezary syndrome

  Primary cutaneous CD30[+] T-cell lymphoproliferative disorder

  Anaplastic large cell lymphoma, *ALK* positive

  Extranodal NK/T cell lymphoma, nasal type

  Enteropathy-associated T-cell lymphoma

  Hepatosplenic T-cell lymphoma

  Adult T-cell leukemia/lymphoma

  Angioimmunoblastic T-cell lymphoma

Hodgkin Lymphoma

Nodular lymphocyte predominant Hodgkin lymphoma

Classical Hodgkin lymphoma

  Nodular sclerosis

  Mixed cellularity

  Lymphocyte-rich

  Lymphocyte-depleted

---

[a]NOS: not otherwise specified

plasma cells, the T-cell malignancies are more often named by location or clinical presentation and have neither been divided into the T-cell subsets (beyond sometimes CD4 vs. CD8 cells) nor related to their products such as their distinct cytokine profiles. In addition, few T-cell malignancies have defined genetic abnormalities. Overall, we still rely on their clinical presentations to distinguish among the T-cell neoplasms; however, we can expect the classification of T-cell malignancies to undergo changes in the near future.

A designation that is often puzzling to the student is Hodgkin lymphoma. The malignant cell, the Reed–Sternberg cell or variant, is actually a B cell gone awry somewhere within, or when just emerging from, the germinal center. For many decades the lineage of this cell eluded investigators. For one thing, being morphologically bizarre, it resembles no normal cell and it does not express lineage-specific markers. Its isolation is difficult since there are usually few malignant cells in the involved lymph node comprised of numerous reactive cells. Microdissection of the malignant cells followed by DNA amplification techniques and analysis was required to finally classify the Reed–Sternberg cell as a B cell. However, since physicians have been successfully treating this malignancy for about 40 years, it is counterproductive to suddenly group Hodgkin lymphoma with B-cell lymphomas, which receive different treatment and have different prognoses. Thus the separate category of Hodgkin lymphoma remains; in fact, the universe of lymphomas is still divided into Hodgkin and non-Hodgkin lymphomas.

If we review the normal differentiation of B and T cells, we can relate the lymphoid malignancies (non-Hodgkin) to specific stages in their development based on their surface markers or CD molecules and on events occurring in their genome (Figs. UIV.1 and UIV.2). Thus the precursor B-cell leukemia/lymphomas (B-ALL—acute lymphoblastic leukemia) and precursor T-cell leukemia/lymphoma

(T-ALL) can be related to the development of B cells in the bone marrow and T cells in the thymus, respectively (see Cases 1–3). Similarly, the peripheral lymphoid neoplasms can be related to their mature normal counterparts based on their surface markers and the result of events in their nucleus (such as somatic hypermutation and isotype switching in B cells; see Case 4). In myeloid malignancies, the malignant cells will be frozen in or accumulate at a particular stage of differentiation or activation; however, the initial transforming event may occur in an earlier cell that continues to mature up to a certain point. In contrast, for several peripheral B-cell malignancies there is evidence that the transforming event is truly in the mature cell stage rather than in an earlier cell. Three of the peripheral B-cell neoplasms—follicular, mantle cell, and Burkitt lymphomas—are characterized by translocations placing a protooncogene under the control of an immunoglobulin gene promoter, usually the heavy-chain gene (Fig. UIV.3). This results in constitutive activation of the respective oncogene. In follicular lymphoma, the position of the breakpoint in the immunoglobulin gene and the evidence from the adjacent nucleotide sequence suggest that the translocation occurs during VDJ rearrangement in the precursor B cell in the bone marrow (see Cases 1, 2 and 25). In other lymphomas, such as endemic Burkitt lymphoma, the position of the breakpoint suggests that the translocation (which contributes to the transformation of the cell) occurs during somatic hypermutation or heavy chain isotype switching, processes that take place in the periphery (see Case 4).

As with any neoplasm, those of lymphoid origin are the outgrowth of a single aberrant clone. This principle of the monoclonal origin of tumors is perhaps easiest to demonstrate in the lymphoid system, where rearrangements of the genes for the B- or T-cell receptor result in different sizes and electrophoretic properties of the resulting productive

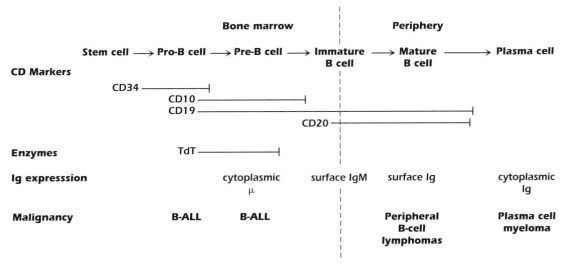

Figure UIV.1. Correlation of B-cell development with B-cell malignancies.

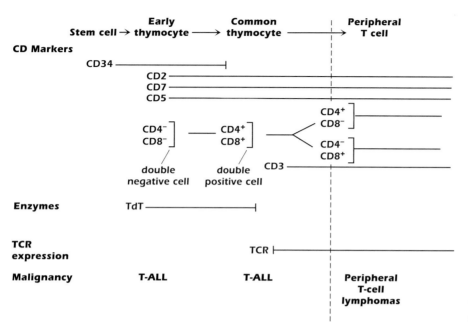

Figure UIV.2. Correlation of T-cell development with T-cell malignancies.

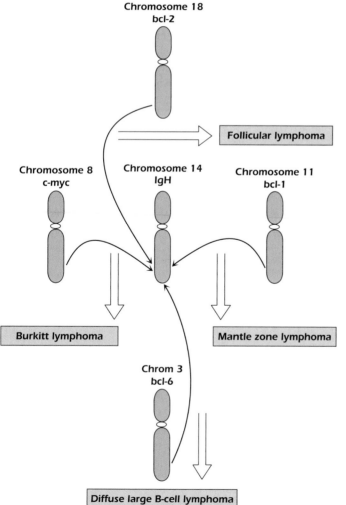

Figure UIV.3. Translocation partners frequently observed in lymphoma development.

genes. Extraction of DNA and evaluation by Southern blot analysis will reveal a single band for the immunoglobulin in the case of B-cell malignancy or T-cell receptor genes for T-cell malignancies. This single band demonstrates that all the cells of the tumor have the same rearrangement of those genes as opposed to the indistinct banding pattern expected of genes rearranged as the result of normal processing.

THE LYMPHOID MALIGNANCIES DISCUSSED IN THIS UNIT

From this vast array of lymphoid neoplasms we have selected a handful to discuss in detail. Our selection is based on what the lymphoma may teach us (or allow us to teach you) about the normal counterpart and/or about the neoplastic process. Lymphoid malignances associated with viral infections such as the Epstein–Barr virus (EBV), which are increased in incidence in immunodeficiency diseases such as AIDS (Case 9) and X-linked lymphoproliferative disease (Case 7), are described in those chapters. Here we have selected chronic lymphocytic leukemia/small lymphocytic lymphoma (Case 24), follicular lymphoma (Case 25), and plasma cell neoplasms (Case 26). Rather than using the cases to study the diseases themselves as we did in the preceding chapters, clinical features will be discussed only as they reflect alterations in the immune system. Treatment also will only be detailed when it makes use of our knowledge of the immune system. Unfortunately, even today many of the therapies for all cancers, including those described here, are nonspecific toxic agents; however, this is changing rapidly, and we can hopefully look forward to the development of more specific biologic agents to control disease in the near future.

Presentation of chronic lymphocytic leukemia/small lymphocytic lymphoma (Case 24) allows us to relate this malignant population(s) to normal B1 and marginal zone B cells. In addition, this malignancy is characteristically associated with an array of autoimmune phenomena, demonstrating once again the generalized derangement of the immune system that results even when only one portion or cell subtype is aberrant or uncontrolled. Follicular lymphoma (Case 25) provides us with a framework to discuss normal events in the follicle and is a continuation of the discussion of B-cell activation which began in Unit I on the immunodeficiency diseases. Plasma cell neoplasms (Case 26) give us an opportunity to describe the ultimate product of the B cell, immunoglobulin, and the havoc wreaked by its overproduction. The study of myeloma has allowed scientists both to decipher the structure of immunoglobulins by providing this monoclonal product in abundance and to provide proof for the clonal origin of tumors. Not insignificantly, cell lines from these tumors have been manipulated to provide monoclonal antibody products to an array of targets and have had far-reaching applications outside of medicine. Lastly, recent work on plasma cell neoplasms and their treatment has opened up the whole area of cross-talk or cross-communication between cells of the immune system (in fact, the entire hematopoietic system) and supporting elements; in this case the supporting elements are the bone marrow stroma and bone itself. This field has great significance and potential for understanding embryonic and stem cell development.

In closing, presentation of a well-selected group of neoplastic diseases of the immune system will allow us to fulfill the paradigm of teaching presented in the introduction to this book, namely a tricornered collection of diseases of the immune system that rests securely on the three legs of immunodeficiency, immune dysregulation and autoimmunity and malignancy.

24

CHRONIC LYMPHOCYTIC LEUKEMIA/SMALL LYMPHOCYTIC LYMPHOMA

SUSAN R. S. GOTTESMAN

 CASE REPORT

"I've been promoted!"

"Normal" Checkup

Bob, a 58-year-old long-time patient of yours, has just been promoted to executive vice president of global marketing for his company. He requires a complete physical examination for the new position.

All physical findings are within normal limits. In fact, Bob, who is weight and exercise conscious, is in fine shape and full of enthusiasm about his new responsibilities. You send off the required laboratory tests: urine analysis, complete blood count (CBC), and chemistries, requesting copies for your files.

A few days later, you look at Bob's lab results, expecting them to be normal. His CBC is as follows:

	Result	Reference Range
Red Blood Cells (RBC)	$4.3 \times 10^6/\mu L$	4.3–$5.7 \times 10^6/\mu L$
Hemoglobin (Hgb)	13.6 g/dL	13.5–17.8 g/dL
Hemocrit (Hct)	40%	(38.8–50%)
Mean corpuscular volume (MCV)	90 fL	80–94 fL

RBC distribution wideth (RDW)	12.5	11.5–14.5
White blood cells (WBC)	16,000/μL	4800-10,800/μL
Platelets (PLT)	160,000/μL	130,000–400,000/μL

What finding is aberrant given Bob's normal physical presentation?

Bob's WBC count is above the normal range. Although not of great concern, it seems an anomaly since he had no signs of infection to account for the leukocytosis (increase in WBC). Since no differential was ordered, there is no breakdown of the percentage of each type of WBC. The red cell count is toward the lower end of normal and slightly lower than in a routine CBC done one year prior as part of Bob's routine physical at that time.

You record a note to repeat a CBC with differential in six months.

Follow-Up and Diagnosis

Repeat CBC. Six months later, Bob is perplexed as to why your office called him, asking him to return for a

---

Immunology: Clinical Case Studies and Disease Pathophysiology, By Warren Strober and Susan R. S. Gottesman
Copyright © 2009 John Wiley & Sons, Inc.

checkup and repeat laboratory tests. He admits to feeling a little tired with frequent colds but he blames both on his extensive business travel. He is still confident that he can handle the demands of his new job. His physical exam now is within normal limits, except for a mild cold.

CBC results are as follows:

	Result	Reference Range
RBC	$4.1 \times 10^6/\mu L$	$4.3-5.7 \times 10^6/\mu L$
Hgb	13.1 g/dL	13.5–17.8 g/dL
Hct	39%	38.8–50%
MCV	90 fL	80–94 fL
RDW	12.5	11.5–14.5
WBC	21,000/μL	4800–10,800/μL
PLT	170,000/μL	130,000–400,000/μL
WBC differential		
Neutrophils	25%	40–74%
Lymphocytes	70%	19–48%
Monocytes	4%	3.4–9%
Eosinophils	1%	0–7%
Basophils	0%	0–1.5%

What additional information do you have by virtue of repeating and comparing the CBC results and evaluating the composition of the white cells in the circulation?

The leukocytosis is shown to be chronic over a period of at least six months, has increased further in magnitude, and is now found to be due primarily to lymphocytes. A reactive lymphocytosis due to a viral infection will cause an increase in T cells, primarily of the CD8 $^+$ or cytotoxic cell subset. (Note that this might invert the CD4/CD8 T-cell ratio, but the inversion would be due to an increase in cytotoxic T cells rather than to a decrease in CD4$^+$ T cells, as is found in HIV infections.) An increase of such magnitude due to increased numbers of B cells must be investigated as a possible monoclonal or malignant proliferation. Malignancies of mature small T cells, albeit less common, are also a consideration. Of concern is the further slight decrease in his red cell numbers. Anemia, particularly in a male or postmenopausal female, must be investigated thoroughly. One possible cause could be an infiltrate replacing or crowding out the cells in the bone marrow.

Phenotype of Lymphocytes.   You decide to identify the lymphocytes in the peripheral blood. How do you proceed?

Peripheral blood samples are sent for microscopic examination of morphology and for "immunophenotyping" of the lymphocytes. ***Immunophenotyping****: Using*

immunologic methods to determine the character or phenotype of the cell. In this case, the phenotype would be determined using antibodies, usually monoclonal antibodies, which bind to molecules on the cell surface. These molecules serve as surface markers which are designated by the letters CD (clusters of differentiation) and a unique number, and characterize lymphocytes with respect to lineage [T, B, natural killer (NK)] and stage of differentiation. Many are found on other hematopoietic and nonhematopoietic cells. They function as receptors and ligands and in general determine how the cell interacts with its environment.

For phenotyping cells in the peripheral blood, the antibodies are tagged with a fluorescent dye and their binding is detected in a flow cytometer (see Unit V for detailed assay description).

Examination of the peripheral smear reveals abundant lymphocytes, which are approximately normal in appearance (Fig. 24.1). They show no signs of activation, as would be expected in an infection (increase in size due to increase in cytoplasm, which decreases the nuclear/cytoplasmic ratio), or show no evidence of being early or immature cells, as in acute leukemias.

Immunphenotyping results as percent of total lymphocytes are as follows:

	Result	Reference Range
CD3	15%	55–82%
CD4	10%	25–58%
CD8	4%	12–43%
CD19	82%	5–26%
CD20	84% (dim)	5–26%
CD10	<2%	<2%
CD23	80%	(see interpretation)
CD38	15%	(see interpretation)
Kappa	90% (dim)	(see interpretation)
Lambda	10%	(see interpretation)
IgM	85% (dim)	(see interpretation)
IgD	80% (dim)	(see interpretation)
IgG	1%	(see interpretation)
IgA	1%	(see interpretation)
CD2	12%	55–82%
CD7	13%	55–82%
CD5	95%	55–82%
CD5/CD19	70%	1–4%

What is the normal subset distribution of peripheral blood lymphocytes?

Normally, T cells, as evidenced by their expression of CD3, constitute 55–82% of the circulating lymphocytes. They are

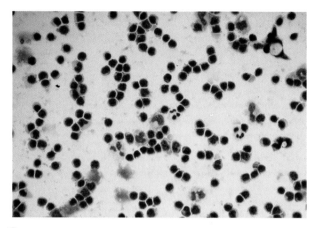

Figure 24.1. Peripheral blood demonstrating CLL cells. The vast majority of the cells present are small lymphocytes.

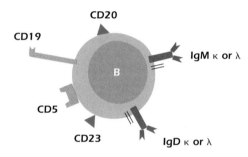

Figure 24.2. Surface markers of B-CLL cell

distributed between helper T cells (CD4$^+$) and cytotoxic T cells (CD8$^+$) in a ratio of approximately 2:1. The remaining 20–45% of the lymphocytes are B cells and NK cells.

What is the predominant cell population seen in Bob's blood? Which result seems to be an anomaly at first glance?

The majority of the cells are B cells, as evidenced by their expression of the B-lineage markers, CD19 and CD20 (Fig. 24.2). Additionally, as suggested by their morphologic appearance, they are mature B cells expressing CD20 and surface immunoglobulin; however, the density of expression is lower than normal as reflected by the dim staining.

The cells express both μ and δ heavy chains, which are the two heavy chains that are normally expressed together on the B-cell surface at a certain stage of development (see below). The organization of the heavy-chain gene makes this feasible (see Case 4; see also Coico and Sunshine, Chapter 4).

The expression of CD5, which is frequently used as a pan T-cell marker, is not an anomaly but is found on certain normal B cells and at specific stages of activation (see below). However, it is this cell population that is obviously increased.

The results are consistent with a monoclonal proliferation of CD5$^+$ B cells, characteristic of **chronic lymphocytic leukemia (CLL)/small lymphocytic lymphoma (SLL)**.

What is the evidence that this proliferation is monoclonal? What is meant by clonality? How could you prove clonality of the cells if necessary?

The B cells may be assumed to be monoclonal by their expression of surface immunoglobulin of a single light chain, κ, as opposed to a mixture of κ and λ light chains. A monoclonal population is defined as a population of cells originating from a single cell such that all the progeny are identical or are derived from the original founder clone. If necessary, clonality of the cells in question can be proven by Southern blot analysis of extracted, cut DNA (see Unit V). The DNA fragments will show a single rearranged band for the heavy chain and a single rearranged band for the light-chain immunoglobulin genes when reacted with the appropriate probes. The DNA from a polyclonal proliferation of B cells will have multiple rearrangements, differing in each cell, so that a spectrum of cut DNA sizes will be evident as a smear rather than as a single band when separated on a gel.

Prognostic Indicators: Cytogenetics and Molecular Studies. You ask Bob and his wife to come to your office to discuss the results, obtain additional samples for cytogenetic and molecular studies, stage him (determine the extent of the disease), and begin the discussion of his options. In disclosing to Bob that he has CLL, you emphasize that this leukemia is usually slowly progressive, having a low proliferation rate, but that the malignant cells are not very susceptible to standard chemotherapy. Bone marrow transplantation is discussed for the future; however, Bob has no siblings and comes from a small family.

Karyotype is found to be normal; additionally there is no evidence of trisomy 12, deletion 11q, or deletion 17p by FISH (fluorescence in situ hybridization) analysis (see Unit V). Abnormality is found at chromosome 13q14 by FISH and the IGH region is hypermutated.

What is the significance of these cytogenetic results?

CLL has been divided into two prognostic groups based on their cytogenetic and phenotypic characteristics. The more aggressive group correlates with an unmutated V$_H$ region, trisomy 12, 11q$^-$, 17p$^-$, and high positivity for CD38 and ZAP-70, an intracellular tyrosine kinase. The less aggressive subgroup has a mutated V$_H$ region (bcl-6 mutations correlate with the V-region mutations), lacks the chromosomal abnormalities of the aggressive group, but has a chromosome 13q14 abnormality and expresses only low levels of CD38 and ZAP-70. Although these findings started only as correlations, the pathophysiologic explanations are now being unraveled (see below).

Bob's results indicate that he falls into the good prognosis group; he does not express CD38, has an abnormality at 13q14, and has hypermutated IGH region genes. Bone

TABLE 24.1. Clinical Staging of Chronic Lymphocytic Leukemia

Stage 0	Bone marrow and blood lymphocytosis only: Absolute lymphocytes $\geq$ 15,000/μL; $\geq$ 40% lymphocytes in bone marrow
Stage I	Lymphocytosis with enlarged lymph nodes
Stage II	Lymphocytosis with enlarged spleen and/or liver
Stage III	Lymphocytosis with anemia Hgb <11g/dL or Hct <33% (organomegaly may or may not be present)
Stage IV	Lymphocytosis with thrombocytopenia: Platelets <100,000/ μL (organomegaly and anemia may or may not be present)

marrow analysis and evaluation of lymph nodes and spleen by radiographic studies places Bob at stage 0 (Table 24.1). A wait-and-watch approach is adopted.

Early Symptoms

Over the next two years Bob's course is uneventful and he is able to conduct his life and work normally. However, evaluation at the end of this period discloses that he now has a WBC count of 38,000/μL and some cervical lymphadenopathy (enlargement of lymph nodes). He is increasingly anemic, and a bone marrow evaluation demonstrates diffuse infiltration by small lymphocytes. He is considered stage III CLL/SLL (Table 24.1). A decision is made to start chemotherapy with low-dose leukeran (an alkylating agent) and prednisone (a steroid) under the care of a hematologist.

Complications and Progression

Several months later Bob comes to your office complaining of extreme fatigue and has slight yellowing of the whites of his eyes. On physical examination, you detect diffuse lymphadenopathy, splenomegaly (enlarged spleen), and slight tachycardia (increased heart rate). His sclerae are indeed slightly yellow. His peripheral blood shows a rising lymphocytosis and a decreasing RBC count with a hemoglobin of 9 and a hematocrit of 27%. The smear confirms these findings of severe anemia and shows spherocytes. A direct Coombs test is positive. Serum bilirubin is elevated.

What does this constellation of results indicate?

These results are consistent with **autoimmune hemolytic anemia** *(AIHA). In CLL, AIHA is caused by the production of antibodies reactive to the patient's own red cells either by the CLL cells themselves or, more commonly, by other B cells whose activity is no longer properly controlled. In the latter case, the antibodies are usually polyclonal IgG antibodies. When antibodies are present on the patient's red cells, they agglutinate when antiglobulin is added; this is a positive direct Coombs test (see Unit V). In the body these antibody-coated red cells are usually phagocytized by macrophages in the spleen and liver; however, some may be eliminated by NK cells via antibody-dependent cell cytotoxicity (ADCC). When a macrophage ingests only pieces of red cell membrane with the antibody attached, smaller spherical red blood cells, called spherocytes, are formed. Jaundice is due to an increase in unconjugated*

bilirubin as a result of hemoglobin released from red cell breakdown. Uncommonly, lysis of red cells occurs within the vasculature, usually the result of an IgM, rather than an IgG, autoantibody. This leads to the release of hemoglobin in the vasculature and excretion of hemoglobin in the urine (dark urine).

Within a few days Bob calls, relating symptoms of herpes zoster reactivation. This is not uncommon in patients with incipient immunodeficiency. He is becoming increasingly uncomfortable. A serum electrophoresis shows a small M spike in a background of hypogammaglobulinemia. Immunofixation electrophoresis (IFE; see Unit V) identifies the spike as monoclonal IgMκ and verifies the paucity of the other immunoglobulin classes (see Case 26).

Is a monoclonal spike an indication of a second neoplasm, a plasma cell malignancy?

CLL is often characterized by the production of a small amount of monoclonal antibody, usually of the IgM class. IFE identifies the immunoglobulin classes and clonality of the abnormal immunoglobulin production. Although the CLL cells could be the source of this antibody and the antibody could be an autoantibody against the patient's own cells (such as RBC or platelets), in this case it is neither. The concurrence of monoclonal antibody, autoantibodies, and decreased antibody production to exogenous antigens is often seen in any derangement of the immune system and results in humoral immunodeficiency along with autoimmune phenomena.

Increasing the dosage of chemotherapy and a more aggressive regimen are begun in an effort to control the leukemic proliferation and thereby control the anemia and immunodeficient state which are causing the clinical symptoms.

Over the next seven years, despite various chemotherapeutic regimens, Bob's condition gradually worsens with overall increasing lymphocytosis, lymphadenopathy, splenomegaly, weight loss, autoimmune hemolysis, and recurrent infections, particularly bacterial infections. These infections are due to progressive neutropenia, resulting both from CLL cells crowding the bone marrow and from the chemotherapy. Bob is able to continue working, although he has had to change to a position with a less strenuous schedule.

Bob now presents with a new finding: One lymph node group has increased rapidly in size over a one-week period, while his other lymph nodes maintain their usual, albeit enlarged size. A biopsy of this lymph node discloses diffuse large B-cell lymphoma with areas of necrosis (cell death). Any remaining scattered small lymphocytes are characterized as his CLL cells. Over the next few months the large cell lymphoma progresses despite aggressive chemotherapy. Bob requests care at home and dies a few days later, approximately 11 years after first presenting with initially silent CLL.

 DIFFERENTIAL DIAGNOSIS

As discussed in the case report, the differential diagnosis at presentation is first between a reactive leukocytosis and leukemia. Bacterial infections will result in an increase in neutrophils, whereas viral infections cause a greater rise in lymphocytes. Acute leukemias will show the presence of immature cells or blasts in the peripheral blood. In chronic leukemias, a clonal population of mature cells circulates. In this case, the predominant circulating population consists of lymphocytes with the phenotype of a subset of mature B cells, classical for CLL.

 PATHOGENESIS/IMMUNOGENESIS

Normal B-Cell Subsets and Their Responses to Antigenic Stimulation

In considering the B-cell response to antigen (humoral response), it is clear that different subpopulations of B cells respond to different types of antigens: T-dependent antigens and T-independent antigens.

Antigen Type. *Thymus-dependent (TD) antigens* are protein antigens that require T-cell help to enable the B cell to effectively produce antibody. These antigens bind to the B cell via their B-cell receptor (BCR), are internalized and degraded, and their derived peptides are expressed on the surface of that B cell. The small peptide fragments are presented in the context of MHC class II to the antigen-specific T helper cell via its T-cell receptor (TCR). This cognate interaction between the antigen-specific helper T cell and the B cell includes additional interaction between CD40 on the B cell and CD40 ligand (CD40L or CD154) on the T cell. These cooperative interactions between the antigen-specific T and B cells occur on the way into and within a newly formed germinal center and result in the production of T-cell cytokines that affect both B-cell proliferation and differentiation (see Case 25). These B cells are designated B2 cells, conventional B cells, or follicular precursor and

follicular center cells and are the cells predominantly responsible for the adaptive humoral immune response (see introduction to Unit I and below). This response is characterized by its ability to evolve with the formation of high-affinity antibodies (affinity maturation) and antibodies of different isotypes: IgG, IgA, and IgE. For a review of isotype switching, see Case 4.

T-independent (TI) antigens can be subdivided into two types. *TI-1 antigens* are simply B-cell mitogens, proliferation-inducing agents, which, at high doses, can directly stimulate B-cell division in an antigen-nonspecific manner. One example is lipopolysaccharide (LPS). *TI-2 antigens* have highly repetitive structures or epitopes and are typically polysaccharides, usually ones which are part of bacterial capsules, but also include DNA, RNA, and flagellin. These TI-2 antigens stimulate B cells in a T-independent but antigen-specific manner and only activate mature B cells. Presumably their structure allows them to cross-link a critical number of BCR molecules stimulating the specific B cell to produce IgM. In addition, these antigens may bind both the BCR and coreceptors, such as Toll-like receptors (TLRs), generating the second signal on their own. Cytokines from T helper cells may further stimulate these B cells to respond and to isotype switch in some instances, but T-cell-derived cytokines are not necessary for the IgM response. Obviously, the ability to respond to TI-2 antigens is determined by the specificity of the BCR and is a central part of our innate immune response. B1 cells (also called CD5$^+$ B cells) and marginal zone B cells are found to be the populations responsive to TI-2 antigens (see below).

B-Cell Subpopulations. If you analyze the immune system by characterizing the B cells which occupy different locations within the peripheral lymphoid organs (lymph nodes and spleen), blood, and fluid cavities, you can subdivide B cells into several groups based on functional capacity, morphology, and phenotype (Table 24.2).

The *B1 cells*, forming part of our innate immune system, have been further subdivided into *B1-a* and *B1-b* cells, based on the presence or absence of CD5 on their surface. Much of the work on B1 cells comes from mouse studies. B1 cells are produced early in ontogeny and predominantly populate the mouse peritoneal cavity, where they are capable of self-renewal and are thus independent of the bone marrow. B1 cells typically respond to T-independent type 2 (TI-2) antigens without T-cell help and without prior sensitization to produce IgM. The antibody produced is polyspecific, binding to several ligands but preferentially to the stimulating antigen, usually bacterial polysaccharides. Only a limited set of variable (V) region genes is used. This is a rapid, broad response, similar to innate immunity rather than adaptive immunity. It is proposed that this response controls the bacterial infection early after

TABLE 24.2. Mature B-Cell Subpopulations

B2 cells (conventional): CD5$^-$, CD19$^+$, CD20$^+$, CD23$^-$, sIg$^+$ (all isotypes)	Present in peripheral blood, lymph nodes, and spleen; responsible for adaptive immunity to TD Ag; travel through germinal center, hypermutate, isotype switch, form memory cells
B1-a cells: CD5$^+$, CD19$^+$, CD20^{dim}, CD23$^+$, sIgM±IgD	Present in body cavities with small numbers in peripheral blood; responsible for innate immunity to TI-2 Ag, produce cross-autoreactive antibody
B1-b cells: CD5$^-$, CD19$^+$, CD20^{dim}, sIgM$^+$	Respond to TI Ag, form long-lived memory cells
Mantle cell B cells: CD5$^+$, CD19$^+$, CD20$^+$, sIgM$^+$	Present in zone around germinal centers and in primary unstimulated follicles; have not hypermutated or isotype switched
Marginal zone B cells: CD5$^-$, CD19$^+$, CD20$^+$	Present in mucosal-associated lymphoid tissue and in marginal zone of spleen; splenic population responsible for response to *S. pneumoniae*.

encounter, until more specific and higher affinity antibodies can be produced by conventional B cells. Polysaccharide antigens do not specifically stimulate T cells; therefore B1 cells responding to them do not usually isotype class switch or undergo hypermutation. In addition, no memory B cells are formed. The broadly reactive antibodies produced by B1 cells may have some degree of autoreactivity. Indeed B1-a cells have been implicated in rheumatoid arthritis. Recent work in the mouse suggests that B1-b cells are a distinct and stable subpopulation capable of responding to certain bacterial antigens in a T-independent manner but which form long-lived memory cells.

The conventional B cells, or **B2 cells**, are those responsible for the adaptive immune response. B2 cells are the predominant B cell in the peripheral blood and the lymph nodes, circulating throughout the body. In response to their specific antigen and with T-cell help, they will proliferate and differentiate in germinal centers and may isotype switch and undergo hypermutation of their immunoglobulin genes, the latter process leading to affinity maturation of the antibody response. They may become plasma cells or memory cells or, once antigen is decreased, in the absence of continued stimulation, they may undergo apoptosis (see Case 25). B2 cells originate in the bone marrow, which is capable of producing them throughout the individual's lifespan. In the peripheral blood, these mature circulating B cells express CD19, CD20, and surface Ig with a mixture of κ and λ light-chain-expressing cells. Most express CD45RA, an isoform of CD45 correlated with naive or virgin status with respect to antigen encounter. Additional surface antigens and transcription factors are turned on in the germinal center.

In addition, two other morphologic and immunophenotypic groups of B cells have been identified. The **mantle zone B cells** are believed to occupy the primary follicle in the lymph node and be pushed to the outside of the germinal center once it is formed. These are small, mature resting B cells, which express surface IgM and express CD5, similar to the B1 cells. Mantle zone B cells usually have no evidence of hypermutation of their immunoglobulin genes.

B cells in the **marginal zone** differ morphologically and phenotypically from their relatives mentioned above. They are most prominent in the mucosal-associated lymphoid tissues, particularly those of the gut, and occupy a unique region of the spleen on the outer border of the red pulp. In humans, the marginal zone cells of the spleen are believed to be responsible for the body's response to *Streptococcus pneumonia*. The newborn, with its underdeveloped splenic marginal zone, cannot respond with antibody formation to *S. pneumonia* and is very susceptible to the organism until the appearance of the splenic marginal zone B cells in the spleen. Asplenic patients are similarly susceptible.

How are these subpopulations of B cells related? Are they different and stable subsets or stages of differentiation of one or two populations? As you may guess, these are areas of active investigation. How this discussion relates to (or confuses) our knowledge of CLL/SLL will become apparent below.

Tranformation of B Cells

Malignant transformation of each of these four or five subpopulations of B cells can occur. The transformation results in a distinctly behaving lymphoma that has chromosomal abnormalities, some of which are characteristic of that neoplasm. The phenotype of the malignant cell in all cases parallels the phenotype of the normal cell counterpart (see the introduction to this unit). Thus, transformation of follicular center cells results in follicular lymphoma, transformation of mantle cells results in mantle cell lymphoma, and malignant transformation of marginal zone cells results in marginal zone lymphoma. The cells of each lymphoma have the same phenotype as the normal cell counterpart. Diffuse large B-cell lymphoma has a heterogeneous origin. For some of the lymphomas, characteristic chromosomal translocations have been identified. As discussed in the follicular lymphoma case, these neoplasms are characterized by a translocation between the *bcl-2* gene, an antiapoptotic protein and the immunoglobulin gene, usually the heavy chain, leading to a block in apoptosis. Mantle cell lymphomas, on the other hand, show mostly overexpression of cyclin D1, as the result of either a translocation (also with immunoglobulin genes) or a point mutation. This results in an increase in cell cycle transit from G1 to S and, hence, a more aggressive lymphoma than those associated with an apoptotic defect. Subtypes of marginal zone lymphomas are associated with translocation of the MALT1 gene, leading to dysregulation of the signaling pathway downstream of CD40. Marginal zone lymphomas of the mucosal-associated lymphoid tissue are of particular interest. They are mostly extranodal and a subset is associated with chronic antigenic stimulation in the involved organ. For example, patients with Hashimoto's thyroiditis, an autoimmune disease of the thyroid, have a high incidence of marginal zone lymphoma in the thyroid.

CLL/SLL is considered one malignancy with different presentations in individual patients since the malignant cell is identical. Some patients present with lymph node involvement first, followed by infiltration of the bone marrow and peripheral blood; this is the classic clinical picture of SLL. Others present as Bob did, with blood and marrow involvement first. As the disease progresses, clinical symptoms merge with CLL cells in the circulation, marrow, lymph nodes, spleen, and liver. The normal counterpart of the CLL cell is a recirculating cell and the malignant cell similarly recirculates and accumulates throughout the body. CLL is the most prevalent leukemia of adults in North America and Western Europe but is much less common in Asia and Africa.

CLL cells are characterized by the phenotype discussed: CD19$^+$, CD20$^+$, CD5$^+$, CD23$^+$, sIgM$^+$, sIgD$^{+/-}$. This phenotype is characteristic of B1-a cells in the circulation. The low proliferation rate of CLL cells leads to their accumulation and accounts partially for their resistance to traditional chemotherapy. A small monoclonal spike of IgM is frequently seen in CLL. The reactivity of this IgM is sometimes against the patient's red cells or platelets but is usually unknown.

The parallelism with B1-a cells is not absolute and recent evidence in humans suggests that there are two subsets of CLL in spite of almost identical surface markers. In one, the immunoglobulin genes of the malignant cells show evidence of hypermutation. Since hypermutation normally takes place in the germinal centers, some investigators have suggested that these CLLs originate from a post–germinal center cell. However, these CLLs are still mostly IgM$^+$, not having undergone isotype switching. Normal marginal zone lymphocytes of the spleen have evidence of somatic hypermutation, are often memory cells, and express IgM, although they do not express CD5. Perhaps they are the normal counterpart of the CLLs with hypermutated immunoglobulin genes, and the lack of CD5 simply reflects their activation state. Patients with hypermutated CLLs have a more indolent course. The second group of CLL patients has unmutated V$_H$ genes; their CLL cells more closely resemble normal B1-a cells.

One aspect of the genetic changes in CLL is beginning to be understood. Recall that CLL can be divided into two subgroups depending on the presence or absence of deletion at chromosome 13q14.3. A deletion at that location has been correlated with good prognosis and a longer interval to progression. When efforts were made to identify the protein(s) encoded by this region of the genome, no protein could be found. Instead, the genes mapping to this region code for two microRNAs, miR-15 and miR-16. Both function normally to block Bcl-2 mRNA (Fig. 24.3). Without these microRNAs to down-regulate Bcl-2 at the posttranscriptional level, Bcl-2 is overexpressed. Thus we have a malignancy characterized by nondividing mature cells that fail to die. Although B1 cells are normally long-lived and express bcl-2 protein, in CLL cells with this deletion the bcl-2 is overexpressed. In contrast to follicular lymphoma, the *BCL-2* gene is not itself mutated or translocated. The involvement of microRNAs in the control of protein synthesis in normal and malignant cells is opening up new areas of investigation and the possibility of new therapeutic targets.

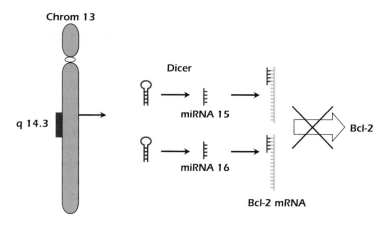

Figure 24.3. Normal function of miRNA-15 and-16 in cell.

CLINICAL ASPECTS OF CHRONIC LYMPHOCYTIC LEUKEMIA

Complications

Autoimmune Hemolytic Anemia. AIHA can occur as a separate entity in a patient, as a result of a drug reaction, or associated with other autoimmune diseases or malignancy. AIHA is frequently seen in CLL. IgG autoantibodies bind to the red cells but, unlike IgM, do not effectively activate the complement cascade. These antibody-coated cells are eliminated from the circulation as a result of either phagocytosis by macrophage of the reticular endothelial system or lysis by NK cells in an ADCC reaction.

IgM autoantibodies are very effective in activating the complement cascade and therefore can lead to intravascular lysis of the red cells. "Cold" agglutinins are usually IgM antibodies (see Case 26). These antibodies only effectively bind to the cells at temperatures of <37°C. Hemolysis is therefore more common in the extremities (fingers and toes) and in cold weather. Peripheral blood smears from these patients show a distinctive three-dimensional agglutination or "sticking together" of the red cells as the colder outside temperature and cold slide allow for IgM binding when the blood sample is removed from the body. For IgM autoantibodies, the indirect Coombs test, which detects antibody in the serum, is positive. Intravascular hemolysis results in the excretion of hemoglobin. Normally the bone marrow will try to compensate for the peripheral destruction of red cells by increasing their production. Therefore, there will be an increase in the peripheral blood of early red cells (reticulocytes) released from the marrow. In the case of CLL and other malignancies occupying the marrow, there is a more profound anemia because there is not appropriate compensation.

Thrombocytopenia. Similar to the red cell anemia, thrombocytopenia (decreased platelets) may result from both platelet destruction by autoantibody and decreased production due to reduced megakaryocytes crowded out of the bone marrow by CLL cells.

Immunodeficient State. The reduced ability of normal B cells to function and the tumor infiltration of the sites of B-cell stimulation and antibody production (the lymph nodes and spleen) lead to a progressively worsening humoral immunodeficient state. The crowding of the bone marrow with malignant cells also results in a progressive neutropenia, which is compounded by the use of myelosuppressive chemotherapeutic agents. The patients are particularly susceptible to *S. pneumoniae, Haemophilus influenza*, and *Neisseria* ssp. In many patients it is the repeated infections and worsening anemia that impact quality of life and may even result in death.

Disease Progression

Large Cell Lymphoma. In 5% of the patients with CLL/SLL, large-cell lymphoma develops, initially at a single location. This has been referred to as a "Richter's transformation." In actuality, these large lymphoma cells may derive from the CLL cells or they may originate from a unique progenitor cell (a second lymphoma) as evidenced by different immunoglobulin gene rearrangements. More rarely, large lymphoma cells may be T-cell lymphomas. The large cell lymphoma is usually resistant to therapy and has a rapid downhill course. Occasionally, patients can develop Hodgkin lymphoma.

Prolymphocytic Leukemia. In CLL, a small percentage of the malignant cells are larger, with more cytoplasm and a single prominent nucleolus. These cells, called prolymphocytes, are derived from the same progenitor as the CLL cells, with the same surface markers. When they predominate, the patient is considered to have prolymphocytic leukemia and experiences a more rapid course.

TREATMENT

Since CLL cells often have their apoptotic pathways turned off by the expression of bcl-2 and have a low mitotic rate, they are relatively resistant to chemotherapeutic agents, most of which target cycling cells. Therefore, treatment is usually not begun until the patient has a significant tumor burden, at least stage 1. The objective of chemotherapy has been to reduce the tumor load rather than cure CLL. Newer treatment for B-cell lymphomas employs monoclonal antibodies against CD20. These are effective in some lymphomas even without toxins linked to them. However, CLL cells have a low density of CD20 on their surfaces. Despite the fact that this makes them less susceptible than other B-cell lymphomas, this is still frequently added to the CLL treatment regimen. A second monoclonal antibody, one directed against CD52 on B cells, is also used as an addition to chemotherapeutic agents.

Bone marrow transplantation, whether allogeneic or autologous, is effective when the patient can be purged of tumor cells. Again the limiting factor is the efficacy with which the CLL cells can be eliminated.

REFERENCES

Alugupalli K, Leong JM, Woodland RT, Muramatsu M, Honjo T, Gerstein RM (2004): B1b lymphocytes confer T cell-independent long-lasting immunity. *Immunity* 21: 379–390.

Chiorazzi N, Ferrarini M (2003): B cell chronic lymphocytic leukemia: Lessons learned from studies of the B cell antigen receptor. *Annu Rev Immunol* 21: 841–894.

Chiorazzi N, Rai KR, Ferrarini M (2005): Chronic lymphocytic leukemia. *New Engl J Med* 352: 804–815.

Cimmino A, Calin GA, Fabbri M, Iorio MV, Ferracin M, Shimizu M, Wojcik SE, Aqeilan RI, Zupo S, Dono M, Rassenti L, Alder H, Volinia S, Liu CG, Kipps TJ, Negrini M, Croce CM (2005): MiR-15 and miR-16 induce apoptosis by targeting BCL2. *Proc Natl Acad Sci USA* 102: 13944–13949.

Hardy R, Hayakawa K (2001): B cell development pathways. *Annu Rev Immunol* 19: 595–621.

Pillai S, Cariappa A, Moran ST (2005): Marginal zone B cells. *Annu Rev Immunol* 23: 161–196.

Rai KR, Sawitsky A, Cronkite EP, Chanana AD, Levy RN, Pasternack BS (1975): Clinical staging of chronic lymphocytic leukemia. *Blood* 46: 219–234.

25

FOLLICULAR LYMPHOMA

SUSAN R. S. GOTTESMAN

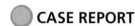 **CASE REPORT**

"I feel a lump."

Initial Presentation and Workup

Sharon, a 40-year-old teacher, discovers a small lump under her right arm during the course of her monthly breast self-examination. It is about 1/2 in. (1 cm) in diameter and nontender. She decides to just watch it for awhile.

The next month Sharon observes that the lump is still there, perhaps slightly larger. After noticing small "lumps" or enlarged "glands" along the side of her neck, she finally decides to make an appointment to see you.

You examine Sharon and palpate 1–2 cm lymph nodes in several nodal groups. Her liver and spleen are normal to palpation. The remainder of the physical examination is normal.

What is the differential diagnosis of peripheral lymphadenopathy?

Lymph node enlargement (adenopathy) is the result of a process intrinsic to the lymph node alone or disease elsewhere in the body. In either case, the differential diagnosis of lymphadenopathy divides into reactive versus malignant processes causing enlargement. Reactive

processes imply that the lymphocytes in the lymph node are responding to stimuli and include but are not restricted to infectious diseases. Frequently, reactive nodes are tender or painful. Localized adenopathy would suggest that the node is draining a localized infection, for example, bacterial infections of the skin, throat, or ear. Sometimes the organism also localizes in that draining node, such as in tuberculosis, cat scratch fever, syphilis, and toxoplasmosis. Generalized lymphadenopathy is seen in systemic infections such as infectious mononucleosis and human immunodeficiency virus (HIV) infection. The lymph nodes also enlarge in autoimmune diseases such as systemic lupus erythematosus, as a result of blocked drainage, and in several processes of unknown etiology such as sarcoidosis and Castleman's disease.

Among the malignant processes, localized lymphadenopathy may be due to metastatic deposits, usually of solid tumors (breast, colon) or to lymphoma, particularly Hodgkin lymphoma or diffuse large cell lymphoma. Diffuse adenopathy is more often a sign of a hematologic malignancy, usually non-Hodgkin lymphoma (see Unit IV introduction).

Sharon denies any constitutional symptoms such as fever, weight loss, and night sweats. You carefully examine her breasts and order a complete blood count (CBC), chemistries, and tests for HIV, infectious mononucleosis, and Epstein–Barr virus (EBV) as well as place a PPD test for tuberculosis (see Unit V). You start her on a six-week

---

trial of broad-spectrum antibiotics but caution her that radiographic studies and a lymph node biopsy (sample of the node) may be necessary.

The PPD test is read as negative at 48 h. All tests for infectious agents are also negative, and CBC and chemistries are all normal. After six weeks there is no decrease in the size of the lymph nodes; there is instead a slight increase. You send Sharon for radiographic studies. A chest X ray shows no evidence of lung disease, but a computerized tomography (CT) scan of the chest shows multiple enlarged nodes. You refer Sharon to a surgeon for a lymph node biopsy.

Definitive Diagnosis

Two weeks later you receive a call from the surgeon and a copy of the pathology report. The pathology report reads: Follicular lymphoma, grade I. What does the pathology report mean?

> *Follicular lymphoma is a malignant transformation of the B cells of the follicle. The normal counterpart is the centrocyte of the germinal center, also called the secondary follicle (see below). Grade I signifies that the lymphoma is composed primarily of small cells and maintains the nodular pattern of follicles of lymph nodes. Grading of any tumor is a microscopic evaluation of how closely the malignant cells resemble their normal counterpart with regard to both the individual cell morphology and tissue structure (Fig. 25.1).*

Immunophenotyping by flow cytometry (see Unit V for detailed description of laboratory tests) reports that 80% of the cells isolated from a sample of the lymph node are CD19$^+$, CD20$^+$, CD10$^+$, CD5$^-$, CD22$^+$, CD23$^-$, sIgG$^+$, sIgκ$^+$. The cells are also positive for bcl-2 protein in the nuclei (Fig. 25.2) and for bcl-6. Cytogenetic analysis demonstrates a translocation between chromosomes 14 and 18. The remainder of the lymph node cells are T cells of both the CD4 and CD8 subsets.

What can you surmise from the phenotype of the lymph node cells?

> *A normal lymph node is comprised of approximately 60–70% T cells divided between CD4 and CD8 subsets. The 30–40% B cells are normally a mixture of κ- and λ-expressing cells in a ratio of 1:1 to 3:1 κ to λ. The B cells of the germinal center are normally CD19$^+$, CD20$^+$, CD10$^+$, CD5$^-$ and express surface Ig. The overwhelming predominance of B cells from the biopsied node suggests an abnormal B-cell proliferation. The phenotype of those B cells suggests that they are derived from the follicular center B cells. The presence of a single immunoglobulin isotype IgG-κ strongly suggests a monoclonal B-cell population.*

What is the significance of the expression of bcl-2 and the translocation between chromosomes 14 and 18?

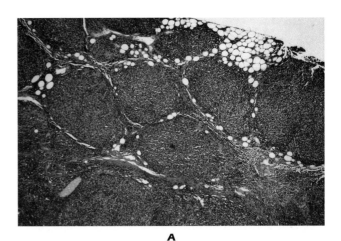

A

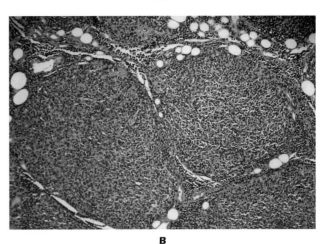

B

Figure 25.1. Histology of follicular lymphoma, grade 1. (**A**) Low power (100×). Notice back-to-back follicles or nodules, absence of tingible body macrophages, and absence or narrowing of surrounding mantle zones. Nodules exist outside of lymph node capsule and in surrounding fat. (**B**) High power (400×). Nodules comprised of mostly small cells leading to grade 1 designation.

> *The translocation between chromosomes 14 and 18, which is found in the vast majority of follicular lymphomas (>90%), places the bcl-2 gene from chromosome 18 next to the J region of the gene for the immunoglobulin heavy chain on chromosome 14 (bcl-2-JH rearrangement see below). This leads to the constitutive expression of bcl-2, an anti-apoptotic protein. Apoptosis is programmed cell death and is an important cellular function in follicular B cells (Fig. 25.3; see also Case 6).*

Treatment Plan

You call Sharon back to your office, explain the disease to her, and stage her (determine the extent of the disease in the body). This involves a PET (positron emission tomography)–CT scan and bone marrow biopsy. From

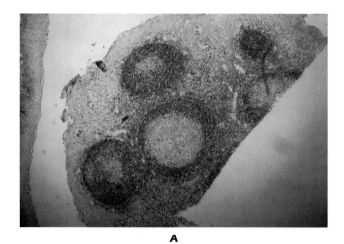

A

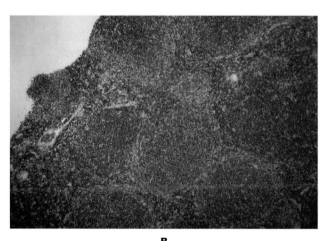

B

Figure 25.2. Immunohistochemical staining for bcl-2 protein (brown color is positive). (**A**) Normal reactive tonsil. Notice negative images of germinal centers where bcl-2 protein expression is turned off. (**B**) Follicular lymphoma. The cells in both the nodules and the interfollicular areas express bcl-2 (brown staining). The interfollicular cells express it normally, whereas the cells in the malignant follicles express bcl-2 as a result of the translocation of the bcl-2 gene to the immunoglobulin gene.

the customary presentation of follicular lymphoma you expect that her bone marrow will be involved and that she will have lymphadenopathy throughout her body. You explain that this lymphoma, untreated, grows slowly but that it is progressive. Partly because it is slow growing, it is not very susceptible to eradication by conventional chemotherapy. Strategies for treatment are discussed: a wait-and-see approach, standard chemotherapy with or without immunotherapy, or high-dose chemotherapy followed by either autologous stem cell transplantation purged of lymphoma cells or allogeneic stem cells. She is a young healthy patient, and in collaboration with an oncologist, you suggest a combination of chemotherapy with the newer immunotherapies as a first approach.

How do you target the lymphoma cells more specifically than using conventional chemotherapy?

Advantage is taken of the B-cell-specific markers on the surface of the lymphoma cells. Antibody to CD20 is used to target these malignant B cells which express CD20 at a high density. This antibody can be used as part of the chemotherapeutic regimen and may be unlabeled or tagged with toxins. The unlabeled antibody, the preparation currently in use, attaches to the cell and the cell is eliminated by complement fixation, by antibody-dependent cell cytotoxicity (ADCC), or by phagocytosis.

Staging shows evidence of lymphoma in multiple lymph node groups throughout Sharon's body, as documented by increased lymph node size on radiographic studies. A bone marrow sample demonstrates focal collections of lymphoma as well as the normal hematopoietic cells. The lymphoma cells occupy approximately 10% of marrow space.

Sharon begins conventional chemotherapy (which is not specific for the lymphoma cells) and anti-CD20 therapy. She initially shows a dramatic response with shrinkage of all enlarged lymph nodes. However, after several weeks Sharon has had only a partial response, and serum tests show the presence of antibody to the anti-CD20. In spite of suppression of essentially all of Sharon's B cells, she was still able to make antibody against the administered anti-CD20 antibody, blocking its effect.

Why is Sharon reacting to the anti-CD20 medication?

Anti-CD20 is a chimeric antibody, with part of the molecule derived from mouse and part from humans (see definitions below), and therefore is immunogenic in humans.

Change of Tactics

Sharon's disease progresses. Given her young age, a decision is made to become more aggressive with therapy. Sharon is to be given intensive chemotherapy followed by stem cell transplant.

What is the difference between an autologous versus an allogeneic stem cell transplant?

In an autologous transplant, Sharon's own stem cells will be returned to her. This can be done if all lymphoma cells in her body are eliminated by intensive immunosuppressive therapy and harvested cells are purged of any lymphoma cells prior to reintroduction. An autologous transplant has the advantage of avoiding immunosuppressive drugs to prevent rejection. An allogeneic transplant would be a transplant from an outside donor. Again the patient must be treated with intensive chemotherapy to eliminate the lymphoma cells. A donor stem cell transplant would be considered if Sharon has a donor matched at the major and minor histocompatibility loci. This is more likely in near relatives. An allogeneic transplant has the advantage of sometimes resulting in a graft-versus-lymphoma effect.

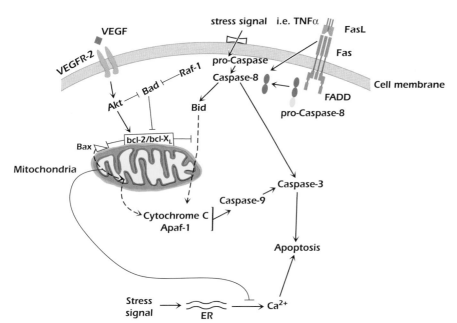

Figure 25.3. Mechanism of apoptosis involving bcl-2. Bcl-2 is present on the outer membrane of the mitochondria and normally interacts with related anti- and proapoptotic proteins which collectively are called the Bcl-2 family of proteins. They regulate mitochondrial permeability and function. Apoptosis may be initiated in a Fas–FasL-dependent fashion (see Case 6) following stress signals or when the cell is deprived of survival signals. With decreased bcl-2 and/or bcl-X_L, increased permeability of the mitochondrial membrane allows leakage of enzymes (especially cytochrome c) which activate the caspase cascade, resulting in apoptosis.

The decision was made to give an autologous transplant. Purging is accomplished by reacting Sharon's harvested marrow cells with monoclonal antibodies against B-cell antigens and sorting using a fluorescent activated cell sorter. This should eliminate any lymphoma cells among the harvested marrow cells. The efficiency of purging is evaluated by looking for cells with bcl-2-JH rearrangement, which is detectable by polymerase chain reaction (PCR) followed by Southern blot analysis (see Unit V). Following purging, no detectable lymphoma cells are found and the transplant is performed. Sharon remains disease free three years after transplant and is followed by annual radiographic exams and bone marrow biopsy with PCR for cells with the identified translocation.

PATHOPHYSIOLOGY

The Normal Lymph Node

Lymph Node Structure.   The lymph node consists of a fibrous capsule with a subcapsular sinus (Fig. 25.4). The cortex has a series of primary follicles which are unstimulated B cells and secondary follicles if stimulated. Secondary follicles consist of a germinal center surrounded by a mantle cell zone composed of small resting cells. Some lymph nodes, particularly those in the gut, have a prominent marginal zone outside the mantle zone. These areas: the germinal center, mantle zone, and marginal zone, are all composed predominantly of B cells, with differences in surface markers and state of activation. The germinal center is often described as polarized with a dark zone of centroblasts, large cells with vesicular nuclei, and a light zone of centrocytes, small cells with irregularly

shaped (cleaved) nuclei. Also present in the germinal center are scattered T cells (to supply help), follicular dendritic cells (to display antigen), and macrophages (to clean up dying cells). The paracortex is the T-cell zone and extends between the follicles. In addition to T cells, the paracortex is comprised of plasma cells, macrophages, dendritic cells, and immunoblasts. The medulla, which consists of the medullary cords and sinuses, contains mostly macrophages and plasma cells. Lymph enters the lymph node through multiple afferent vessels in the subcapsular sinus and leaves through a single efferent lymphatic in the hilum. Blood enters and leaves through the hilum, branching into extensive capillaries and high endothelial venules.

The Germinal Center.   What are the events in the normal germinal centers?

Germinal centers are the sites where antigen-specific B cells respond to antigen with further maturation and antibody production (Fig. 25.5). The founder B cells enter the primary follicle, where they encounter processed antigen presented in the context of major histocompatibility complex (MHC) class II surface molecules on macrophages and follicular dendritic cells. T cells, also specific for the antigen, provide help for the B cells, which themselves become antigen presenting cells (APCs). The B cells bearing surface immunoglobulin [B-cell receptor (BCR)] specific for the antigen, have their BCR engaged and, with a second costimulatory signal, are stimulated to respond. They endocytose the antigen, process it, and present it to the T cell in the context of MHC class II molecules on their surface. The T and B cells therefore interact through processed antigen–MHC class II complex on the B cell and the T-cell receptor (TCR) and CD4 on the T cell, along with several pairs of costimulatory molecules

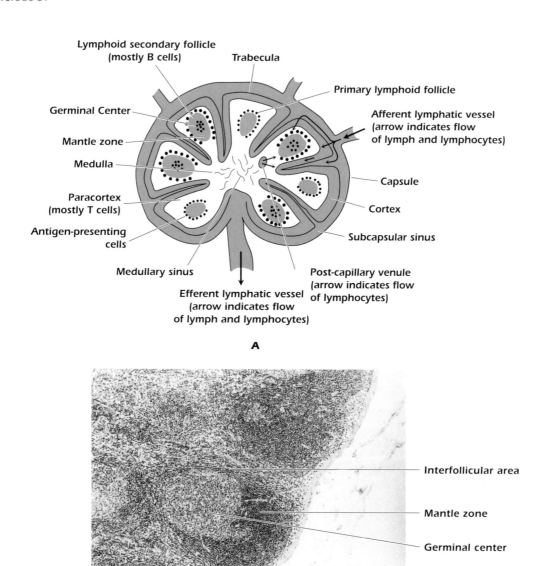

Figure 25.4. (**A**) Diagram of a section of a lymph node. *Arrows:* flow of lymph and lymphocytes. (**B**) Histological section of lymph node.

and ligands, notably CD28 on T cells and CD28L on B cells. The T cells in turn produce cytokines, which further promote the proliferation of the B cells, isotype switching of the heavy chain, and their differentiation into plasma cells or memory cells. In addition, affinity maturation of the antibody response is accomplished by the somatic hypermutation (SHM) of the immunoglobulin variable region and the selective survival advantage of B cells bearing BCR with high affinity for the antigen. These B cells thus proliferate, forming the germinal center (also known as a secondary follicle). It is believed that SHM is occurring in the dark zone of the germinal center, the zone populated by centroblasts. Pushed to the outside of the germinal center are small quiescent B cells which form a collar called the mantle zone. The mantle cells were probably the cells of the primary follicle. They express CD19, CD20, low-density

CD5, CD21, and sIgM and are negative for CD10 and CD23. They have not encountered their specific antigen or trafficked through a germinal center, as evidenced by the absence of hypermutation of their immunoglobulin genes.

How is the immune response turned off?

Stimulation is required for the continued survival of the B cell in the germinal center. Without stimulation, the B cell undergoes an apoptotic death. This allows for the selection of only antigen-specific B cells and the cessation of the B cell response once the concentration of antigen has waned. Thus, the germinal centers are the site of proliferation, differentiation, and cell death. Normally, bcl-2 protein, an antiapoptotic molecule, is not expressed in follicular center

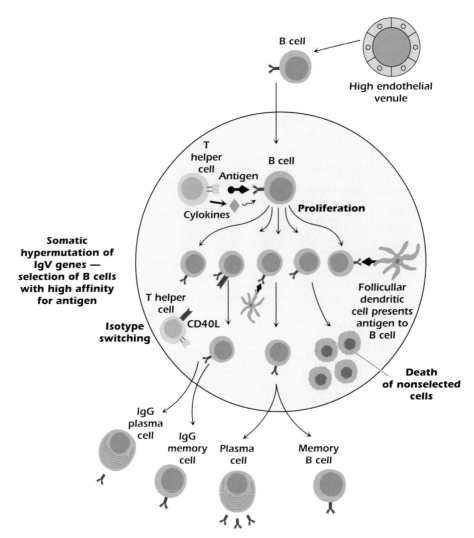

Figure 25.5. Development of B cells in the germinal center: somatic hypermutation, affinity maturation, isotype switching, memory B cell and plasma cell formation, and cell death.

B cells. The constitutive expression of bcl-2 in the lymphoma cells prevents their natural death.

What is the fate of germinal center B cells which are specific for the antigen and which survive?

The B cells which survive as the result of continued stimulation are believed to become the centrocytes of the light zone of the germinal center. The ultimate fate of the cells which do not undergo apoptosis is to become a memory B cell or a plasma cell. These cells will have undergone heavy-chain isotype class switching (as well as SHM) to allow the production of IgG, IgA, or IgE.

Some of the factors determining the alternative fates of these B cells and the transition times through the stages are known. As will be discussed below and further in Case 26, **Bcl-6** is a critical transcription factor which acts to prevent the premature differentiation of the B cell into a plasma cell by inhibiting the transcription of plasma cell-specific genes. In addition to inhibiting plasma cell differentiation, Bcl-6 maintains the B-cell-specific gene expression program, keeping the B cell in the stage of undergoing proliferative expansion and SHM and inhibiting its transition to memory B cells. Overall this allows for the affinity maturation of the antibody response before the B cells go on to become memory cells or plasma cells. A third function of Bcl-6 is to inhibit genes which limit the proliferative capacity of the cell. A fourth and related function is its ability to prevent the sensing and correction of DNA damage by those guardians of the genome operative in all the body's cells. These include p53, a tumor suppressor gene and possibly ATR [ataxia-telangiectasia mutated (ATM) and Rad3 related]. Bcl-6 accomplishes this by suppressing the transcription of these genes.

The usefulness of this latter normal function of bcl-6 is evident from the realization that SHM and isotype class switching will be regarded as DNA damage by these normally protective molecules (see Case 4). If expressed, these molecules will prevent cell division and allow the cell to repair its "damaged" DNA or cause the cell to die.

Characteristic Translocations in B-Cell Lymphomas Contributing to Transformation and Clinical Behavior

During the normal course of B-cell response to antigen, the immunoglobulin genes continue to undergo rearrangement for isotype switching and somatic mutation for affinity maturation. It is hypothesized that this makes the immunoglobulin genes susceptible sites for translocation of other genes (Fig. 25.6).

BCL-2. As discussed above the translocation of *BCL-2*, the gene for the antiapototic protein, to the immunoglobulin gene leads to its overexpression in these B cells and prevents their death. Specifically *BCL-2* translocates to the J region of the immunoglobulin heavy-chain gene coming under the influence of the regulation of the immunoglobulin genes [t(14;18)]. This leads to the continued expression of bcl-2 protein, and this clone of cells with the translocation therefore accumulates. Over time the lymphoma becomes more aggressive, may acquire additional chromosomal abnormalities, and becomes independent of the expression of bcl-2. The position of the breakpoint resulting in the *BCL-2-IGH* translocation suggests that this event occurs in a precursor B cell during VDJ rearrangement in the bone marrow. In this case, the B cell with the traslocated gene must continue to mature and make its way to the periphery.

Transgenic mice, constitutively expressing bcl-2, develop massive follicular lymphoid hyperplasia. Approximately 30% of the mice progress to lymphoma. This finding also suggests that the overexpression of bcl-2 alone is not sufficient for transformation but that a second event is required.

BCL-1. Mantle cell lymphoma resulting from transformation of mantle zone B cells frequently is associated with the translocation of *BCL-1* to the immunoglobulin heavy-chain gene [t(11;14)]. The *BCL-1* gene codes for cyclin D1, which is necessary for the progression of the cell from G1 to S in the cell cycle. Mantle cell lymphomas thus have a higher proliferative rate than follicular lymphomas and a more aggressive clinical course. Some mantle cell lymphomas have point mutations, rather than translocations that result in overexpression of cyclin D1 and the same clinical outcome.

BCL-6. As discussed above, *BCL-6* codes for a DNA binding protein. The gene for bcl-6 is often translocated in diffuse large B-cell lymphomas but only sometimes has an immunoglobulin gene as its translocation partner [t(3;14)]. Alternatively the lymphoma cells may demonstrate point mutations in *BCL-6*. Either scenario leads to overexpression of the transcription factor. An understanding of the functions of this transcription factor in normal germinal center cells and the consequences of its overexpression for lymphomagenesis has contributed to clinical management of these lymphomas (see below).

c-MYC. c-*MYC* codes for a transcription factor required for normal cell proliferation. In its normal state, c-*MYC* is termed a protooncogene. Protooncogenes code for proteins involved in cell growth, proliferation, and differentiation but require tightly controlled regulation.

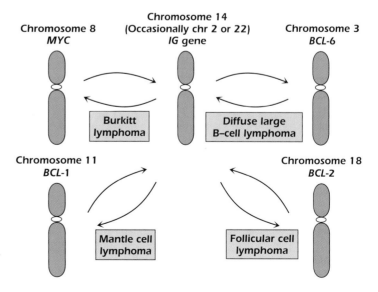

Figure 25.6. Translocation partners with immunoglobulin gene involved in lymphoma development.

The inappropriate expression of these proteins can result in cell transformation. Dysregulation of c-myc is found in many tumors and c-myc is considered an oncoprotein when overexpressed. c-*MYC* is translocated to one of the immunoglobulin genes, most often the heavy-chain gene [t(8;14)], in Burkitt lymphoma, an aggressive B-cell neoplasm. These tumors have a very high proliferation rate, with over 95% of the cells in the cell cycle, and also have a rapid rate of cell death.

Diffuse Large B-Cell Lymphoma

Diffuse large B-cell lymphomas (DLBCLs) are a heterogeneous group of lymphomas about which little was understood until recently. DLBCLs may evolve from a preceding small-cell lymphoid neoplasm such as chronic lymphocytic leukemia/small lymphocytic lymphoma (CLL/SLL) or follicular lymphoma, may develop in an immunodeficient patient in association with a transforming virus such as EBV, or may arise de novo. Among the group of de novo DLBCLs, two prognostic subgroups have been recognized; one that responds well to chemotherapy leading to a cure and another group that responds poorly.

Gene microarray analysis of histologically identical DLBCLs from patients with the same stage of disease allowed classification of two different sets of patients based on the pattern of gene activity. Gene micorarray analysis is used to detect messenger RNA present in the cells and indicate which genes are turned on and being actively transcribed. Complementary DNA (cDNA) copies are made from the RNA extracted from the cells and hybridized with DNA attached to a microchip. The two groups identified correlated well with response to therapy with one group having a five-year survival of 75% and a particular gene expression pattern and a second group having a 15% five-year survival and a different pattern of gene expression. The group with the better survival demonstrated a gene expression profile similar to normal germinal center B cells (GC-like) whereas the group with the poor response to therapy and survival had a gene expression profile similar to normal *in vitro* activated B cells or immunoblasts. In the future it is hoped that this procedure not only will be used to predict the course of the disease but also may identify active genes and their products that could be targeted in therapy. Of the genes differentially expressed in the two prognostic groups, *BCL-6* is believed to have special significance.

Could this correlation to normal germinal center B-cell biology help account for the clinical observation of response to therapy?

The enhanced expression of BCL-6 may contribute to lymphoma formation by preventing the cell from moving beyond the proliferating centroblast stage. This would not explain the response to therapy, however. With continued bcl-6 expression in the lymphoma cells, p53 expression will

remain turned off and the cells' P53 gene will be intact or unmutated. Solid tumors (epithelial neoplasms such as colon cancer) frequently have mutated p53 genes; this is considered to be a major factor in their poor responsiveness to chemotherapy. P53 is a tumor suppressor gene; the function of at least one allele required to prevent the continued proliferation of cells with chromosomal damage. Therefore, a lymphoma with overexpression of bcl-6 and an intact P53 gene (a germinal center cell gene expression profile) may have a better chance of successful treatment. The elimination of bcl-6 by chemotherapeutic agents will release the inhibition of P53 gene expression; the chromosomal damage caused by these agents could then be recognized by the p53, resulting in the initiation of the apoptotic program and elimination of the cell.

CLINICAL FEATURES OF FOLLICULAR LYMPHOMA

Patients usually present with widespread disease (advanced stage), including bone marrow involvement; however, the bone marrow involvement is usually not as extensive as in patients with CLL (see Case 24). Therefore, patients do not present with evidence of bone marrow suppression such as anemia or fatigue. Although follicular lymphoma is slow growing over many years, the malignancy is both progressive and resistant to conventional chemotherapy. The patients initially show a high response rate to standard therapy. After relapse, subsequent remissions in response to different combinations of therapy occur in a progressively lower percentage of patients and are of shorter duration when they do take place. Eventually an aggressive large cell lymphoma evolves in most patients. Median survival is approximately six years.

TREATMENT

Most conventional chemotherapy treatments are not specific for tumor cells and work best against dividing cells. Thus, chemotherapy results in the death of normal cells which naturally continue to divide, such as hair follicles, cells lining the gastrointestinal tract, and nonmalignant cells of the hematopoietic system. Many of the side effects of cancer therapy, including alopecia (hair loss), nausea and vomiting, anemia (decreased red blood cells), easy bruising (due to decreased platelets), and susceptibility to infection (due to decreased neutrophils and decreased normal lymphocytes), are debilitating and some even fatal. An additional problem is that tumors with quiescent cells and/or with low proliferative rates, such as follicular lymphoma, are not well controlled by these treatments. New therapies take advantage of characteristics of the tumor cell that may be lineage specific, such as CD20 in this case, or even tumor specific, in instances when an abnormal protein can be targeted.

High Tech Becomes Therapy

Designer Antibodies. Originally, immunomodulatory antibody treatments in humans used mouse monoclonal antibodies. These antibodies were generated using hybridoma technology. Briefly, mice were immunized with the human antigen, and their antibody-producing cells were isolated, fused *in vitro* with a malignant mouse plasma cell line (myeloma cells), and grown as clones from individual fused cells. Those clones making antibodies of the desired specificity were selected and expanded in culture. The antibodies produced by that clone were thus identical (monoclonal) and directed against a small region (epitope) on the antigen. However, administration of these mouse monoclonal antibodies to humans eventually led to human antimouse antibodies (HAMAs). In addition, the mouse antibodies did not effectively induce elimination of the target cells in the patient. They were not efficient in fixing human complement for complement-mediated lysis, nor did the mouse antibodies react with the Fc receptors on human cells for ADCC or phagocytosis.

Genetic engineering techniques were then applied to the problem. cDNA was made from the RNA for these antibodies and from human antibodies and these DNA segments were cut and recombined *in vitro*. The result was the combination of the DNA coding for the human Fc portion of the immunoglobulin molecule with mouse DNA coding for the Fab portion (antigen-combining site) (see Cases 4 and 26 for immunoglobulin structure). This "chimeric" DNA was then inserted into cultured cells that acted as antibody-producing factories or even into bacteria which served the same function. Anti-CD20 antibody is a chimeric $IgG_1\kappa$ antibody, approximately 25% mouse and 75% human. Approximately 50% of patients receiving these preparations still developed antibodies called human antichimeric antibodies (HACAs). Recently, some therapeutic antibodies have been made by using only the hypervariable portions of the mouse Fab fragment with the remainder of the molecule being human. These "humanized" antibodies induce a lower but still significant incidence of human antihumanized antibodies (HAHAs). This may be the best which can be achieved. Even within an individual, if a large amount of antibody of a single specificity is made, that unique hypervariable region, called the idiotype, can be immunogenic, leading to anti-idiotype antibodies. Reaction against the idiotype is postulated to be a normal control mechanism of the immune response.

CD20 was determined to be the most effective target for antibody-directed therapy since it does not shed or modulate off the surface of the B cells. Being specifically expressed on B cells, treatment against CD20 allows the patients to retain their T-cell immune function, rendering them less susceptible to infection.

Stem Cell Transplant. The toxic effects of chemotherapy on the hematopoietic cells or bone marrow limit the dose that can be administered. Replenishing or rescuing the bone marrow with stem cells has been used in animal models for decades and is now regularly applied as clinical treatment in humans.

Stem cells were originally isolated from bone marrow, requiring multiple aspirations from the donor's marrow. Although this procedure is still used, stem cells can also be harvested from peripheral blood, as small numbers of these cells are present in the circulation. Advantage is taken of the expression of CD34 on the surface of stem cells to isolate them. Granulocyte colony-stimulating factor (G-CSF), granulocyte–monocyte colony-stimulating factor (GM-CSF), or G-CSF plus stem cell factor (SCF) is administered to the donor to increase the number of stem cells in the circulation.

In making a choice between allogeneic and autologous stem cell transplant, several principles of immunology must be considered and applied. For allogeneic transplant, the donor and recipient must be matched at the major and most minor histocompatibility loci, requiring HLA typing (see Case 20 for a discussion of allogeneic renal transplants). Sibling donors are most likely to match the patient. Even with matching, life-long immunosuppression of the recipient is necessary to prevent host-versus-graft disease. This leaves the patient vulnerable to infections and some cancers due to lack of immune surveillance (see Case 9). The transplanted cells that develop into lymphocytes must learn the recipient's MHC as self (see Case 3) to avoid graft-versus-host (GVH) disease and to collaborate with host APCs in the development of an immune response against foreign invaders. Chronic GVH disease is a difficult complication to manage in these patients. On the other hand, in some types of hematologic malignancies, a graft-versus-leukemia (GVL) effect is seen in allogeneic transplants with certain histocompatibility mismatching, and this prevents relapse. The GVL effect is due to the activity of T cells and natural killer (NK) cells in the graft. The NK cells kill without prior sensitization, lysing targets which have reduced levels of MHC class I or inappropriate class I on their surface. Although active in myeloid leukemia, this latter effect is not very prominent in follicular lymphomas.

Autologous stem cell transplant requires elimination or purging of tumor cells. Even after selection of $CD34^+$ stem cells, there is contamination with tumor cells. Purging may be accomplished in several ways, all of which take advantage of tumor cell surface antigens. A "cocktail" of several antibodies against B-cell antigens (CD10, CD19, CD20, CD22) can be incubated with the harvested cells followed by incubation with complement to initiate complement-mediated lysis. Alternatively, the antibodies may be attached to magnetic beads and the reacting cells removed in a magnetic field. The same principle is applied by using these antibodies bound to a column to extract the lymphoma cells or using a fluorescent-activated cell sorter to separate the cells with antibodies bound (see Unit V).

The purity of the preparation may be verified at the molecular level by taking advantage of the ability to detect the lymphoma cells' characteristic translocation, t(14;18). Fluorescent *in situ* hybridization (FISH; see Unit V) can detect abnormal cells by using fluorescent-labeled probes that react with specific DNA segments. Two probes, one for the *BCL-2* gene and a second for the *IGH* gene, can be used and their independent versus combined signals evaluated. Alternatively, a single probe for the translocation site can be employed.

More sensitive for the detection of a very low number of cells is the use of PCR (see Unit V). Briefly, oligonucleotides complementary to the DNA in both the *BCL-2* gene (usually at the major break point) and the consensus J region of *IGH* are used as primers, and repeated copies of that DNA segment are made. Since only the translocation site has this unique junctional complex, amplification of the abnormal gene can be used to quantitate the number of copies. PCR, which has a sensitivity of $1/10^5$ cells, is used to check the purity of marrow cells for transplant and to follow the patient for the first signs of relapse.

REFERENCES

Alizadeh AA, Eisen MB, Davis RE, Ma C, Lossos IS, Rosenwald A, Boldrick JC, Sabet H, Tran T, Yu X, Powell JI, Yang L, Marti GE, Moore T, Hudson J Jr, Lu L, Lewis DB, Tibshirani R, Sherlock G, Chan WC, Greiner TC, Weisenburger DD, Armitage JO, Warnke R, Levy R, Wilson W, Grever MR, Byrd JC, Botstein D, Brown PO, Staudt LM (2000): Distinct types of diffuse large B-cell lymphoma identified by gene expression profiling. *Nature* 405:503–511.

Freedman AS, Neuberg D, Mauch P, Soiffer RJ, Anderson KC, Fisher DC, Schlossman R, Alyea EP, Takvorian T, Jallow H, Kuhlman C, Ritz J, Nadler LM, Gribben JG (1999): Long-term follow-up of autologous bone marrow transplantation in patients with relapsed follicular lymphoma. *Blood* 94:3325–3333.

Hunault-Berger M, Ifrah N, Solal-Celigny P (2002): Intensive therapies in follicular non-Hodgkin lymphomas. *Blood* 100:1141–1152.

Klein U, Dalla-Favera R (2008): Germinal centres: Role in B-cell physiology and malignancy. *Nature Rev Immunol* 8:22–32.

Küppers R (2005): Mechanisms of B-cell lymphoma pathogenesis. *Nature Rev Cancer* 5:251–262.

Phan RT, Dalla-Favera R (2004): The BCL-6 proto-oncogene suppresses p53 expression in germinal centre B cells. *Nature* 432:635–639.

Ranuncolo SM, Polo JM, Dierov J, Singer M, Kuo T, Greally J, Green R, Carroll M, Melnick A (2007): Bcl-6 mediates the germinal center B cell phenotype and lymphomagenesis through transcriptional repression of the DNA-damage sensor ATR. *Nature Immunol* 8:705–714.

Tan P, Mitchell DA, Buss TN, Holmes MA, Anasetti C, Foote J (2002): "Superhumanized" antibodies: Reduction of immunogenic potential by complementarity-determining region grafting with human germline sequences: Application to an anti-CD28. *J Immunol* 169:1119–1125.

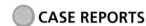

26

PLASMA CELL NEOPLASMS

SUSAN R. S. GOTTESMAN

CASE REPORTS

"Clinic Day": Monday afternoon is myeloma clinic day and you are scheduled to see three patients: Sally, Franny, and Michael.

Presentations

Sally. Sally, a 65-year-old female, is here for her biannual blood tests. She has been coming for 10 years, since she was discovered to have a small *monoclonal spike* in serum protein electrophoresis. The study was conducted following the finding of elevated protein on blood tests during a routine checkup. Although her immunoglobulin level has been slowly increasing, she remains asymptomatic and is not in need of treatment. She carries a diagnosis of *monoclonal gammapathy of undetermined significance (MGUS).*

Franny. Franny is a 47-year-old female also here for her checkup but you see her monthly. Three years ago she presented to the emergency room with back pain and paratheses (numbness) in her legs. Workup at that time included magnetic resonance imaging (MRI) that revealed a paraspinal mass compressing the spinal cord. This necessitated emergency surgery to remove the mass and alleviate pressure on the spinal cord. Upon histologic examination,

the mass proved to be comprised entirely of plasma cells. This finding plus the presence of a large monoclonal spike in the serum and Bence Jones proteins in the urine led to the diagnosis of aggressive *plasma cell myeloma* (multiple myeloma). Franny was subsequently treated with paraspinal region radiation and an aggressive chemotherapy regimen. She has had a stormy course complicated by infections and renal failure. At present she is doing relatively well on a clinical trial of thalidomide.

Michael. Michael is a 60-year-old male who began to experience blurry vision and headaches about four years ago. These symptoms continued and were more recently accompanied by discomfort in his fingers on cold days. He finally saw an ophthalmologist who, upon examination of Michael's eye grounds with an ophthalmoscope, detected dilated tortuous blood vessels accompanied by microinfarcts in both eyes. He also noted that Michael's fingers had a dusky, even purplish shade. The ophthalmologist suspected the presence of a "hyperviscosity" syndrome and sent Michael to a hematologist, who subsequently made the diagnosis of *Waldenström macroglobulinemia* and initiated treatment. Michael is now followed in your clinic.

What is common to all three patients?

All three patients have a proliferation of plasma cells with overproduction and secretion of their product, immunoglobulin. Moreover, these plasma cells are

---

Immunology: Clinical Case Studies and Disease Pathophysiology, By Warren Strober and Susan R. S. Gottesman
Copyright © 2009 John Wiley & Sons, Inc.

337

monoclonal—they originate from a single founder cell and secrete immunoglobulin molecules that are identical in structure and amino acid composition. The three patients have varied presentations and clinical courses ranging from asymptomatic (Sally) to risk of immediate paralysis (Franny) to stroke and possible death (Michael). These differences are due to differences in the rate of accumulation of the plasma cells (proliferation), location of the plasma cells, and characteristics and levels of their immunoglobulin products.

Diagnostic Workup

At presentation, the three patients required many of the same diagnostic tests, albeit with different degrees of urgency. These included identification and quantification of the immunoglobulin product, semiquantification and morphologic examination of the plasma cells in the bone marrow, and *staging* or determination of the extent of disease in the body. Franny, of course, urgently needed a diagnosis of the mass lesion in her spine and immediate treatment to alleviate the spinal pressure.

These histories lead to the consideration of when a physican may suspect that a patient has increased immunoglobulins and how to characterize and quantitate them.

First Hint: Routine Blood Chemistries.
Routine blood chemistries, as illustrated in Sally's case, provide levels of total protein and albumin, the major protein in serum. In addition to albumin, serum proteins include immunoglobulins. When levels of immunoglobulins increase, the difference between albumin level and total protein level is greater than expected.

Quantification: Serum Protein Electrophoresis.
Serum protein electrophoresis (SPEP) separates proteins into broad categories and can thus be used to quantify the total amount of immunoglobulin in the blood (see Coico and Sunshine, Chapter 4; for detailed description of assays see also Unit V). Serum (blood from which cells and clotting factors have been removed) is applied to an acetate strip or to an agarose gel and subjected to an electric field. The proteins in the serum migrate according to their net charge under the pH conditions used during electrophoresis so that, at pH 8.6 (the pH usually employed), five regions are distinguished. Albumin has a relatively negative net charge and migrates near the anode. Moving from anode to cathode, the regions are designated α_1, α_2, β, and γ. After electrophoresis the proteins in the various bands are quantitated using protein-binding dyes and a densitometer. At pH 8.6, immunoglobulins, with their relatively neutral net charge, migrate toward the cathode. Thus the γ region contains most of the immunoglobulin, the exception being IgA, half of which migrates in the β region (Fig. 26.1). (*Note:* The designation γ-globulin here does not refer to IgG; rather it indicates proteins migrating in the γ region on electrophoresis and includes all the immunoglobulin classes.)

In a normal individual, the proteins in the γ region or γ globulin appear as a broad, somewhat diffuse band since each of its constituent immunoglobulins (even those of the same class) has a slightly different charge due to variations in the amino acid sequence of the antigen-binding (variable) region (Fig. 26.1A&C). However, a patient with a monoclonal immunoglobulin will show a sharp band of protein at a particular mobility (Fig. 26.1A&B), designated an M spike (M stands for monoclonal, not IgM).

Definitive Classification: Immunoelectrophoresis or Immunofixation.
To determine which immunoglobulin class comprises the spike, immunoelectrophoresis or immunofixation electrophoresis is commonly used (see Unit V). In immunoelectrophoresis, serum is inserted into a well or hole in an agarose gel and an electric current is applied so that the different serum proteins, including various immunoglobulin classes, migrate to different positions. Antibodies specific for the individual heavy chains and light chains are then applied to a trough situated parallel to the migrating proteins. With normal serum, the antibodies react with the immunoglobulins to form a symmetric arc-shaped immunoprecipitate; with serum containing a monoclonal spike, the antibodies react with one of the immunoglobulins to form an asymmetric and distorted arc (see Coico and Sunshine chapter 5). In immunofixation, serum electrophoresis is performed as for SPEP, but in this case multiple acetate strips or gels are set up. After electrophoresis, polyclonal goat or rabbit antihuman antibodies (detecting antibodies) directed against a specific heavy or light chain class are individually applied to separate strips. This leads to precipitation of an antigen–antibody complex (in a sharply defined zone of equivalence) in the strip containing the antibody specific for the monoclonal spike. The strips are then washed to remove protein that has not been precipitated and the complexes are detected using a protein-binding dye as above (Fig. 26.2).

If light chains and heavy chains have different molecular weights and charges, why does the band developed with the specific anti-light-chain antibody (i.e., anti-κ) occupy the same position in its strip as the band developed with the specific anti-heavy-chain antibody (i.e., anti-γ)?

When the serum is run, the immunoglobulins are intact and are not broken down into their composite chains. The monoclonal immunoglobulin molecule (i.e., IgGκ) is therefore migrating to the same position in each strip. Different detecting antibodies (anti–light chain or anti–heavy chain) react with the intact immunoglobulin, which is in the same position in the individual strips.

A: M spike 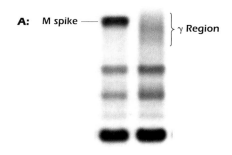 γ Region

B: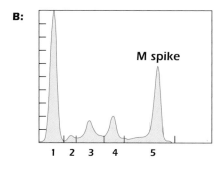

M spike

1 2 3 4 5

Fraction	%	% Ref. Range	g/dL	g/dL Ref. Range
1. Albumin	45.42–	52.00–65.00	3.82	3.20–5.60
2. Alpha 1	2.41–	2.50–5.00	0.20	0.10–0.40
3. Alpha 2	12.06	7.00–13.00	1.01	0.40–1.20
4. Beta	10.52	8.00–14.00	0.88	0.50–1.10
5. Gamma	29.60+	12.00–22.00	2.49+	0.50–1.60
Total			8.40+	6.00–8.30

Restricted Band	%	g/dL		
Gamma	23.49	1.97		

Ratio				
A/G	0.83			

C:

1 2 3 4 5

Fraction	%	% Ref. Range	g/dL	g/dL Ref. Range
1. Albumin	46.37–	52.00–65.00	3.66	3.20–5.60
2. Alpha 1	2.71	2.50–5.00	0.20	0.10–0.40
3. Alpha 2	16.52+	7.00–13.00	1.30+	0.40–1.20
4. Beta	14.73+	8.00–14.00	1.16+	0.50–1.10
5. Gamma	19.67	12.00–22.00	1.55	0.50–1.60
Total			7.90	6.00–8.30

Ratio				
A/G	0.86			

Figure 26.1. (**A**) Serum protein electrophoresis: Left column shows M spike, presumed monoclonal band in gamma region. Right column shows polyclonal pattern. (**B**) Densitometer tracing and measurements of SPEP sample showing M spike in part A (left column). (**C**) Densitometer tracing and measurement of SPEP sample showing polyclonal pattern in part A (right column). +: above reference range −: below reference range

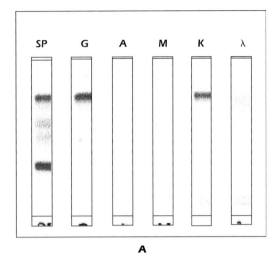

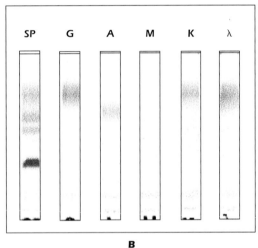

🔵 Figure 26.2. (**A**) Immunofixation electrophoresis of serum showing M spike in Figures 26.1A (left column) and 26.1B. Monoclonal immunoglobulin of IgGκ is documented. Notice the bands appear in the same location in the gel developed with anti-γ chain and the gel developed with anti-κ chain. Serum is run with immunoglobulins intact, resulting in their precipitation in the same location in the electrophoretic field. (**B**) Immunofixation electrophoresis (IFE) of serum showing polyclonal pattern in Figures 26.1A (right column) and 26.1C. IFE confirms the polyclonal pattern. Most of the serum immunoglobulin is IgG with a small amount of IgA. The κ and λ light chains are approximately equivalent.

Quantification of Plasma Cells: A Window into the Body. Although plasma cell proliferations sometimes form mass lesions as in Franny's case, plasma cells generally "home" (migrate) to the bone marrow. Thus, a sample of bone marrow is taken in an attempt to quantify the plasma cell burden in the body. In addition, these malignant plasma cells affect the bone structure, causing breakdown or lysis of bone and releasing calcium.

Lytic lesions are detected on radiographic skeletal survey as part of the workup. This information is added to the data collected on the level of immunoglobulin product.

Diagnosis of Plasma Cell Dyscrasias

Plasma cell myeloma is a clinical pathologic diagnosis that involves specific criteria based on the tests described above. In addition to multiple myeloma or plasma cell myeloma and MGUS, there are solitary plasmacytoma and smoldering myeloma designations.

Review of Presentations and Clinical Courses

Sally has a clone of plasma cells whose product, a monoclonal immunoglobulin, was an incidental finding. Although the number of these cells may be slowly increasing, it is not now and may never cause her any difficulty. In other words, her disease may never progress to multiple myeloma. Nevertheless, it is important to follow her to verify that her disease has not progressed to the point where it meets the diagnostic criteria for multiple myeloma or smoldering myeloma as outlined in Table 26.1. Sally is considered to have a plasma cell dyscrasia or MGUS.

Franny, in contrast, has a clone of plasma cells that has a more dangerous biologic behavior, even though it may be producing the same immunoglobulin subclass as Sally's cells. Franny has symptoms relating to the accumulation of those malignant cells and to the production of high levels of immunoglobulin. The former can lead to mass effects (such as her paraspinal plasmacytoma); the latter can lead to various types of organ dysfunction, the most serious of which is renal dysfunction and failure. The malignant plasma cells can also have marrow suppressive effects leading to anemia and can have suppressive effects on normal B cells that produce protective antibodies, leading to susceptibility to infections. Franny fulfills the diagnostic criteria for plasma cell myeloma and required immediate treatment. Although her age at diagnosis is younger than usual for plasma cell myeloma, this could be due to the fact that Franny is African-American, an ethnic group recognized to develop aggressive plasma cell myeloma at an earlier age.

Michael, although he also has a malignant clone of plasma cells, has a different entity, most likely a lymphoma producing excessive amounts of IgM and causing macroglobulinemia. He presented with blurry vision, headaches, and changes in the extremities, all indications of circulatory problems in small vessels. The underlying pathophysiology leading to these symptoms was revealed by the fact that exposure to cold caused pain in his hands; this pointed to the presence of circulating immunoglobulin that precipitates from solution upon exposure to cold: cryoglobulin (also see Case 23). In many patients with Waldenström macroglobulinemia, the

TABLE 26.1. World Health Organization Criteria of Plasma Cell Dyscrasias

Multiple Myeloma Diagnostic Criteria

1. Plasma cells: ≥10% monoclonal plasma cells in bone marrow (or ≥30% if nonsecretory) *and/or* plasmacytoma (mass of plasma cells)

2. Monoclonal immunoglobulin in serum or urine: serum IgG ≥ 3.0 g/dL, serum IgA ≥ 2.0 g/dL, or urine light chain >1g/24 h

3. Myeloma-related organ dysfunction: elevated serum calcium, renal insufficiency, anemia, *and/or* lytic bone lesions

MGUS Diagnostic Criteria

1. Plasma cells: ≤10% monoclonal plasma cells in bone marrow

2. Low monoclonal immunoglobulin in serum or urine

3. Normal serum calcium, hemoglobin, and creatinine (renal function); no bone lesions, no evidence of amyloidosis or light-chain disease

Waldenström Macroglobulinemia Diagnostic Criteria

Monoclonal IgM (or rarely, IgA) level >3 g/dL. This is usually found in patients with lymphoplasmacytic lymphoma but may also be seen in individuals with marginal zone lymphoma of mucosa-associated lymphoid tissue (MALT) type.

IgM has autoantibody activity and thus may also cause complications based on the autoantigen it is directed against, for example, myelin, clotting factors, or platelets.

 PATHOPHYSIOLOGY OF INCREASED IMMUNOGLOBULIN LEVELS

Normal Immunoglobulin Structure

The basic immunoglobulin molecule consists of two light chains and two heavy chains connected by disulfide bonds (Fig. 26.3). If the molecule is cut by the enzyme papain, it is divided into two fragments with different biologic functions. The ***Fab portion***, which contains the complete light chains and the variable portion of the heavy chains, is the antigen-binding region of the molecule. The ***Fc fragment*** (crystallizable fragment) contains the remaining constant region of the heavy chains and governs the molecule's biologic properties. This portion of the immunoglobulin molecule controls how it functions in the body, such as whether it can bind complement, whether it can cross the placenta, and which cells it can bind to via their Fc receptors. The immunoglobulin molecule derives its heavy-chain subclass designation from the constant regions it uses for its Fc portion.

What is the structure of the different immunoglobulin subclasses?

IgG is a monomeric immunoglobulin molecule with two light chains and two heavy chains linked by disulfide bonds; it therefore has two antigen-binding sites. IgD and IgE have similar structures. IgA, in its secreted serum form, is a dimeric immunoglobulin consisting of two basic immunoglobulin molecules held together by a J chain. In addition, at mucosal surfaces IgA binds to a secretory component to facilitate its transport through epithelial cells and retains a portion of this molecule as it is released onto the mucosal surface. The IgM molecule is a pentamer of a

basic immunoglobulin molecule and therefore has a total of 10 light chains, 10 heavy chains, and 10 binding sites. The five units are held together by J chains. The molecular weight of IgM is 900,000, while that of IgG is 150,000 daltons.

Consequences of Increased Serum Immunoglobulin

Any large increase in the concentration of positively charged protein in the serum, including immunoglobulins, will tend to neutralize the normal negative charges on the red blood cells and cause them to stick together rather than repel each other. As a result, peripheral blood smears of patients with high levels of IgG or monomeric IgM will exhibit ***rouleaux formation***, i.e. stacking of the red blood cells like coins. In contrast, high levels of pentameric IgM will cause the red cells to agglutinate in large three-dimensional structures which are seen on peripheral blood smears.

How might IgM cause circulatory problems?

The large size of IgM (900,000 Da) leads to the retention of IgM in the intravascular compartment, in contrast to IgG, which is distributed between the intra- and extravascular compartments. This high level of IgM in the circulation plus the large size of the molecule itself results in hyperviscosity and sluggish blood flow, causing capillary perfusion blockade and microinfarction. When circulating in a dimeric form, IgA may also cause hyperviscosity with similar consequences.

What is cryoglobulin?

Cryoglobulin is an immunoglobulin molecule which precipitates at low temperature—hence its ability to cause circulatory difficulties in the fingertips exposed to the cold. It may be composed of a single monoclonal immunoglobulin, IgM, as occurs in Waldenström macroglobulinemia (type I), or it may be mixed, formed by a reaction between an autoreactive immunoglobulin and a second immunoglobulin

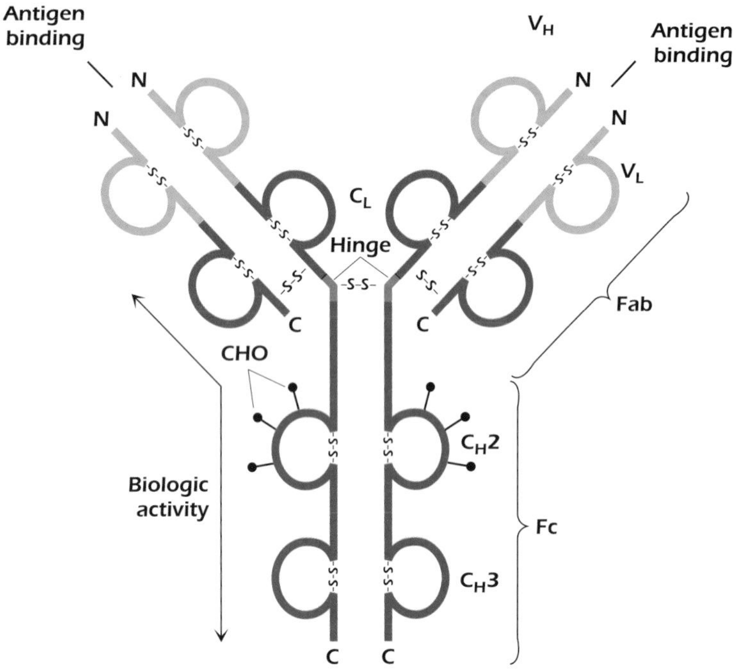

Figure 26.3. Immunoglobulin molecule showing immunoglobulin fold domains formed by intrachain disulfide bonds.

(types II and III). In either case, precipitation occurs below 37° C.

How do you explain Michael's presentation?

Hyperviscosity and cryoglobulinemia together account for at least some of Michael's symptoms. Hyperviscosity probably caused the disturbances in the retinal microcirculation and led to blurred vision and findings on opthalmolopathic exam. This symptom leads to concern that other organs commonly involved by small-vessel disease, the brain and kidney, will be affected. The reported headache therefore leads to a sense of urgency for immediate action to lower the level of IgM (see plasmapheresis below). In contrast, the symptoms of pain, discoloration, and parathesias in Michael's hands are probably the result of the tendency of his monoclonal IgM to cryoprecipitate, since it is clearly related to exposure to lower temperature.

Renal Failure Due to Excess Immunoglobulin Production and Amyloidosis

Hyperviscosity is not the only cause of renal damage in plasma cell dyscrasias. More commonly, renal damage or even failure can be due to hypercalcemia (increased calcium) as a result of bone breakdown or to the detrimental effects of plasma cell products passing through the kidneys. These products, which may consist of either whole immunoglobulin molecules or, more frequently dimers of light chains, known as **Bence Jones proteins**, may collect in the tubules. Bence Jones proteins are secreted in the urine of those myeloma patients making excess light chains. This

occurs more commonly in patients producing λ-containing immunoglobulin than in those producing immunoglobulins containing κ chains.

Light chains, also usually λ type, may deposit in the renal tubules and in the walls of small vessels in numerous organs as a special protein structure called amyloid. **Amyloid** is a general term for extracellular deposits of amorphous, homogeneous proteinaceous material that stain with metachromatic dyes. These deposits cause necrosis (death) of the neighboring cells by pressure atrophy. Although amyloid may be comprised of a variety of glycoproteins depending on the disease situation, they share a fibrillary structure that forms β-pleated sheets. This structure is appreciated on electron microscopy and X-ray crystallography and accounts for their properties upon staining with metachromatic dyes and examination using polarized light microscopy. Amyloidosis associated with plasma cell dyscrasias is composed of light chains, usually λ, and is called systemic **primary amyloidosis**.

Amyloidosis may also be seen in patients with chronic inflammatory diseases and is designated systemic **secondary amyloidosis**. In rheumatoid arthritis and chronic infections such as tuberculosis, the amyloid is composed of serum amyloid-associated protein (SAA), a protein synthesized by the liver. In patients with chronic renal failure from causes other than a plasma cell disorder, the amyloid is composed of SAA or proteins such as β_2-microglobulin. **Localized amyloidosis** is restricted to one organ and occurs in endocrine glands in association with endocrine tumors, in the heart as an isolated inherited entity due to a mutation in the transthyretin gene, and in the cerebral plaques in Alzheimer's disease.

PATHOPHYSIOLOGY OF PLASMA CELL DYSCRASIAS

Up to this point we have been discussing the products of the plasma cells and the havoc those products wreak rather than the biologic basis or the spectrum of plasma cell diseases. Strictly speaking, some of the clinical consequences of markedly increased immunoglobulin do not require that it be monoclonal. High levels of polyclonal immunoglobulins, such as that occasionally occurring in acquired immunodeficiency syndrome (AIDS), can cause similar problems.

Plasma Cell Biology

What is the job of a plasma cell?

The job of the plasma cell is to synthesize and secrete large amounts of its specific antibody. It is a high-output factory with a single product (Fig. 26.4). The manipulations of its DNA (rearrangement, isotype switching, somatic hypermutation for affinity maturation) happened at an earlier stage, when it was a B cell, usually in the germinal center (see Case 25).

To accomplish the task of mass producing its protein product, immunoglobulin, the cell changes from a B cell to a plasma cell. Like all cells with the primary function of producing large amounts of secreted protein, the amount of cytoplasm and rough endoplasmic reticulum increases, and the Golgi region, where the protein is folded and packaged, becomes prominent. In addition to becoming a high-production Ig factory, the cell must alter the immunoglobulin produced to the secreted, rather than the membrane-bound, form. This is accomplished by differential splicing of the RNA message so that the transmembrane piece is no longer translated. Lastly, as is seen everywhere in cell development, during the plasma cell's differentiation, it loses its high proliferative potential as it increases its productive capacity.

Accompanying these alterations of form and purpose, the plasma cell also changes its expression of the surface molecules that control its function. It no longer requires T-cell help and down-regulates its major histocompatibility complex (MHC) class II molecules. It is also no longer receiving signals through its B-cell receptor (BCR), and the expression of surface molecules (CD19, CD21, CD22, CD45) and intracellular messengers that modulate the signal from the BCR decreases. Chemokine receptors, CXCR5 and CCR7, which maintain the B cell's presence in the germinal center, are also no longer expressed. The plasma cell instead expresses the chemokine receptor CXCR4, which helps its trafficking from the germinal center to the splenic red pulp and bone marrow and begins to express Syndecan-1, which recognizes bone marrow extracellular matrix and stromal cells. It also expresses the integrin VLA-4 (very

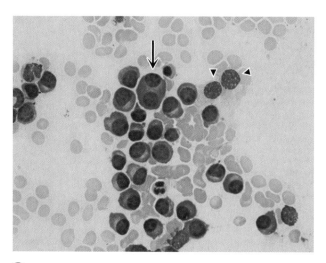

Figure 26.4. Bone marrow aspirate of patient with plasma cell myeloma (magnification 1000×). This would be typical of a patient like Franny at the time of diagnosis. The majority of cells present are plasma cells with typical plasma cell morphology. One binucleate plasma cell (arrow) (not a feature diagnostic of malignancy), two osteoblasts in the upper right side (arrow heads), two erythroid precursors, and three developing myeloid cells are seen.

late antigen 4), which increases its ability to contact bone marrow stromal cells. This contact is needed for the plasma cells to receive IL-6 produced from these supporting cells (Fig. 26.5).

The above changes in cell surface antigen expression, which result in new trafficking and signaling patterns, are orchestrated by the transcription factors operating within the cell. These include bcl-6 and pax5, factors which are required to maintain the cell as a B cell and block plasma cell differentiation, and Blimp-1, XBP-1 and IRF4, transcription factors needed to activate genes important in plasma cell formation and feedback to inhibit the B-cell transcription factors (bcl-6 and pax5).

Bcl-6 is required for the germinal center reaction and represses *PRDM1*, the gene encoding Blimp-1, thereby preventing plasma cells from developing prematurely. *Pax5*, B lineage-specific activator protein, activates a group of genes whose products are required for BCR signaling (CD19, CD79a, Syk, and BLNK) and represses those for Ig secretion (XBP-1, J chain, and IgH).

When the B cell receives a strong signal through its BCR, bcl-6 decreases, releasing *PRDM1* and allowing the synthesis of Blimp-1. Blimp-1 is also increased by cytokine signals from T helper cells; these include IL-2, IL-5, IL-6, and IL-10, all of which signal through Stat3. *Blimp-1* then represses Pax, thus releasing the expression of genes for Ig secretion, and represses bcl-6, ensuring plasma cell differentiation. The loss of Pax repression and the stimulation by IL-6 lead to expression of *XBP-1*, a factor required

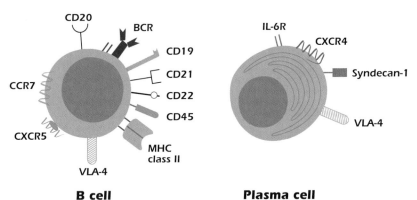

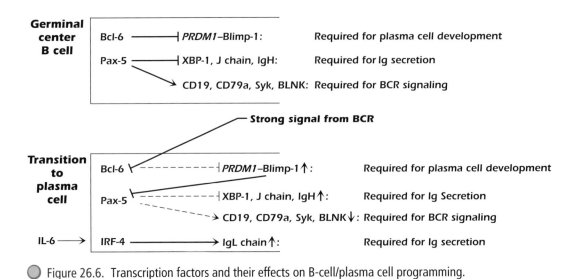

Figure 26.5. B cell with surface markers; plasma cell with surface markers.

for plasma cell development by an as-yet-unknown mechanism. Finally, *IRF4*, a member of the interferon regulatory factor family, is expressed when the germinal center B cell makes the commitment to become a plasma cell and, among other effects, activates enhancers of the immunoglobulin light-chain genes (Fig. 26.6).

Having made the above changes, the cell, now in the form of a "plasmablast," leaves the germinal center and migrates to various tissue sites. Although some of these cells are still producing IgM antibodies, many have undergone class switching in the germinal center (see Case 25). Thus, the majority of plasma cell myelomas are IgG- or IgA-secreting cells.

Some plasmablasts migrate to areas repeatedly stimulated by the same antigen. However, others migrate to the bone marrow and are maintained there for years under the influence of stromal cells that provide survival signals, notably IL-6. This interaction with the bone marrow stromal cells is similar to the situation with all the hematopoietic cells which also depend on the bone marrow microenvironment. The plasma cells will divide and finish their differentiation to mature plasma cells independent of antigen. This accumulation of Ig-secreting plasma cells in the

marrow increases with age, thus providing a cellular substrate for the development of myeloma.

Where Does Waldenström Macroglobulinemia Fit In?

Although it is clear that the normal counterparts of myeloma cells are the terminally differentiated plasma cells that have homed to the bone marrow, the analogy to normal is murkier in macroglobulinemia. In Waldenström macroglobulinemia, the cells producing the monoclonal IgM are often a mixture of lymphocytes, plasma cells, and something in between called lymphoplasmacytoid cells. The short answer to the question regarding the normal counterpart to the malignant cell in Waldenström macroglobulinemia is "not known." The longer answer is that it may depend on the underlying lymphoma producing this IgM. Sometimes macroglobulinemia is associated with marginal-zone lymphomas. Marginal-zone lymphocytes are particularly numerous in mucosa-associated lymphoid tissue (MALT). These cells, along with B1 cells (see Case 24), generate the body's first humoral response to organisms and are capable of developing into plasma cells

Figure 26.6. Transcription factors and their effects on B-cell/plasma cell programming.

and secreting antibody in a T-cell-independent fashion. These cells normally undergo apoptosis after a few days. However, if they are first activated by a T-cell-dependent antigen, they can traffic to the germinal center.

In other patients, the IgM is produced by a lymphoplasmacytic lymphoma. This lymphoma is composed of B cells that have gone through the germinal center and have undergone somatic hypermutation but have not isotype switched. In either case, the production of macroglobulin often arises from malignant cells straddling the transition from B lymphocyte to plasma cell, whether or not they have transited the germinal center.

A Vicious Cycle

The gradually increasing population of plasma cells in the bone marrow requires a series of genetic events to undergo malignant transformation into myeloma cells (see below). The latter, however, are still not cell autonomous and require two-way interactions with stromal cells for their survival and expansion. In fact, a vicious cycle of cross-talk between the myeloma and stromal cells takes place that leads to ever-increasing support for myeloma cell growth (Fig. 26.7).

The myeloma cells produce tumor necrosis factor α (TNF-α), which stimulates the expression of adhesion molecules on both the myeloma cells and stromal cells through its activation of NF-κB. The malignant plasma cells express leukocyte function-assisted antigen 1 (LFA-1), intercellular and vascular adesion molecules (ICAM-1, VCAM-1), and mucin-1 (MUC-1) and the bone marrow stromal cells express ICAM-1 and VCAM-1. This increases the adhesion of the myeloma cells to the stromal cells and both the direct cell–cell contact and TNF-α stimulate IL-6 production by the stromal cells. IL-6 then acts as a survival and growth factor for the malignant plasma cells. Although TNF-α acting alone can induce apoptosis, its role in increasing IL-6 production causes an overall antiapoptotic effect. In addition, the plasma cells, particularly the malignant ones, produce cytokine

products that affect the cells involved in bone formation (osteoblasts) and turnover (osteoclasts). In the malignant situation, the effect on the latter cells, the osteoclasts, is dominant and the net effect is the development of lytic bone lesions that are characteristic of multiple myeloma.

The Genetic Abnormalities Identified in Multiple Myeloma

Obviously since the progeny of a single founder cell proliferates and accumulates in myeloma, there must be an event that initiates it, presumably a genetic mutation. As is the case with many other malignancies, however, no single genetic mutation has been identified to account for the development of multiple myeloma. Only approximately one-half the patients evaluated show a detectable abnormality by standard karyotype analysis. These include trisomies of chromosomes 3, 5, 9, and 15 and monosomies of 13 and 16. Monosomy 13 has been correlated with a poor prognosis. Translocations involving the heavy-chain gene have been found in some patients. In patients with Waldenström macroglobulinemia associated with lymphoplasmacytic lymphoma, 50% have been found to have rearrangement or translocation of the *PAX-5* gene. In multiple myeloma, 30% have been found to have activating point mutations in a *RAS* gene.

TREATMENT OF PLASMA CELL DYSCRASIAS

Overall Objectives of Treatment

It is immediately apparent that the behavior of the plasma cell neoplasms in each of the three patients described above is sufficiently unique to require different treatment plans. Nevertheless, there are certain general (and interrelated) treatment goals: lowering the immunoglobulin product, killing the malignant cells, and dealing with the secondary consequences of both. For MGUS, as the name implies, no

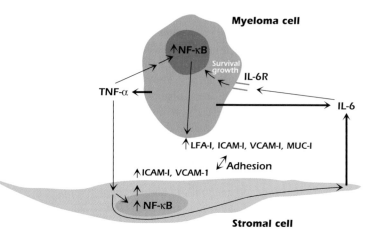

Figure 26.7. Interaction between myeloma cells and bone marrow stromal cells. (Thick arrows denote production of cytokines; thin arrows denote effect.)

treatment is necessary, and watchful waiting is the rule of thumb. In contrast, lowering the level of immunoglobulin is extremely important in Waldenström macroglobulinemia and may be required on an emergency basis. This is usually accomplished by plasmapheresis, a rapid but temporary treatment modality in which the patient is subjected to removal of several units of blood and subsequent return of their red blood cells without the plasma. More sustained therapy addressing all three goals consists of cytotoxic chemotherapy possibly combined with autologous stem cell transplant (similar to that undertaken in cases of follicular lymphoma). These procedures are particularly applicable to Franny's aggressive plasma cell myeloma. However, success rates have been disappointing and recurrence of tumor has been almost inevitable. Alternative strategies take advantage of what is known about the biology of the myeloma cells and their need for support from bone marrow stromal cells. Here the approach is to combine standard chemotherapy with agents designed to disrupt the cellular interactions necessary for sustaining expansion of the myeloma cells.

Immunomodulatory Strategies

Cytokine Interference. Why didn't anti-IL-6 work?

One very logical (but perhaps naive) strategy was to treat patients with anti-IL-6 antibodies. If the myeloma cells need IL-6 as a growth factor, whether made by stromal cells or the myeloma cells themselves, why not just disrupt that stimulation pathway? This was in fact one of the first immunomodulatory strategies tried. However, this treatment was unsuccessful for two important reasons. First, while cytokines may have very specific actions in the immune system, most affect cells in other organ systems in the body. IL-6 has a particularly broad range of activities and therefore anti-IL-6 therapy had significant side effects. In addition, although it is an important cytokine for plasma cell growth, IL-6 is not the sole agent promoting myeloma cell survival and proliferation.

Back to Basics. Several more strategic lines of attack have been developed and are still being evaluated. Among the immunomodulatory drugs (ImiDs) is thalidomide. Thalidomide is perhaps best known for its marked teratogenic actions, which are probably the result of its significant antiangiogenic effects. It holds promise as an effective agent in myeloma because thalidomide modulates the adhesion molecules on both the myeloma and stromal cells and thus inhibits their interaction and their production of cytokines. In addition, it decreases NF-κB activity and thus the effects of production of TNF-α, the stimulus for the expression of adhesion molecules important to myeloma cell–stromal cell crosstalk.

Proteosome inhibitors and arsenic trioxide have also been found to have inhibitory clinical effects on myeloma. All have in common the inhibition of NF-κB activity and may also affect myeloma cell growth by turning off TNF-α production.

An additional target being investigated is Ras. A significant number of myeloma patients have activating mutations in one *RAS* gene, and Ras proteins are important in signal transduction, thus researchers have sought ways to counteract the constitutive activity of this gene. One candidate agent is an inhibitor of farnesyl transferase, the enzyme required for posttranslational lipid modification of Ras protein.

Treatment of one of the serious complications of myeloma, the lytic bone lesions, has been found to affect myeloma cell growth itself. Bisphosphonates are used in the treatment of many malignancies to prevent the bone breakdown that occurs in the situation of bone marrow metastases. These drugs, which suppress osteoclast activity, also disrupt the interaction of the stromal and myeloma cells and may have direct benefits in decreasing tumor cell growth.

Thus, while current therapy for myeloma is not very effective, new agents being developed as a result of our increasing knowledge of the biology of these cells have created a more hopeful outlook for the future.

● MAKING THE BEST OF A BAD SITUATION: RESEARCH TOOLS

The diagnosis of a plasma cell dyscrasia is usually a devastating, life-threatening development for the individual patient. Nevertheless, these plasma cell neoplasms have proved useful in providing material to study the normal immune system and have also been exploited for the development of techniques used in a variety of fields. Thus, our knowledge of the structure of immunoglobulins comes from studying the monoclonal products of myeloma cells. This is particularly true for Bence Jones proteins, which, by virtue of their secretion into the urine, provide a solution of pure monoclonal light chain that allowed the elucidation of light chain structure. Even the concept of monoclonality as applied to an understanding of cancer biology in general owes much to the study of myeloma.

In 1975, the behavior of myeloma cells was adapted by Köhler and Milstein to produce hybridomas. Hybridomas, which manufacture large amounts of monoclonal antibody of a known specificity, are maintained as cell lines, and use of these products has revolutionized medicine in all areas as well as other diverse fields, such as agriculture (see Unit V; see also Coico and Sunshine, Chapter 5).

REFERENCES

Calame KL, Lin KI, Tunyaplin C (2003): Regulatory mechanisms that determine the development and function of plasma cells. *Annu Rev Immunol* 21:205–230.

Köhler G, Milstein C (1975): Continuous cultures of fused cells secreting antibody of predefined specificity. *Nature* 256:495–497.

Durie BGM, Kyle RA, et al. (2003): Myeloma management guidelines: A concensus report from the scientific advisors of the International Myeloma Foundation. *Hematol J* 4:379–398.

Jaffe ES, Harris NL, Stein H, Vardiman JW (2001): *Tumours of Haematopoietic and Lymphoid Tissues*. Lyon, France: IARC Press.

Ludwig H (2005): Advances in biology and treatment of multiple myeloma. *Ann Oncol* 16(Suppl 2):ii106–ii112.

Unit V

LABORATORY TESTS USED IN THE WORKUP OF PATIENTS WITH IMMUNOLOGIC DISEASES*

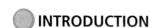

INTRODUCTION

Numerous techniques and assays indispensable for analysis of the underlying defects in immunologic diseases have been referred to in various case studies in this text. Some of these are antibody-based (serologic) methods. Others include molecular methods, cell culture techniques, and analyses of human disease states through the study of animal models. Recently, genome sequence and protein databases have become widely available. A brief summary of the major techniques and assays is included here to enable you to understand their applicability and to help you appreciate the specificity and sensitivity of each test.

METHODS FOR ANALYSIS OF ANTIBODY–ANTIGEN INTERACTIONS

General Considerations

The reaction between antigen and serum antibodies (*serology*) serves as the basis for many immune assays. Because of the exquisite specificity of the immune

response, the interaction between antigen and antibody *in vitro* is widely used for diagnostic purposes for the detection and identification of either antigen or antibody.

Antigen–antibody interactions may result in a variety of consequences, including ***precipitation*** (if the antigen is soluble), ***agglutination*** (if the antigen is particulate), and ***activation of complement***. It should be noted, however, that these outcomes are not primary phenomena due to the simple interaction between antibody and antigen; rather they are secondary phenomena that require the extensive cross-linking that only occurs between multivalent antibodies and antigens, each with at least two combining sites per molecule (Fig. UV.1).

Primary Interactions between Antibody and Antigen

No covalent bonds are involved in the interaction between antibody and an epitope. The relatively weak binding forces consist mainly of ***van der Waals forces, electrostatic forces***, and ***hydrophobic forces***, all of which require the interacting moieties to be in very close proximity. This very close fit is often compared to that between

*Adapted from Chapter 5 of R. Coico, G. Sunshine, and E. Benjamini (2003): *Immunology: A Short Course*, 5th ed. New York: John Wiley & Sons.

Immunology: Clinical Case Studies and Disease Pathophysiology, By Warren Strober and Susan R. S. Gottesman
Copyright © 2009 John Wiley & Sons, Inc.

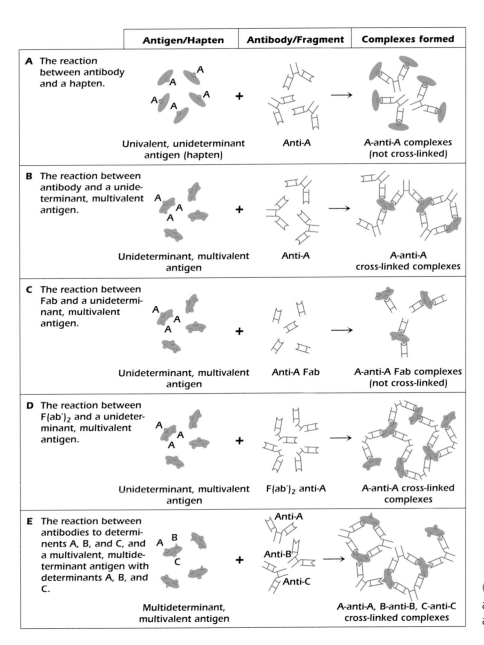

	Antigen/Hapten	Antibody/Fragment	Complexes formed

A The reaction between antibody and a hapten.

Univalent, unideterminant antigen (hapten) + Anti-A → A-anti-A complexes (not cross-linked)

B The reaction between antibody and a unideterminant, multivalent antigen.

Unideterminant, multivalent antigen + Anti-A → A-anti-A cross-linked complexes

C The reaction between Fab and a unidetermi-nant, multivalent antigen.

Unideterminant, multivalent antigen + Anti-A Fab → A-anti-A Fab complexes (not cross-linked)

D The reaction between F(ab')$_2$ and a unideter-minant, multivalent antigen.

Unideterminant, multivalent antigen + F(ab')$_2$ anti-A → A-anti-A cross-linked complexes

E The reaction between antibodies to determi-nents A, B, and C, and a multivalent, multide-terminant antigen with determinants A, B, and C.

Multideterminant, multivalent antigen + Anti-A, Anti-B, Anti-C → A-anti-A, B-anti-B, C-anti-C cross-linked complexes

Figure UV.1. Reactions between antibody or antibody fragments and antigens or hapten.

a lock and key. Because of the low levels of energy involved in the interaction between antigen and antibody, antigen–antibody complexes can be readily dissociated by low or high pH, high salt concentrations, or chaotropic ions such as cyanates, which efficiently interfere with the hydrogen bonding of water molecules.

Association Constant

The reaction between an antibody and an epitope of an antigen is exemplified by the reaction between antibody and a univalent hapten (small antigen with one determinant). Because an antibody molecule is symmetric, with two identical antigen-binding sites per Fab (fragment antigen binding) region, one antibody molecule binds with two identical

monovalent hapten molecules; each binding site reacts in an independent fashion with one hapten molecule (Fig. UV.2).

The *association constant K* is a measure of the affinity of the antibody for the hapten or an epitope of the antigen. When all of the antibody molecules that bind a given hapten or epitope are identical (as in the case of monoclonal antibodies), then K represents the intrinsic association constant. However serum antibodies are normally heterogeneous, therefore, even when they bind to a single epitope, the association constant is an average of association constants of all the antibodies binding to the epitope and is referred to as K_0. The interaction between antibodies and each epitope of a multivalent antigen follows the same kinetics and energetics as those involved in the interaction between antibodies and haptens because each epitope of the

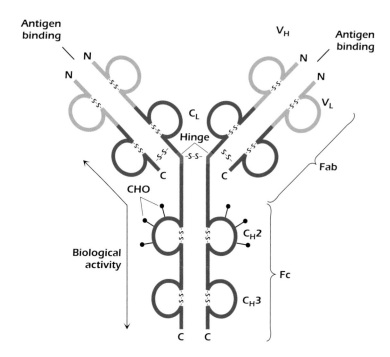

Figure UV.2. The basic antibody molecule.

antigen reacts with its corresponding antibody in the same manner described above.

Affinity and Avidity

The intrinsic association constant that characterizes the binding of an antibody with an epitope or a hapten is termed *affinity*. When the antigen consists of many repeating identical epitopes or when antigens are multivalent, the association between the entire antigen molecule and antibodies depends not only on the affinity between each epitope and its corresponding antibody but also on the sum of the affinities of all the epitopes involved. For example, the affinity of binding of anti-A with multivalent A (shown in Fig. UV.1B) may be four or five orders of magnitude higher than binding between anti-A and univalent A (Fig. UV.1A) because the pairing of anti-A with multivalent A is influenced by the increased number of sites with which anti-A can react.

The term *avidity* is used to denote the overall binding energy between antibodies and a multivalent antigen. Thus, in general, because IgM has 10 binding sites in contrast to IgG (which has two), IgM antibodies are of higher avidity than IgG antibodies, although the binding with ligand of each Fab in the IgM antibody may be of the same affinity as that of the Fab in IgG.

Secondary Interactions between Antibody and Antigen

Agglutination Reactions. Referring again to Figure UV.1, the reactions of antibody with a multivalent antigen that is a *particulate* (i.e., an insoluble particle)

results in the cross-linking of the various antigen particles by the antibodies (Fig. UV.1D and UV.1E). This cross-linking eventually causes clumping or agglutination of the antigen particles by the antibodies.

When the antigen is a natural constituent of a particle, the agglutination reaction is referred to as *direct agglutination*. When the agglutination reaction takes place between antibodies and soluble antigen attached to an insoluble particle, the reaction is referred to as *passive agglutination*.

Titer. The ability of an antibody to cause antigens to agglutinate requires an optimal proportion of antibody relative to antigen. A method sometimes used to measure the level of serum antibody specific for a particulate antigen is the agglutination assay. More sensitive quantitative assays (such as enzyme-linked immunosorbent assay (ELISA), which is discussed later in this unit) have largely replaced the agglutination assay for measuring antibody levels in serum. Indeed, the agglutinating titer is only a semiquantitative expression of the antibodies present in the serum; it is not a quantitative measure of the concentration of antibody (weight/volume). It does, however, provide information on the behavior of antigen–antibody reactions (see below).

The assay is performed by mixing twofold serial dilutions of serum with a fixed concentration of antigen. High dilutions of serum usually do not result in antigen agglutination because there are not enough antibodies to cause appreciable, visible agglutination. The highest dilution of serum that still causes agglutination, but beyond which no agglutination occurs, is termed the *titer*. It is a common observation that agglutination may not occur at high concentrations of antibody (low dilutions), even though it does take place at higher dilutions of serum. The tubes with high concentrations of serum, where agglutination does not occur, represent a *prozone*. In the prozone, antibodies are present in excess. The reason for the absence of agglutination in the prozone is that every epitope on a single particle of antigen may bind to only a single antibody molecule, preventing cross-linking between different particles.

Because of the prozone phenomenon, in testing for the presence of agglutinating antibodies to a certain antigen, it is imperative that the antiserum be tested at several dilutions. Testing serum at only one concentration may give misleading conclusions if no agglutination occurs because the absence of agglutination might reflect either a prozone effect or a lack of antibody.

Zeta Potential. The surfaces of certain particulate antigens may possess an electrical charge, such as the net negative charge on the surface of red blood cells caused by the presence of sialic acid. When such charged particles are suspended in saline solution, an electrical potential termed the *zeta potential* is created between particles, preventing them from getting very close to one another. This makes the agglutination of charged particles by antibodies more difficult, particularly the agglutination of red blood cells by IgG antibodies. The distance between the Fab arms of the IgG molecule, even in its most extended form, is too short to allow effective bridging between two red blood cells across the zeta potential. Thus, although IgG antibodies may be directed against antigens on the charged erythrocyte, agglutination may not occur because of the repulsion by the zeta potential. On the other hand, some of the Fab areas of IgM pentamers are far enough apart and can bridge red blood cells separated by the zeta potential. The zeta potential of IgM antibodies, along with their pentavalence, is a major reason for their effectiveness as agglutinating antibodies.

Through the years attempts have been made to improve agglutination reactions by decreasing the zeta potential in various ways, none of which has proved universally applicable or effective. However, an ingenious method to overcome this problem was devised in the 1950s by Coombs. This method, described below, facilitates the agglutination of erythrocytes by IgG antibodies specific for erythrocyte antigens. It is also useful for the detection of nonagglutinating antibodies present on the surface of patients' erythrocytes.

Coombs Test. The *Coombs test* uses antibodies from a different species that are made to react against human immunoglobulins (heterologous antibodies). These heterologous antibodies detect the presence of autoantibodies on the surface of red blood cells. Hence, The Coombs test is also referred to as the *anti-immunoglobulin test*. It is based on two important facts: (1) immunoglobulins of one species (e.g., human) are immunogenic when injected into another species (e.g., rabbit) and lead to the

production of antibodies against the immunoglobulins and (2) many of the anti-immunoglobulins (e.g., rabbit antihuman Ig) bind to antigenic determinants present on the Fc (fragment crystallizable) portion of the antibody and leave the Fab portions free to react with antigen. For example, if human IgG autoantibodies are attached to erythrocytes, rabbit–antihuman Ig will bind to the Fc portion of the human Ig and form bridges (cross-links) between the red cells, thus causing agglutination.

There are two versions of the Coombs test: the *direct Coombs test* and the *indirect Coombs test*. Although the two versions differ somewhat in mechanics, both are based on the same principle: using heterologous anti-immunoglobulins to detect a reaction between immunoglobulins and antigen. In the direct Coombs test, anti-immunoglobulins are added to the particles (e.g., red blood cells) that are suspected of having antibodies bound to them. In the indirect Coombs test, the patient serum is incubated with test cells and antibodies in the serum are detected by the ability of added antihuman immunoglobulin to result in agglutination. For example, hemolytic disease of the newborn (HDN) is caused by maternal anti-Rh IgG antibodies bound to the baby's erythrocytes. If a newborn baby is suspected of having HDN, the addition of antihuman immunoglobulin to a suspension of the baby's erythrocytes (the direct Coombs test) would cause red blood cell agglutination to occur. In some cases, the direct Coombs test fails due to the zeta potential. The indirect Coombs test can then be used to determine whether the mother's serum contains anti-Rh antibodies. In the indirect Coombs test, the anti-immunoglobulin reagents are added only after the woman's serum is combined with Rh^+ erythrocytes. Thus, the direct Coombs test measures bound antibody and the indirect test measures serum antibody.

Passive Agglutination. The agglutination reaction can be used with soluble antigens provided that the soluble antigen can be firmly attached to an insoluble particle. For example, the soluble antigen thyroglobulin can be attached to latex particles; then, when antibodies to thyroglobulin antigen are added, agglutination of latex particles coated with thyroglobulin will occur. The addition of soluble antigen to the antibodies before the introduction of the thyroglobulin-coated latex particles will inhibit agglutination because the antibodies will combine with the soluble antigen. If the soluble antigen is present in excess of the number of available binding sites, the unbound soluble antigen will block the binding of the antibodies to the particulate antigen; this phenomenon is referred to as *agglutination inhibition*. Passive agglutination can be used to verify the specificity of the antibodies present and to determine the concentration of antibody.

Agglutination reactions are widely used in clinical applications. In addition to the examples already given, major applications include erythrocyte typing in blood banks, diagnosis of immunologically mediated hemolytic diseases such as drug-induced autohemolytic anemia, tests for rheumatoid factor (human IgM antihuman IgG; see Chapter 21), the confirmatory test for syphilis, and the latex test for pregnancy, which involves the detection of human chorionic gonadotropin (HCG) in the urine of pregnant women.

Precipitation Reactions

Reaction in Solutions.   In contrast to the agglutination reaction, which takes place between antibodies and particulate antigen, the **precipitation reaction** takes place when antibodies and soluble antigen are mixed. As in the case of agglutination, precipitation of antigen–antibody complexes occurs because the divalent antibody molecules cross-link multivalent antigen molecules to form a lattice. When it reaches a certain size, this antigen–antibody complex loses its solubility and precipitates out of solution. The phenomenon of precipitation is termed the **precipitin reaction**.

Figure UV.3 depicts a qualitative precipitin reaction. Increasing concentrations of antigen are added to a series of tubes that contain a constant concentration of antibodies, causing variable amounts of precipitate to form. The weight of the precipitate in each tube may be determined by a variety of methods. If the amount of the precipitate is plotted against the amount of antigen added, a precipitin curve like the one shown in Figure UV.3 is obtained.

There are three important areas under the curve shown in Figure UV.3: (1) the zone of antibody excess (prozone), (2) the equivalence zone, and (3) the zone of antigen excess. In the equivalence zone, the proportion of antigen to antibody is optimal for maximal precipitation; in the zones of antibody excess or antigen excess, the proportions of the reactants do not lead to efficient cross-linking and formation of precipitate.

It should be emphasized that the zones of the precipitin curve are based on the amount of antigen–antibody complexes precipitated. However, the zones of antigen or antibody excess may contain soluble antigen–antibody complexes; this is particularly true of the zone of antigen excess, where a minimal amount of precipitate is formed but large amounts of antigen–antibody complexes are present in the supernatant. Thus, the amount of precipitate formed is dependent on the proportions of the reactant antigens and antibodies: The correct proportion of the reactants results in maximal formation of precipitate; excess of antigen (or antibody) results in soluble complexes.

Precipitation Reactions in Gels.   Precipitation reactions between soluble antigens and antibodies can take place not only in solution but also in semisolid media such as agar gels. This occurs when soluble antigen and antibody are placed in wells cut in a gel (Fig. UV.4A) and the antibody and antigen are allowed to diffuse toward and eventually interact with each other. In this "double-diffusion" arrangement, the diffusion creates concentric concentration gradients that result in the formation of a visible precipitate in the zone where the reactants are present at concentrations that facilitate precipitation (Fig. UV.4B).

Radial Immunodiffusion.   The radial immunodiffusion test, depicted in Figure UV.5, is a variation of the double-diffusion test. The wells contain antigen at different concentrations, and the antibodies are distributed uniformly in the agar gel. This results in the formation of a precipitin ring around the well. The distance the precipitin ring migrates from the center of the antigen well is directly proportional to the concentration of antigen in the well. The relationship between concentration of antigen in a well and the diameter of the precipitin ring can be plotted as shown in the graph in Figure UV.5. If wells such as F and G

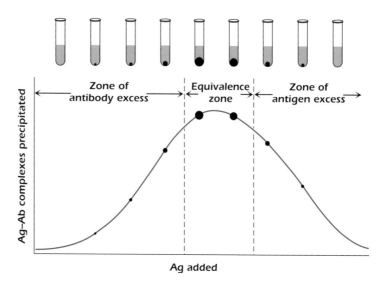

Figure UV.3. Precipitin reaction.

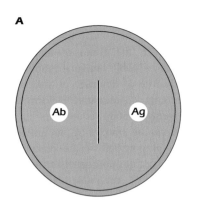

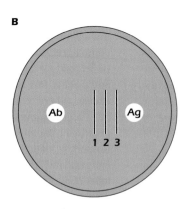

Figure UV.4. (**A**) Gel diffusion by antibodies and a single antigen. (**B**) Gel diffusion by antibodies to antigens 1, 2, and 3.

contain unknown amounts of the same antigen, the antigen concentration can be determined by comparing the diameter of the precipitin ring with the diameter of the ring formed by a known concentration of the antigen.

An important application of radial immunodiffusion is clinical measurement of concentrations of serum proteins. Antiserum to various serum proteins is incorporated in the gel; concentration of a particular protein in a serum sample is determined by comparing the diameter of the resulting precipitin ring with those obtained using known concentrations of the protein.

Immunoassays

Immunoelectrophoresis. Electrophoresis involves separation of a mixture of proteins added to a poly-acrylamide gel through the use of an applied electric field followed by the detection of these proteins with a protein-binding dye. This method is commonly used to characterize and quantitate human serum proteins as a first step since the serum proteins separate into their various components according to their mobilities in the electrical field. By applying specific antibodies to the gel after electrophoretic separation, a method termed *immunoelectrophoresis* or *immunofixation*, the proteins can be more specifically identified and quantitated. The

antibodies diffuse in the agar, as do the separated serum proteins. At an optimal antigen–antibody ratio, each antigen and its corresponding antibodies form precipitin lines. Comparison of the pattern and intensity of lines of normal human serum with the results obtained with sera of patients may reveal an absence, overabundance, or other abnormality of one or more serum proteins. This methodology is used to detect the production of a monoclonal antibody and to quantitate it in patients with plasma cell neoplasms (see Case 26).

Western Blots (Immunoblots). In the **Western blot (immunoblot) technique**, antigen (or a mixture of antigens) is first separated in a gel. The separated material is transferred onto protein-binding sheets (e.g., nitrocellulose) using an electroblotting method. Antibody is then applied to the nitrocellulose sheet and binds with its specific antigen. The antibody may be labeled (e.g., with radioactivity) or a labeled anti-immunoglobulin may be used to localize the antibody and the antigen to which it is bound. These Western blots are used widely in research and clinical laboratories for the detection and characterization of antigens. A particularly useful example is the confirmatory diagnosis of HIV infection (see Case 9) by the application of a patient's serum to the nitrocellulose sheets on which HIV antigens are bound. The finding of specific antibody is strong evidence of infection by the virus (Fig. UV.6).

Radioimmunoassays. The first type of immunoassay developed to detect and quantitate small amounts of antigen, antibody, or antigen–antibody complex was the radioimmunoassay. However, because this assay required the use of radiolabeled molecules and thus a panoply of special procedures that are necessary for the safe use of such molecules, it has been replaced by the solid-phase nonradioactive immunoassay described below or other nonradioactive techniques.

Solid-Phase Immunoassays. Solid-phase immunoassay, one of the most widely used immunologic techniques, is now automated and in clinical medicine is applied to the detection of antigen or antibody. An example is the

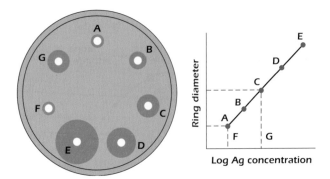

Figure UV.5. Radial diffusion. A, B, C, D, and E represent known concentrations of antigen; F and G represent unknown concentrations that can be determined from the graph.

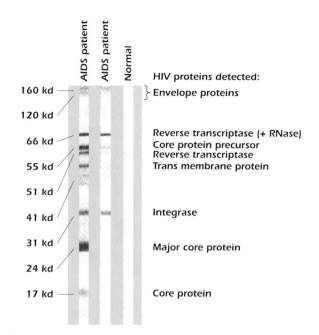

AIDS patient
AIDS patient
Normal

HIV proteins detected:

160 kd — } Envelope proteins

120 kd —

66 kd — Reverse transcriptase (+ RNase)
Core protein precursor
Reverse transcriptase
55 kd — Trans membrane protein

51 kd —

41 kd — Integrase

31 kd — Major core protein

24 kd —

17 kd — Core protein

Figure UV.6. Western blots of serum samples from two HIV-infected individuals and one control subject.

use of solid-phase immunoassay for the detection of antibodies to HIV (see Case 9).

Solid-phase immunoassays employ the ability of plastics such as polyvinyl or polystyrene to adsorb monomolecular layers of proteins onto their surface. Although the adsorbed molecules may lose some of their antigenic determinants, enough of them are still available to their corresponding antibodies such that the presence of these antibodies may be detected by the use of anti-immunoglobulins (Fig. UV.7). These anti-immunoglobulins are labeled with a radioactive tracer or an enzyme. Using an enzyme tag, the presence of anti-immunoglobulins can be detected by adding a substrate that gives a color reaction. This assay is called an *enzyme-linked immunosorbent assay (ELISA)*.

After coating the plastic surface with antigen, any uncoated plastic surface must be blocked to prevent it from absorbing the other reagents, most importantly the labeled reagent. Such blocking is achieved by coating the plastic surface with a high concentration of an unrelated protein, such as gelatin, after the application of the antigen.

Since the plastic wells are usually coated with relatively large amounts of antigen, high concentrations of antibodies can be bound. Therefore large amounts of labeled anti-immunoglobulin may be needed to bind to all the antibodies. Thus, it is important to always use an excess of labeled anti-immunoglobulin to ensure saturation.

Solid-phase immunoassay may also be used for qualitative or quantitative evaluations of antigen. Such determinations are performed by mixing known antiserum with dilutions of soluble antigen before adding the antiserum

to the antigen-coated plastic wells. This preliminary procedure results in the binding of the antibodies with the soluble antigen, decreasing the availability of free antibodies. The higher the concentration of the soluble antigen that reacts with antibodies before the addition of the antibody to the wells, the lower the number of antibodies that are available to bind with the antigen on the plate and the lower the number of labeled anti-immunoglobulins that can bind to the antigen–antibody complexes bound to that plate. The decrease in the amount of labeled antibody as a function of the concentration of antigen used can be plotted on a graph. The amount of antigen in an unknown solution can be determined from the graph by comparing the decrease in bound label caused by the unknown solution to the decrease caused by known concentrations of pure antigen (standard curve).

IMMUNOFLUORESCENCE AND IMMUNOHISTOCHEMISTRY

General Considerations

Both immunofluorescence and immunohistochemistry are designed to characterize cells by making use of antibodies specific for molecules on the surface or in the interior of the cells. In immunofluorescent techniques, the bound antibody is detected using a fluorescent dye either bound directly to that antibody (direct immunofluorescence) or bound to a second immunoglobulin that reacts against the first specific antibody (indirect immunofluorescence). In immunohistochemistry, the bound antibody is detected using an enzymatic reaction leading to a colored product.

A fluorescent compound absorbs light at one wavelength and reemits it at a longer wavelength. Thus the difference between incident light and emitted light can be distinguished. Antibodies can be covalently linked to fluorescent groups in a manner that does not cause any appreciable change in antibody activity.

One widely used fluorescent compound is fluorescein isothiocyanate (FITC), which fluoresces with a visible greenish color when excited by ultraviolet light. FITC is easily coupled to free amino groups. Another widely used fluorescent compound is phycoerythrin (PE), which fluoresces red and is also easily coupled to free amino groups. Fluorescence microscopes equipped with an ultraviolet (UV) light source permit visualization of fluorescent antibody on a microscopic specimen. Fluorescent-labeled antibodies are commonly used in conjunction with a flow cytometer (see below).

Direct Immunofluorescence. Direct immunofluorescence involves reacting the target tissue (or microorganism) with specific, fluorescent labeled antibodies. It is widely used for clinical purposes such as identifying lymphocytic subsets and confirming the presence and pattern

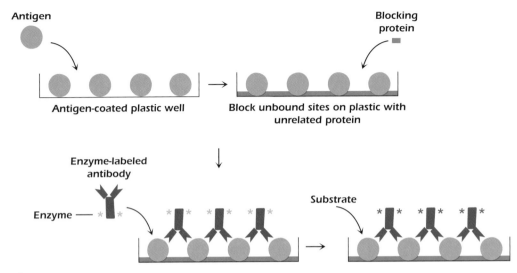

Figure UV.7. Representative ELISA using a well coated directly with antigen.

of deposition of specific protein and antigen–antibody complexes in tissues such as kidney and skin in autoimmune diseases. However to combine with histology, it requires that the tissue be frozen.

Indirect Immunofluorescence. Indirect immuno-fluorescence involves reacting the target first with unlabeled specific (primary) antibodies and then with fluorescently labeled (secondary) anti-immunoglobulin antibody. This method has the advantage of using a single anti-Ig antibody preparation to localize primary antibodies of many different specificities. In addition, since the anti-immunoglobulins contain antibodies to many epitopes on the primary antibody, the use of fluorescent anti-immunoglobulins significantly amplifies the fluorescent signal. An excellent example of the use of indirect immunofluorescence is the screening of patients' sera for anti-DNA antibodies in cases of systemic lupus erythematosus (SLE; see Case 22). Applications to tissue again require frozen samples.

Flow Cytometry

Flow cytometry is a very powerful tool that combines a flow cell apparatus with direct or indirect immunofluores-cence to specifically identify cell surface or intracellular antigens. A cell suspension is passed through an apparatus that causes the formation of a stream of small droplets, each containing a single cell. These droplets are passed between a laser beam of UV light and detectors. The detectors directly opposite the light source (0° angle) detect light that passes through undisturbed (forward scatter; Fig. UV.8). The amount of forward scatter correlates with cell size. Detectors at right angles (90°) from the light source detect light that is scattered after it has hit the cell or particle (side scatter). This correlates with cell

complexity—nuclear contour, granularity. Each cell type has a characteristic range of forward and side scatter. For example, lymphocytes can easily be distinguished from neutrophils by comparing these ranges.

Typically, the cells have first been reacted with an antibody with a fluorescent tag. If the cells have bound antibody, they will emit light of a characteristic wavelength when hit by the laser light beam. A detector, which allows only light of a specified wavelength through, picks up emitted fluorescence from labeled cells and is thus able to determine if the cell has attached antibody. In addition, from the intensity of the signal, the density of the target antigen on the cell is indicated. Very low levels of antigen can be detected, and many cells (10,000–20,000) can be analyzed within minutes. Currently, flow cytometers can be equipped with multiple lasers and can detect up to eight different fluorescent dyes simultaneously on a single cell. All parameters—forward scatter, side scatter, and staining—are measured for each individual cell as it passes through and is analyzed.

In addition, some instruments are equipped with a "sorting" capacity. The signal emitted from the detector is passed to an electrode that charges the droplet, leading to its deflection in an electromagnetic field (Fig. UV.9). As the droplets pass through the laser beam, they are counted and can be sorted according to whether they emit a signal (i.e., whether they are labeled or unlabeled).

With this type of apparatus it is now possible to rapidly develop a profile of a pool of lymphocytes based on their differential expression of cell surface molecules, the relative amount of cell surface molecule expressed on each cell, and the size distribution and numbers of each cell type. It is also possible to use the apparatus to sort a collection of cells stained with five or more different fluorescent labels and to obtain a relatively homogeneous sample of a specific cell

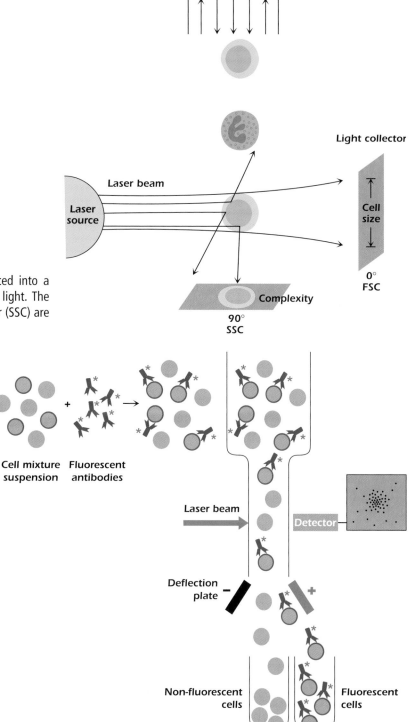

Figure UV.8. Flow cytometry: Cells are forced into a stream as single cells and are hit by a beam of light. The forward scatter of the light (FSC) and side scatter (SSC) are characteristic of cell type.

Figure UV.9. Flow cytometric analysis and cell sorting based on reaction with fluorescent antibody.

type. A variation of this technique uses fluorescent antibodies coupled to magnetic beads to separate cell populations. Cells that bind to the fluorescent antibody can be separated from unstained cells by a magnet. Both separation methods result in the isolation and concentration of rare cells, such as hematopoietic stem cells used for transplantation.

The most common method for phenotyping and sorting cells involves the use of antibodies that react with cell surface proteins identified as *clusters of differentiation (CD) antigens*. The CD nomenclature originates from studies using monoclonal antibodies (discussed later in this chapter) to characterize cells phenotypically. It was found that cell surface markers (CD antigens) are associated with distinct stages of cell development. In addition, these proteins have important biologic functions required for normal cell physiology. The developmental stages of B cells and T cells and their functional subsets can now be phenotyped based on their expression of CD markers. However, surface expression of a particular molecule may not be specific for just one cell or even for a cell lineage. Nonetheless, cell surface expression can be exploited for purification and characterization of cells. CD antigens are identified by a number that specifies a unique cell surface protein; for example, CD4 and CD8 are unique CD antigens. Newly discovered cell surface proteins are assigned CD numbers by the Nomenclature Committee of the International Union of Immunologic Sciences.

Characterization of molecules within the cell requires that the cell membrane be made permeable to allow the antibodies into the cell. The treatment must be such that it does not cause lysis of the cell or allow the antibody (with antigen) to leak back out. For both surface markers and internal antigens, staining is done on live cells that are fixed with formaldehyde following reaction with antibody.

Immunohistochemistry on Tissue Sections

Immunohistochemical staining is generally used to characterize cells on slides, either as single cells affixed to slides or as cut sections from blocks of tissue. The tissues have been preserved or fixed, usually with formalin, embedded in paraffin (wax mold), and cut into 3–5 micron sections onto slides. Antibodies to cell constituents such as keratin or to surface markers such as CD molecules are reacted with the tissue. Their binding is detected in one of two ways: by a secondary antibody with a bound enzyme (horseradish peroxidase or alkaline phosphatase) or by linkage of the primary antibody to biotin and detection by reaction of the bound enzyme with streptavidin. A chromogen is added and converted to a colored product by the enzyme. This color product is visualized under light microscopy. This technique has the advantage of allowing assessment of tissue architecture by showing the distribution and morphologic characteristics of the labeled cells.

IMMUNOABSORPTION AND IMMUNOADSORPTION

Because of the specific binding between antigen and antibody, it is possible to trap, or selectively remove, an antigen against which an antibody is directed from a mixture of antigens in solution. Similarly, it is possible to selectively remove antigen-specific antibodies from a mixture of antibodies using the specific antigen.

There are two general, related methods of removal. In one method, the absorption is done with both the antigen

and antibody in solution (*immunoabsorption*). In the other, it is performed with one attached to an insoluble support (*immunoadsorption*). Immunoadsorption is of particular value because the adsorbed material can then be recovered from the complex by careful treatments that dissociate antigen–antibody complexes, such as lowering the pH (HCl–glycine or acetic acid, pH 2–3) or adding chaotropic ions. These procedures allow the effective purification of antigens or antibodies of interest.

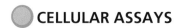 CELLULAR ASSAYS

General Considerations

Several methods are used to assess leukocyte function. In this section we will concentrate on assays of lymphocyte function. Assays designed to measure responses of B cells to antigenic or mitogenic stimulation are sometimes used to assess humoral immunocompetence. In experimental settings, these assays clarify the regulatory and molecular mechanisms associated with B-cell activation. Similarly, assays for measuring T-cell function are used both clinically and experimentally to measure T-cell proliferative responses, T-cell effector responses, and T-cell cytokine profiles. T-cell assays have contributed significantly to our understanding of T-cell functional diversity and to the identification of the many cytokines produced by cells belonging to a particular subset.

Assessment of Lymphocyte Function

Assays used to assess lymphocyte function generally attempt to answer one of the following questions: (1) Do the B cells or T cells respond normally to mitogenic stimuli that activate cells to undergo a proliferative response? (2) Does mitogenic or antigen-driven stimulation result in antibody production (for B cells) or cytokine production (for T cells)? In addition, given the functional heterogeneity of T cells, T-cell assays can also be used to evaluate the functional integrity of a specific subset. This is particularly useful in the clinical evaluation of patients with suspected immunodeficiency diseases. In the case of T helper cell assays, the target cell receiving the T-cell help generally determines the functional parameter to be measured. For example, the target population might be B cells in an assay designed to test the ability of T cells to help induce antibody responses. In this example, the assay would quantitate the level of antibody produced. Similarly, in studies to determine whether T cells provide the help needed for optimal activation of macrophages, the parameters would focus on functional properties associated with these phagocytic cells. Many of the assays used to assess T helper cell function also rely on the measurement of specific cytokines, since the cells receiving help may be activated to produce cytokines themselves.

B- and T-Cell Proliferation Assays

Mitogen-stimulated lymphocyte activation triggers biochemical signaling pathways that lead to gene expression, protein synthesis, cell proliferation, and differentiation. Mitogens that selectively stimulate either B- or T-cell populations have been identified; however, the proliferative responses generated in response to mitogens are polyclonal in nature. Unlike immunogens, which activate only the lymphocyte clones bearing the appropriate antigen receptor, polyclonal activators stimulate many B- or T-cell clones regardless of their antigenic specificity. Mitogens that selectively activate B cells, such as the *lipopolysaccharide (LPS)* component of Gram-negative bacterial cell walls, will cause polyclonal stimulation of B cells. The magnitude of cell proliferation occurring in response to mitogenic stimulation can be measured by adding radiolabeled nucleosides (e.g., tritiated thymidine) to the medium during cell culture and then quantitating its incorporation into the DNA of dividing cells using a liquid scintillation counter. Similarly, several sugar-binding proteins called lectins, including *concanavalin A (Con A)* and *phytohemagglutinin (PHA)*, are very effective T-cell mitogens. *Pokeweed mitogen (PWM)* is another example of a lectin with potent mitogenic properties, especially effective for human B cells. However, unlike Con A and PHA, it also activates human T cells.

Antibody Production by B Cells

Mitogenic stimulation of B and T cells results in the proliferation and differentiation of many clones. In the case of B cells, the polyclonal activators LPS or PWM can be used to assess the ability of a population of B cells to produce antibody. ELISA is the most commonly used quantitative assay for measuring antibody levels. Alternatively, B cells can be stimulated with mitogens or specific antigens *in vitro*, then temporarily cultured in chambers directly on nitrocellulose membranes in a so-called *ELISPOT* assay. The protein-binding property of nitrocellulose facilitates the capture of secreted antibody by individual B cells. This yields discrete foci of antibody bound to the nitrocellulose that can be detected using a secondary, enzyme-labeled antibody specific for the bound antibody.

Effector Cell Assays for T and Natural Killer Cells

As noted above, the selection of an effector cell assay depends on the questions that need to be answered. T-cell assays are as varied as the functionally diverse T-cell subsets known to exist. Thus, assays for B cells, macrophages, and even other T cells have been developed that evaluate the T helper cell activity. Similarly, several assays that measure cytotoxic activity of CD8$^+$ T cells are available.

One such assay, called the *cytotoxicity assay*, measures the ability of cytotoxic T cells or natural killer (NK) cells to kill radiolabeled target cells expressing an antigen to which the cytotoxic T cells have been sensitized. In a related assay, NK cells are cultured with radiolabeled target cells to which target cell-specific antibodies are bound. This approach is based on the fact that NK cells express membrane Fc receptors that bind to the Fc region of certain immunoglobulin isotypes and measures an important functional property of NK cells known as **antibody-dependent cell-mediated cytotoxicity (ADCC)**.

 ## CELL CULTURE

General Considerations

Several experimental systems have revolutionized our ability to investigate a multitude of questions about the development of the immune system, its functional and regulatory properties, and the pathologic mechanisms associated with immunodeficiency and autoimmune diseases. Many of these experimental systems depend on cell culture methods used to maintain cells *in vitro*. Cell culture systems have facilitated several major scientific breakthroughs, including the development in the 1970s of B-cell hybridoma/monoclonal antibody technology by Kohler and Milstein (see Case 26). Knowledge of the growth factors required to maintain lymphoid cells has made it possible to clone and grow functionally competent cells *in vitro*. In addition, recombinant DNA techniques have permitted the transfer of genes to cloned cell lines, thereby allowing researchers to answer many questions related to the gene under investigation. Similarly, recombinant DNA techniques have made it possible to develop genetically engineered immune molecules and receptors. When expressed by the transfected cell, these molecules and receptors can be used to elucidate the biologic consequences of receptor expression and receptor triggering (e.g., ligand binding). These *in vitro* systems continue to be used to advance our knowledge of the immune system and, in some cases, to develop new biologic therapies and vaccines for clinical use.

Primary Cell Cultures and Cloned Lymphoid Cell Lines

The ability to culture primary lymphoid cells consisting of heterogeneous populations of T cells and/or B cells (albeit for limited periods of time) has allowed immunologists to study the biochemical and molecular mechanisms controlling many important biologic features of B and T cells, including gene rearrangement. Advances in cell culture systems have led to the development of cell cloning techniques. Transformation of B and T cells derived from a specific parent cell to generate cloned, immortal cell lines has been achieved using a variety of methods. These include exposure of cells to certain carcinogens or viruses, such as exposure to the Epstein–Barr virus in the case of B cells and human T-cell leukemia virus type 1 for T cells. Cell lines may also be derived from tumors that arise either spontaneously or experimentally (as a result of carcinogen exposure or virus infection). The major advantage of using cloned cell lines is that large numbers of cells can be generated. A disadvantage is that they are, by definition, abnormal. Indeed, many transformed cells have abnormal numbers of chromosomes and often display phenotypic and functional properties not seen in normal cells. A major advance in the generation of cloned lymphoid cells came in the late 1970s with the discovery that nontransformed antigen-specific T-cell lines and antigen-specific T-cell clones could be grown indefinitely when a T-cell growth factor (interleukin-2) was included in the culture along with a source of antigen and antigen-presenting cells. This approach offered several advantages over the use of transformed cells, since the cells derived from such cultures were, for all intents and purposes normal, allowing the generation of large numbers of nontransformed antigen-specific T cells for investigation. Indeed, many of these cloned T-cell lines have been used in the identification and biochemical characterization of cytokines, leading to the ultimate cloning of genes that encode these proteins.

In short, cell culture systems have served as a gateway for research endeavors attempting to shed light on both the physiologic and pathophysiologic properties of lymphoid cells. As will be discussed below, cell culture systems have also been exploited productively in the development of many useful diagnostic and therapeutic reagents, such as monoclonal antibodies.

B-Cell Hybridomas and Monoclonal Antibodies

The specificity of the immune response has served as the basis for serologic reactions in which antibody specificity is used for the qualitative and quantitative determination of antigen. However, the discriminating power of serum antibody is not without limitations; the immunizing antigen, which usually has many epitopes, leads to production of antisera that contain a mixture of different antibodies with specificity for a collection of epitopes. Indeed, even antibodies to a single epitope are usually mixtures of immunoglobulins with different fine specificities and therefore different affinities for the determinant. Furthermore, immunization with an antigen expands various populations of antibody-forming lymphocytes. These cells can be maintained in culture for only a short time (on the order of days), so it is impractical, if not impossible, to grow normal cells and obtain clones that produce antibodies of a

single specificity in significant amounts. A quantum leap in the resolution and discriminating power of antibodies took place in the 1970s with the development of methods for the generation of monoclonal antibodies by Kohler and Milstein, who shared the Nobel Prize for this discovery. *Monoclonal antibodies* are homogeneous populations of antibody molecules derived from the progeny of a single antibody-producing cell in which all antibodies are identical and of the same precise specificity for a given epitope.

Malignant non-immunoglobulin-producing plasma cells (myeloma cells, which are immortal in cell culture) are used in the production of monoclonal antibodies. The cells are engineered to be deficient in an enzyme [hypoxanthine guanine phosphoribosyl transferase (HGPRT)] and therefore will not survive in culture unless this enzyme is added to the media in which the cells are grown. These cells are fused (hybridized) with a source of freshly harvested B cells (e.g., spleen cells) from a mouse recently immunized with antigen to form *B-cell hybridomas* (Fig. UV.10). The cell fusion is often accomplished by the use of polyethylene glycol (PEG). Following fusion, the cells are cultured in media lacking HGPRT. Since the antibody-producing B cells produce HGPRT, hybridoma cells will survive in the absence of supplemented HGPRT in the culture medium. Within days, nonfused HGPRT-negative malignant plasma cells die, as do all nonfused B cells, which have a limited lifespan in culture on their own. Those hybrid cells synthesizing specific antibody are selected by testing for antigen reactivity of the supernatant (e.g., ELISA) and then cloned from single cells and propagated in tissue culture; each clone synthesizes antibodies of a single specificity. The cells can be propagated indefinitely because cells of one fusion partner, the myeloma, are malignant. The highly specific monoclonal antibodies are used for numerous procedures, ranging from specific diagnostic tests to biologic agents used in immunotherapy of cancer. In immunotherapy, various drugs or toxins are conjugated to monoclonal antibodies; in turn, the monoclonal antibodies deliver these substances to the tumor cells against which they are directed.

T-Cell Hybridomas

Hybridoma technology is not limited to the production of monoclonal antibodies. In the late 1970s, methods were also developed for the production of T cell hybridomas. This involved fusing lines of malignant T cells with nonmalignant, antigen-specific T lymphocytes, following expansion of the T-lymphocyte populations by immunization with antigen. T-cell hybridomas have been very useful in analysis of the relationship between T cells of a single specificity and a corresponding epitope.

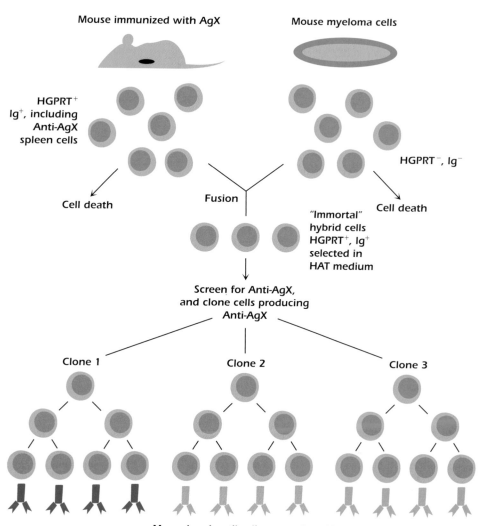

Mouse immunized with AgX   Mouse myeloma cells

HGPRT⁺
Ig⁺, including
Anti-AgX
spleen cells

HGPRT⁻, Ig⁻

Cell death   Fusion   Cell death

"Immortal"
hybrid cells
HGPRT⁺, Ig⁺
selected in
HAT medium

Screen for Anti-AgX,
and clone cells producing
Anti-AgX

Clone 1   Clone 2   Clone 3

Figure UV.10. Production of monoclonal antibodies.

Monoclonal antibodies to antigen X

GENETICALLY ENGINEERED ANTIBODIES AND RECEPTORS

To date, most monoclonal antibodies have been created using mouse cells, which are suitable for diagnostic purposes and many other functions. However, their administration in humans carries with it the potential complication of the formation of antibodies to the mouse immunoglobulins. By and large, attempts to develop *in vitro* human monoclonal antibodies have not been very successful.

Human monoclonal antibodies are currently being produced by genetic engineering using several approaches. One method utilizes the technology of recombinant DNA to produce a chimeric mouse–human monoclonal antibody. These so-called **humanized antibodies** consist of the constant region of human immunoglobulin and the variable region of a mouse immunoglobulin. A similar method is used to construct humanized antibodies that consist of a human constant region and a variable region containing a mouse hypervariable region. Yet another method utilizes the

polymerase chain reaction (PCR) to generate gene libraries of heavy and light chains from B-cell hybridomas or plasma cell DNA (see below). With this technology, it is now possible to produce millions of clones of different specificities, screen them rapidly for the desired specificity, and generate the desired monoclonal Fab constructs (antigen-binding regions) without immunization and without the difficulties encountered in the production of monoclonal antibodies.

Genetic engineering of immune proteins is not limited to the production of monoclonal antibodies. Many genes encoding membrane receptors expressed on lymphoid and nonlymphoid cells have been cloned and, in some cases, genetically engineered to allow for gene transfer to cells that do not normally express these receptors. The expression of certain costimulator molecules facilitates cell–cell interactions, such as the physical contact between cytotoxic T cells and target cells, which results in the killing of the target cells. The expression of such costimulator molecules (e.g., CD80) on tumor cells through gene transfer significantly enhances the ability of T cells to recognize and kill target cells. Experimental vaccination strategies have demonstrated that immunization of tumor-bearing animals with their own tumor cells, which have been removed and transfected with the CD80 gene, can potentiate T cells to recognize and destroy the parent tumor cells (a form of immunotherapy). A similar strategy using tumor cells transfected with certain cytokine genes has been used with some success in animal models.

 # EXPERIMENTAL ANIMAL MODELS

General Considerations

Several important *in vivo* animal models have been developed, with experimental value and clinical payoffs similar to those emerging from the use of the *in vitro* systems noted above. These *in vivo* systems rely on the use of inbred mouse strains with a variety of genetic profiles, some of which are genetically engineered. Some inbred strains have an innate predisposition for developing a particular disease [e.g., mammary cancer, leukemia, autoimmune disease, severe combined immunodeficiency disease (see Case 2)]. Genetically altered animals have also been developed that either express a particular cloned foreign gene (transgenic mice) or interfere with the expression of targeted genes (knockout mice). Such strains are useful in the study of the expression of the transgene or in determining the consequences of gene silencing. We begin with a discussion of inbred strains of animals.

Inbred Strains

Many of the classic experiments in the field of immunology have been performed using inbred strains of animals such as mice, rats, and guinea pigs. Selective inbreeding of littermates for more than 20 generations usually leads to the production of an inbred strain. All members of that inbred strain are genetically identical. Therefore, like identical twins, they are said to be *syngeneic*. Immune responses of inbred strains can be studied in the absence of variables associated with genetic differences between animals. Organ transplants between members of inbred stains are always accepted because their major histocompatibility complex (MHC) antigens are identical. Indeed, knowledge of the laws of transplantation and the identification of the MHC as the major genetic barrier to transplantation came from research using inbred strains. These experiments led to the identification of class I and class II MHC genes. It also explained their main function, the delivery of peptide fragments of antigen to the cell surface, which allows the antigen to be recognized by antigen-specific T cells.

Adoptive Transfer

Protection against many diseases is conferred through cell-mediated immunity by antigen-specific T cells, rather than through antibody-mediated (humoral) immunity. The distinction between these two arms of the immune response can be demonstrated readily by adoptive transfer of T cells or by passive administration of antiserum or purified antibodies. *Adoptive transfer* of T cells is usually performed using genetically identical donors and recipients (e.g., inbred strains) and results in long-term adoptive immunization following antigen priming. By contrast, transfer of antibody-containing serum, which can be performed across MHC barriers and is effective as long as the transferred antibodies remain active in the recipient, is called passive immunization.

SCID and RAG-Deficient Mice

Severe combined immunodeficiency disease (SCID) is a disorder in which B cells and T cells fail to develop, causing the individual to be compromised with respect to lymphoid defense mechanisms (see Case 2). In the 1980s, an inbred strain of mice spontaneously developed an autosomal recessive mutation in the DNA repair gene, *Prkdc*, resulting in SCID in homozygous *scid/scid* mice. Because of the absence of functional T and B cells, SCID mice are able to accept cells and tissue grafts from other strains of mice or even other species. SCID mice can be engrafted with human hematopoietic stem cells to create *SCID-human chimeras*. Such chimeric mice develop mature, functional T and B cells derived from the infused human stem cell precursors. This animal model has become a valuable research tool, since it allows immunologists to manipulate the human immune system *in vivo* and to investigate the development of various lymphoid cells. Moreover, SCID-human mice can be used to test candidate vaccines, including those that might be useful in protecting humans from HIV infection.

RAG (Recombination Activating Protein)-deficient mice are deficient in either the *RAG1* or *RAG2* genes that encode enzymes essential for immunoglobulin and T-cell receptor recombination (see Case 2); thus, like SCID mice they lack functional B and T cells and can be used in much the same way as SCID mice.

Thymectomized and Congenically Athymic (Nude) Mice

The importance of the thymus in the development of mature T cells can be demonstrated by using mice that have been neonatally thymectomized, irradiated, and then reconstituted with syngeneic bone marrow. Such mice fail to develop mature T cells. Similarly, mice homozygous for the recessive nude mutation also fail to develop mature T cells because the mutation results in an athymic (and hairless, hence the term *nude*) phenotype (see Case 3). In both situations, T-cell development can be restored by grafting these mice with thymic epithelial tissue. Like SCID mice, these animal models have been useful in the study of T-cell development. They have also been useful for the *in vivo* propagation of tumor cell lines and freshly harvested tumor tissue from other strains and other species due to the absence of T cells required for the rejection of foreign cells.

Transgenic and Gene-Targeted Mice

Transgenic Mice. Another significant animal system used extensively in immunologic research is the transgenic mouse. *Transgenic mice* are made by injecting a cloned gene (*transgene*) into fertilized mouse eggs. The eggs are then microinjected into mice rendered pseudopregnant using hormone therapy (Fig. UV.11). The success rate of this technique is rather low, with approximately 10–30% of the offspring expressing the transgene. Since the transgene is integrated into both somatic and germline cells, it is transmitted to the offspring as a Mendelian trait. By constructing a transgene with a particular promoter, it is possible to control its expression. Some promoters function only in certain tissues; for example, the insulin promoter only functions in the pancreas. Others function in response to biochemical signals that can be supplied as a dietary supplement. Transgenic mice have been used to study genes that are not usually expressed *in vivo* (e.g., oncogenes) as well as the effects of particular immunoglobulin molecules, T-cell receptors, MHC class I or class II molecules, and a variety of cytokines. In some transgenic mice, the entire mouse immunoglobulin locus has been replaced by human immunoglobulin genes. These are useful in generating "human" antibodies in the mouse. However, the transgenic method has two disadvantages. First, the transgene integrates randomly within the genome. Second, it is unphysiologic to express high quantities of transgenes in the wrong tissues, so investigators must use great care in interpreting their results.

Gene-Targeted Mice (Knockout Mice). Sometimes it is of interest to determine how the removal of a particular gene product affects the immune system. Using a *gene-targeting* method, it is possible to replace a normal gene with one that has been mutated or disrupted to thus generate so-called *knockout mice*. Unlike transgenic mice, knockout mice express transgenes that integrate at specific endogenous gene sites through a process known as homologous recombination. Virtually any gene for which a mutated or altered transgene exists can be targeted this way. Knockout mice have been generated by using mutated or altered transgenes that target, and therefore silence, the expression of a variety of important genes, including those encoding particular cytokines and MHC molecules. Knockout mice have also been used to identify the parts of genes essential for normal gene function. In order to identify the responsible part of the gene, different mutated copies are introduced back into the genome by transgenesis to see which one restores normal function.

MOLECULAR TECHNIQUES

Analysis of DNA and RNA by PCR

PCR is a method of amplifying DNA and thereby gaining access to the sequence of the DNA for mutational analysis. The amplified DNA can be used to create plasmids to be inserted into cells for functional studies of the DNA, for the construction of transgenes to obtain transgenic animals, and for the construction of targeting vectors to obtain animals lacking a particular gene (knockout mice) or containing a mutated gene (knock-in mice).

First, short priming oligonucleotides (oligos for short) are synthesized that are complementary to stretches of DNA flanking opposite ends of the DNA to be amplified. One oligo is complementary to one strand of DNA and the second one is complementary to the other strand of DNA. In the first step of the actual PCR, the priming oligos are incubated with the target DNA, which has been heated to separate the two DNA strands. This takes place in a solution that imposes a high level of binding specificity between the priming oligos and the DNA; a thermostable polymerase and free nucleotides are also added. In the second step of the PCR, the temperature is lowered to allow the polymerase to synthesize a new strand of DNA complementary to each DNA strand. The initial replication of the DNA of interest is now completed.

The temperature is then raised to again separate the double-stranded DNA, and the process is repeated. Initially the polymerase will produce strands that "overshoot" the portion of the DNA delimited by the priming oligos, but the delineated portion soon becomes the dominant species because the primers begin the polymerization at the same site on each strand. With each repeat (cycle), the amount of replicated DNA doubles, so that the amount of the DNA fragment increases rapidly. Very soon, enough DNA is obtained so that it can be analyzed on ethidium bromide gel and/or subjected to various other types of analysis. In practice, the multiple-cycle PCR is carried out automatically by a PCR device that varies the temperature according to a predetermined schedule.

The basic PCR technique is also used to amplify RNA. This is accomplished by converting the RNA to DNA with a reverse transcriptase and then treating the resulting DNA as discussed above.

Southern and Northern Blotting

Southern and Northern blotting are basic molecular techniques for the analysis of the DNA and RNA, respectively. In Southern blotting (named for Dr. Southern), the genomic DNA to be analyzed is first digested with a restriction enzyme into thousands of small fragments of varying size. A *restriction enzyme* is an enzyme that cuts DNA at sites containing short target sequences that occur at random

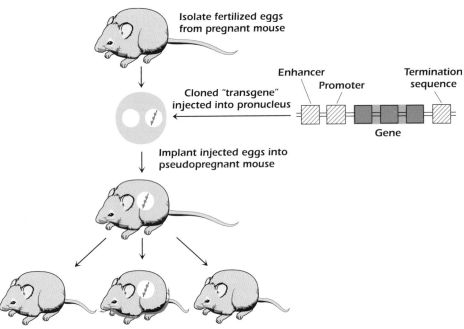

Figure UV.11. General procedure for producing transgenic mice.

within the genome, hence the variation in the size of fragments obtained during digestion. The digested DNA is then electrophoresed on an agarose gel to organize the fragments according to size and transferred to a nylon filter where it is bound in place. The filter is then hybridized with a labeled (denatured) DNA probe that specifically binds to the DNA of the gene of interest and washed to remove unbound probe. One or more discrete bands can be visualized, with sizes specified by the restriction enzyme used initially to cut the DNA since different enzymes cut the gene of interest in different places. Probes are usually labeled with ^{32}P or with chemiluminescence labels. Southern blotting of the DNA of plasma cells of myeloma patients will yield discrete bands because the cells contain large amounts of uniform DNA encoding immunoglobulin. In contrast, those from normal individuals will yield a smear reflecting the variability of their immunoglobulin genes from cell to cell. Likewise, genes with mutations can be distinguished from normal genes because the mutations introduce changes in restriction enzyme cutting patterns. An advantage of Southern blot analysis over PCR is that the former allows scanning of thousands of genes and is not affected by complexities in the primary sequence of the genes.

Northern blots are similar to Southern blots, except that they use undigested mRNA rather than digested genomic DNA as the starting material. For best results, affinity-purified mRNA rather than whole RNA is used, and the RNA is isolated under denaturing conditions to avoid self-hybridization.

Fluorescence *In Situ* Hybridization

Fluorescence in situ hybridization (*FISH*) is a technique used to detect genes in cellular chromosomes. It is therefore useful for the analysis of chromosomal translocations or other chromosomal disorders. This technique also relies on hybridization; it consists of incubation of cells with labeled probes that specifically bind to certain genes. These probes are typically labeled with biotin- or digoxygenin-tagged nucleotides, which are then detected with flourescence-labeled antibodies. The cells examined are in an early metaphase state so that the condensed chromatin can be visualized. Positive results yield two labeled dots representing genes on sister chromatids. Appropriate synthesis of the probes and application of two different probes with different signals allow the detection of translocations.

Microarray Analysis of RNA Expression (Gene Chip Analysis)

Microarrays, or *gene chips*, are powerful tools for examining the level of expression of thousands of genes simultaneously. The microarray comprises thousands of DNA fragments, each with a unique sequence, attached in an ordered arrangement to a glass slide or other surface. These DNA fragments, in the form of complementary DNA (cDNA; generally 500–5000 base pairs long) or oligonucleotides (20–80 base pairs long), can represent genes from all parts of the genome. Alternatively, specialized microarrays can

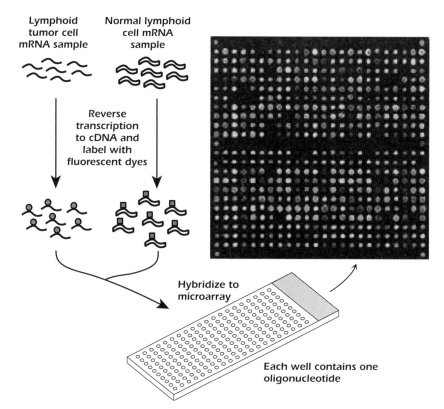

Lymphoid tumor cell mRNA sample

Normal lymphoid cell mRNA sample

Reverse transcription to cDNA and label with fluorescent dyes

Hybridize to microarray

Each well contains one oligonucleotide

Figure UV.12. Microarray assay comparing samples of mRNA from lymphoid tumor cells and normal lymphoid cells.

be prepared that use DNA from genes of particular interest. To perform a microarray assay, a sample of total mRNA (the product obtained from transcription of all active genes) from a cell or tissue is commonly tested with a reference sample to compare gene expression among various samples. For example, different cell types or tissues can be compared, cells can be compared at different stages of differentiation, or tumor cells can be compared with their normal counterparts. The samples added to the microarray are generally not mRNAs; rather, the total mRNA is reverse transcribed into cDNA, which is then labeled with a fluorescent material (a fluorochrome). Different-colored fluorochromes are used to label the different sources of cDNAs distinctly. Figure UV.12 illustrates how microarrays are used to compare gene expression in a lymphoid tumor cell population with that of a normal cell population. A red fluorochrome is used to label experimental tumor cell cDNAs, and a green fluorochrome is used for cDNAs prepared from the control normal counterparts. The labeled cDNAs are washed over the microarray and allowed to

hybridize by base pairing with matching fragments. cDNA samples derived from both samples are combined so that they compete for binding to the microarray. Unhybridized material is washed away, leaving pockets of fluorescence where matching has occurred. At the end of the hybridization reaction, the microarray is laser scanned to reveal red, green, or yellow spots, indicating higher levels of the experimental tumor cell cDNA (red), higher levels of the control cDNA (green), or equal levels of DNA in the two samples (yellow). To interpret the results, a fluorescence scanner examines each spot on the slide for the precise level of fluorescence. The data are then analyzed by a computer program that typically combines the fluorescence information with a genetic database to determine which genes are overexpressed or underexpressed in the tested samples. Characterization of the pattern and amount of binding to the microarray has many potential uses in the field of immunology, including clinical diagnosis of lymphoid tumors, drug development, prediction of responsiveness to drugs, and new gene discovery.

Index

Abatacept, 282
Aberrant clones, lymphomas and, 313–315
ABO mismatch, 261
Acetylcholine receptor (AChR), 184. *See also* AChR entries;
　　Anti-AChR entries
Acetylcholinesterase inhibitors, in myasthenia gravis,
　　193–194
AChR antibodies/autoantibodies, 188. *See also* Acetylcholine
　　receptor (AChR)
　levels of, 185
　in myasthenia gravis, 190–192
AChR-reactive T cells, 192
Acquired agammaglobulinemia, 69
Acquired angioedema (AAE), 103–104
Acquired immunodeficiency syndrome (AIDS), 2, 82,
　　111–124, 315. *See also* AIDS entries; Human
　　immunodeficiency virus (HIV)
　CNS symptoms, 120
　debilitating illnesses, AIDS-associated, 120
　epidemiology and clinical features of, 117–120
　HIV infection and AIDS, 117
　Kaposi sarcoma (KS), 119
　Mycobacterial infections, 119–120
　NAT test, 112, 114–115
　p17 matrix protein, 116
　phases of
　Pneumocystis jiroveci, 54, 57, 120, 170. *See also* PCP
　　(*Pneumocystis carinii* pneumonia)
　p24 core antigen, 116

　p24 virion, 114
　Rev protein, 116–117
　T cell lysis, in HIV, 121
　Toxoplasmosis, 57, 92, 93
　treatment of, 122–123
　tropic HIV, 116
　Trypanosomiasis, 92
　window period, 112
ACR criteria, for SLE classification, 287–289. *See also*
　　American College of Rheumatology (ACR)
Activation-induced apoptosis, 83. *See also*
　　Activation-induced cell death (AICD)
Activation-induced cell death (AICD), 87
Activation-induced cytidine deaminase (AID), 59–60, 75
Activation-induced cytidine deaminase mutations,
　　64–65
　treatment for, 122–123
Acute lymphoblastic leukemia (ALL), 92, 313
　B-ALL 313
　T-ALL 38
Acute retroviral syndrome, signs and symptoms associated
　　with, 118
Acute tubular necrosis (ATN), 266
Acyclovir, 94, 98
ADA-deficient SCID, 13, 29 *See also* Adenosine deaminase
　　(ADA); Adenosine deaminase (ADA) deficiency;
　　Severe combined immunodeficiency disease (SCID)
　gene therapy for, 37.
Adalumimab, 281

ADAM33 gene, 156

Adaptive immune system, 6–7

Adenosine deaminase (ADA) deficiency, 13. *See also* ADA-deficient SCID

Adenosine deaminase (ADA), mutations in, 31–32

Adoptive transfer, in experimental animal models, 364

Adult T-cell leukemia/lymphoma, 312

Aeroallergen-related allergic disease, 140

Affinity, in antigen–antibody interactions, 353

Affinity maturation, of germinal center B cells, 332

Agglutination
  assays, 353–355
    Latex, passive agglutination with thyroglobulin, 354
    Latex pregnancy test, passive agglutination in, 355
  Coombs test and, 354
  direct, 353
  inhibition, 354–355
  passive, 353, 354–355
  types and nature of antigen–antibody, 353–355
  via antigen–antibody interactions, 351
  zeta potential in, 354

AIDS-associated illnesses, 118–120. *See also* Acquired immunodeficiency syndrome (AIDS)

AIDS-associated malignancy, 119

AIDS enteropathy, 120

AIDS phases, 117, 118–120

AIRE gene defect, 202. *See also* Autoimmune regulator (AIRE)

AIRE transcription factor, 181

Airway hyperreactivity (AHR), 153, 155
  in asthma, 152

Airway obstruction, 103
  in asthma, 148

Akin, Cem, xi, 129

Alanine aminotransferase (ALT), 93, 112, 162, 163

Albumin, 256, 257, 260, 338, 339

Albuterol, 148, 158
  Nebulized albuterol inhalation, 149

Albuterol inhalation, 149

Albuterol inhaler, 147

Alefacept, 253

Alkaline phosphatase, in immunohistochemistry, 360

Allergen immunotherapy, 158

Allergens, antigens as, 127–128

Allergic angioedema, 103

Allergic reactions, 103, 127, 129–130

Allergies, environmental, 148

Allergy shots, 158

Allergy testing, 139–141, 150

Allogeneic hematopoietic stem cell transplantation (SCT), 37

Allogeneic skin graft rejection, 11

Allorecognition, 263

$\alpha_4\beta_7$ integrin receptor, 116

Amyloid, renal failure and, 342
  Primary amyloidosis, 342

Amyloidosis, 303
  primary and secondary, 342
  renal failure due to, 342

Anakinra, 281–282

Anaphylaxis, 128, 137–146
  anaphylactic reactions, 129–130
  definitive diagnosis of, 138
  pathogenesis of, 145–146
  pathophysiology of, 143–146
  skin testing, 139–140, 141, 150
  symptoms of, 138
  systemic anaphylactic reaction, 145–146
  treatment plan for, 141–143
  workup completion related to, 138–141

Anaplastic large cell lymphoma, 312

ANCA-associated vasculitides, 169–172.
    See also Antineutrophil cytoplasmic antibody (ANCA)

Anemia
  in chronic lymphocytic leukemia/small lymphocytic lymphoma, 318, 320, 324
  in follicular lymphoma treatment, 334
  iron deficiency anemia, 236, 237
  in lupus, 288
  megaloblastic, 220
  microcytic, 71

Anergic B cells, 290

Aneurysms, 168, 169

Angioedema, 138. *See also* Hereditary angioedema (HAE)
  acquired angioedema, 103–104
  cardiovascular collapse, 138
  drug-induced angioedema, 103

Angiogenesis, in rheumatoid arthritis, 279

Angioneurotic edema, 103

Angiotensin II antagonist, 303

Angiotensin-converting enzyme (ACE) inhibitors, 103, 258, 260

Angiotensin receptor blockers (ARBs), 260

Animal models, 364–365. *See also* Mice (mouse)

Anti-AChR, 186, 190, 193. *See also* Acetylcholine receptor (AChR)

Antibodies. *See also* Autoantibodies
  agglutinating titers of, 353–354
  basic molecules of, 353
  biological functions of,
  collagen-specific, 275
  in chronic lymphocytic leukemia/small lymphocytic lymphoma, 318, 321, 324
  in flow cytometry, 358–360
  in follicular lymphoma treatment, 329, 335–336
  genetically engineered, 363–364
  humanized, 363
  in immunofluorescence and immunohistochemistry, 357–360
  placental transmission, 54

plasma cells and, 343
in plasma cell neoplasm diagnosis, 338–340
removal via immunoabsorption and immunoadsorption, 360
role in MS, 204–205
Antibody–antigen complexes, 180. *See also* Antigen-antibody complexes
Antibody–antigen interactions, methods for analyzing, 351–357
Antibody-based assays, 351
Antibody-dependent cell-mediated cytotoxicity (ADCC), 361
in chronic lymphocytic leukemia/small lymphocytic lymphoma, 320, 324
in follicular lymphoma treatment, 329
Antibody excess zone, in precipitin reactions, 355
Antibody fragments, antigen/hapten complexes with, 352–353
Antibody responses, CD19 deficiency and, 79
Antibody targets, monoclonal, 315
Anti-CCP antibodies, 273, 276
Anti-CD3/anti-CD28, 56
stimulation by, 18
Anti-CD3 monoclonal antibody (OKT3), 265
Anti-CD4 monoclonal antibodies, 193
Anti-CD20 antibody, 94, 98, 262
in follicular lymphoma treatment, 329, 335
Anti-CD25 (anti-IL-2R) antibody therapy, 265
Anti-CD40 stimulation, 18
Anticytokines, 244
Anti-dsDNA antibodies, 284
Antiendomesial antibody tests, 222
Antifibrinolytic agents, 110
Antifibrotic therapies, 307–308
Anti-G6P isomerase antibodies, 276
Antigen–antibody complexes, 352
in immunoabsorption and immunoadsorption, 360
in plasma cell neoplasm diagnosis, 338
in precipitation reactions, 355
in solid-phase immunoassays, 357
Antigen–antibody interactions
in immunoassays, 356–357
primary, 351–352
secondary, 353–356
Antigen-driven stimulation, cellular assays and, 360
Antigen excess zone, in precipitin reactions, 355
Antigenic challenge, specific antibody responses to, 17
Antigenic diversity, lymphoid malignancies and, 311
Antigen presentation, in systemic lupus erythematosus, 293–294
Antigen-presenting cells (APCs), 56, 120, 199, 211, 292
β cells functioning as, 213
B cells as, 293–294
in the CNS, 204
of lymph node, 330, 331

surrogate, 260
T cell activation by, 293
Antigen receptor gene rearrangement, 32
Antigens
as allergens, 127–128
in CLL/SLL pathogenesis/immunogenesis, 321
in disease delay/prevention, 216
exogenous antigens, 175, 247, 290
in flow cytometry, 358–360
in immunofluorescence and immunohistochemistry, 357–360
in monoclonal antibody production, 363
plasma cells and, 344
removal via immunoabsorption and immunoadsorption, 360
stimulation and response of T cells to, 247–248
Antigen sequestration defects, 181
Antigen-specific B cells, of lymph node, 330, 331
Antigen-specific T-cell lines, 362
Antigen-specific T-cell receptors, 247
Antigen-specific T cells, adoptive transfer and, 364
Antigen-specific T_{reg} cell dysfunction, 202
Anti-gliadin antibody test, 222
Anti-glomerular basement membrane (anti-GBM) antibody disease, 170
Antihistamines, 132, 140
Anti-HLA antibody, 262
Antihuman IgE, 141–142. *See also* Immunoglobulin E (IgE)
Anti-IgE monoclonal antibody, 160
Anti-IL-4 mAb antibody, 160. *See also* Interleukin 4 (IL-4)
Anti-IL-6 antibodies, in plasma cell neoplasm treatment, 346. *See also* Interleukin 6 (IL-6)
Anti-IL-12p40 monoclonal antibody, 240, 244, 253. *See also* Interleukin 12 (IL-12)
Anti-immunoglobulins, in solid-phase immunoassays, 357
Anti-immunoglobulin test, in antigen–antibody interactions, 354
Anti-inflammatory drugs, 103
Anti-matrix metalloprotease 1 (MMP-1), 306
Anti-metabolite agents, 265
Anti-myeloperoxidase antibody, 172
Anti-neutrophil cytoplasmic antibody (ANCA), 163, 170, 172. *See also* ANCA-associated vasculitides
Wegener's granulomatosis and, 171–172
Anti-nuclear antibodies (ANAs), 163, 273, 302
SLE-specific, 284
Anti-platelet-derived growth factor (PDGF) receptor, 306
Anti-reticular antibody, 222
Anti-retroviral therapy, highly active, 122–123
Anti-Scl-70 antibody, 306
Anti-SSA/Ro antibodies, 273
Anti-SSB/La antibodies, 273
Anti-TGF-β antibody therapy, 307. *See also* Transforming growth factor β (TGF-β)

Anti-thymocyte globulin (ATG), 265

Anti-TNF-α, agents, 236, 243, 244, 308. *See also* Tumor necrosis factor-α (TNF-α)

APC cytokines, in psoriasis, 249–250. *See also* Antigen-presenting cells (APCs) and Psoriasis

Aphthous ulcers, 287

Aplastic anemia, 95

Apoptosis 83–85
    assay of, 84
    in follicular lymphoma diagnosis, 328, 330
    immune response and, 331–333
    lymphocyte, 83–85
    mitochondria, in apoptosis, 330

Apoptosis assay, *in vitro*, 84

Apoptotic blebs, 292

A proliferation-inducing ligand (APRIL), 75, 79

Arsenic trioxide, in plasma cell neoplasm treatment, 346

Arteritis, 166
    giant cell, 167–169

Arthralgia, 117–118

Arthritis, 181. *See also* Rheumatoid arthritis (RA)
    infectious arthritis, 270
    inflammatory arthritis, 270
    noninflammatory arthritis, 270
    osteoarthritis, 270
    palindromic arthritis, 270
    psoriatic, 251, 252, 253
    septic arthritis, 270
    subtypes of, 270

Arthropathies, insidious-onset, 270

Aspartate aminotransferase (AST), 93, 112, 162, 163

Association constant (K), in antigen–antibody interactions, 352–353

Asthma, 128, 147–160
    allergy link, 157
    case report of, 147–150
    chronic asthma, 150
    defined, 148
    diagnosis of, 148–149
    effector phase in, 151
    exercise-induced, 149
    extrinsic asthma, 148
    factors in exacerbation of, 149–150
    genetics of, 156
    in asthma, 148
    IgE responses, 152
    immediate and late phase responses, 150
    immediate phase response (IPR), in asthma, 150
    immunologically mediated, 148–149
    immunologically mediated asthma, subtypes of, 148–149
    immunologic basis of, 148, 152
    immunomodulation, 160
    incidence of, 156
    intermittent asthma, 157–158
    intrinsic asthma, 149

late-phase response (LPR), in asthma, 150

long-acting bronchodilators, 158

medical history related to, 147

Natural Killer T cells (NKT) in, 154

nebulized albuterol inhalation, 149

novel therapies, 160

pathophysiology of, 150–156

persistent/chronic, 158

pharmacotherapies, 159, 160

physical exam for, 148

precipitated by gastroesophageal reflux disease, 149

precipitated by NSAIDs, 149

pulmonary structure and pathogenesis of, 152

social and family history related to, 148

in the T_H2 inflammatory response, 154

tolerogenic mechanisms in, 155–155

treatment of, 150, 156–160

triggers of, 149

workup and management for, 149–150

Ataxia telangiectasia, 32

Athymic mice, 364–365

Athymic patients *See* DiGeorge Syndrome

Atopy, genetics of, 156

Auspitz sign, 246

Autoantibodies, 171
    AChR, 190–192
    against β-cell-associated antigens, 211
    cell destruction and, 215
    in chronic lymphocytic leukemia/small lymphocytic lymphoma, 320
    to glucose-6-phosphate isomerase, 276
    in Graves disease, 184
    in myasthenia gravis, 190–192
    in rheumatoid arthritis, 271, 276
    role in scleroderma, 301–302, 306
    in SLE, 284, 289
    SSc-specific, 302
    in ulcerative colitis, 241

Autoantibody disease, 182

Autoantibody-mediated tissue injury, complement in, 294

Autoantibody production, cellular interactions leading to, 292–293

Autoantigens
    autoimmune disease caused by, 237–238
    in plasma cell neoplasm presentations and clinical courses, 341
    release of, 179
    in systemic autoimmune states, 292

Autohemolytic anemia, passive agglutination and, 355

Autoimmune cytopenias, 72–73

Autoimmune disease(s), 1, 35, 71, 80, 175–182. *See also* Tolerance and individual diseases
    caused by autoantigens in nonpathogenic mucosal microflora, 237–238
    in CVID, 78–79

in DiGeorge syndrome, 45, 52
general features of, 178–180
genetic basis of, 179
immunologic mechanisms, leading to tissue damage in autoimmune diseases, 180
loss of tolerance in, 180–182
multiple sclerosis as, 204
nonhematologic, 86
thymomas and, 192
tissue damage in, 180
Autoimmune encephalomyelitis, 22
Autoimmune hemolytic anemia (AIHA), 82, 85
in chronic lymphocytic leukemia/small lymphocytic lymphoma, 320, 324
Autoimmune lymphoproliferative syndrome (ALPS), 81–89
case report of, 81–86
clinical course of, 85–86
clinical features and course of, 86
diagnosis of, 82–85
differential diagnosis and initial workup for, 81–82
history and physical examination for, 81
immunosuppressive therapy, 86
malignancy and, 88
molecular basis of, 87–88
pattern of inheritance of, 85
types of, 88
Autoimmune mouse models, 179
Autoimmune polyendocrinopathy-candidiasis-ectodermal dystrophy (APECED), 51
Autoimmune regulator (AIRE), 51, 176, 178. *See also* AIRE entries
Autoimmune regulator mutations, 212
Autoimmune thrombocytopenia (ITP), 82
in inflammatory bowel diseases, 232
Autoimmunity
in ALPS, 86
B-cell, 181
in CVID, 72–73
Autologous stem cell transplantation, in follicular lymphoma treatment, 329–330, 335
purging, in follicular lymphoma treatment, 330, 335
Autoreactive B cells, 292
Autoreactive cells, 177–178
deletion of, 176
Autoreactive T cells, 50–51, 193
Avidity, in antigen–antibody interactions, 353
Axonal damage, 205
Azathioprine, 188, 236, 243–244, 265
Azidothymidine (AZT), 122

B1-a cells, in CLL/SLL pathogenesis/immunogenesis, 321–322, 323
B1-b cells, in CLL/SLL pathogenesis/immunogenesis, 321–322

B1 cells, 176, 315
in CLL/SLL pathogenesis/immunogenesis, 321–322
in respiratory mucosa, 152–155
in SLE, 291–292
Waldenström macroglobulinemia and, 344–345
B2 cells, 176
in CLL/SLL pathogenesis/immunogenesis, 321, 322
in SLE, 291–292
B7 costimulatory molecule, 177
B7 gene, genetic engineering and, 364
Bacterial infections
in complement deficiency, 109, 110
high grade, 19
Neisseria, 109, 110
BAFF-R, 74. *See also* B-cell activation factor of TNF family (BAFF)
mutations, 79–80
signaling, 79
Baid, Smita, xi, 207
B- and T-cell development flow chart, 13
Bare lymphocyte syndrome (BLS) type I, 36
Bare lymphocyte syndrome (BLS) type II, 35–36
Basiliximab, 265
Basophils, 145
activated, 127
Basta, Milan, xi, 101
B-cell abnormalities, 71
in CVID, 76–78
distinction among, 20–21
B-cell activation, 315
B-cell activation factor of TNF family (BAFF), 74, 75, 176, 290, 292, 306. *See also* BAFF entries
B-cell anergy/induction, in SLE, 290–292
B-cell antigen receptors (BCRs), 74
B-cell antigens, in follicular lymphoma treatment, 335
B-cell autoimmunity, 87
B cell clonality, in chronic lymphocytic leukemia/small lymphocytic lymphoma diagnosis, 319
B-cell deficiencies, 10, 17
B-cell development, 22–23, 77
B-cell malignancies and, 313
in SLE, 290
B-cell functional assays, 10, 18, 42, 55–56, 70–71, 361
B-cell hybridoma/monoclonal antibody technology, cell cultures and, 361, 362
B-cell lineage
Hodgkin lymphoma and, 313
neoplasms of, 311
B-cell lymphomas, 95
aggressive, 119
classification of, 312–313
CLL/SLL pathogenesis/immunogenesis, 322–323
diffuse large B-cell lymphomas, 334
follicular lymphoma, 327–337

B-cell malignancies, B-cell development and, 313
  classification of, 312–315
B-cell maturation, defect in, 55
B-cell maturation antigen (BCMA), 75, 79
B cell maturation phases, 58–59
B-cell proliferation, 95, 319
B-cell receptor signaling, 176
B-cell receptors (BCRs), 10
  cross-linking of, 290
  in CLL/SLL pathogenesis/immunogenesis, 321
  in lymph node, 330–331
  plasma cells and, 343
B-cell receptor signaling complex, 75
B-cell responses, 6, 7
  in CVID, 70–71
  T-cell-independent, 120
B cells, 9, 46. *See also* B lymphocytes
  activation in SLE, 293
  antibody production by, 74–76, 361
  autoantibody production and, 292–293
  cellular assays of, 360, 361
  central tolerance, 181
  in chronic lymphocytic leukemia/small lymphocytic
    lymphoma, 318, 321–323
  cultures of, 361–362
  development checkpoints, 290
  EBER-positive, 96
  effector cell assays and, 361
  in follicular lymphoma diagnosis, 328, 329
  functional assay, 17–18, 58–61,
  Hodgkin lymphoma and, 313
  memory B cells, 73–76, 78, 79, 332
  neoplasms of, 311
  normal distribution of, 319
  plasma cells and, 343–344
  role in scleroderma, 306
  SCID mice and, 364
  subset distribution, abnormalities of, 76
  subtypes of, 291
  synovial, 277
  terminal differentiation, 74
  tolerance, 176
  Waldenstrom macroglobulinemia and, 345
  with latent EBV virus, 94
B cell lymphoma, 72, 78, 118, 311–315, 317–325, 327–336,
    337–347
  See also: diffuse large B cell lymphoma, chronic
    lymphocytic leukemia, Burkitt lymphoma, follicular
    lymphoma, Lymphoid maligancics
BCL-1 gene, in lymphoma development, 333
bcl-1 protein, in lymphoma development, 333
BCL-2 gene
  in CLL/SLL pathogenesis/immunogenesis, 323
  in follicular lymphoma pathogenesis and treatment, 333,
    336

bcl-2 protein
  in apoptosis, 330, 331–332, 333
  in CLL/SLL pathogenesis/immunogenesis, 323
  in follicular lymphoma diagnosis, 328, 329
BCL-6 gene
  diffuse large B-cell lymphomas and, 334
  in lymphoma development, 333
bcl-6 protein
  in germinal center B cells, 332
  in lymphoma development, 333
  plasma cells and, 343
B-CLL cells, 319 *see* chronic lymphocytic
    leukemia
bcl-XL protein, in apoptosis, 330
bcr–abl oncogene product, 135
BCR expression defect, 24
BCR gene rearrangement, 33
BCR signaling, plasma cells and, 343, 344
Bence Jones proteins
  in plasma cell neoplasm research, 346
  plasma cell myeloma and, 337s
  renal failure and, 342
β-cell destruction, in diabetes mellitus type 1, 210–211,
    213–215
β-hemolytic streptococcus, 248, 249
Bilirubin, in chronic lymphocytic leukemia/small
    lymphocytic lymphoma, 320
Bisphosphonates, 133
  in plasma cell neoplasm treatment, 346
Blimp-1 transcription factor, plasma cells and,
    343
Blocking cytokines, 296
Blood-brain barrier, 204
Bloom syndrome, 32
B lymphocytes, *See also* B cell entries
Bone breakdown
  in plasma cell neoplasm, treatment of, 346
  in rheumatoid arthritis, 280
Bone marrow biopsy, 85–86, 131
  in follicular lymphoma, 328–329, 330
Bone marrow failure, 98
  stromal cells, in plasma cell dyscrasias, 345
Bone marrow stroma, lymphomas and, 315
Bone marrow transplantation, 52, 65 *See also* Stem cell
    transplantation
  in chronic lymphocytic leukemia/small lymphocytic
    lymphoma treatment, 319, 324
  in hematologic disease, 133
Bradykinin, 107
Bronchiectasis, 57, 67
Bronchodilators, long-acting, 158
Bronchospasms, 148, 149, 150, 152
Brudzinski's sign, 15
Bruton's agammaglobulinemia, 43. *See also* X-linked
    agammaglobulinemia (XLA)

Bruton's agammaglobulinemia (BTK) deficiency, 71
Bruton's tyrosine kinase (Btk), 21
    activation of, 23, 24
BTK gene, 24
Buckley, Camilla, xi, 183
^{125}I-α-Bungarotoxin–AChR complexes, 185
Burkitt lymphoma, 91–92, 95, 119, 312, 313, 314
    c-MYC gene and, 334
    endemic Burkitt lymphoma, 313
    translocation partners in, 333

C-peptide measurement, 208–209
C1 complex proteins, in SLE, 294
C1 esterase inhibitor (C1-INH), 102, 103. *See also* C1-INH entries
    interaction with non-complement proteases, 106
    intravenous, 109–110
    major function of, 104
C1-INH deficiency, 103, 104, 107, 128. *See also* C1 esterase inhibitor (C1-INH)
C1-INH gene mutation, 104
C1-INH protein, 106
C1 molecules, 104
C2 level, 103
C3bBb complexes, 105–106
C3BNBB (C3b)nBb complexes, 106
C3 tick-over, 105
C4 level, 103
C5a molecule, 295
C5 convertase, 104
Cachexia, 120
Calcineurin inhibitors (CNIs), 158, 264–265
Candotti, Fabio, xi, 27
CARD15 gene mutation, 237–238, 243
Cardiac arrhythmias, in anaphylaxis, 137
Caspases, in apoptosis, 330
Cat scratch disease, 92
CCR5 chemokine receptor, 116, 120
CCR7 chemokine receptor, 47
CD1d molecule, 241–242
CD3 chain deficiencies, 37
CD3 chain mutations, 35
CD3ζ expression, 293
CD4:CD8 T-cell ratios, 70, 115, 118
CD4 coreceptor, 49
CD4$^+$ markers, 319
CD4$^+$ T cells, 9, 10, 36, 37, 46
    autoimmune diseases and, 180
    in CVID, 78
    depletion, probable causes of, 121–122
    in HIV 114, 115
    in the MS inflammatory response, 204
CD5 marker, 319
    in CLL/SLL pathogenesis/immunogenesis, 322

CD8$^+$ cells, as effector cells, 250
CD8 coreceptor, 49
CD8$^+$ IELs, 227. *See also* Intraepithelial lymphocytes (IELs)
CD8 lineage, 46
CD8$^+$ markers, 319
CD8$^+$ T cells, 9, 37
    antigen-specific stimulation of, 247–248
    β-cell destruction and, 213–215
    in CVID, 78
    effector cell assays and, 361
    in the MS inflammatory response, 204
    role in disease, 180
    target cell destruction by, 214
CD16/56$^+$ cells, 28
CD19$^+$CD34$^+$ B cells, 24
CD19$^+$ cells, 28
CD19 deficiency, 79
CD19 marker, 74–75, 319
    in CLL/SLL pathogenesis/immunogenesis, 322
CD20 marker, 319
    in chronic lymphocytic leukemia/small lymphocytic lymphoma treatment, 322, 324
    in follicular lymphoma treatment, 329, 334, 335
CD21 marker, 79
CD25 marker, 178
CD27$^+$/IgD$^-$ B cells, reduced number of, 70
CD27 marker, 62, 76–78, 79
CD28 marker, lymph nodes and, 331
CD28 signaling, 214
CD38 marker, 319–320
CD40–CD40L (CD40L–CD40) interaction, 56, 57, 61–62, 65
CD40 defect, 71
CD40 ligand (CD40L), 55, 56, 60, 76
    in CLL/SLL pathogenesis/immunogenesis, 321, 323
    expression, in SLE, 293–294
    gene mutation, 57, 60, 62, 176
    in psoriasis, 249
CD45 mutations, 35
CD45RA marker, 57, 324
CD52 marker, in chronic lymphocytic leukemia/small lymphocytic lymphoma treatment, 324
CD55 decay-activating factor, 109
CD59 molecule, 109
CD79 transmembrane signal-transducing molecules, 23
CD80 molecule, 260
CD86 molecule, 260
CD103$^+$ dendritic cells, 239
CD117 stem cell factor receptor, 47, 135
CD150 receptor, 97
CDC cross-match, 262
CD coreceptor complex, 74–75

CD markers
  in chronic lymphocytic leukemia/small lymphocytic
        lymphoma, 318–319, 321, 322, 323
  in follicular lymphoma diagnosis, 328, 335
  lymph nodes and, 331
  lymphomas and, 313, 314
  nomenclature, 360
  plasma cells and, 343, 344
Celecoxib, 301
Celiac disease, 182, 219–229
  antibody tests, 221–222
  case report of, 219–223
  clinical features of, 224–225
  clinical history and physical exam, 219–221
  defined, 221
  differential diagnosis of, 223–224
  epithelial cell factors in, 227–228
  genetic factors underlying, 226
  HLA-DQ alleles, celiac disease and, 226
  HLA genes, celiac disease and, 226
  HLA phenotyping, celiac disease and, 222
  "latent" celiac disease, 224
  long-term consequences of, 225
  microscopic features diagnostic of, 222–223
  morphologic evidence of, 222–223
  nondietary approaches to, 229
  oral tolerance and mucosal immunity in, 225–226
  pathophysiology of, 226–228
  silent, 224
  specific workup for, 221–223
  treatment of, 223, 228–229
Cell cultures
  primary, 361–362
Cell lysis, spontaneous, 109.
Cell-mediated immunity, 6, 7, 9, 30, 42
  studies, 18, 56
Cell-mediated lysis (CML) cytotoxicity assays, 11
Cell phenotyping, via flow cytometry, 359–360
Cell proliferation, chronic inflammation and, 311
Cell sorting, with flow cytometers, 358, 359–360
Cell types, in lymphoid neoplasm classification,
        312
Cellular assays, 360–361
Cellular crescents in renal glomeruli, 286
Cellular interactions, in psoriasis, 249–251
Centers for Disease Control (CDC), AIDS-associated
        diseases defined by, 119
Central nervous system (CNS), enteroviral infection of,
        22, 72. *See also* CNS entries; Primary CNS
        lymphoma
Central tolerance, 50, 175–177, 212
  B cell, 181
Centroblasts, of lymph node, 330, 331
Centrocytes, of lymph node, 330
Cerebrospinal fluid (CSF) exam, 15–16, 196

Cervical cancer, 119
c-FLIP molecule, 87
CH50 assay, 12
Chemokine (C–C motif) 2 (CCL2), 306
Chemokines, 180, 279
  in asthma, 150
  defective functioning of, 7
  in RA pathogenesis, 278
  in the T_H2 inflammatory response, 154
Chemotherapy
  in chronic lymphocytic leukemia/small lymphocytic
        lymphoma treatment, 320–321, 324
  in follicular lymphoma treatment, 329–330, 334
  in plasma cell neoplasm treatment, 346
Chimeric DNA, in follicular lymphoma treatment, 335
Chimeric monoclonal antibody, 281
Chlamydia organisms, 149
2-Chlorodeoxyadenosine, 133
Cholera toxin, 239
Chromagen, in immunohistochemistry, 360
Chromosomal analysis –FISH, 366
Chromosomes
  diffuse large B-cell lymphomas and, 334
  in FISH analysis, 366
  in follicular lymphoma diagnosis, 328
  in lymphoma development, 333–334
  lymphomas and, 314
  multiple myeloma and, 345
Chronic inflammation, neoplasia and, 311
Chronic lymphocytic leukemia (CLL)/small lymphocytic
        lymphoma (SLL), 92, 312, 315, 317–325
  autoreactivity, in CLL/SLL pathogenesis/immunogenesis,
        322
  case report of, 317–321
  chromosomal abnormalities in, 319–320
  clinical aspects of, 324
  clinical staging of, 320
  differential diagnosis of, 321
  diffuse large B-cell lymphomas and, 334
  early symptoms of, 320
  hypermutation, in, 322, 323
  karyotyping in, 319
  pathogenesis/immunogenesis of, 321–323
  phenotype of, 323
  prognostic indicators of, 319–320
  treatment of, 324
Chronic myelomonocytic leukemia, 82
Churg–Strass syndrome, 171
CIA mouse model, 275
Circulating immune complex (CIC) levels, 102
c-Kit stem cell factor receptor, expression of, 135 *See*
        CD117
CLA (cutaneous lymphocyte-associated antigen), 250,
        253
Class II transactivator (CIITA), 36

Class switching, structural basis of, 59–61
Class switch recombination, 61
CLL (chronic lymphocyte leukemia) cells, 319 *See also*
 Chronic Lymphocytic Leukemia
Clonality, in chronic lymphocytic leukemia/small
 lymphocytic lymphoma diagnosis, 319
Cloned lymphoid cell lines, 361–362
Clotting factors, 94
Clusters of differentiation (CD). *See also* individual CD
 entries
 detected by flow cytometry, 359–360
c-MYC gene, in lymphoma development, 333–334
CNS-specific macrophages, 204
Coagulation factors, inactivation of, 106
Cohen, Jeffrey I., xi, 91
Copitis, *See* Ulcerative colitis, Crohn's disease, and
 Inflammatory bowel disease
 indeterminate, 237
 indiscriminate, 235
Collagen-induced arthritis (CIA), 275
Collagen-vascular diseases, 92
Colon cancer, inflammatory bowel disease and, 237, 242
Colonoscopy, 235–236
Common γ chain (γc), 29
 gene transfer of, 38
 mutation, 34
Common lymphoid progenitor (CLP), 46, 47
Common variable immunodeficiency (CVID), 20, 57, 67–80,
 223, 224
 B-cell responses in, 70–71
 case report of, 67–72
 cellular abnormalities in, 76–78
 clinical aspects of, 71–73
 chronic infection in, 80
 genetic factors in, 78–80
 pathogenesis of, 76–80
 phenotype, 76
 prognosis and treatment for, 80
 structural, 72
 T-cell abnormalities in, 78
 T-cell responses, in CVID, 70
 villous atrophy in, 73
 workup for diagnosis, 69–71
Complement(s), 61
 abnormalities of, 102, 103
 activation pathways, 104–106
  alternative pathway, 104–106
  classical pathway, 104–105
  Rectin pathway, 104–105
 activation via antigen–antibody interactions, 351
 deficiencies, 7
 early complement components, deficiencies of, 109
 functional assay, 12
 functions of, 107–108
 hypocomplementemia, 165

inherited complement deficiencies, 110
nonspecific immunity assays, 18–19
role in SLE, 284, 294
in the T$_H$2 inflammatory response, 155
components, 10
 activation of, 104
 C5-C9, 106
 in immune complexes, 164
 reduced levels of, 104
Complement-dependent cytotoxicity (CDC) assay,
 262
Complement deficiency conditions, 107–109
 prevalence of, 109
Complementary DNA (cDNA), 116
 diffuse large B-cell lymphomas and, 334
 in follicular lymphoma treatment, 335
 microarray analysis and, 366–367
Concanavalin A (ConA), 18
 in B-cell and T-cell proliferation assays, 361
Congenically athymic mice, 364–365
Congenital immunodeficiency diseases, 1
Congenital thymic aplasia, 30, 41–52. *See also* DiGeorge
 syndrome
 pathophysiology of, 51–52
Congenital X-linked T-cell immunodeficiency, 82
Connective tissue disease, 301, 303
Connective tissue mast cells, 133
Coombs test, 85
 in antigen–antibody interactions, 354
 in chronic lymphocytic leukemia/small lymphocytic
  lymphoma, 320, 324
 direct Coombs test, 85
 indirect Coombs test, 85
Coronary artery vasculitis, 167
Cortical epithelial cells of thymus, 49
Corticosteroids, 86, 156–157, 158, 260
 in inflammatory bowel disease, 236, 243
 in MS treatment, 206
 in myasthenia gravis, 187–188, 194
 in rheumatoid arthritis, 281
 in SLE, 296
 side effects of, 187–188
Costimulator(y) molecules, 296–297
 activation of, 76
 genetic engineering and, 363–364
 signaling, 263
Coxsackie virus, 81
Craniofacial anomalies, 52 *See also* DiGeorge syndrome
Creatine phosphokinase (CPK), 303
Creatinine, differential diagnosis of an elevation in transplant,
 266
Creatinine clearance, 256, 259
CREB transcriptional activator, 293
CREM transcriptional repressor, 293
Crescenteric diseases of kidney, 257

Crohn's disease, 232
    CARD15 gene mutation in, 237–238
    character of inflammation in, 240
    clinical features of, 236–237
    colitis, 182
    discontinuous inflammation, 233
    mucosal immune response underlying, 238
    pathophysiology of, 240–241
    T_H1 and T_H17 responses in, 241
    T_H1 T-cell-mediated process, in Crohn's disease,
        240
    versus ulcerative colitis, 233–235
Cromones, 158
Cross-linking, in antigen–antibody interactions, 353
Cross match test, 262
Cross-reactive T cells, 213
Cryoglobulin
    associated with high immunoglobulin levels, 341–342
    in plasma cell neoplasm presentations and clinical courses,
        340–341
Cryoglobulinemia, essential mixed, 161–164, 165
Cryoprecipitates, circulating, 165
Crystal-induced arthritis, 270
Crystalline fragment (Fc), 143, 341 *See also* Immunoglobulin
        structure
CTLA-4 (cytotoxic T-lymphocyte-associated antigen)
        molecule, *See also* Cytotoxic T-lymphocyte-associated
        antigen 4-lmmunoglobulin (CTLA4-lg)
    expression of, 214
    genetic variants of, 212
Cutaneous anaplastic large cell lymphoma, 312
Cutaneous lupus erythematosus (CLE), 287
    subacute cutaneous lupus erythematosus (SCLE),
        287
CVID. *See* Common variable immunodeficiency
CXCR4 chemokine receptor, 116
    plasma cells and, 343
Cyclic adenosine monophosphate (cAMP) levels, 158
Cyclophosphamide (CYC), 172, 287, 296, 302
    in scleroderma, 306
Cyclosporin(e) A, 158, 193, 253, 264
Cytochrome C, in apoptosis, 330
Cytogenetics, in chronic lymphocytic leukemia/small
        lymphocytic lymphoma, 319–320
Cytokine
    assays, 11, 360
    antigen-specific T-cell lines and, 362
    B-cell production and, 215
    biological effects of, 35
    "cytokine network," 251
    defective functioning of, 7
    γ chain, 29
    γ chain gene transfer, 38
    γ chain mutation, 34
    genes, genetic engineering and, 364

gene-targeted mice and, 365
    in IgA nephropathy, 260
    inflammatory cytokines, 204, 227
    "master" cytokines, 199, 240
    mechanisms terminating signal, 35
    in plasma cell neoplasms, 345, 346
    products of mast cells, 135
    profiles, 180
    in RA pathogenesis, 278
    release, $CD4^+$ and $CD8^+$ cell stimulation and, 248
    role in SLE, 294
    T_H1/T_H17 cytokine synthesis, 240
    T_H2 family of, 127
    T cell differentiation, 201–202
    transcription of, 74
    transgenic mice and, 365
Cytomegalovirus (CMV), 29, 57, 120
    infection, 93
    scleroderma and, 304
Cytopenias, autoimmune, 71, 72–73, 85, 86
Cytoplasmic ANCA (cANCA), 170. *See also* Antineutrophil
        cytoplasmic antibody (ANCA)
Cytoreductive therapies, 133
Cytotoxic chemotherapy, in plasma cell neoplasm treatment,
        346
Cytotoxic function, decrease in, 97
Cytotoxicity assays, for T and NK cells, 361
Cytotoxic T cells, *see* Cytotoxic T lymphocytes
Cytotoxic T-lymphocyte-associated antigen
        4-lmmunoglobulin (CTLA4-lg), 282. *See also*
        CTLA-4 entries
Cytotoxic T lymphocytes (CTLs), 94–95, 210
    cytotoxic capability of, 215
    genetic engineering and, 363–364
    normal distribution of, 319

D816V *c-kit* mutation, 135
Daclizumab, 265
Danazol, 103
Darier's sign, 129
Death domain, 87
Death-inducing signaling complex (DISC), 87, 88
Delayed-type hypersensitivity (DTH) reaction, 11, 36, 42
    assay, 18, 56, 210
    in MS, 199–201
    T_H1/T_H17 T-cell subset differentiation and,
        199–202
Deletional tolerance, 239
Demyelination, 205
    immune-mediated demyelinating diseases, 205
Dendritic cells
    abnormalities, in CVID, 78
    in HIV infection, 120
    in RA synovium, 277
    of the thymic medulla, 51

subpopulations, 293
T cell interaction with, 199–201
Depolarization block, 188
Dermal fibrosis, 306
Dermatitis herpetiformis, 224–225
Dermographism, 140
Designer antibodies, in follicular lymphoma treatment, 335
Diabetes Control and Complications Trial (DCCT), 215
Diabetes mellitus type 1, 207–217
    clinical features of, 209
    continuous subcutaneous insulin infusion (CSII) in, 215
    defined, 208
    genes versus environment in, 212–213
    immunologic tolerance in, 212–213
    immunomodulation, 216
    immunopathologic mechanisms underlying, 210
    nonobese diabetic, 179, 276
    predicting and preventing, 216
    treatment of, 209, 215–216
Diabetes mellitus type 2, 303
Diabetes Prevention Trial Type 1 Diabetes (DPT-1), 216
Diabetic ketoacidosis (DKA), 208, 209
Dialysis, versus kidney transplantation, 261
Diarrhea
    bloody, 231–232
    persistent, 219
Diffuse large B-cell lymphomas (DLBCL), 95, 312, 314, 334
    BCL-6 gene and, 333
    clinical features of, 303–304
    translocation partners in, 333
    HIV, 119
DiGeorge syndrome, 30, 41–52
    cardiac malformations and complications, 43, 45, 52
    case reports of, 41–43
    clinical features of, 44–45
    congenically athymic, 364–365
    differential diagnosis of, 43–44
    facial structures, abnormal development of, 45
    gene rearrangement, 22–23, 33, 46–47, 48, 49, 58, 60, 61, 62
    history of, 41–43
    immune dysfunction, in DiGeorge syndrome, 45
    infants with, 43
    neurologic abnormalities in, 52
    nude mice, 51, 364–365
    palate, abnormal development of, 45
    pathophysiology of, 51–52
    thymectomized, 364–365
    thymic aplasia, pathophysiology of, 51–52
    thymic transplants in, 51
    treatment of, 52
    versus SCID, 44
Digoxygenin, in FISH analysis, 366
Dihydrorhodamine assay, 12, 19

Diphenhydramine, 102
Diphtheria and tetanus (DT) antigens, 17
Diplopia, 183, 186
Direct allorecognition, 263
    in antigen–antibody interactions, 354
    in chronic lymphocytic leukemia/small lymphocytic lymphoma treatment, 320
Discoid lupus erythematosus, 287
DNA damage, in germinal center B cells, 333
DNA rearrangement enzymes, mutations in, 32
DNA repair defects, multisystem disorders resulting from, 32–34
DNA repair gene, SCID mice and, 364
DNA viruses, oncogenic, 119
Double diffusion test, in precipitation reactions, 355
DPP10 gene, 156
DR3/DR4 haplotypes, 212
Dx-88 peptide, 110
Dysarthria, 186, 187
Dyspnea, 169
    exertional, 304

EBV See also Epstein–Barr virus (EBV)
    acute EBV infection, pathology of, 96
    EBV-encoded RNAs (EBERs), 96.
    infection, acute, 93
    infection, severe, 94
    infection, systemic, 94
    latency-associated genes, 94
    viral capsid antigen (VCA) tests, 93
Echovirus type II, 72
Ectodermal dysplasia (ED), 64
Edema
    causes of, 101–102
    localized, 104
    nonpitting putting, 300
Edrophonium, 194
Efalizumab, 253
Electrophoresis, assays via, 356
Electrophysiologic tests, 185–186, 188
Electrostatic forces, between antibodies and antigens, 351
ELISPOT assay, 361
Enanthem, 117
Encephalomyelitis
    autoimmune, 22
    experimental allergic, 204
Encephalopathy, in XHIGM patients, 58
Environmental allergies, 148
Environmental factors
    in diabetes mellitus type 1, 212–213
    in MS, 205
    in rheumatoid arthritis, 274–275
    role in autoimmunity, 179
    in scleroderma, 304
    in SLE susceptibility, 290

Enzyme linked immunosorbent assay (ELISA), 17, 112, 222, 357, 358, 361. *See also* HIV-ELISA test;
Eosinophilia, 86, 149, 224
Eosinophilic fasciitis, 303
Eosinophils, 144
Eotaxin, 150, 154
Epidermal hyperplasia, 248
Epinephrine, 102, 132, 138, 156
Epi-Pen, 142
Epithelial barrier function, in inflammatory bowel disease, 242–243
Epithelial cell factors, in celiac disease, 227–228
Epithelial growth factor (EGF), 152
Epitopes, 179, 185
    acetylcholine receptor, 190
    autoimmune response to, 189–190
    epitope spreading, 182, 213
    shared epitopes, 274
Epstein–Barr nuclear antigen (EBNA), 94, 95
Epstein–Barr virus (EBV), 81, 91, 315. *See also* EBV entries
    antibodies to, 95
    B-cell lymphomas and, 119
    body's natural response to, 94–95
    primary cell cultures for, 362
    serdogical testing for, 93
Equivalence zone, in precipitin reactions, 355
Erythema, 139, 166
Erythematous exanthema, 117
Erythrocytes. *See also* Red blood cell entries
    Coombs test and, 354
    dysmorphic, 256, 258–259
    passive agglutination and, 355
    zeta potential and, 354
Erythrocyte sedimentation rate (ESR), 82, 162, 163
Erythrodermic psoriasis, 252
Erythrophagocytosis, 96
E-selectin molecule, 253
Esophageal disease, in scleroderma, 304
Essential mixed cryoglobulinemia, 163, 165, 172
Etanercept, 253
European Nicotinamide Diabetes Trial (ENDIT), 216
Evoked potentials (EP) test, 196
Exanthems, 166
Exocytosis, 133
Experimental allergic encephalomyelitis (EAE), 204
    autoimmunity studies on, 179
Extracellular matrix (ECM), 279
Extracellular matrix protein, 304
Exudate, 15

Fab (antigen binding) fragment, 143, 341 *See also* Fragment antigen binding

Failure to thrive, 27, 28, 42, 58
Fanconi anemia, 32
Fanconi syndrome, 208
Farnesyl transferase inhibitor, in plasma cell neoplasm treatment, 346
Fas pathway
    Fas-associated protein with death domain (FADD), 87
    FAS–FADD complex, 87
    Fas–FasL pathway, 214–215
    Fas ligand (FasL), 87
    Fas-mediated apoptotic pathway, 87
    Fas molecules, 87
    malfunctions of, 87–88
Fat excretion study, 220
Fc receptors, 61, 144, 176
FcεR receptors, 61, 133, 144
Fcγ receptors (FcγRs), 294–295
    classes of, 294–295
    FcγRI receptor, 294
    FcγRIIb receptor, 292
    FcγRII receptor family, 294
    FcγRIII receptor, 295
Felty's syndrome, 272
Fibrillin-1, 304
Fibrillin gene, 306
Fibroblast cytokines, 278–279
Fibronectin, 260
Fibrosing alveolitis, 304
FISH (fluorescence *in situ* hybridization) analysis, 319, 366
    in follicular lymphoma, 336
Fish oil, 260
Fistulae, 231, 233
    Enterocutaneous fistula, 233
    Enteroenteric fistula, 233
    Enterovesicular fistula, 233
Fleischer, Thomas, xi, 81
Flow cytometric analysis, 357, 358–359
    and cell sorting, in follicular lymphoma treatment, 336
    in follicular lymphoma diagnosis, 328
    immunophenotyping by, 83
    of PMA-stimulated neutrophils, 19
    quantitative studies by, 17
Fluorescein isothiocyanate (FITC), in immunofluorescence, 357
Fluorescent dyes
    in flow cytometry, 358
    in immunofluorescence, 357
Follicle, *see* Germinal center
Follicular center cells, in CLL/SLL pathogenesis/immunogenesis, 321 *See also* Germinal center B cells
Follicular lymphoma, 312–313, 314, 327–336
    case report of, 327–330
    clinical features of, 334
    definitive diagnosis of, 328

diffuse large B-cell lymphomas and, 334
histology of, 328
immunophenotyping, 328
pathophysiology of, 330–334
translocation partners in, 333
treatment of, 328–329, 329–330, 334–336
Food allergy, 146, 219
Forkhead box transcription factor, *See* Fox transcription
    factors
Forward scatter (FSC), in flow cytometry, 359
Fox (forkhead box) Transcription Factors
    Foxn1, 51
    Foxp3 intracellular transcription factor, 155, 178, 182, 225,
      293
Fragment antigen binding (Fab), 143
    in antigen–antibody complexes, 352–353
    in follicular lymphoma treatment, 335
    in plasma cell neoplasm pathophysiology, 341
    of neutrophils, 18–19
    zeta potential with, 354
Fungal infections, 28, 119
    Histoplasmosis, 92

Gag gene, 117
γδ T cells, 47–48, 259 *See also* T cells
γ globulin, in plasma cell neoplasm diagnosis, 338
Gastric acid hypersecretion, 132
Gastroesophageal reflux disease (GERD)
    asthma precipitated by, 149
    therapies for, 158
Gastrointestinal (GI) disorders
    bleeding, 94, 231–232
    chronic, 20
    CVID-associated, 71–72, 73
    in hyper-IgM syndrome, 58
    infection of, 72, 120
    malignancy, 225, 237
    mucosal inflammation, 73
    opportunistic infections of, 120
    symptomatology, 67, 69, 138
Gaucher's disease, 92
Gene chips, 366–367
Gene microarray analysis,
    of diffuse large B-cell lymphomas, 334
    lymphomas and, 313–315
Gene-targeted mice, 365
Gene therapy, for SCID and X-SCID, 37–38
Genetically engineered antibodies, 363–364
Genetically engineered receptors, 363–364
Genetic basis, of autoimmune diseases, 179
Genetic factors
    in celiac disease, 226
    in CVID, 78–80
    in diabetes mellitus, 211, 212
    in inflammatory bowel disease, 243

    in multiple sclerosis, 205
    in psoriasis, 251–252
    in scleroderma, 304
    in SLE susceptibility, 290
Gene transfection, 37–38
Genome sequence databases, 351
Germinal center B cells
    diffuse large B-cell lymphomas and, 334
    fates of, 332
Germinal center (GC), 7–9, 61–62, 74, 75, 83,
    330–333
    immune response and, 331–332
    Waldenström macroglobulinemia and, 345
Giant cell arteritis, 167–169, 172
    clinical features of, 169
    pathophysiology of, 168–169
    treatment of, 169
Giardia lamblia, 72
Glatiramer acetate, 206
Gliadin, 222
    peptides, T-cell response to, 228
Glomerular disease, 256, 259
Glomerular filtration rate (GFR), 257
Glomerular sclerosis, 118
Glomerulonephritis, 165, 170–171, 172, 257
Glucocorticoid-induced tumor necrosis factor receptor
    (GITR), 178
Glucocorticoids, 132–133, 169
Glucocorticoid therapy, long-term, 264
Glucose-6-phosphate dehydrogenase (G6PD) isozyme, 25
Glucose-6-phosphate (G6P) isomerase, autoantibodies to,
    276
Glucosuria, 208
Glutamic acid decarboxylase (GAD), 216
Glutamic acid decarboxylase tests, 209
Glutamine deamination, 227
Gluten-free diet, 222, 223, 228
Gluten peptide antigen-causing disease, 226–227
Gluten peptides, binding ability of, 227
Gluten tolerance, 221–222
Glycosylation defect, 259
Goodpasture's disease/symdrome, 170, 257
Gottesman, Susan R. S., xi, 5, 15, 41, 311, 317, 327, 337
gp41 glycoprotein, 116
gp120 glycoprotein, 116
Graft rejection mechanisms, 263–264
    accelerated acute, 264
    acute rejection, 264
    chronic rejection, 264
    hyperacute rejection, 262, 263
Graft-versus-host (GVH) disease (GvHD), 37, 224
    in follicular lymphoma treatment, 335
Graft-versus-lymphoma/lymphoma (GVL) effect, in follicular
    lymphoma treatment, 329, 335

Gram-negative bacteria, in B-cell and T-cell proliferation
     assays, 361
Granulocyte colony-stimulating factor (G-CSF), 86
  in follicular lymphoma treatment, 335
  as therapy, 57
Granulocyte-macrophage colony-stimulating factor
     (GM-CSF), 133, 153
  in follicular lymphoma treatment, 335
Granulocytosis, 16
Granuloma, 120
  formation of, 168–169
  inflammation, 172, 227
  in vasculitis, 168
Graves disease, 184
Growth factors, 279
  in IgA nephropathy, 260
  in RA pathogenesis, 278
Guillain–Barré syndrome, 181
Guttate psoriasis, 246, 249, 252

H2 receptor blockers, 132
Haemophilus influenzae, in chronic lymphocytic
     leukemia/small lymphocytic lymphoma, 324
Hairlessness, 64
Hairy cell luekemia, 312
Hamilton, Robert G., xi, 137
Haplotypes, extended, 78
Haptenating agent, 42, 237
Haptens, antibody/antibody fragment complexes with,
     352–353
Hashimoto's thyroiditis, 323
Hassall's corpuscles, 46
Heavy-chain, antibodies to, in plasma cell neoplasm
     diagnosis, 338–340
Heavy-chain genes, "C-region," 58
Heavy-chain immunoglobulin portions, 137, 319, 341, 342
Heavy-chain isotype-class switching, 58, 60, 61, 62, 70, 75,
     76, 79, 290
  of germinal center B cells, 332
  lymphomas and, 313
Helper T cells, 9, 115. *See also* T_H entries
  cellular assays of, 361
  collagen-specific, 275
  role of, 144
  subsets, 199–202
Hematologic disorders, 131, 133
Hematologic malignancy, 82, 130, 311–347
Hematopoiesis, 22, 43
Hematuria, 256, 258, 259
Hemoglobin A_1C, determination of, 208
Hemolytic anemia, autoimmune, 82, 85
  in chronic lymphocytic leukemia/small lymphocytic
     lymphoma, 324
Hemolytic disease of the newborn (HDN), Coombs test and,
     354

Hemoptysis, 169, 170
HEp2 cells, 301, 302
Hepatitis, 58, 81, 98
  viral, 93
Hepatitis A virus (HAV), TIM-1 protein relationship to, 156
Hepatitis C virus (HCV) infection, 165
  chronic, 163–164
Hepatomegaly, 96
Hepatosplenic γ, δ T-cell lymphoma, 312
Hepatosplenomegaly, 16, 91
Hereditary angioedema (HAE), 101–110 *See also*
     Angioedema
  case report of, 101–103
  clinical course of, 104
  clinical presentation and workup for, 101–102
  diagnosis of, 102–103
  differential diagnosis of, 103–104
  incidence of, 106
  pathophysiology of, 106–109
  symptoms of, 104
  treatment of, 103, 109–110
  Type I hereditary angioedema, 106
  Type II hereditary angioedema, 106–107
Herpes virus, 119
Herpes zoster reactivation, in chronic lymphocytic
     leukemia/small lymphocytic lymphoma, 320
HGPRT (hypoxanthine guanine phosphoribosyl transferase),
     B-cell hybridomas and monoclonal antibodies and,
     362
Highly active antiretroviral therapy (HAART), 114,
     122–123
HIGM-I syndrome. *See* Hyper-IgM syndrome; X-linked
     hyper-IgM (XHIGM) syndrome
HIGM-II syndrome, 64–65, *See also* Hyper-IgM syndrome
HIGM-III syndrome, 63. *See also* Hyper-IgM syndrome
HIGM-IV syndrome, 64, *See also* Hyper-IgM syndrome
HIGM-V syndrome, 65, *See also* Hyper-IgM syndrome
HIGM syndrome, 71. *See also* Hyper-IgM syndrome
Histamine (H1, H2) antagonists, 138
Histocompatibility testing, 262
Histoplasmosis infection, 92
  Acute disseminated histoplasmosis, 92
HIV-1, 116, *See also* Human immunodeficiency virus (HIV)
  acute infection, 117
  chronic HIV infection, 113–114
  crisis HIV phase, 114, 117, 118–120
  drug resistance, 122
  ELISA antibody test, 112, 114. *See also* Enzyme-linked
     immunosorbent assay (ELISA)
  genome, 116–117
  immune depletion, in HIV, 121
  structure of, 115
  Western blot, 113, 114
HIV-2 virus, 116. *See also* HIV-1 virus; HIV virus
Hives, 138

HIV infection
  acute phase of, 112, 117
  chronic, 113–114
  crisis phase, 114, 117, 118–120
  diagnosis of, 118
  epidemiology and clinical features of, 117–120
  highly active antiretroviral therapy and, 122–123
  immunodeficiency due to, 224
  immunopathophysiology of, 120–122
  laboratory testing of, 115, 118
  neonatal, 54
  psoriasis and, 252
  RNA levels, 115
  tests for diagnosis and monitoring of, 112, 113, 114–115
  time course of, 112
  treatment in the acute stage of, 122–123
  typical screening for, 114
HIV, *See also* HIV-1, HIV infection
  acute HIV infection, 117–118
  blood donations, HIV and, 123
  chronic "latent" HIV phase, 114, 117, 118
  dissemination of, 121
  HIV infection and AIDS, 117
  long terminal repeat (LTR), 116–117
  revprotein, 116–117
  vaccine, 123
  variants, 116
  viral load testing, 113
  viral replication, 120
  virion, 114
HLA alleles, *See* Human leukocyte antigens (HLAs)
HLA-B gene, 252
HLA-C gene, 252
  HLA-Cw6 allele, 250, 252
HLA class I molecules, 211, *See also* Major
    Histocompatibility Complex and MHC
HLA class II molecules, 211, *See also* Major
    Histocompatibility Complex and MHC
HLA delineation, 261–262
HLA-DQ alleles, celiac disease and, 226
HLA-DR4, in RA pathogenesis, 274
HLA genes, celiac disease and, 226
HLA-identical grafts, 261–262
HLA phenotyping, celiac disease and, 222
Hodgkin lymphomas, 91, 119
  Classical Hodgkin lymphoma, 312
  classification of, 312
  Nodular lymphocyte predominant Hodgkin lymphoma, 312
Homograft response studies, 42
Hormone-secreting tumor, 130
Hormone therapy, transgenic mice and, 365
Horseradish peroxidase, in immunohistochemistry, 360
Host-versus-graft (HVG) disease, in follicular lymphoma
    treatment, 335
Hull, Keith, xi, 283

Human antichimeric antibodies (HACAs), 281
  in follicular lymphoma treatment, 335
Human antihumanized antibodies (HAHAs), in follicular
    lymphoma treatment, 335
Human antimouse antibodies (HAMAs), in follicular
    lymphoma treatment, 335
Human herpes virus 6 (HHV-6), 93
Human herpes virus 8 (HHV-8), 119
Human immunodeficiency virus (HIV), 6, 81, 92, 111–113.
    See also HIV entries
  acute infection, 111–113
  control of the spread of, 123
  clinical history and initial evaluation for, 111–112
  effects on the immune system, 118
  follow-up and initiation of therapy for, 112–113
  life cycle of, 116–117
  mode of transmission of, 119
  Western blots for, 356, 357
Human immunoglobulin genes, transgenic mice and, 365
Humanized antibodies
  production of, 363
  mouse monoclonal antibody (mAb), 160, 265
Human leukocyte antigens (HLAs), 20, 37, 72, 179–180,
    181, 211, 212, 261, 263, 274.
  B8 class I antigen, 212
  B15 class I antigen, 212
  B27 antigen, 181
Human papillomavirus (HPV), 119
Human T-cell leukemia virus type I, primary cell cultures
    for, 362
Humoral immunity, 6, 9, 42, 72
  studies of, 17, 360–361
Hybridization
  in FISH analysis, 366
  microarray analysis and, 367
Hybridoma
  development, 346
  monoclonal antibody technology, cell cultures and, 361,
    362
Hydrophobic forces, between antibodies and antigens, 351
Hygiene hypothesis, 155–156
Hymenoptera venom
  sensitivity, 145
  skin testing, 139, 140
Hypercalcemia, 208
  renal failure and, 342
Hyper-IgA (HIGA) mouse, 259
Hyper-IgM syndrome, 43, 53–65. *See also* HIGM entries
  alternative forms of, 63–65
  case report of, 53–57
  clinical features of, 57–58
  clinical history and initial evaluation of, 53–54
  defects in, 62, 63
  diagnosis and classification of, 57

Hyper-IgM syndrome (*continued*)
    due to activation-induced cytidine deaminase (AID)
        mutations, 64–65
    due to CD40 mutations, 63
    due to NEMO mutations, 64
    due to uracil–DNA glycosylase mutations, 65
    hematologic manifestations, in hyper-IgM syndrome,
        58
    medical course of, 57
    pathogenesis of, 61–65
    Pneumocystis jiroveci pneumonia in, 54, 57,
        (*Pneumocystis carinii* pneumonia)
    treatment of, 65
    workup and diagnosis of, 54–57
    XHIGM-ED, 64. *See also* X-linked hyper-IgM (XHIGM)
        syndrome
    X-linked hyper-IgM (XHIGM) syndrome, 57
Hypersensitivity, delayed-type, 11
Hypersensitivity test, delayed-type, 56
Hyperviscosity syndrome, 120
    high immunoglobulin levels and, 341, 342
    renal failure and, 342
    Waldenström macroglobulinemia and, 337
Hypoalbuminemia, 73
Hypocalcemia, 43, 45
Hypodontia, 64
Hypoesthesia, 195
Hypogammaglobulinemia, 17, 29, 94, 95, 98, 192
    in chronic lymphocytic leukemia/small lymphocytic
        lymphoma, 320
Hypohydrosis, 64
Hypohydrotic ectodermal dysplasia (ED), 64
Hypoparathyroidism, 41, 44, 45
Hypotension, 138
^{125}I-α-bungarotoxin–AChR complexes, 185

Icatibant, 110
ICOS gene defects, 79. *See also* Inducible costimulator
    (ICOS)
ICOS-L molecule, 79. *See also* Inducible costimulator
    molecule-ligand (ICOS-L)
IFN-α production. *See* Interferon α (IFN-α)
IgA structure, 68
IgA antiendomesial antibody test, 222. *See also* Hyper-IgA
    (HIGA) mouse; Immunoglobulin A (IgA)
IgA deficiency (IgAD), 24,56, 68, 70, 80, 224
    pathogenesis of, 76–80
IgA-fibronectin aggregates, 259–260
IgA/IgG antigliadin antibody assay, 222
IgA nephropathy, 182, 255–261
    case reports of, 255–258, 260–267
    clinical features and monitoring of, 258–259
    clinical history and initial evaluation of, 255–256
    diagnosis of, 256–258
    pathophysiology of, 259–260

    structural defect in IgA, 259
    treatment of, 260
Ig class switch differentiation, 59–61. *See also*
    Immunoglobulins (Igs), Class Switching
IgE antibodies, 138, 139–140. *See also* Immunoglobulin E
    (IgE)
    allergens bound to, 127
    antivenom serology panel, 140
    in anaphylaxis, 141
    in asthma, 152
    biology/function, 143–144
    as mediators of allergic response, 148
    synthesis, control of, 144
IgG antibodies, 10, 93. *See also* Immunoglobulin G (IgG)
    affinity and specificity for AChR, 190, 193. *See also*
        Acetylcholine receptor (AChR)
    anti-dsDNA antibodies, 294
    antivenom levels, 142–143
    blocking, 158
    in chronic lymphocytic leukemia/small lymphocytic
        lymphoma, autoantibodies 324
    index, 196–197
    levels, 56, 68, 69, 70–71
    in myasthenia gravis, 184
    stimulating, 144–145
    subclass deficiency, 70
    synthesis, control of, 144
    zeta potential with, 354
IGH gene,
    in B cell lymphomas, 314
    in chronic lymphocytic leukemia/small lymphocytic
        lymphoma diagnosis, 319
    in follicular lymphoma, 336
IgM (immunoglobulin M) antibodies, 10, 93
    autoantibodies, nonpathogenic, 291–292
    in chronic lymphocytic leukemia/small lymphocytic
        lymphoma, 324
    responses, 71
    zeta potential with, 354
IgM$^+$/IgD$^+$ B cells, 62
Ig replacement therapy, 62, 69., IVIG
IL-2 production, 87. *See also* Interleukin 2 (IL-2)
IL-2Rα mutations, 34
IL2RA gene, 34
IL2RG gene, 29
IL-4 receptor, 306. *See also* Interleukin 4 (IL-4)
IL-7Rα mutations, 34. *See also* Interleukin 7 (IL-7)
IL7RA gene, 34
IL-12p70 monoclonal antibody, 275. *See also* Interleukin 12
    (IL-12)
IL-12 production, 62
IL-15 secretion, epithelial- cell, 227. *See also* Interleukin 15
    (IL-15)
IL-17 cytokine family, in the T_H2 inflammatory response,
    153. *See also* Interleukin 17E (IL-17E)

Illei, Gabor, xi, 283
Imatinib, 135
Immediate hypersensitivity response, 127, 134, 144
Immune complex
  deposition, 295
  diseases, 164
  formation, 164–165
  intravascular immune complex, 164
  vasculitis, pathophysiology of, 164–165, 172
Immune surveillance
  defect, 73
  mechanism, 214
Immune system
  adaptive, 6–7
  arms, interactions among, 12
  cell mediated, 9
  dysregulation of, 2
  humoral, 9
  innate, 6
Immunoablative chemotherapy, 297
Immunoabsorption, 360
Immunoadsorption, 360
Immunoblots, immunoassays via, 356
Immunodeficiencies, 3–124, 224
  acquired immunodeficiency syndrome (AIDS),
    111–124
  autoimmune lymphoproliferative syndrome, 81–89
  common variable immunodeficiency disorders,
    67–80
  complement deficiencies, 107–109
  defining, 71
  differential diagnosis of and workup of, 5–13,
    16–22, 30
  DiGeorge syndrome, 41–52
  hyper-IgM syndrome, 53–65
  in chronic lymphocytic leukemia/small lymphocytic
    lymphoma, 324
  lymphoid malignancies and, 311
  severe combined immunodeficiency disorders, 27–39
  X-linked agammaglobulinemia (Bruton's
    agammaglobulinemia, 15–25
  X-linked lymphoproliferative syndrome, 91–99
Immunodysregulation, polyendocrinopathy, enteropathy
  X-linked (IPEX) syndrome, 178, 182
Immunoelectrophoresis
  assays via, 356
  in plasma cell neoplasm diagnosis, 338–340
Immunofixation electrophoresis (IFE)
  assays via, 356
  in chronic lymphocytic leukemia/small lymphocytic
    lymphoma treatment, 320
  in plasma cell neoplasm diagnosis, 338–340
Immunofluorescence, 357–360
  direct immunofluorescence, 357–358
  indirect immunofluorescence, 357, 358

Immunoglobulin A (IgA). *See also* IgA entries
  deficiency, 67–80
  DiGeorge syndrome and, 42
  high levels of, 341
  molecular structure of, 341
  nephropathy, 255–267
  structure of, 68
Immunoglobulin class switching, 59–62, 70, 75, 76, 79, 290,
    313, 332 *See also* class switching and heavy chain
    isotype class switching
Immunoglobulin constant regions, purpose of, 61
Immunoglobulin D (IgD), molecular structure of, 341. *See
    also* CD27$^+$/IgD$^-$ B cells; IgM$^+$/IgD$^+$ B cells
Immunoglobulin E (IgE). *See also* IgE entries;
  contrast with IgG, 144
  molecular structure of, 341
Immunoglobulin G (IgG). *See also* IgG entries
  high levels of, 341
  molecular structure of, 341
  zeta potential with, 354
Immunoglobulin gene promoter, lymphomas and, 313
Immunoglobulin genes
  in CLL/SLL pathogenesis/immunogenesis, 323
  in hyper-IgM syndrome, 58–60
  in lymphoma development, 333–334
  in severe combined immunodeficiency disorders, 32–33
  switch regions, 59
  transgenic mice and, 365
  in X-lined agammaglobulinemia, 22–23
Immunoglobulin isotypes, important features of, 61
Immunoglobulin M (IgM)
  antibody avidity of, 353
  in CLL/SLL pathogenesis/immunogenesis, 321, 323, 324
  in hyper-IgM syndrome, 53–65
  high levels of, 341, 342
  molecular structure of, 341
  in plasma cell neoplasm presentations and clinical courses,
    340–341
  Waldenström macroglobulinemia and, 345
  zeta potential with, 354
Immunoglobulins (Igs), 315. *See also* Ig entries
  in chronic lymphocytic leukemia/small lymphocytic
    lymphoma, 318–319, 320
  Coombs test and, 354
  disulfide bonds, 143, 341, 342
  Fab (antigen binding) fragment, 143, 341 *See also*
    Fragment antigen binding
  Fc (crystallizable) fragment, 143, 341
  in follicular lymphoma diagnosis, 328, 329
  in follicular lymphoma treatment, 335
  lymph nodes and production of, 331
  in plasma cell neoplasm research, 346
  in plasma cell neoplasms, 338
  produced by germinal center B cells, 332
  plasma cells and, 343, 344

Immunoglobulins (Igs) (*continued*)
   production of, 74–76
   quantification, 338–340
   structure, 143, 341
   studies, 42
   synthesis, 22–23
Immunohistochemistry, 82, 357–360
   peroxidase, 360
   on tissue sections, 360
Immunologic workup
   for immunodeficiency investigation, 5–14
   laboratory tests in, 351–367
Immunomodulation
   in asthma, 160
   drugs (ImiDs), in plasma cell neoplasm treatment, 346
   in diabetes mellitus, 216
   in multiple sclerosis, 205–206
   in rheumatoid arthritis, 282
   topical in psoriasis, 246
Immunophenotypic studies, 28, 44, 83, 358–360
   in chronic lymphocytic leukemia/small lymphocytic
      lymphoma, 318–319
   in follicular lymphoma diagnosis, 328
Immunosuppression therapy
   in autoimmune lymphoproliferative syndrome, 86
   for cryoglobulinemia, 165
   in diabetes mellitus, 215–216
   in kidney transplantation, 263–265
   in inflammatory bowel disease, 243
   in scleroderma, 306
   in XLPS, 98
   sirolimus, 265
   steroid sparing, 188, 194
   tacrolinus, 264, 267
Immunotherapy
   allergen, 158
   allergen injections, 144–145
   as an approach to allergic disease, 142
   for asthma, 150
   in follicular lymphoma treatment, 329
   stimulating antigen-specific IgG antibodies by, 144–145
Indirect allorecognition, 263
   in antigen–antibody interactions, 354
   in chronic lymphocytic leukemia/small lymphocytic
      lymphoma treatment, 324
Inducible costimulator (ICOS), 74. *See also* ICOS gene
   defects
Inducible costimulator molecule-ligand (ICOS-L), 74. *See
   also* ICOS-L molecule
Induction therapy, 264, 265
Infections
   AIDS-associated, 119–120
   chronic, 27
   in CVID, 72
   in complement deficiency, 109, 110

   opportunistic, 7, 29, 35, 36, 43, 45, 118–120, 122
   recurrent, 7
   with follicular lymphoma treatment, 334
Infectious arthritis, 270
Infectious mononucleosis (IM), 92
   EBV-associated, 93
Infertility, cyclophosphamide-induced, 296
Inflammation
   from Crohn's disease versus ulcerative colitis, 233–235
   dendritic cell–T cell interaction and, 199–201
   granulomatous, 172, 227
   in multiple sclerosis, 202
   mucosal, 237
   neoplasia and, 311
Inflammatory arthritis, 270
Inflammatory bowel disease (IBD), 182, 220, 231–244
   biologic agents, in inflammatory bowel disease, 244
   blood work results for, 232
   case report on, 231–236
   causes of, 232
   clinical course and treatment of, 236
   clinical features of, 236–237
   colitis, 182
   diagnostic workup in, 232–236
   discontinuous and continuous inflammation, 233
   effector versus regulatory cell defects in, 238–240
   effector cell defects, 238–240
   epithelial barrier function and innate immunity in,
      242–243
   genetic factors in, 243
   histologic features, 234–235
   idiopathic inflammatory bowel diseases, 232
   immunopathogenesis of, 237
   immune homeostasis, in regulatory cells, 239
   in inflammatory bowel disease, 242–243
   oral tolerance to, 240
   pathogenesis of, 237–243
   pathophysiology of, 240–243
   psoriasis and, 253
   relapsing pattern, 236
   symptoms of, 232
   treatment of, 243–244
Inflammatory cells, across the blood-brain barrier, 204
Infliximab, 281
Influenza vaccines, 158
Innate immune system, 6
   influence of, 189
   in inflammatory bowel disease, 242–243
INS gene, 212
Insulin, 211
   continuous subcutaneous insulin infusion (CSII), 215
   C-peptide, measurement in serum, 208–209
   multiple subcutaneous injections (MDIs), 215
   preproinsulin, 211
   proinsulin, 211

pump, 215
treatment with, 215
Insulin gene (*INS*), 212
Insulinlike growth factor 1 (IGF-1), 305
Insulin-secreting pancreatic β cells, immune attack of, 210
Insulin-specific T$_{reg}$ cells, 212
Integrins, plasma cells and, 343
Intercellular adhesion molecules (ICAM, ICAM-1, ICAMs), 133, 150
    in plasma cell dyscrasias, 345
Interferon α (IFN-α), 133, 215, 293. *See also* IFN-α production
    in SLE, 294
Interferon γ (IFN-γ), 60, 62, 87, 144, 213
    in celiac disease, 227
    production of, 56
Interferons (IFNs), plasma cells and, 343, 344
Interfollicular cells of lymph node, in follicular lymphoma, 329
Interleukin-1 (IL-1), 167
Interleukin 1 family, 279
Interleukin 1β inhibition, in rheumatoid arthritis, 281–282
Interleukin 2 (IL-2), 144, 178, 248. *See also* IL-2 entries
    antigen-specific T-cell lines and, 362
    production, 87
    signaling in severe combined immunodeficiency disorders, 34, 35, 38
Interleukin 4 (IL-4), 60, 180, 202. *See also* IL-4 mAb; IL-4 receptor
    in the T$_H$2 inflammatory response, 152–153
Interleukin 5 (IL-5), in the T$_H$2 inflammatory response, 153
Interleukin 6 (IL-6), 178, 202, 279. *See also* IL-6 antibodies blockade, 282
    in plasma cell neoplasm mechanism and treatment, 345, 346
Interleukin 7 (IL-7), 36. *See also* IL-7 entries
Interleukin 8 (IL-8), keratinocyte-derived, 251
Interleukin 9 (IL-9), in the T$_H$2 inflammatory response, 153
Interleukin 10 (IL-10), 178
Interleukin 12 (IL-12), 56, 62, 78, 237, 238, 250. *See also* Anti-IL-12p40 monoclonal antibody; IL-12 entries
Interleukin 13 (IL-13), 180, 241, 242, 305
    in the T$_H$2 inflammatory response, 153
Interleukin 15 (IL-15), 225, 227, 279. *See also* IL-15 secretion
Interleukin 17E (IL-17E), 153. *See also* IL-17 cytokine family
Interleukin 23 (IL-23), 250
Interleukin 25 (IL-25), in the T$_H$2 inflammatory response, 154
Interstitial fibrosis, 304
Intestinal epithelial cell defect, 221
Intestinal nodular lymphoid hyperplasia, 58, 73
Intestinal T-cell lymphoma, 312
Intradermal skin testing, 139–140, 141, 142
Intraepithelial lymphocytes (IELs), 222–223, 227

Intravenous drug use (IVD), 119
Intravenous immunoglobulin (IVIG) therapy, 19, 25, 57, 65, 69, 72, 80, 86, 94, 98, 166, 167, 194,
In vitro assay systems, 361
    apoptosis assay, 84
    B-cell responses, in CVID, 70–71
    immunoglobulin production, 55–56
    proliferation studies, 18
    specific antibody production, 11
    T-cell functional assays, 11
In vivo assay systems, 364–365
    specific antibody production, 10–11
    T-cell functional assays, 11, 18
IRF4 transcription factor, plasma cells and, 343, 344
Islet β cells, 211
    antigen 512 (ICA512) tests, 209
    destruction, immunologic mechanisms of, 213–215
    organ-specific autoimmune diseases, 179
    progressive destruction of, 210
    transplantation, 215–216
Islets of Langerhans, 211
Isohemagglutinins, 10, 42
Isotype switching, 59, 144, *See also* class switching, heavy chain class switching, immunoglobulin class switching
    in germinal center B cells, 332
    signal for, 60–61

Jaccoud's arthropathy, 288
JAK3 (Janus-associated kinase 3) deficiency, 29
JAK3 gene, mutations in, 24, 34–35
Jaundice, 85
    in chronic lymphocytic leukemia/small lymphocytic lymphoma, 320
J chains, in plasma cell neoplasm pathophysiology, 341
Juvenile idiopathic arthritis (JIA), 270
Juvenile rheumatoid arthritis (JRA), 45, 92

Kallikrein–bradykinin pathway, 107
Kaposi sarcoma (KS), 119
Kawasaki disease, 165–166, 172
    cardiac disease in, 167
    clinical features and complications of, 167
    pathophysiology of, 166–167
    principal diagnostic criteria for, 167
    treatment of, 167
K/BxN mice, 276
Keratinocyte, in Psoriasis
    damage, 249
    proliferation, 248, 251
Kernig's sign, 15
Ketanserin, 303
Kidney, *See also* Nephr- entries; Renal entries, Transplantation
    biopsy, 257–258, 286. *See also* Renal biopsy

Kidney (*continued*)
  electron microscopy of, 258
  fluorescent microscopic examination of, 258
  glomerular disease, 256, 259
  immune complex deposition in, 287
  renal disease, 256–257, 285–288
Kidney donors, 261–262
Kidney transplantation, 182, 255, 261–267
  early follow-up after, 262–263, 266–267
  in the United States, 261–262
  versus dialysis, 261
Kitani, Atsushi, xi, 299
KL-6 glycoprotein, 303
Knockout mice, 365
  as experimental animal models, 364

Lactose intolerance, 221
LAG-3 (lymphocyte activation gene 3), 178
λ5 deficiency, 24
λ chains, renal failure and, 342
Lambert–Eaton myasthenic syndrome (LEMS), 183,
      184–185
Langford, Carol A., xi, 161
Large bowel biopsy, 232–235
Large B cell lymphoma
  in chronic lymphocytic leukemia/small lymphocytic
      lymphoma, 324
  molecular mechanisms of, 333, 334
Larsen classification of SLE, 274
Laryngeal edema, 110, 138, 146
Lasers, in flow cytometers, 358, 359
Latent membrane protein (LMP), 94, 95
Leukemia
  Acute Lymphoblastic Leukemia (ALL), pre-B,
      313
  Acute Lymphoblastic Leukemia (ALL), pre-T,
      313
  chronic Lymphocytic Leukemia/Small Lymphocytic
      Lymphoma, 371–325
  hairy cell luekemia, 312
  juvenile myelomonocytic leukemia, 92
  lymphoma versus, 312
  mast cell, 136
  prolymphocytic leukemia, 312
  T-cell large granulocytic leukemia, 312
Leukocyte common antigen (LCA), 35
Leukocyte function-associated/assisted antigen 1 (LFA-1),
      116
  in plasma cell dyscrasias, 345
Leukocytes, cellular assays of, 360
Leukocytosis, 169
  in chronic lymphocytic leukemia/small lymphocytic
      lymphoma, 318, 321
Leukopenia, 85
Leukophagocytosis, 96

Leukotriene
  antagonists, 158
  sulfidopeptide, 150
Lhermitte's sign, 198
Libman–Sacks endocarditis, 288
Lichen planus, 246
Ligand-receptor signaling cascades, 79
Light chain antibodies, in plasma cell neoplasm diagnosis,
      338–340
Light chain of immunoglobulin molecule
  in plasma cell neoplasm pathophysiology, 341, 342
  plasma cells and, 344
  renal failure and, 342
  structure, 137
LIM-domain-only (*LMO2*) oncogene, 38
  clinical features of, 303–304
Linkage dysequilibrium, 78, 211, 226
Lipid rafts, 293
Lipopolysaccharides (LPSs), 237
  in B-cell and T-cell proliferation assays, 361
  in CLL/SLL pathogenesis/immunogenesis, 321
Lisinopril, 258
Liver complications
  failure, in XLPS, 96
  in hyper-IgM syndrome, 58
Long terminal repeat (LTR), 116–117
Losartan, 303
Lumbar puncture (LP), 196
Lung disease as complications of
  common variable immunodeficiency disorder, structural,
      72
  common variable immunodeficiency disorder, chronic
      infection, 80
  scleroderma, 304, 307
Lupus. *See* Systemic lupus erythematosus (SLE)
  Subacute cutaneous lupus erythematosus (SCLE), 287
Lupus nephritis, 257, 285, 288
  treatment of, 296–297
  WHO classification and histologic features of, 286
Lymphadenitis, 92
Lymphadenopathy, 16, 73, 81–82, 85, 86, 118
  in chronic lymphocytic leukemia/small lymphocytic
      lymphoma, 320
  differential diagnosis of, 91–92, 327
  diffuse lymphadenopathy, 91
  follicular lymphoma diagnosis and, 327
  in HIV, 111–112
  infectious causes of, 92
  in X-linked lymphoproliferative syndrome, 91
Lymph nodes
  germinal centers of, 330–333
  histopathologic findings in, 83
  in chronic lymphocytic leukemia/small lymphocytic
      lymphoma, 321
  in follicular lymphoma diagnosis, 327

in follicular lymphoma treatment, 329
medulla, of lymph node, 330, 331
normal structure, 330–333
primary follicles, of lymph node, 330, 331
Lymphocyte(s)
  apoptosis, 83–85
  cellular functional assays of, 360
  clones, in B-cell and T-cell proliferation assays,
    361
  in CLL/SLL differential diagnosis, 321
  cultures of, 361–362
  flow cytometry of, 358–359
  in follicular lymphoma diagnosis, 327
  phenotyping and subset analysis, 18, 28, 55, 70, 318,
    357–359
  proliferation studies, 18, 29, 42, 55, 70, 361
  thymic, 45
Lymphocytopenia, in chronic lymphocytic leukemia/small
    lymphocytic lymphoma, 320
Lymphocytosis, in chronic lymphocytic leukemia/small
    lymphocytic lymphoma, 318, 320
Lymphoid malignancies/neoplasms (Lymphoma), 309–347,
    315
  adult T cell leukemia/lymphoma, 312
  AIDS associated, 119
  ALPS and, 86, 88
  anaplastic large cell lymphoma, 312
  chronic lymphocytic leukemia, 312, 315, 317–325
  classification of, 311, 312–315
  celiac disease and, 225
  CNS lymphoma, 119
  common variable immunodeficiency disorders associated,
    73
  diffuse large B cell, 324
  follicular lymphoma, 327–336
  hepatosplenic γ, δ T-cell lymphoma, 312
  hyper-IgM disorder associated, 58
  intestinal T, 312
  large cell, 324, 333, 334
  lymphoplasmacytic, 312
  mantle cell lymphoma, 312, 313, 314, 322–323, 333
  marginal zone lymphoma, 312, 323
  primary effusion, 119
  plasma cell neoplasms, 337–347
  pymhoplasmacytic lymphoma, 312
  small lymphocytic lymphoma, 312, 315, 317–325
  severe combined immunodeficiency diseases associated,
    38
  thyroid associated, 323
  translocation partners in, 333–334
  versus leukemia, 312
  in XLPS, 95
Lymphoid organs, primary, 20
Lymphoma, *see* Lymphoid malignancies
Lymphomatoid granulomatosis, 95, 312

Lymphoplasmacytic lymphoma, 312
Lymphoplasmacytoid cells, Waldenström macroglobulinemia
    and, 344
Lymphoproliferative disorders, 73, 82
Posttransplant lymphoproliferative disorders, 312
Lymphotoxin α (LT-α), 215
Lysosomal storage disorders, 92

Mac-1 integrin, 133
Macroglobulinemia, in plasma cell neoplasm presentations
    and clinical courses, 340–341. *See also* Waldenström
    macroglobulinemia
Macrophages
  cellular assays and, 360
  cytokine products, 278–279
  in follicular lymphoma, 328
  in giant cell arteritis, 169
  of lymph node, 330–331
  in multiple sclerosis, 200
  in RA synovium, 277
  R5 macrophage variant, 116, 120
  R5X4 macrophage variant, 116
  in the skin DTH reaction, 200
  in synovial tissue, 278
  X4 macrophage variant, 116
Maculopapular lesions, 129
Major histocompatibility complex (MHC), 211. *See also*
    Human leukocyte antigen (HLA), MHC entries;
    Peptide–MHC complex; Self-MHC molecules
  CVID and, 78–79
  in follicular lymphoma treatment, 335
  haplotype, 211
  influence on autoimmune disease occurrence, 179–180
  interaction with TCR, 48
  in T cell activation, 293
Malabsorption, 58, 71, 73, 220, 221
Malar rash, 283, 287
Maldarelli, Frank, xi, 111
Malignancies (malignancy)
  AIDS-related, 119
  ALPS and, 88
  celiac disease and, 225
  hematologic, 82, 309–347
  lymphadenopathy- and splenomegaly-associated, 91
  in X-linked agammaglobulinemia patients, 25
Malignant transformation
  B-cell proliferation and, 95
  in CLL/SLL pathogenesis/immunogenesis, 322–323
  in ulcerative colitis, 242
MALT1 gene, in CLL/SLL pathogenesis/immunogenesis, 323
Mannan-binding protein (MBP), 260
Mannon, Peter, xii, 231
Mannon, Roslyn B., xii, 255
Mannose-binding lectin (MBL), 105. *See also* MBL
    deficiencies

Mantle cell lymphomas, 312, 313, 314
  BCL-1 gene and, 333
  in CLL/SLL pathogenesis/immunogenesis, 322–323
  translocation partners in, 333
Mantle zone, of lymph node, 330, 331
Mantle zone B cells
  in CLL/SLL pathogenesis/immunogenesis, 321–322
  in follicular lymphoma, 328
Marginal zone, of lymph node, 330
Marginal zone B cells (MZ B cells), 176, 291, 292, 315
  in CLL/SLL pathogenesis/immunogenesis, 321–322, 323
  Waldenström macroglobulinemia and, 344
Marginal zone lymphomas, 312, 323
  Nodal marginal zone lymphoma, 312
  Splenic marginal zone lymphoma, 312
Martin, Roland, xii, 195
MASP1–3 serine proteases, 105
Mast cell(s)
  activated, 135
  in anaphylaxis, 145
  biology, normal, 133–135
  clustered, 131
  degranulation, 145
  excess, 130
  neoplastic, 135, *See also* mastocytosis
  in RA synovium, 277
  response to allergen, 134
  subsets of, 133
  tryptase, 130–131
Mast cell leukemia, 136
Mast cell sarcoma, 136
Mast cell tryptase analysis, 138
Mastocytosis, 127, 129–136
  aggressive systemic mastocytosis, 136
  case report of, 129–133
  categories of, 135–136
  cutaneous mastocytosis, 130, 136
  definitive diagnosis and workup, 130–132
  diagnostic criteria in, 131–132
  differential diagnosis of, 129–130
  extracutaneous mastocytoma, 136
  history and physical examination, 129
  indolent systemic mastocytosis, 132, 136
  pathophysiology of, 135–136
  signs and symptoms of, 130
  treatment for, 132–133
  World Health Organization classification of, 131–132
  with associated clonal hematologic non-mast cell lineage, 136
Matrix metalloproteases (MMPs), 280
MBL deficiencies, 109. *See also* Mannose-binding lectin (MBL)
Mean corpuscular volume (MCV), of red blood cell, 317, 318

Megakaryocytes, 86
Megaloblastic anemia, 220
Membrane attack complex (MAC), 104
  formation of, 106, 109
Membranous lupus nephritis, 285, 286–287
Memory B cells, 79
  class-switched, 78
  formation of, 73–76, 332
Meningoencephalitis, chronic, 72
Mesalamine, 236, 243
Mesna, 302
Messenger RNA (mRNA)
  microarray analysis and, 367
  in Northern blotting, 366
Methotrexate, 247, 253
Methylprednisolone, 172, 287
MHC (HLA) alleles, *See also* Major histocompatibility complex (MHC) and Human leukocyte antigen (HLA)
  celiac disease and, 226
  genetic influence on rheumatoid arthritis, 274
MHC antigen expression, 20
MHC class I genes, transgenic mice and, 365
MHC class I molecules, 211, 247–248
MHC class II antigen expression, 193, 213
MHC class II genes, 247
  plasma cells and, 343
  transgenic mice and, 365
MHC class II immunodeficiency, clinical presentation of, 36
MHC class II molecules, 211, 247–248
  defective expression of, 35
MHC genes, 212
Mouse Models. *See also* Animal models
  gene-targeted, 365
  hyper-IgA, 259
  K/BxN, 276
  knockout, 364, 365
  MRL mouse strain, 87
  nonobese diabetic, 179, 276
  nude, 51, 364–365
  RAG-deficient, 364
  SCID, 364
  SLE models, 292
  thymectomized, 364–365
  tight-skinned (Tsk-1), 306
  transgenic, 364, 365, 366
  xid mouse, 24
MIC expression, 227–228
Microarrays, 366–367
Microbial antigens, T_{reg} cells generated against, 239
Microcytic anemia, 71
Microflora antigens, 237–238
Microglial cells, 204
MicroRNAs, in CLL/SLL pathogenesis/immunogenesis, 323
Microscopic polyangiitis, 171

Milk intolerance, 223

Mitochondria, in apoptosis, 330

Mitogen-activated protein kinases (MAPKs), 79
  activation of, 134
  pathways, 23

Mitogenic stimuli,
  B-cell and T-cell proliferation assays, 361
  cellular assays and, 360

Mittleman, Barbara, xii, 269

Mixed lymphocyte culture (MLC) assays, 11

Molecular mimicry, 179, 181–182,
  in myasthenia gravis, 193
  role in multiple sclerosis pathogenesis, 202–203
  in scleroderma 304

Molecular techniques, 365–367

Monoclonal antibodies
  B-cell hybridomas and, 362
  in chronic lymphocytic leukemia/small lymphocytic
    lymphoma, 318, 324
  hybridoma technology, cell cultures and, 361, 362
  in immunoelectrophoresis, 356
  in plasma cell neoplasm, 363
  T-cell hybridomas and, 362
  targets, 315

Monoclonal B cell proliferation, in chronic lymphocytic
    leukemia/small lymphocytic lymphoma diagnosis,
    319, 320

Monoclonal gammapathy of undetermined significance
    (MGUS)
  diagnosis criteria for, 341
  plasma cell neoplasms and, 337, 340
  presentation and clinical course of, 340
  treatment of, 345–346

Monoclonality, in plasma cell neoplasm, 337, 340–341,
    346

Monoclonal plasma cells
  B-cell hybridomas and, 362
  in plasma cell neoplasms, 337–338, 340–341, 346

Monoclonal (M) spike
  in chronic lymphocytic leukemia/small lymphocytic
    lymphoma, 320
  plasma cell neoplasms and, 337, 338, 339, 340

Monocyte chemotactic protein 1 (MCP-1), 306

Monocyte(s) *See also* macrophage
  cytokine production, 56
  in RA synovium, 277–278
  Staphylococcus aureus Cowan (SAC) strain 1, 56

Monospot test, 93, 112

Montelukast, 158

Morse, Caryn G., xii, 111

Mouse–human monoclonal antibody, genetic engineering of,
    363.

μ chain deficiency, 24

Mucocutaneous lesions, differential diagnosis in children,
    166

Mucosal-associated lymphoid tissue (MALT)
  marginal zone lymphoma, 312
  Waldenström macroglobulinemia and, 344–345

Mucosal immunity, 72, 225–226, 239
  abnormality of, 259
  IgA response, magnitude of, 259
  inflammation, animal models of, 240
  mast cells, 133
  nonpathogenic mucosal microflora, autoimmune disease
    caused by autoantigens in, 237–238
  suppressor cells, 239–240

Multiallergen screen, 140

Multiple myeloma *See also* plasma cell myeloma
  diagnosis criteria for, 341
  genetic abnormalities in, 345
  plasma cell dyscrasias and, 340

Multiple sclerosis (MS), 180, 182, 195–206
  "At risk for MS" category, 198
  case report of, 195–198
  clinical features of, 198
  defined, 196
  definite MS, 198
  differential diagnosis for, 197–198
  environmental factors in, 205
  genetic factors in, 205
  immunity in, 205
  immune-mediated demyelinating diseases, 205
  immunologic dysfunction, 202–203
  immunomodulation, 205–206
  immunopathogenesis of, 204–205
  inflammatory cascade in, 203
  initial presentation and evaluation of, 195–196
  initiation of immunologic dysfunction in, 202–203
  Interferon β (IFN-β), in MS treatment, 206
  "Leaky" thymic negative selection, 202
  major pathology of, 196
  in multiple sclerosis, 201–202
  Myelin basic protein (MBP), 203, 204
  Myelin basic protein-specific helper T cells,
    202
  Myelinoligodendrocyte glycoprotein (MOG),
    204
  Myelin-specific autoreactive cells, 202
  primary progressive, 198
  pathophysiology of, 202–205
  treatment, 198, 205–206
  workup for diagnosis of, 196–197

Multivalent antigens, 352–353

Muramyl dipeptide (MDP), 238

Murine experimental models, 204. *See also* Mouse models

Muscle-specific tyrosine kinase (MuSK), 188. *See also*
    MuSK antibodies

MuSK antibodies, in myasthenia gravis, 192. *See also*
    Muscle-specific tyrosine kinase (MuSK)

Myalgia, 118

Myasthenia gravis (MG), 179, 180, 181, 182, 183–194
   autoantibodies in, 190–192
   autoimmune responses, 189
   case report of, 183–188
   clinical course and evaluation of, 186–188, 189
   crisis, 189
   diagnosis of, 185
   differential diagnosis of, 184
   history and initial evaluation of, 183–186
   immune therapies, in myasthenia gravis, 194
   immunopathologic mechanisms underlying,
      189–193
   MuSK antibodies in, 192
   neuromuscular junction damage in, 190–191
   role of thymus in, 192–193
   seronegative, 188, 194
   subgroups of, 189
   T-cell responses in, 192–193
   thymoma and, 192–193
   treatment of, 193–194
Mycobacterial infections, 119–120
Mycophenolate mofetil (MMF), 86, 265, 296
Mycoplasma organisms, 149
Mycosis fungoides, 303, 312
MYC overexpression, 95
Myelin basic protein (MBP), 203, 204
Myelin basic protein-specific helper T cells, 202
Myelinoligodendrocyte glycoprotein (MOG), 204
Myelin-specific autoreactive cells, 202
Myelodysplastic syndrome, childhood-onset, 82
Myeloid malignancies, 313
Myeloma cells
   B-cell hybridomas and monoclonal antibodies and,
      362
   in plasma cell dyscrasias, 345
Myelomas, *See* plasma cell myeloma and multiple myeloma
Myelomonocytic leukemia, juvenile, 92
Myocarditis, 167
Myoid cells, 192
Myositis, 303

Nadeau, Kari C., xii, 147
Nail disease, psoriasis and, 252
NAT test in HIV infection, 112, 114–115
Natural antibody studies, 42
Natural killer cell neoplasms, classification of, 312–315
Natural killer (NK) cells, 28, 152, 214. *See also* Natural
      killer T (NKT) cells; NK entries
   function, evaluation of, 12.
   cellular assays of, 361
   in chronic lymphocytic leukemia/small lymphocytic
      lymphoma, 318, 320
   in follicular lymphoma treatment, 335
   in the T_H2 inflammatory response, 154

Natural killer T (NKT) cells, in the T_H2 inflammatory
      response, 154. NKT cell response in ulcerative colitis,
      241–242
Natural regulatory T cells, 214, 225–226
Natural suppressor cells, 239
NBT test, 12, 18
Negative selection, 46, 50–51, 176
   "Leaky" thymic negative selection, 202
Neisseria
   in chronic lymphocytic leukemia/small lymphocytic
      lymphoma, 324
   in complement deficiency, 109, 110
Neonatal HIV infection, 54
Neoplasia. *See also* Malignancy
   lymphoid, 311–315
   plasma cell, 337–347
   in XHIGM patients, 58
Nephritic syndrome, definition of, 257 *See also* Renal and
      Kidney
Nephritis. *See*, Lupus nephritis, 285–287
Nephropathy. *See* IgA nephropathy
Nephrotic syndrome, definition of 257 *See also* Renal and
      Kidney
Neuraminidase inhibitors, 158
Neuromuscular junction (NMJ), 184, 185
   impaired transmission at, 183, 185
   mechanisms of damage to, 190–191
Neutropenia, 57, 58, 85
   in chronic lymphocytic leukemia/small lymphocytic
      lymphoma, 320
   treatment of, 65
Neutrophils
   ANCA-activated, 172
   in CLL/SLL differential diagnosis, 321
   functional assays of, 18–19
   in synovial tissue, 278
Niemann–Pick disease, 92
Nifedipine, 303
Nitroblue tetrazolium (NBT) assay, 12, 18
NK cell *See* Natural Killer (NK) cells
   effector cell assays, for T and NK cells, 360, 361
NK cell leukemia, 312
NK/T cell lymphoma, 312
NKG2D receptor, 227
NKT cell response
   in ulcerative colitis, 241–242
NOD2. *See also* Nonobese diabetes (NOD) mice
   mutations, 243
   protein, 238
Non-complement proteases, C1-INH interaction with,
      106
Non-Hodgkin lymphomas, 91
   classification of, 312, 313
Nonobese diabetic (NOD) mice, 179, 212, 213,
      276

Nonsteroidal anti-inflammatory drugs (NSAIDs), 271, 270, 280–281, 301
  asthma precipitated by, 149
Northern blotting, 365–366
Notarangelo, Luigi D., xii, 27
NTBA receptor, 97
Nuchal rigidity, 15
Nuclear factor κB (NF-κB), 79, 116, 238
  in plasma cell dyscrasias, 345
  in plasma cell neoplasm treatment, 346
Nuclear factor κB essential modulator (NEMO), 64
Nuclear factor of activated T cells (NFAT), 264
Nude mice, 51, 364–365
Nurse-like cells, in RA synovium, 277
Nutritional deficiencies
  chronic, 224
  in inflammatory bowel disease, 236

Obliterative vasculopathy, 304
Oligoclonal bands (OCBs), 196–197
Oligonucleotides
  microarray analysis and, 366–367
  in polymerase chain reactions, 365
Omalizumab, 160
Omega-3 fatty acids, 260
Oncogenes, transgenic mice and, 365
Oncogenic viruses,
  DNA, 119
  lymphoid malignancies and, 311
OPG (Osteoprotegerin), 280
Opportunistic infections, 7, 29, 43, 65, 119
  Histoplasmosis, 92
  Pneumocystis jiroveci, 54, 57, 119, 120, 170. See also
    PCP (Pneumocystis carinii pneumonia)
  Trypanosomiasis, 92
Opportunistic pathogens, 54, 58, 72, 119
Optic neuritis, 195–196
Oral antigen administration, 216
Oral tolerance, 225–226, 239
  mediation of, 240
Organ-specific autoimmune diseases, 178–179, 180
Osteoarthritis, 270
OX40/OX40L, 62
Oxidative burst, 12

p17 matrix protein, 116
p24 core antigen, 116
p24 virion, 114
p53 expression, diffuse large B-cell lymphomas and, 334
P53 gene, diffuse large B-cell lymphomas and, 334
p53 mutations, 95
Palindromic arthritis, 270
Pancreatic polypeptide (PP) cells, 211
Pancytopenia, 85

Panel-reactive antibody (PRA) level, 262
Pannus formation, in rheumatoid arthritis, 280
Paracortex, of lymph node, 330, 331
Paraneoplastic diseases, 192
Paraproteins, 276
Parasites
  IgE defense against, 144
  Toxoplasmosis, 57, 92, 93
  Trypanosomiasis, 92
Park, Deric M., xii, Deric M., 195
Paroxysmal nocturnal hemoglobinuria, 109
Particulates, agglutination of, 353
Passive agglutination, 353, 354–355
Passive tolerance, 178
Pathogen-associated molecular patterns (PAMPs), 6
Pathogens, "high-grade," 72
  Leishmaniasis, 92
  Neisseria, 109, 110
  Pneumocystis jiroveci, 54, 57, 120, 170. See also PCP
    (Pneumocystis carinii pneumonia)
  Trypanosomiasis, 92
  Toxoplasmosis, 57, 92, 93
Pattern recognition molecules, 6
Pattern recognition receptors (PRRs), 292
Pauci-immune glomerulonephritis, 170–171
Pax5 protein, plasma cells and, 343–344
PCP (Pneumocystis carinii pneumonia), 119, 120. See also
    Pneumocystis jiroveci
  treatment, prophylactic, 122
Peptide–MHC complex, 48. See also Major
    histocompatibility complex (MHC)
Peptidoglycan, 238
Perforin, 214
Perianal fistula, 233
Pericarditis, 167
Perinuclear ANCA (pANCA), 170. See also Antineutrophil
    cytoplasmic antibody (ANCA)
Periodic acid Schiff (PAS) stain, 163
Peripheral blood lymphocytes
  analysis of lymphocyte subsets in, 17
  cell type, quantitation of, 28
  in chronic lymphocytic leukemia/small lymphocytic
    lymphoma, 320, 321, 323, 324
  normal subset distribution of, 318–319
  phenotyping of, 318–319
Peripheral tissue antigens (PTA), 51
Peripheral tolerance, 175, 177–178
  breaching, 181–182
Peroxidase, in immunohistochemistry, 360
Petechiae, 162
Phagocytes, 18 See also macrophage
  cellular assays and, 360
  deficiency of, 7
  functional assays, 11–12
Phagocytosis, 11, 86

Pharyngeal infection, psoriasis and, 249

Phenotyping, via flow cytometry, 359–360

PHF11 gene, 156

Phosphatidylinositol bisphosphate (PIP$_2$), 134

Phosphatidylinositol (PI3) kinase, 75

Phosphodiesterase inhibitors, 158

Phycoerythrin (PE), in immunofluorescence, 357

Phytohemagglutinin (PHA), 11, 18, 29
  in B-cell and T-cell proliferation assays, 361

Pityriasis rosea, 246

Pityriasis rubra pilaris, 246

Placentally transmitted antibodies, 54

Plaquenil, 287

Plasmablasts, 344

Plasma cell dyscrasias *See also Plasma cell myeloma*
  diagnosis of, 340
  pathophysiology of, 343–345
  presentations and clinical courses of, 340
  treatment of, 345–346

Plasma cell myeloma/neoplasm, 337–347, 312, 313, 315,
    337, 340, 343, 344
  case reports of, 337–341
  diagnostic workups for, 338–340
  immunomodulatory drugs (ImiDs), 346
  increased immunoglobulin levels and, 341–342
  karyotype analysis, 345, 346
  presentation and clinical course of, 340–341
  pathophysiology of, 341–342, 343–345
  plasma cell dyscrasias, 340, 343–345, 345–346
  research tools from, 346
  smoldering myeloma, plasma cell dyscrasias and, 340
  solitary plasmacytoma, 340
  stromal cells, in plasma cell dyscrasias, 345
  treatment of, 345–346

Plasma cells
  analysis of by Southern blotting, 366
  B-cell hybridomas and monoclonal antibodies and,
    362
  biology of, 343–344
  formation of, 332
  infiltration in celiac disease, 223
  quantification of, 340
  Waldenström macroglobulinemia and, 344–345

Plasmapheresis, 165, 187, 190, 194

Platelet-derived growth factor (PDGF), 154, 279

Platelets (PLT), in chronic lymphocytic leukemia/small
    lymphocytic lymphoma, 317, 318

PMA-stimulated neutrophils, flow cytometric analysis of,
    19

Pneumocystis jiroveci, 54, 57, 120, 170. *See also* PCP
    (*Pneumocystis carinii* pneumonia)

Pokeweed mitogen (PWM), 10, 18, 29
  in B-cell and T-cell proliferation assays, 361

Pol gene, 117

Polyarteritis nodosa, 164

Polyclonal activators, in B-cell and T-cell proliferation
    assays, 361

Polyclonal B cell proliferation, in chronic lymphocytic
    leukemia/small lymphocytic lymphoma diagnosis,
    319

Polyclonal hypergammaglobulinemia, 120

Polyclonal T-cell stimulation, 55–56

Polydipsia, 209

Polyethylene glycol (PEG), B-cell hybridomas and
    monoclonal antibodies and, 362

Polymerase chain reactions (PCRs), 365
  in follicular lymphoma, 330, 336
  multiple-cycle PCR, 365
  Southern blotting versus, 366

Polymyalgia rheumatica, 169

Polyphagia, 209

Polysaccharides, response to, 321, 322

Polyuria, 209

Positive selection, 46, 48–49, 176 *See also*
    Thymus

Poststreptococcal glomerulonephritis, 257

Posttransplant lymphoproliferative disorders, 312

PPD (Purified Protein Derivative) tuberculosis test,
    327–328

PRDM1 gene, plasma cells and, 343, 344

Pre-B-cell receptor (pre-BCR), 23
  activation of, 24

Precipitation
  in gels, 355
  lattices, in precipitation reactions, 355
  precipitin ring, in radial immunodiffusion test, 355–356
  types and nature of, 355–356
  via antigen–antibody interactions, 351

Precursor B cell leukemia/lymphomas (B-ALL), 312,
    313

Precursor T cell leukemia/lymphomas (T-ALL), 312,
    313, 314

Prednisolone/Prednisone, 302 168, 169, 170, 172
  therapy, 73, 102, 132–133
  treatment, in myasthenia gravis, 187–188

Pregnancy test, passive agglutination in, 355

Pregnant women, HIV$^+$, 123

Preproinsulin, 211

Primary amyloidosis, 342

Primary antigen–antibody interactions, 351–352

Primary cell cultures, 361–362

Primary effusion lymphoma, 119

Primary follicles, of lymph node, 330, 331

Primary immunodeficiency diseases, definition of, 5

Primary progressive MS, 198. *See also* Multiple sclerosis
    (MS)

Privileged sites, 177

Prkdc gene, SCID mice and, 364

Pro-B cells, 22

Progenitor T cells
  commitment to the T-cell lineage, 46
  travel through the thymus, 46–51
Programmed cell death, 83. *See also* Apoptosis
Proinflammatory cytokines, 295
Proinflammatory T cells, 202
Proinsulin, 211
Proliferation assays, 10, 11
  B-cell and T-cell, 361
  in hyper-IgM syndrome, 55–56
  in vitro, 29, 361
Proliferative lupus nephritis, 285, 286–287
Prolymphocytic leukemia, 312
  in chronic lymphocytic leukemia/small lymphocytic
    lymphoma, 324
Proteases, as allergens, 127
Proteinase 3, 171
Protein databases, 351
Protein kinase C (PKC), 134
Proteinuria, 255–256, 260, 266
  detection of, 259
Proteosome inhibitors, 132
  in plasma cell neoplasm treatment, 346
Protooncogenes
  in lymphoma development, 333–334
  lymphomas and, 313
Prozone
  in agglutinating titers, 354
  in precipitation reactions, 355
Pseudopolyps, 237
Psoriasis, 181, 182, 245–254
  case report of, 245–247
  cellular interactions resulting in, 249–251
  chronic plaque psoriasis, 246, 252
  clinical features and course of, 252–253
  costimulatory interactions in, 249
  definitive diagnosis of, 246–247
  effector cells causing, 249
  genetic factors in, 251–252
  immunomodulation, topical, 246
  immunopathogenesis of, 248–251
  induction of inflammation in, 251
  intertriginous areas, 253
  nail disease, 252
  plaque, histopathologic features of, 246–247
  presentation and initial workup of, 245–246
  pustular psoriasis, 252
  susceptibility regions in, 251–252
  treatment of, 253–254
  types of, 252
  vulgaris, 246
PTCH1 receptor, 48
Ptosis, 183, 186
Pulmonary disease, 92
  in asthma, 152

  in hyper-IgM syndrome, 57–58
  hypertension, 304
  inflammation, 157
  insufficiency, 72, 80
  respiratory failure, preventing, 156
  respiratory infections, 21–22, 35, 68
  symptoms in common variable immunodeficiency
    disorders, 67
Pulmonary function markers, 303
Pulmonary function tests, 149, 150
  nephelometry assay, 17
  peak respiratory flow, 149
  spirometer studies, 149
Pulmonary-renal syndromes, differential diagnosis of,
    170–171
Puncture skin testing, 139
Purging, in follicular lymphoma treatment, 330, 335
Purine "salvage" pathway, 31
Purine nucleoside phosphorylase (PNP)
  deficiency in, 29
  mutations in, 32
Purpura, 162, 163
Purulent nasal discharge, 147
Pyogenic bacteria, 7
Pyridostigmine, 186, 194
Pyrimethamine-sulfadiazine therapy, 57
Pyuria, 256

Quantitative vs Qualitative assays, 9–12
  analysis of, 10

R5 macrophage variant, 116, 120
R5X4 macrophage variant, 116
Race, HLA associations and, 212
Radial immunodiffusion test, precipitin reactions and,
    355–356
Radioactive labeling, immunoassays via, 356
Radioimmunoassays (RIAs), 17, 356
Radiosensitivity-SCID (RS-SCID), 32. *See also* Severe
    combined immunodeficiency disease (SCID)
RAG1/2 genes, 32, 364 *See also* Recombination enzymes
    (Rag 1 and 2)
RAG (Recombination Activating Protein)-deficient mice, 364
RANKL (Receptor Activation of NF-κB Ligand), 280
RANK ligand system, 280
RANTES cells, 150, 154
Rapid plasma regain (RPR), 246
RAS gene, in plasma cell neoplasm treatment, 346
Rash. *See also* Skin rash
  "Butterfly" rash, 283, 287
  in HIV, 111–112
  in mastocytosis, 129
  invasculitis, 161
  lupus-associated, 283
  malar, 283, 287

Rash (*continued*)
    pityriasis rosea, 246
    pityriasis rubra pilaris, 246
    scaly, differential diagnosis of, 245–246
Ras proteins, in plasma cell neoplasm treatment, 346
RAST-type assays, 140
RA synovium, cells in, 277
Raynaud's phenomenon, 287, 300, 303, 304, 306
Reactive center loop (RCL) of C1INH, 106
Receptor editing in B cells, 176, 290
Receptor molecule mutations, in CVID, 76
Receptors
    genetic engineering and, 363–364
    transgenic mice and, 365
Recombinant DNA techniques
    cell cultures and, 361
    for genetically engineered antibodies, 363
Recombination enzymes (Rag 1 and 2), 23. *See also* RAG
    entries
Recurrent infections, 7
Red blood cells (RBCs)
    count, 28
    distribution wideth (RDW) 317, 318
    in chronic lymphocytic leukemia/small lymphocytic
        lymphoma, 317, 318, 320
    in urine, 256
Red cell agglutination, in chronic lymphocytic
        leukemia/small lymphocytic lymphoma, 324
Red cell anemia, in chronic lymphocytic leukemia/small
        lymphocytic lymphoma, 324
Red cell aplasia, 192
Red cell casts, 256
Reed–Sternberg cells, Hodgkin lymphoma and, 313
Regulatory cell(s). *See also* T regulatory (T$_{reg}$) cells
    defects, in inflammatory bowel disease, 238–240
    immune homeostasis in, 239
    Natural regulatory T cells, 214, 225–226
Regulatory factor X (RFX) factors, 36
Regulatory mechanisms, in respiratory mucosa and asthma,
    155
Regulatory T cells, failure of, 182. *See also* T regulatory
    (T$_{reg}$) cells
    Natural suppressor cells, 239
Reiter's syndrome, 252–253
Renal biopsy, 266. *See also* Kidney entries; Nephr- entries
Renal disease
    due to excess immunoglobulin production and amyloidosis,
        342
    end-stage renal disease (ESRD), treatment
        recommendations for, 261
    etiology of, 257–258
    glomerular sclerosis, 118
    glomerulonephritis, 165, 172, 257
    in HIV-infected patients, 118
    insufficiency, 170, 259

nephritic syndrome, 257
nephrotic syndrome, 257
pauci-immune glomerulonephritis, 170–171
poststreptococcal glomerulonephritis, 257
proliferative lupus nephritis, 285, 286–287
proteinuria, 255–256, 260, 266
red cell casts, 256
in scleroderma, 304
in SLE, glomerulonephritis, 294–295
Renal ultrasound, 266
Respiratory failure, preventing, 156 *See also*
    pulmonary
Respiratory infections, 21–22, 35, 68
    IgA deficiency and, 68
    viral infections, 149–150
Respiratory mucosa
    immune response in, 152–155
    in hyper-IgM syndrome, 54
    T-cell responses in, 156
    tolerogenic mechanisms in, 155
Respiratory syncytial virus (RSV), 150
Restriction enzymes, in Southern blotting,
    365–366
Reticulocytes, 85
Retinoids, oral, 253
Retrovirus, 116
Rev protein, 116–117
RF serologic marker, 272–273
Rheumatic heart disease, 181
Rheumatoid arthritis (RA), 180, 182, 269–282,
    303
    American Rheumatism Association criteria for, 272
    biologic therapies, 281–282
    bone breakdown in, 280
    cartilage destruction, 279–280
    case report of, 269–271
    cellular response in, 276–278
    clinical features and diagnosis of, 271–274
    collagen-specific immunity, 275
    constitutional symptoms of, 270
    disease-modifying antirheumatic drugs (DMARD), 271,
        281
    environmental influences on, 274–275
    experimental models of, 275–276
    genetic susceptibility toward, 274
    history and initial evaluation of, 269–270
    HLA-DR4 human leukocyte antigen, in RA pathogenesis,
        274
    immune effectors in, 276–279
    immunomodulation, 282
    immunopathogenesis of, 274–280
    infectious arthritis, 270
    inflammatory arthritis, 270
    Interleukin 1β inhibition in, 281–282
    ischemia in, 279

joint damage and destruction caused by, 279–280

joint damage, 279–280

Juvenile idiopathic arthritis (JIA), 270

Juvenile rheumatoid arthritis (JRA), 45, 92

K/BxN, 276

laboratory features in, 272, 273

nurse-like cells, in RA synovium, 277

pannus formation in, 280

radiographic features of, 273–274

RA synovium, cells in, 277

seropositive, 271

synovial cells, 276–277

as a systemic disease, 272

TNF-α inhibitors, 281. *See also* Tumor necrosis factor α
(TNF-α)

treatment of, 271, 280–282

Rheumatoid factor (RF), 276

passive agglutination and, 355

serologic marker, 272–273

Rituximab, 86, 94, 98, 282

RNA editing molecules, 60

RNA expression, microarray analysis of, 366–367

Rother, Kristina I., xii, 207

Rouleaux formation, in high immunoglobulin levels, 341

Rubella, 92

Runting, 42. *See also* Failure to thrive

SAP

deficiency, 97

gene, function of, 96

immunologic function, impact of SAP mutations
on, 97

mutations, 96–98

protein, 97, 98

Sarcoidosis, 92

Sarcoma, mast-cell, 136

Scaly rash, differential diagnosis of, 245–246

SCID-human chimeras, 364. *See also* Severe combined
immunodeficiency disease (SCID)

SCID transplant model, 275–276

Sclerodactyly, 299

Scleroderma (SSc), 299–308

case report of, 299–303

clinical features of, 304

complications, 304

cutaneous manifestations of, 304

definitive diagnosis and treatment plan for, 302–303

diagnostic workup and evaluation of, 301–302

diffuse scleroderma, 302, 303

effector mechanisms in, 306

fibroblasts, role in scleroderma, 306

fibrosis, 307–308

genetic and environmental factors in, 304

history and initial evaluation of, 299–301

immunopathology of, 304–306

interstitial pulmonary fibrosis, 304

limited scleroderma, 302, 303

pathophysiology of, 304–306

role of B cells and autoantibodies in, 306

tight-skinned mouse model, 306

treatment of, 306–308

Sclerosing cholangitis, 58

Secondary antigen–antibody interactions, 353–356

Secondary follicles, of lymph node, 330, 331

Secondary immunodeficiencies, definition of, 6, 7

Secondary lymphoid organs, 7

Second signal, in breaching peripheral tolerance, 181

Self-antigen, structure of, 189

Self-antigen expressing epithelial cells, 51

Self-antigen targets, 213

Self-MHC molecules, 176. *See also* Major histocompatibility
complex (MHC)

Self-peptides, expression of, 51

Self-tolerance, breakdown in, 182

Sepsis, 112

postsplenectomy, 86

Septic arthritis, 270

Serine protease inhibitors (SERPINs), 106

Serine proteases, 105

Serological assays/tests, 351

EBV-specific, 93

in inflammatory bowel diseases, 235

in scleroderma, 301

Serotonin antagonist, 303

Serum amyloid-associated (SAA) protein, renal failure and,
342

Serum antibodies/immunoglobulins, 10

agglutinating titers of, 353–354

laboratory tests using, 351–357

quantitative assay, 17

Serum protein electrophoresis (SPEP), for plasma cell
neoplasm diagnosis, 337, 338, 339

Serum proteins, radial immunodiffusion test for, 356

Serum sickness, 164

Severe combined immunodeficiency disease (SCID), 27–39.
See also ADA-deficient SCID; SCID entries; X-linked
SCID (X-SCID)

case report of, 27–30

disorders in, 30

family history, 27

gene therapy, for SCID and X-SCID, 37–38

hematopoietic stem cell transplantation, for SCID, 37

immunophenotypic analysis, of X-SCID and IL7Rα SCID
patients, 34

initial management of, 29

"leaky" phenotype, 37

mouse model of, 364

molecular biology of, 30–37

RAG-deficient, 364

subtypes of, 29–37

Severe combined immunodeficiency disease (SCID)
　　(*continued*)
　　T⁻B⁺NK⁻ SCID subgroup, 29
　　T⁻B⁻ SCID subgroup, 31–34
　　T⁻B⁺ SCID subgroup, 34–35
　　T⁺B⁺ SCID subgroup, 35–36
　　treatment of, 30, 37–38
　　versus DiGeorge syndrome, 44
Sezary syndrome, 312
SH2D1A gene, 96
Side scatter (SSC), in flow cytometry, 359
Signaling lymphocyte activation molecule (SLAM) receptor
　　family, 97. *See also* SLAM-associated protein (SAP)
　　test
Simian immunodeficiency virus (SIV), 123
Single-fiber electromyography, 186
Single-nucleotide polymorphisms (SNPs), 243, 304
　　RA-associated, 274
Sinus infection, 150
Sinusitis, 147
Sirolimus, 265 *See also* Immunosuppressive therapy and
　　Transplantation
Sjögren's syndrome, 271, 272, 273
Skin biopsy
　　in mastocytosis, 130
　　in scleroderma, 301, 302
Skin DTH reaction, 199–201. *See also* Delayed-type
　　hypersensitivity (DTH) reaction
　　use in clinical evaluation, 200–201
Skin rash, in vasculitis, 161. *See also* Rash
Skin sclerosis, treatment of, 307 *See also* Scleroderma
Skin testing, 139–140, 141, 150
Skin ulcers, scleroderma-related, 307
SLAM-associated protein (SAP) test, 94. *See also* SAP
　　entries; Signaling lymphocyte activation molecule
　　(SLAM) receptor family
SLE classification, clinical features and ACR criteria for,
　　287–289. *See also* Systemic lupus erythematosus
　　(SLE)
SLP-65 adaptor protein, 23
Small lymphocytic lymphoma (SLL), 312, 315, 317–325 *See
　　also* Chronic lymphocytic leukemia
　　autoreactivity in, 322
　　case report of, 317–321
　　differential diagnosis of, 321
　　diffuse large B-cell lymphomas and, 334
　　early symptoms of, 320
　　hypermutation in, 322, 323
　　karyotyping in, 319
　　pathogenesis/immunogenesis of, 321–323
　　prognostic indicators of, 319–320
　　treatment of, 324
Small vessel vaculitides, 163, 170
SMO expression, 48
Sneller, Michael C., xii, 161

Solid-phase immunoassays, 262, 356–357
Solitary plasmacytoma, 340
Soluble IL-4 receptor (sIL-4R), 160
Somatic hypermutation (SHM), 62, 65
　　in CLL/SLL pathogenesis/immunogenesis, 323
　　in germinal centers, 331, 332–333
Sonic hedgehog (SHH) protein, 48
Sorting, with flow cytometers, 358, 359–360
Southern blotting, 365–366
　　in chronic lymphocytic leukemia/small lymphocytic
　　　lymphoma diagnosis, 319
　　in follicular lymphoma treatment, 330
Spherocytes, in chronic lymphocytic leukemia/small
　　lymphocytic lymphoma, 320
Spirometer studies, 149
Splenectomy, 86
Splenic marginal zone lymphoma, 312
Splenomegaly, 73, 81, 86, 93
　　in chronic lymphocytic leukemia/small lymphocytic
　　　lymphoma, 320
　　infectious causes of, 92
Spondyloarthropathies, 270
Sprue, refractory, 225
Sputum production, chronic, 69
Squamous cell carcinoma, 119
src homology-2 (SH2) domain, 97
Staphylococcus aureus Cowan (SAC) strain 1, 56
Stat4 expression, 274
STAT transcription factors, 35
Stem cell factor (SCF), 47, 135
　　in follicular lymphoma treatment, 335
Stem cell transplantation (SCT)
　　allogeneic hematopoietic, 37
　　in follicular lymphoma treatment, 329–330, 335–336
　　in XLPS, 98
"Steroid-sparing" immunosuppressive agents, 188, 194
Steroid therapy, 73, 102, 132–133 *See also* prednisone
　　in myasthenia gravis, 187–188
Still's disease, 270
Stinging insect
　　hypersensitivity to, 139
　　medically important, 139
Stool,
　　blood in, 231
　　examination, results of, 232
　　fat excretion study, 220
Streptavidin, in immunohistochemistry, 360
Streptococcal
　　exotoxin, 249
　　M proteins, 249
　　pyrogenic exotoxins (SPE), 248
　　superantigen (SSA), 248
Streptococcus, β-hemolytic, 248, 249
Streptococcus pneumoniae

in chronic lymphocytic leukemia/small lymphocytic lymphoma, 324
String sign, 234
Strober, Bruce, xii, 245
Strober, Warren, xii, 5, 53, 67, 219
Stromal cells, in plasma cell dyscrasias, 345
Subcapsular sinus, of lymph node structure, 330, 331
Sulfidopeptide leukotrienes, 150
Superantigen hypothesis, 165–166
Superantigens, 166–167
    evolutionary benefit of, 248
    stimulation and response of T cells to, 248
Suppressor cell-mediated oral tolerance, 239
Suppressor T cells, 78, 115, 239–240 *See also* Regulatory T cell and Treg cells
Swiss-type agammaglobulinemia, 43
Switch regions of immunoglobulin genes, 59
Syk tyrosine kinase, 293
Sympathetic ophthalmoplegia, 181
Syndecan-1, plasma cells and, 343
Syngeneic strains, as experimental animal models, 364
Synovial cells, in rheumatoid arthritis, 276–277
Synovial fluid analysis, 272
Synovitis, 169
Syphilis
    passive agglutination and, 355
    secondary, 246
Systemic autoimmune diseases, 179–178, 182
Systemic inflammatory disorder, 271
Systemic inflammatory reactions, 104
Systemic lupus erythematosus (SLE), 87, 92, 179, 283–297, 303. *See also* Lupus nephritis; SLE entries
    antigen presentation and lymphocyte response in, 293–294
    autoantibodies in, 285
    autoantibody induction in, 290–293
    cardiopulmonary involvement in, 288
    clinical course and treatment of, 287
    dermatologic symptoms of, 287
    diagnostic criteria for, 288
    drug-induced lupus, 287
    hematologic manifestations of, 288
    history and initial evaluation of, 283–284
    hormonal influences, on SLE suisceptibility, 290
    immunopathogenesis of, 289–296
    indirect immunofluorescence assay for, 358
    influences on susceptibility to, 290
    ischemic heart disease, 288
    Larsen classification, 274
    lupus nephritis, 257, 285, 288
    malar rash, 283, 287
    membranous lupus nephritis, 285, 286–287
    models of, 292
    mouse models of, 292
    musculoskeletal symptoms of, 288
    neuropsychiatric symptoms of, 288
    organ involvement in, 296
    proliferative lupus nephritis, 285, 286–287
    renal complications in, 288
    tissue injury in, 294–295
    treatment of, 296–297
Systemic sclerosis, 180, 182
Systemic smoldering mastocytosis, 136
Systemic vasculitis syndromes, 164 *See also* vasulidities

TACI, 75 *See also* Transmembrane activator and calcium-modulating cyclophilin ligand interactor (TACI)
    mutations, 79–80
    signaling, 79
Tacrolimus, 264, 267
TARC cells, 150, 154
Target of rapamycin (TOR) protein, 265
Tat protein, 116–117
T-B-cell collaboration 11
    in hyper-IgM syndrome, 55–56
    studies of 44
T-cell abnormalities, in CVID, 72, 78
T-cell activation, signals in, 263
T-cell acute lymphoblastic leukemia, 38
T-cell antigen receptors (TCRs), 74. *See also* T-cell receptor(s) (TCRs)
T-cell cytokine profiles, cellular assays of, 360
T-cell cytokines, 278
T-cell deficiency, 17, 43
    in DiGeorge syndrome, 45, 52, 72
T-cell development, lymphomas and, 314
T-cell differentiation, 77, 201–202
    normal, 36–37
T-cell dysfunction, in SLE, 295
T-cell function
    assays, 11, 360, 18
    defective, 35–36, 72
    disruption of, 30
    dysfunction in SLE, 295
T-cell hybridomas, 362
T-cell "ignorance," 177
T-cell large granular cell leukemia, 312
T-cell leukemia virus type I, primary cell cultures for, 362
T-cell lineages, 199
T-cell lymphomas (neoplasms), classification of, 312–315
    extranodal NK/T cell lymphomas, 312
    Mycosis fungoides, 303, 312
T cell lysis, in HIV, 121
T-cell maturation ALSO see Thymus
    defect in, 55
    extrathymic, 45
T-cell-mediated immunity, defective, 7, 54
T-cell proliferative responses, cellular assays of, 360

T-cell receptor(s) (TCRs), 154, 248. *See also* T-cell antigen receptors (TCRs); TCR gene rearrangement
  antigen-specific, 247
  β (TCR β), 48
  in CLL/SLL pathogenesis/immunogenesis, 321
  generation in thymus, 46–49
  gene rearrangement, 33, 46–48
  genes, 46
  interaction with MHC, 48
  stimulation, 18, 36
  transgenic mice and, 365
T-cell responses, 7, 71
  assays of, 17–18, 360
  in CVID, 70
  in myasthenia gravis, 192–193
  in rheumatoid arthritis, 274
  MHC molecules in, 211
T cells, 6–7. *See also* T lymphocytes
  alloreactive, 263
  anergy of, 181
  autoreactive, 193
  cellular assays of, 360, 361
  in chronic lymphocytic leukemia/small lymphocytic lymphoma, 318
  cultures of, 361–362
  defective function, immunodeficiencies due to, 35–36
  delayed-type hypersensitivity reaction and, 199–202
  in follicular lymphoma, 328, 335
  functional assays, 11, 18
  genetic engineering and, 363–364
  Hodgkin lymphoma and, 313
  islet-infiltrating, 213
  of lymph node, 330–331
  normal distribution of, 318–319
  nude mice and, 364–365
  plasma cells and, 343
  proliferative responses, assays of, 360
  role in scleroderma, 304–305
  SCID mice and, 364
  in SLE patients, 293
  stimulation, 55–56
  stimulation and response to antigens and superantigens, 247–248
  subset analysis, 114
  subset differentiation, 199–202
  synovial, 276–277, 278
  tolerance, 176
  Waldenström macroglobulinemia and, 345
  with MBP specificity, 204
T-cell subpopulation, autoimmune defect in, 292
TCR *See* T-cell receptor(s)
Telangiectasia, 299
Tensilon test, 188
Terminal deoxynucleotidyl transferase (TdT), 32
TG2-mediated deamination, 227

T_H1 cells, 60, 144
  allergen-specific, 158
  differentiation, 201
  to gluten peptides, 227
  responses, 97, 98, 169, 180
T_H1 T-cell-mediated process, in Crohn's disease, 240
T_H1/T_H17 cytokine synthesis, 240
T_H1/T_H17 T-cell-mediated lesions, 240–241
T_H1/T_H17 T-cell subset differentiation
  delayed-type hypersensitivity reaction and, 199–202
  in multiple sclerosis, 201–202
T_H1-type autoimmune diseases, 294
T_H2 cells, 60–61, 144
  differentiation, 202
  immune response, 152–155
  mediated hypersensitivity diseases, 127
  in ulcerative colitis, 241
T_H2 cytokines
  in asthma, 148
  role in scleroderma, 304–305
T_H2-type autoimmune diseases, 294
T_H17 cytokine responses, 180
T_H17 effector cell, 178
T_H17 T-cell differentiation, 201
T helper cells, 9, 115. *See also* T_H entries
  cellular assays of, 361
  collagen-specific, 275
  in chronic lymphocytic leukemia/small lymphocytic lymphoma, 318, 321
  normal distribution of, 319
  role of, 144
Thiopurine methyltransferase (TPMT) level, 194
Thrombocytopenia, 35, 85, 92, 162
  autoimmune, 82
  in chronic lymphocytic leukemia/small lymphocytic lymphoma, 324
Thrombocytosis, 169
Thymectomized mice, 364–365
Thymectomy, 45, 186–187
  for myasthenia gravis, 194
Thymic alymphoplasia, 43
Thymic aplasia, pathophysiology of, 51–52
Thymic epithelial cells, 46, 51
Thymic events, in loss of tolerance, 181
Thymic stromal lymphopoietin (TSLP), 127
  in the T_H2 inflammatory response, 154
Thymocytes
  education, 47, 51
  fate of, 50
  lineage commitment, 48
  lymphomas and, 314
  maturation of, 48, 49
  selection, negative and positive, 46, 48, 50–51
  survival of, 48
  trafficking pattern of, 49

Thymomas, 186, 187, 194
    myasthenia gravis and, 192–193
Thymus
    absence of, 41, 51–52
    as a black box, 45–51
    cellular organization of, 47
    congenital absence of, 43
    education in, 46, 48, 50–51
    epithelial cells of, 46, 51
    hyperplasia, 192
    lymphomas and, 313
    in myasthenia gravis, 187, 192–193
    Neonatal period, thymectomy during, 45–46
    normal function, 45–51
    normal T-cell differentiation in, 36–37
    selection in, negative and positive, 46, 48, 50–51,
        212
    tolerance induction in, 181
    transplantation, 52
Thymus-dependent (TD) antigens, 321
Thymus-independent (TI) antigens, 321
    TI-1 antigens, 321
    TI-2 antigens, 321
Thyroglobulin, passive agglutination of, 354
Thyroiditis, Hasimoto's, 323
Tight-skinned mouse (Tsk-1 mouse), 306
Tim-1 gene, 156
Tingible body macrophages, 328
Tissue transglutaminase (tTG), 222
Titer, via antigen–antibody interactions, 353–354
T lymphocytes, *See* T-cell entries
TNBS colitis, 237, 238–239, 240
TNF-α inhibitors, in rheumatoid arthritis, 281. *See also*
        Tumor necrosis factor α (TNF-α)
TNF receptor 1 (TNFR1), 215. *See also* Tumor necrosis
        factor (TNF)
TNFRSF6 gene, 87, 88
TNF superfamily receptors, 79–80
Toclizumab, 282 *See also* immonosuppressive therapy
Tolerance
    active, 178
    breaching tolerance, 181–182
    central, 175–177
    central B cell, 181
    loss in autoimmune diseases, 180–182
    immune nonreactivity, 175–176
    passive, 178
    peripheral, 175, 177–178, 181–182
    peripheral tolerance, 175, 177–178
    in respiratory mucosa and asthma, 155
    oral, 239
    suppressor cell-mediated oral tolerance,
        239
    T-cell "ignorance," 177
    thymic events, in loss of tolerance, 181

Toll-like receptors (TLRs), 6, 158, 238
    activation of, 292
    in CLL/SLL pathogenesis/immunogenesis,
        321
Tonsils, 329
    plasma cell maturation and, 43
    underdeveloped, 44, 54, 57
Toxic megacolon, 237
Toxic shock syndrome toxin 1 (TSST-1), 248
Toxoplasmosis, 57, 92, 93
Tr-1 T$_{reg}$ cells, *See* T regulatory cells
Trabecula, of lymph node structure, 330, 331
Transcription factors, 23
    in CD4$^-$ T cells, 201, 275
    plasma cells and, 343, 344
    in thymocytes, 48
    in T reg cells, 178
Transforming growth factor (TGF), 152
Transforming growth factor β (TGF-β), 75
    as a suppressor cytokine, 239–240
Transforming growth factor β$_1$ (TGF-β$_1$), 178, 226,
        304
    role in scleroderma, 305–306
    signaling, 228
Transgenes, 365, 366
Transgenic mice, 365, 366
    as experimental animal models, 364
Transglutaminase inactivation, 229
Translocations
    in CLL/SLL pathogenesis/immunogenesis, 322–323
    in follicular lymphoma diagnosis, 328
    lymphomas and, 313, 314, 333–334
Transmembrane activator and calcium-modulating cyclophilin
        ligand interactor (TACI), 75. *See also* TACI
Transplantation
    flow cross-match, 262
    histocompatibility testing for, 262
    immunosuppressive drugs in, 263–265
    rejection, 263–264
    renal (kidney), 182, 255, 261–267
    sirotimus, 265
    stem cell, allogeneic, 329, 335
    stem cell, autologous, 329
    "steroid-sparing" immunosuppressive agents, 188, 194
    Tacrolimus, 264, 267
Transporters of peptides (TAPs), 36
T regulatory (T$_{reg}$) cells, 51, 155, 158, 176, 201–202, 239
    action of, 178
    differentiation from naive T cells, 201–202
    natural, 214, 225–226
    near thymic germinal centers, 192
    oral tolerance resulting from, 225–226
Trinitrobenzene sulfonic acid (TNBS), 237. *See also* TNBS
        colitis
Trypanosomiasis, 92

Tryptase, mast-cell, 138
 immunohistochemical staining, 131, 132
 levels, in mastocytosis, 130–131
TTG2 t'TG2 antigens, 225
Tuberculosis, 92
 Disseminated (miliary) tuberculosis, 92
Tumor cell lines, 315
Tumor necrosis factor (TNF), 167. *See also* B-cell activation
   factor of TNF family (BAFF); TNF entries
Tumor necrosis factor α (TNF-α), 56, 210–211, 215, 279.
   See also Anti-TNF-α entries; TNF-α inhibitors
 in plasma cell dyscrasias, 345, 346
Tumor necrosis factor β (TNF-β), 144
22q11.2 deletion syndrome, 52
2B4 receptor, 97
Type 1 acquired angioedema, 103–104
Type 1 diabetes mellitus (T1DM), 182, 207, 208. *See also*
   Diabetes mellitus type 1
Type I hereditary angioedema, 106
Type I immediate hypersensitivity reaction, 144
Type 2 acquired angioedema, 104
Type 2 diabetes mellitus (T2DM), 208. *See also* Diabetes
   mellitus type 2
Type II hereditary angioedema, 106–107
Type IV hypersensitivity reaction, 199
Tyrosine kinase inhibitors, 135
Tyrosine kinases, 35

Ulcerative colitis, 180, 232 *See also* Inflammatory bowel
   disease
 clinical features of, 237
 colitis, 182
 model of, 237, 238–239, 240
 pathophysiology of, 241–242
 surgical approach to, 236, 237
 T$_H$2 responses, in ulcerative colitis, 241
 tissue damage in, 242
 versus Crohn's disease, 233–235
Ultraviolet (UV) light
 in flow cytometry, 358
 in immunofluorescence, 357
Ultraviolet phototherapy, for psoriasis, 247
Umetsu, Dale T., xii, 147
Unideterminant antigens, 352–353
Upper respiratory infection, IgA nephropathy and, 259
Uracil-DNA glycosylase mutations, 65
Uremia, 261
Urinalysis, 258–259
 abnormal, 256
 in diabetes mellitus, 208
 quantitation of protein excretion in, 259
 red cell casts, 256
 spun urine, 256
Urticaria, 102, 138
Urticaria pigmentosa, 129, 130, 131

Vaccines, HIV, 123
van der Waals forces, between antibodies and antigens, 351
Variable (V) region genes, in CLL/SLL
   pathogenesis/immunogenesis, 321–322
Vascular cell adhesion molecules (VCAMs)
 in plasma cell dyscrasias, 345
 VACM-1, 152, 204
Vascular endothelial growth factor (VEGF), 251, 279
Vascular inflammation, 168–169
Vascular injury, in scleroderma, 306
Vasculitides (vasculitis), 95, 128, 161–172
 acute-onset, 165–166
 affecting skin, differential diagnosis of, 164
 ANCA-associated, 169–172
 by pathophysiology, 162
 categories of, 164
 definitive diagnosis of, 163
 due to immune complex deposition, 161–164
 infectious-agent vasculitis, 164
 skin rash, in, 161
 small vessel, 163, 170
 syndromes, 162, 164–165
 treatment plan for, 163–164
 of unknown etiology, 167–169
 vasculitis, pathophysiology of, 164–165, 172
Vβ domain, 248
V(D)J gene rearrangements, 32
VDJ segments, 58
Venom immunotherapy, 142
Venom-specific IgE antibodies, 141. *See also*
   Immunoglobulin E (IgE)
Very late antigen 4 (VLA-4), 204. *See also* VLA-4 (very late
   antigen 4) integrin
Villous atrophy, 222, 223, 224, 227
Vincent, Angela, xii, 183
Viral "setpoint," HIV, 121
Viral replication, HIV, 116–117
Viral vectors, 37
Virus-reactive T cells, 213
 Rubella, 92
Visual disturbances
 high immunoglobulin levels and, 342
 in myasthenia gravis, 183–186
 Waldenström macroglobulinemia and, 337, 340–341
VLA-4 (very late antigen 4) integrin, plasma cells
   and, 343
V-region mutations, in chronic lymphocytic leukemia/small
   lymphocytic lymphoma diagnosis, 319

Waldenström macroglobulinemia, 337, 340–341
 diagnosis criteria for, 341
 high immunoglobulin levels and, 341–342
 multiple myeloma and, 345
 plasma cells and, 344–345
 treatment of, 346

Wasting syndrome, 120
Wegener's granulomatosis, 169–172, 257
    clinical features of, 171–172
    definitive diagnosis of, 170
    pathophysiology of, 171–172
    physical examination and initial workup for,
        169–170
    treatment, 170, 172
Western blots, immunoassays via, 356, 357. *See also* HIV-1
        Western blot
Wheals, 139
Wheezing, 147, 148
Window period, 112
Wiskott–Aldrich syndrome, 32

X4 macrophage variant, 116
XBP-1 transcription factor, plasma cells and,
    343–344
XHIGM-ED, 64. *See also* X-linked hyper-IgM (XHIGM)
    syndrome
xid mouse, 24
X-linked agammaglobulinemia (XLA), 15–25, 71 *See also*
    Bruton's agammaglobulinenia
    BCR gene rearrangement in, 32
    case report of, 15–19
    clinical aspects of, 21–22
    differential diagnosis of, 19–21
    female carrier of, 25
    initial diagnosis of, 16
    pathogenesis of, 23–25
    treatment of, 25

X-linked hyper-IgM (XHIGM) syndrome, 57 *See also*
    Hyper-IgM syndrome
    clinical features of, 57–58
    contrast with severe combined
        immunodeficiency
    molecular basis of, 61–62
X-linked lymphoproliferative syndrome (XLPS), 91–99,
    315
    case report of, 91–94
    clinical features of, 95–96
    defined, 94
    differential diagnosis of, 91–93
    follow-up care for, 94
    hospital course and rationale for treatment, 94
    immunologic abnormalities associated with, 97
    major genetic defect in, 96–98
    pathologic features of, 96
    treatment, 98
X-linked SCID (X-SCID), 29 *See also* Severe combined
    immunodeficiency disorders
    gene therapy for, 37–38
    hematopoietic stem cell transplantation for, 37
    mutation, 34
D-Xylose absorption test, 220

ZAP-70 (ζ-chain-associated protein) deficiency,
    36
ZAP70 gene, mutations in, 24
ZAP-70 tyrosine kinase, 319
Zeta potential, in antigen–antibody interactions,
    354